Lippincott
Illustrated Reviews:
Biochemistry

Seventh Edition

Lippincott Illustrated Reviews: Biochemistry

Seventh Edition

Denise R. Ferrier, PhD

Professor

Department of Biochemistry and Molecular Biology

Drexel University College of Medicine

Philadelphia, Pennsylvania

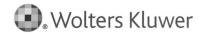 Wolters Kluwer

Philadelphia • Baltimore • New York • London
Buenos Aires • Hong Kong • Sydney • Tokyo

Acquisitions Editor: Shannon Magee
Product Development Editor: Christine Fahey
Editorial Assistant: Brooks Phelps
Marketing Manager: Mike McMahon
Production Project Manager: David Orzechowski
Design Coordinator: Stephen Druding
Manufacturing Coordinator: Margie Orzech
Prepress Vendor: SPi Global

Seventh edition

9 8 7 6 5 4 3 2

Printed in China

Library of Congress Cataloging-in-Publication Data
Names: Ferrier, Denise R., author.
Title: Biochemistry / Denise R. Ferrier.
Other titles: Lippincott's illustrated reviews.
Description: Seventh edition. | Philadelphia : Wolters Kluwer, [2017] | Series: Lippincott illustrated reviews | Includes index.
Identifiers: LCCN 2016035958 | ISBN 9781496344496
Subjects: | MESH: Biochemistry | Examination Questions | Outlines
Classification: LCC QP514.2 | NLM QU 18.2 | DDC 612.3/9—dc23 LC record available at https://lccn.loc.gov/2016035958

LWW.com

Acknowledgments

I am grateful to my colleagues at Drexel University College of Medicine who generously shared their expertise to help make this book as accurate and as useful to medical (and biomedical graduate) students as possible. I am particularly appreciative of the support and encouragement provided by my departmental colleagues Jane Clifford, PhD (Chair); Bradford Jameson, PhD; and Michael White, PhD. As usual, Ms. Barbara Engle was an invaluable sounding board throughout the process.

I am thankful for the efforts of the editors and production staff of Lippincott Williams & Wilkins. Many, many thanks are due to freelancer Kelly Horvath for her assistance in the editing (and many other aspects) of this book. I also want to thank Remya Divakaran at SPi Global for her work in the assembly of the seventh edition.

Contributing Editor, Online Unit Review Questions

Bradford A. Jameson, PhD
Professor
Department of Biochemistry and Molecular Biology
Drexel University College of Medicine
Philadelphia, Pennsylvania

Dedication

This book is dedicated to my grandchildren, Charlie and Isabella, with the promise that I will not write another, and to my students, past and present, with deep gratitude for 25 years of opportunities to teach and learn.

Contents

UNIT VII: Storage and Expression of Genetic Information

Bonus chapter online! Chapter 35: Blood Clotting (*Use your scratch-off code provided in the front of this book for access to this and other free online resources on* thePoint®.) 1/2016

Amino Acids

1

I. OVERVIEW

Proteins are the most abundant and functionally diverse molecules in living systems. Virtually every life process depends on this class of macromolecules. For example, enzymes and polypeptide hormones direct and regulate metabolism in the body, whereas contractile proteins in muscle permit movement. In bone, the protein collagen forms a framework for the deposition of calcium phosphate crystals, acting like the steel cables in reinforced concrete. In the bloodstream, proteins, such as hemoglobin and albumin, transport molecules essential to life, whereas immunoglobulins fight infectious bacteria and viruses. In short, proteins display an incredible diversity of functions, yet all share the common structural feature of being linear polymers of amino acids. This chapter describes the properties of amino acids. Chapter 2 explores how these simple building blocks are joined to form proteins that have unique three-dimensional structures, making them capable of performing specific biologic functions.

II. STRUCTURE

Although >300 different amino acids have been described in nature, only 20 are commonly found as constituents of mammalian proteins. [Note: These standard amino acids are the only amino acids that are encoded by DNA, the genetic material in the cell (see p. 411). Nonstandard amino acids are produced by chemical modification of standard amino acids (see p. 45).] Each amino acid has a carboxyl group, a primary amino group (except for proline, which has a secondary amino group), and a distinctive side chain (R group) bonded to the α-carbon atom. At physiologic pH ($\sim$7.4), the carboxyl group is dissociated, forming the negatively charged carboxylate ion ($-COO^-$), and the amino group is protonated ($-NH_3^+$) (Fig. 1.1A). In proteins, almost all of these carboxyl and amino groups are combined through peptide linkage and, in general, are not available for chemical reaction except for hydrogen bond formation (Fig. 1.1B). Thus, it is the nature of

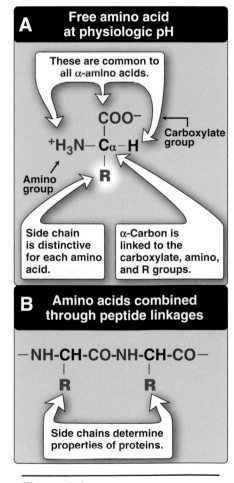

A Free amino acid at physiologic pH

These are common to all α-amino acids.

COO^-

Carboxylate group

$^+H_3N - C\alpha - H$

Amino group

R

Side chain is distinctive for each amino acid.

α-Carbon is linked to the carboxylate, amino, and R groups.

B Amino acids combined through peptide linkages

$-NH\text{-}CH\text{-}CO\text{-}NH\text{-}CH\text{-}CO-$

R   R

Side chains determine properties of proteins.

Figure 1.1
A, B. Structural features of amino acids.

the side chains that ultimately dictates the role an amino acid plays in a protein. Therefore, it is useful to classify the amino acids according to the properties of their side chains, that is, whether they are nonpolar (have an even distribution of electrons) or polar (have an uneven distribution of electrons, such as acids and bases) as shown in Figures 1.2 and 1.3.

A. Amino acids with nonpolar side chains

Each of these amino acids has a nonpolar side chain that does not gain or lose protons or participate in hydrogen or ionic bonds (see Fig. 1.2). The side chains of these amino acids can be thought of as "oily" or lipid-like, a property that promotes hydrophobic interactions (see Fig. 2.10, p. 19).

1. **Location in proteins:** In proteins found in aqueous solutions (a polar environment), the side chains of the nonpolar amino acids tend to cluster together in the interior of the protein (Fig. 1.4). This

NONPOLAR SIDE CHAINS

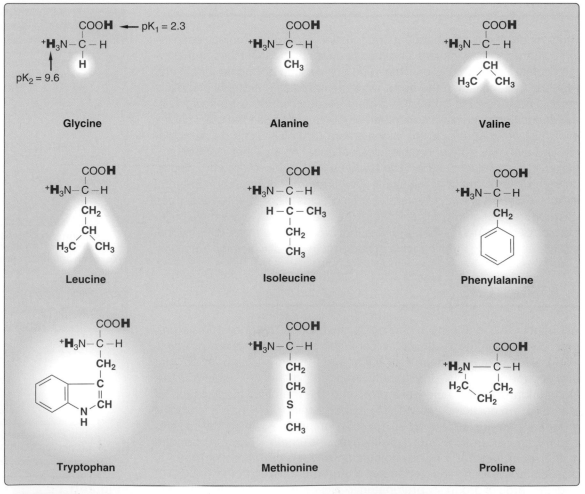

Figure 1.2

Classification of the 20 standard amino acids, according to the charge and polarity of their side chains at acidic pH, is shown here and continues in Figure 1.3. Each amino acid is shown in its fully protonated form, with dissociable hydrogen ions represented in red. The pK values for the α-carboxyl and α-amino groups of the nonpolar amino acids are similar to those shown for glycine.

UNCHARGED POLAR SIDE CHAINS

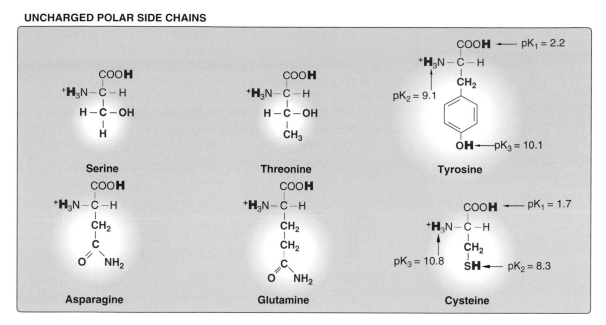

ACIDIC SIDE CHAINS

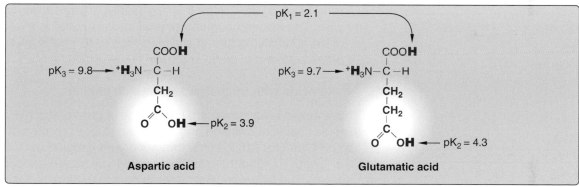

BASIC SIDE CHAINS

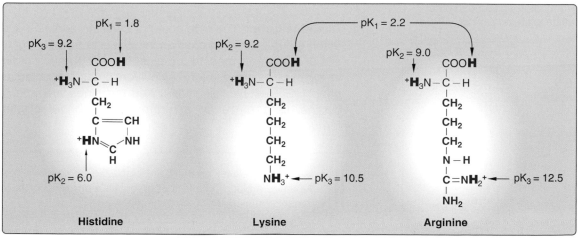

Figure 1.3

Classification of the 20 standard amino acids, according to the charge and polarity of their side chains at acidic pH (continued from Fig. 1.2). [Note: At physiologic pH (7.35 to 7.45), the α-carboxyl groups, the acidic side chains, and the side chain of free histidine are deprotonated.]

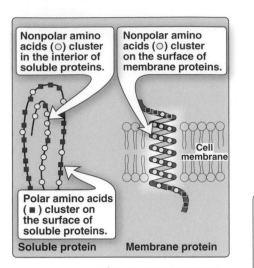

Figure 1.4
Location of nonpolar amino acids in soluble and membrane proteins.

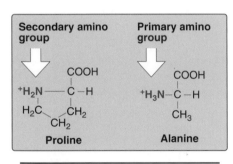

Figure 1.5
Comparison of the secondary amino group found in proline with the primary amino group found in other amino acids such as alanine.

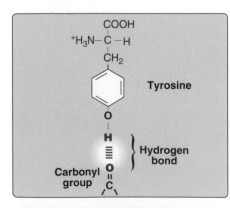

Figure 1.6
Hydrogen bond between the phenolic hydroxyl group of tyrosine and another molecule containing a carbonyl group.

phenomenon, known as the hydrophobic effect, is the result of the hydrophobicity of the nonpolar R groups, which act much like droplets of oil that coalesce in an aqueous environment. By filling up the interior of the folded protein, these nonpolar R groups help give the protein its three-dimensional shape. However, for proteins that are located in a hydrophobic environment, such as a membrane, the nonpolar R groups are found on the outside surface of the protein, interacting with the lipid environment (see Fig. 1.4). The importance of these hydrophobic interactions in stabilizing protein structure is discussed on p. 19.

> Sickle cell anemia, a disease of red blood cells that causes them to become sickle shaped rather than disc shaped, results from the replacement of polar glutamate with nonpolar valine at the sixth position in the β subunit of hemoglobin A (see p. 36).

2. **Proline:** Proline differs from other amino acids in that its side chain and α-amino nitrogen form a rigid, five-membered ring structure (Fig. 1.5). Proline, then, has a secondary (rather than a primary) amino group. It is frequently referred to as an "imino acid." The unique geometry of proline contributes to the formation of the fibrous structure of collagen (see p. 45), but it interrupts the α-helices found in globular proteins (see p. 16).

B. Amino acids with uncharged polar side chains

These amino acids have zero net charge at physiologic pH, although the side chains of cysteine and tyrosine can lose a proton at an alkaline pH (see Fig. 1.3). Serine, threonine, and tyrosine each contain a polar hydroxyl group that can participate in hydrogen bond formation (Fig. 1.6). The side chains of asparagine and glutamine each contain a carbonyl group and an amide group, both of which can also participate in hydrogen bonds.

1. **Disulfide bond:** The side chain of cysteine contains a sulfhydryl (thiol) group (–SH), which is an important component of the active site of many enzymes. In proteins, the –SH groups of two cysteines can be oxidized to form a covalent cross-link called a disulfide bond (–S–S–). Two disulfide-linked cysteines are referred to as cystine. (See p. 19 for a further discussion of disulfide bond formation.)

> Many extracellular proteins are stabilized by disulfide bonds. Albumin, a blood protein that functions as a transporter for a variety of molecules, is an example.

2. **Side chains as attachment sites for other compounds:** The polar hydroxyl group of serine, threonine, and (rarely) tyrosine can serve as a site of attachment for structures such as a phosphate group. In addition, the amide group of asparagine, as well as the hydroxyl group of serine or threonine, can serve as a site of attachment for oligosaccharide chains in glycoproteins (see p. 165).

C. Amino acids with acidic side chains

The amino acids aspartic acid and glutamic acid are proton donors. At physiologic pH, the side chains of these amino acids are fully ionized, containing a negatively charged carboxylate group (–COO⁻). The fully ionized forms are called aspartate and glutamate.

D. Amino acids with basic side chains

The side chains of the basic amino acids accept protons (see Fig. 1.3). At physiologic pH, the R groups of lysine and arginine are fully ionized and positively charged. In contrast, the free amino acid histidine is weakly basic and largely uncharged at physiologic pH. However, when histidine is incorporated into a protein, its R group can be either positively charged (protonated) or neutral, depending on the ionic environment provided by the protein. This important property of histidine contributes to the buffering role it plays in the functioning of such proteins as hemoglobin (see p. 30). [Note: Histidine is the only amino acid with a side chain that can ionize within the physiologic pH range.]

E. Abbreviations and symbols for commonly occurring amino acids

Each amino acid name has an associated three-letter abbreviation and a one-letter symbol (Fig. 1.7). The one-letter codes are determined by the following rules.

1. **Unique first letter:** If only one amino acid begins with a given letter, then that letter is used as its symbol. For example, V = valine.

2. **Most commonly occurring amino acids have priority:** If more than one amino acid begins with a particular letter, the most common of these amino acids receives this letter as its symbol. For example, glycine is more common than glutamate, so G = glycine.

3. **Similar sounding names:** Some one-letter symbols sound like the amino acid they represent. For example, F = phenylalanine, or W = tryptophan ("twyptophan" as Elmer Fudd would say).

4. **Letter close to initial letter:** For the remaining amino acids, a one-letter symbol is assigned that is as close in the alphabet as possible to the initial letter of the amino acid, for example, K = lysine. Furthermore, B is assigned to Asx, signifying either aspartic acid or asparagine; Z is assigned to Glx, signifying either glutamic acid or glutamine; and X is assigned to an unidentified amino acid.

F. Amino acid isomers

Because the α-carbon of an amino acid is attached to four different chemical groups, it is an asymmetric (chiral) atom. Glycine is the exception because its α-carbon has two hydrogen substituents. Amino acids with a chiral α-carbon exist in two different isomeric forms, designated D and L, which are enantiomers, or mirror images (Fig. 1.8). [Note: Enantiomers are optically active. If an isomer, either D or L, causes the plane of polarized light to rotate clockwise, it is designated the (+) form.] All amino acids found in mammalian proteins are of the L configuration. However, D-amino acids are found in some antibiotics and in bacterial cell walls (see p. 252). [Note: *Racemases* enzymatically interconvert the D- and L-isomers of free amino acids.]

1 Unique first letter:

Cysteine	=	Cys =	**C**
Histidine	=	His =	**H**
Isoleucine	=	Ile =	**I**
Methionine	=	Met =	**M**
Serine	=	Ser =	**S**
Valine	=	Val =	**V**

2 Most commonly occurring amino acids have priority:

Alanine	=	Ala =	**A**
Glycine	=	Gly =	**G**
Leucine	=	Leu =	**L**
Proline	=	Pro =	**P**
Threonine	=	Thr =	**T**

3 Similar sounding names:

Arginine	= Arg =	**R**	("a**R**ginine")
Asparagine	= Asn =	**N**	(contains **N**)
Aspartate	= Asp =	**D**	("aspar**D**ic")
Glutamate	= Glu =	**E**	("glut**E**mate")
Glutamine	= Gln =	**Q**	("**Q**-tamine")
Phenylalanine	= Phe =	**F**	("**F**enylalanine")
Tyrosine	= Tyr =	**Y**	("t**Y**rosine")
Tryptophan	= Trp =	**W**	(double ring in the molecule)

4 Letter close to initial letter:

Aspartate or asparagine	=	Asx =	**B** (near A)
Glutamate or glutamine	=	Glx =	**Z**
Lysine	=	Lys =	**K** (near L)
Undetermined amino acid	=		**X**

Figure 1.7
Abbreviations and symbols for the standard amino acids.

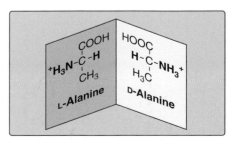

Figure 1.8
D and L forms of alanine are mirror images (enantiomers).

III. ACIDIC AND BASIC PROPERTIES

Amino acids in aqueous solution contain weakly acidic α-carboxyl groups and weakly basic α-amino groups. In addition, each of the acidic and basic amino acids contains an ionizable group in its side chain. Thus, both free amino acids and some amino acids combined in peptide linkages can act as buffers. Acids may be defined as proton donors and bases as proton acceptors. Acids (or bases) described as weak ionize to only a limited extent. The concentration of protons ($[H^+]$) in aqueous solution is expressed as pH, where pH = log $1/[H^+]$ or $-\log [H^+]$. The quantitative relationship between the pH of the solution and concentration of a weak acid (HA) and its conjugate base (A^-) is described by the Henderson-Hasselbalch equation.

A. Equation derivation

Consider the release of a proton by a weak acid represented by HA:

$$HA \quad \rightleftarrows \quad H^+ \quad + \quad A^-$$

weak acid   proton   salt form or conjugate base

The salt or conjugate base, A^-, is the ionized form of a weak acid. By definition, the dissociation constant of the acid, K_a, is:

$$K_a = \frac{[H^+][A^-]}{[HA]}$$

[Note: The larger the K_a, the stronger the acid, because most of the HA has dissociated into H^+ and A^-. Conversely, the smaller the K_a, the less acid has dissociated and, therefore, the weaker the acid.] By solving for the $[H^+]$ in the above equation, taking the logarithm of both sides of the equation, multiplying both sides of the equation by -1, and substituting pH = $-\log [H^+]$ and $pK_a = -\log K_a$, we obtain the Henderson-Hasselbalch equation:

$$pH = pK_a + \log \frac{[A^-]}{[HA]}$$

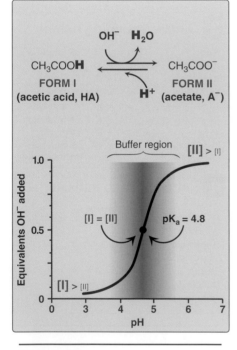

Figure 1.9
Titration curve of acetic acid.

B. Buffers

A buffer is a solution that resists change in pH following the addition of an acid or base. A buffer can be created by mixing a weak acid (HA) with its conjugate base (A^-). If an acid such as HCl is added to a buffer, A^- can neutralize it, being converted to HA in the process. If a base is added, HA can likewise neutralize it, being converted to A^- in the process. Maximum buffering capacity occurs at a pH equal to the pK_a, but a conjugate acid-base pair can still serve as an effective buffer when the pH of a solution is within approximately ± 1 pH unit of the pK_a. If the amounts of HA and A^- are equal, the pH is equal to the pK_a. As shown in Figure 1.9, a solution containing acetic acid (HA = $CH_3 - COOH$) and acetate ($A^- = CH_3 - COO^-$) with a pK_a of 4.8 resists a change in pH from pH 3.8 to 5.8, with maximum buffering at pH 4.8. At pH values less than the pK_a, the protonated acid form ($CH_3 - COOH$) is the predominant species in solution. At pH values greater than the pK_a, the deprotonated base form ($CH_3 - COO^-$) is the predominant species.

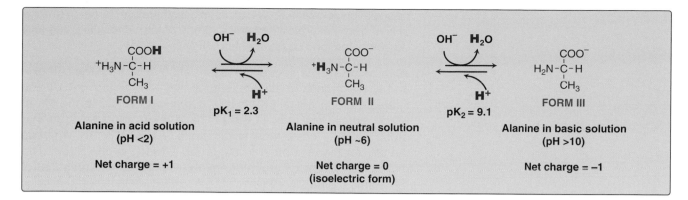

Figure 1.10
Ionic forms of alanine in acidic, neutral, and basic solutions.

C. Amino acid titration

The titration curve of an amino acid can be analyzed in the same way as described for acetic acid.

1. **Carboxyl group dissociation:** Consider alanine, for example, which contains an ionizable α-carboxyl and α-amino group. [Note: Its –CH$_3$ R group is nonionizable.] At a low (acidic) pH, both of these groups are protonated (Fig. 1.10). As the pH of the solution is raised, the –COOH group of form I can dissociate by donating a H$^+$ to the medium. The release of a H$^+$ results in the formation of the carboxylate group, –COO$^-$. This structure is shown as form II, which is the dipolar form of the molecule (see Fig. 1.10). This form, also called a zwitterion (from the German word for "hybrid"), is the isoelectric form of alanine, that is, it has an overall (net) charge of zero.

2. **Application of the Henderson-Hasselbalch equation:** The dissociation constant of the carboxyl group of an amino acid is called K$_1$, rather than K$_a$, because the molecule contains a second titratable group. The Henderson-Hasselbalch equation can be used to analyze the dissociation of the carboxyl group of alanine in the same way as described for acetic acid:

$$K_1 = \frac{[H^+][II]}{[I]}$$

where I is the fully protonated form of alanine and II is the isoelectric form of alanine (see Fig. 1.10). This equation can be rearranged and converted to its logarithmic form to yield:

$$pH = pK_1 + \log \frac{[II]}{[I]}$$

3. **Amino group dissociation:** The second titratable group of alanine is the amino (–NH$_3^+$) group shown in Figure 1.10. Because this is a much weaker acid than the –COOH group, it has a much smaller

dissociation constant, K_2. [Note: Its pK_a is, therefore, larger.] Release of a H^+ from the protonated amino group of form II results in the fully deprotonated form of alanine, form III (see Fig. 1.10).

4. **Alanine pKs:** The sequential dissociation of H^+ from the carboxyl and amino groups of alanine is summarized in Figure 1.10. Each titratable group has a pK_a that is numerically equal to the pH at which exactly one half of the H^+ have been removed from that group. The pK_a for the most acidic group ($-COOH$) is pK_1, whereas the pK_a for the next most acidic group ($-NH_3^+$) is pK_2. [Note: The pK_a of the α-carboxyl group of amino acids is ~2, whereas that of the α-amino group is ~9.]

5. **Alanine titration curve:** By applying the Henderson-Hasselbalch equation to each dissociable acidic group, it is possible to calculate the complete titration curve of a weak acid. Figure 1.11 shows the change in pH that occurs during the addition of base to the fully protonated form of alanine (I) to produce the completely deprotonated form (III). Note the following:

   a. **Buffer pairs:** The $-COOH/-COO^-$ pair can serve as a buffer in the pH region around pK_1, and the $-NH_3^+/-NH_2$ pair can buffer in the region around pK_2.

   b. **When pH = pK:** When the pH is equal to pK_1 (2.3), equal amounts of forms I and II of alanine exist in solution. When the pH is equal to pK_2 (9.1), equal amounts of forms II and III are present in solution.

   c. **Isoelectric point:** At neutral pH, alanine exists predominantly as the dipolar form II in which the amino and carboxyl groups are ionized, but the net charge is zero. The isoelectric point (pI) is the pH at which an amino acid is electrically neutral, that is, in which the sum of the positive charges equals the sum of the negative charges. For an amino acid, such as alanine, that has only two dissociable hydrogens (one from the α-carboxyl and one from the α-amino group), the pI is the average of pK_1 and pK_2 (pI = [2.3 + 9.1]/2 = 5.7) as shown in Figure 1.11. The pI is, thus, midway between pK_1 (2.3) and pK_2 (9.1). pI corresponds to the pH at which the form II (with a net charge of zero) predominates and at which there are also equal amounts of forms I (net charge of +1) and III (net charge of −1).

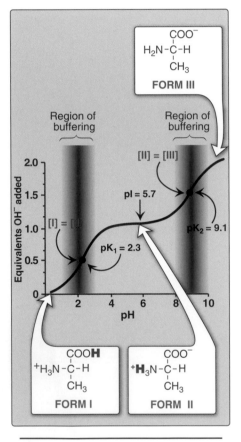

Figure 1.11
The titration curve of alanine.

> Separation of plasma proteins by charge typically is done at a pH above the pI of the major proteins. Therefore, the charge on the proteins is negative. In an electric field, the proteins will move toward the positive electrode at a rate determined by their net negative charge. Variations in the mobility pattern are suggestive of certain diseases.

6. **Net charge at neutral pH:** At physiologic pH, amino acids have a negatively charged group ($-COO^-$) and a positively charged group ($-NH_3^+$), both attached to the α-carbon. [Note: Glutamate, aspartate, histidine, arginine, and lysine have additional potentially

charged groups in their side chains.] Substances such as amino acids that can act either as an acid or a base are defined as amphoteric and are referred to as ampholytes (amphoteric electrolytes).

D. Other applications of the Henderson-Hasselbalch equation

The Henderson-Hasselbalch equation can be used to calculate how the pH of a physiologic solution responds to changes in the concentration of a weak acid and/or its corresponding salt form. For example, in the bicarbonate buffer system, the Henderson-Hasselbalch equation predicts how shifts in the bicarbonate ion concentration, $[HCO_3^-]$, and the carbon dioxide concentration $[CO_2]$ influence pH (Fig. 1.12A). The equation is also useful for calculating the abundance of ionic forms of acidic and basic drugs. For example, most drugs are either weak acids or weak bases (Fig. 1.12B). Acidic drugs (HA) release a H^+, causing a charged anion (A^-) to form.

$$HA \rightleftarrows H^+ + A^-$$

Weak bases (BH^+) can also release a H^+. However, the protonated form of basic drugs is usually charged, and the loss of a proton produces the uncharged base (B).

$$BH^+ \rightleftarrows B + H^+$$

A drug passes through membranes more readily if it is uncharged. Thus, for a weak acid, such as aspirin, the uncharged HA can permeate through membranes, but A^- cannot. Likewise, for a weak base, such as morphine, the uncharged B form permeates through the cell membrane, but BH^+ does not. Therefore, the effective concentration of the permeable form of each drug at its absorption site is determined by the relative concentrations of the charged (impermeant) and uncharged (permeant) forms. The ratio between the two forms is determined by the pH at the site of absorption and by the strength of the weak acid or base, which is represented by the pK_a of the ionizable group. The Henderson-Hasselbalch equation is useful in determining how much drug is found on either side of a membrane that separates two compartments that differ in pH, for example, the stomach (pH 1.0–1.5) and blood plasma (pH 7.4).

IV. CONCEPT MAPS

Students sometimes view biochemistry as a list of facts or equations to be memorized, rather than a body of concepts to be understood. Details provided to enrich understanding of these concepts inadvertently turn into distractions. What seems to be missing is a road map—a guide that provides the student with an understanding of how various topics fit together to "tell a story." Therefore, in this text, a series of biochemical concept maps have been created to graphically illustrate relationships between ideas presented in a chapter and to show how the information can be grouped or organized. A concept map is, thus, a tool for visualizing the connections between concepts. Material is represented in a hierarchic fashion, with the most inclusive, most general concepts at the

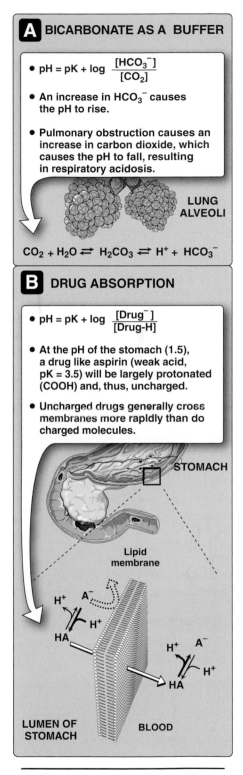

A   BICARBONATE AS A BUFFER

- $pH = pK + \log \dfrac{[HCO_3^-]}{[CO_2]}$

- An increase in HCO_3^- causes the pH to rise.

- Pulmonary obstruction causes an increase in carbon dioxide, which causes the pH to fall, resulting in respiratory acidosis.

LUNG ALVEOLI

$$CO_2 + H_2O \rightleftarrows H_2CO_3 \rightleftarrows H^+ + HCO_3^-$$

B   DRUG ABSORPTION

- $pH = pK + \log \dfrac{[Drug^-]}{[Drug-H]}$

- At the pH of the stomach (1.5), a drug like aspirin (weak acid, pK = 3.5) will be largely protonated (COOH) and, thus, uncharged.

- Uncharged drugs generally cross membranes more rapidly than do charged molecules.

STOMACH

Lipid membrane

H^+ A^-

H^+

HA

H^+ A^-

H^+

HA

LUMEN OF STOMACH   BLOOD

Figure 1.12
The Henderson-Hasselbalch equation is used to predict: (A) changes in pH as the concentrations of bicarbonate (HCO_3^-) or carbon dioxide (CO_2) are altered and (B) the ionic forms of drugs.

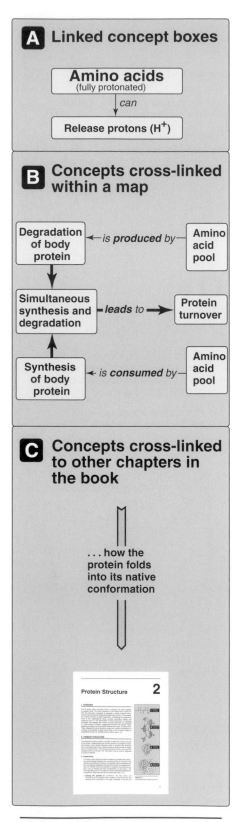

Figure 1.13
A–C. Symbols used in concept maps.

top of the map, and the more specific, less general concepts arranged beneath. The concept maps ideally function as templates or guides for organizing information, so the student can readily find the best ways to integrate new information into knowledge they already possess. Concept map construction is described below.

A. Concept boxes and links

Educators define concepts as "perceived regularities in events or objects." In the biochemical maps, concepts include abstractions (for example, free energy), processes (for example, oxidative phosphorylation), and compounds (for example, glucose 6-phosphate). These broadly defined concepts are prioritized with the central idea positioned at the top of the page. The concepts that follow from this central idea are then drawn in boxes (Fig. 1.13A). The size of the type indicates the relative importance of each idea. Lines are drawn between concept boxes to show which are related. The label on the line defines the relationship between two concepts, so that it reads as a valid statement (that is, the connection creates meaning). The lines with arrowheads indicate in which direction the connection should be read (Fig. 1.14).

B. Cross-links

Unlike linear flow charts or outlines, concept maps may contain crosslinks that allow the reader to visualize complex relationships between ideas represented in different parts of the map (Fig. 1.13B) or between the map and other chapters in this book (Fig. 1.13C). Crosslinks can, thus, identify concepts that are central to more than one topic in biochemistry, empowering students to be effective in clinical situations and on the United States Medical Licensure Examination (USMLE) or other examinations that require integration of material. Students learn to visually perceive nonlinear relationships between facts, in contrast to cross-referencing within linear text.

V. CHAPTER SUMMARY

Each amino acid has an **α-carboxyl group** and a primary **α-amino group** (except for **proline**, which has a **secondary amino group**). At physiologic pH, the α-carboxyl group is dissociated, forming the negatively charged carboxylate ion ($-COO^-$), and the α-amino group is protonated ($-NH_3^+$). Each amino acid also contains one of 20 distinctive **side chains** attached to the α-carbon atom. The chemical nature of this **R group** determines the function of an amino acid in a protein and provides the basis for classification of the amino acids as **nonpolar**, **uncharged polar**, **acidic (polar negative)**, or **basic (polar positive)**. All free amino acids, plus charged amino acids in peptide chains, can serve as **buffers**. The quantitative relationship between the pH of a solution and the concentration of a weak acid (HA) and its conjugate base (A^-) is described by the **Henderson-Hasselbalch equation**. Buffering occurs within ±1 pH unit of the pK_a and is maximal when pH = pK_a, at which $[A^-] = [HA]$. Because the α-carbon of each amino acid (except glycine) is attached to four different chemical groups, it is asymmetric (**chiral**), and amino acids exist in D- and L-isomeric forms that are optically active mirror images (**enantiomers**). The L-form of amino acids is found in proteins synthesized by the human body.

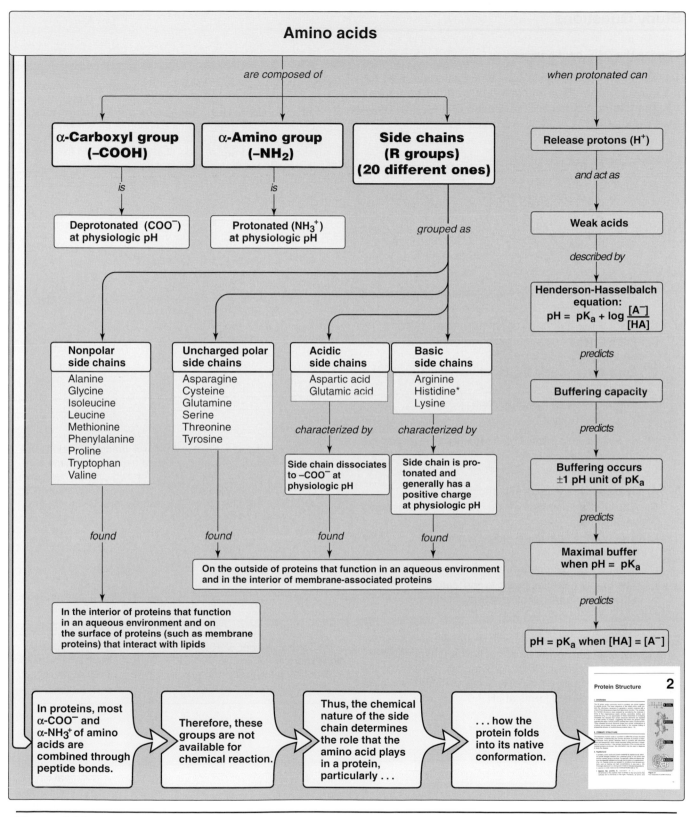

Figure 1.14
Key concept map for amino acids. [Note: *Free histidine is largely deprotonated at physiologic pH, but when incorporated into a protein, it can be protonated or deprotonated depending on the local environment.]

Study Questions

Choose the ONE best answer.

1.1 Which one of the following statements concerning the titration curve for a nonpolar amino acid is correct? The letters A through D designate certain regions on the curve below.

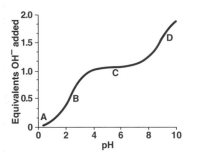

A. Point A represents the region where the amino acid is deprotonated.

B. Point B represents a region of minimal buffering.

C. Point C represents the region where the net charge on the amino acid is zero.

D. Point D represents the pK of the amino acid's carboxyl group.

E. The amino acid could be lysine.

Correct answer = C. Point C represents the isoelectric point, or pI, and as such is midway between pK_1 and pK_2 for a nonpolar amino acid. The amino acid is fully protonated at Point A. Point B represents a region of maximum buffering, as does Point D. Lysine is a basic amino acid, and free lysine has an ionizable side chain in addition to the ionizable α-amino and α-carboxyl groups.

1.2 Which one of the following statements concerning the peptide shown below is correct?

Val-Cys-Glu-Ser-Asp-Arg-Cys

A. The peptide contains asparagine.

B. The peptide contains a side chain with a secondary amino group.

C. The peptide contains a side chain that can be phosphorylated.

D. The peptide cannot form an internal disulfide bond.

E. The peptide would move to the cathode (negative electrode) during electrophoresis at pH 5.

Correct answer = C. The hydroxyl group of serine can accept a phosphate group. Asp is aspartate. Proline contains a secondary amino group. The two cysteine residues can, under oxidizing conditions, form a disulfide (covalent) bond. The net charge on the peptide at pH 5 is negative, and it would move to the anode.

1.3 A 2-year-old child presents with metabolic acidosis after ingesting an unknown number of flavored aspirin tablets. At presentation, her blood pH was 7.0. Given that the pK_a of aspirin (salicylic acid) is 3, calculate the ratio of its ionized to unionized forms at pH 7.0.

Correct answer = 10,000 to 1. $pH = pK_a + \log [A^-]/[HA]$. Therefore, $7 = 3 + x$ and $x = 4$. The ratio of A^- (ionized) to HA (unionized), then, is 10,000 to 1 because the log of 10,000 is 4.

Protein Structure

2

I. OVERVIEW

The 20 amino acids commonly found in proteins are joined together by peptide bonds. The linear sequence of the linked amino acids contains the information necessary to generate a protein molecule with a unique three-dimensional shape that determines function. The complexity of protein structure is best analyzed by considering the molecule in terms of four organizational levels: primary, secondary, tertiary, and quaternary (Fig. 2.1). An examination of these hierarchies of increasing complexity has revealed that certain structural elements are repeated in a wide variety of proteins, suggesting that there are general rules regarding the ways in which proteins achieve their native, functional form. These repeated structural elements range from simple combinations of α-helices and β-sheets forming small motifs to the complex folding of polypeptide domains of multifunctional proteins (see p. 19).

II. PRIMARY STRUCTURE

The sequence of amino acids in a protein is called the primary structure of the protein. Understanding the primary structure of proteins is important because many genetic diseases result in proteins with abnormal amino acid sequences, which cause improper folding and loss or impairment of normal function. If the primary structures of the normal and the mutated proteins are known, this information may be used to diagnose or study the disease.

A. Peptide bond

In proteins, amino acids are joined covalently by peptide bonds, which are amide linkages between the α-carboxyl group of one amino acid and the α-amino group of another. For example, valine and alanine can form the dipeptide valylalanine through the formation of a peptide bond (Fig. 2.2). Peptide bonds are resistant to conditions that denature proteins, such as heating and high concentrations of urea (see p. 20). Prolonged exposure to a strong acid or base at elevated temperatures is required to break these bonds nonenzymically (see p. 14).

1. **Naming the peptide:** By convention, the free amino end (N-terminal) of the peptide chain is written to the left and the free carboxyl end (C-terminal) to the right. Therefore, all amino acid

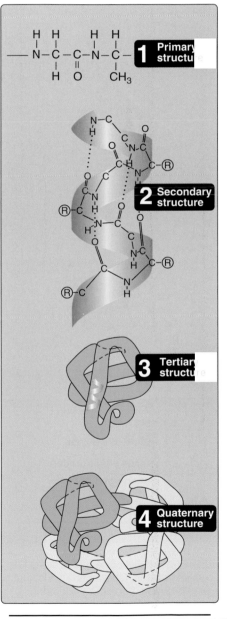

Figure 2.1
Four hierarchies of protein structure.

13

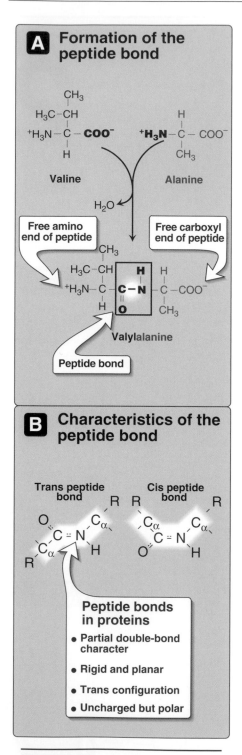

A Formation of the peptide bond

Valine

Alanine

H₂O

Free amino end of peptide

Free carboxyl end of peptide

Valylalanine

Peptide bond

B Characteristics of the peptide bond

Trans peptide bond

Cis peptide bond

Peptide bonds in proteins

- Partial double-bond character
- Rigid and planar
- Trans configuration
- Uncharged but polar

Figure 2.2
A. Formation of a peptide bond, showing the structure of the dipeptide valylalanine. B. Characteristics of the peptide bond. [Note: Peptide bonds involving proline may have a cis configuration.]

sequences are read from the N- to the C-terminal end. For example, in Figure 2.2A, the order of the amino acids in the dipeptide is valine, alanine. Linkage of ≥50 amino acids through peptide bonds results in an unbranched chain called a polypeptide, or protein. Each component amino acid is called a residue because it is the portion of the amino acid remaining after the atoms of water are lost in the formation of the peptide bond. When a peptide is named, all amino acid residues have their suffixes (-ine, -an, -ic, or -ate) changed to -yl, with the exception of the C-terminal amino acid. For example, a tripeptide composed of an N-terminal valine, a glycine, and a C-terminal leucine is called valylglycylleucine.

2. **Peptide bond characteristics:** The peptide bond has a partial double-bond character, that is, it is shorter than a single bond and is rigid and planar (Fig. 2.2B). This prevents free rotation around the bond between the carbonyl carbon and the nitrogen of the peptide bond. However, the bonds between the α-carbons and the α-amino or α-carboxyl groups can be freely rotated (although they are limited by the size and character of the R groups). This allows the polypeptide chain to assume a variety of possible conformations. The peptide bond is almost always in the trans configuration (instead of the cis; see Fig. 2.2B), in large part because of steric interference of the R groups (side chains) when in the cis position.

3. **Peptide bond polarity:** Like all amide linkages, the −C=O and −NH groups of the peptide bond are uncharged, and neither accept nor release protons over the pH range of 2–12. Thus, the charged groups present in polypeptides consist solely of the N-terminal (α-amino) group, the C-terminal (α-carboxyl) group, and any ionized groups present in the side chains of the constituent amino acids. The −C=O and −NH groups of the peptide bond are polar, however, and are involved in hydrogen bonds (for example, in α-helices and β-sheets), as described on pp. 16–17.

B. Determining the amino acid composition of a polypeptide

The first step in determining the primary structure of a polypeptide is to identify and quantitate its constituent amino acids. A purified sample of the polypeptide to be analyzed is first hydrolyzed by strong acid at 110°C for 24 hours. This treatment cleaves the peptide bonds and releases the individual amino acids, which can be separated by cation-exchange chromatography. In this technique, a mixture of amino acids is applied to a column that contains a resin to which a negatively charged group is tightly attached. [Note: If the attached group is positively charged, the column becomes an anion-exchange column.] The amino acids bind to the column with different affinities, depending on their charges, hydrophobicity, and other characteristics. Each amino acid is sequentially released from the chromatography column by eluting with solutions of increasing ionic strength and pH (Fig. 2.3). The separated amino acids contained in the eluate from the column are quantitated by heating them with ninhydrin (a reagent that forms a purple compound with most amino acids, ammonia, and amines). The amount of each amino acid is determined spectrophotometrically by measuring the amount of light absorbed by the ninhydrin derivative. The analysis described above is performed using an amino acid analyzer, an automated machine whose components are depicted in Figure 2.3.

C. Sequencing the peptide from its N-terminal end

Sequencing is a stepwise process of identifying the specific amino acid at each position in the peptide chain, beginning at the N-terminal end. Phenylisothiocyanate, known as Edman reagent, is used to label the amino-terminal residue under mildly alkaline conditions (Fig. 2.4). The resulting phenylthiohydantoin (PTH) derivative introduces an instability in the N-terminal peptide bond such that it can be hydrolyzed without cleaving the other peptide bonds. The identity of the amino acid derivative can then be determined. Edman reagent can be applied repeatedly to the shortened peptide obtained in each previous cycle. Automated sequencers are now used.

D. Cleaving the polypeptide into smaller fragments

Many polypeptides have a primary structure composed of >100 amino acids. Such molecules cannot be sequenced directly from end to end. However, these large molecules can be cleaved at specific sites and the resulting fragments sequenced. By using more than one cleaving agent (enzymes and/or chemicals) on separate samples of the purified polypeptide, overlapping fragments can be generated that permit the proper ordering of the sequenced fragments, thereby providing a complete amino acid sequence of the large polypeptide (Fig. 2.5). Enzymes that hydrolyze peptide bonds are termed *peptidases* (*proteases*). [Note: *Exopeptidases* cut at the ends of proteins and are divided into *aminopeptidases* and *carboxypeptidases*. *Carboxypeptidases* are used in determining the C-terminal amino acid. *Endopeptidases* cleave within a protein.]

E. Determining a protein's primary structure by DNA sequencing

The sequence of nucleotides in a protein-coding region of the DNA specifies the amino acid sequence of a polypeptide. Therefore, if the nucleotide sequence can be determined, knowledge of the genetic code (see p. 447) allows the sequence of nucleotides to be translated into the corresponding amino acid sequence of that polypeptide. This indirect process, although routinely used to obtain the amino acid sequences of proteins, has the limitations of not being able to predict

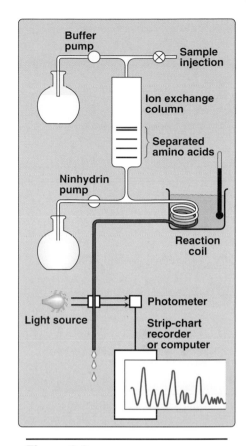

Figure 2.3
Determination of the amino acid composition of a polypeptide using an amino acid analyzer.

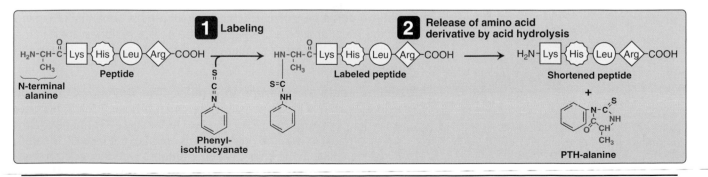

Figure 2.4
Determination of the amino (N)-terminal residue of a polypeptide by Edman degradation. PTH = phenylthiohydantoin.

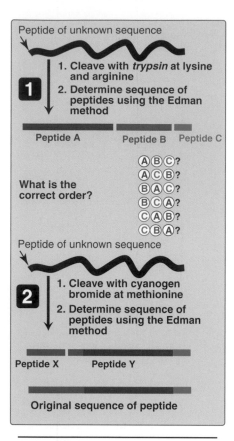

Figure 2.5
Overlapping of peptides produced
by the cleavage action of *trypsin* and
cyanogen bromide.

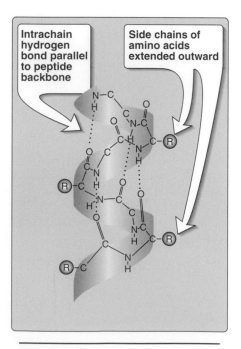

Figure 2.6
Structure of an α-helix.

the positions of disulfide bonds in the folded chain and of not identifying any amino acids that are modified after their incorporation into
the polypeptide (posttranslational modification; see p. 459). Therefore,
direct protein sequencing is an extremely important tool for determining the true character of the primary sequence of many polypeptides.

III. SECONDARY STRUCTURE

The polypeptide backbone does not assume a random three-dimensional
structure but, instead, generally forms regular arrangements of amino acids
that are located near each other in the linear sequence. These arrangements are termed the secondary structure of the polypeptide. The α-helix,
β-sheet, and β-bend (or, β-turn) are examples of secondary structures
commonly encountered in proteins. Each is stabilized by hydrogen bonds
between atoms of the peptide backbone. [Note: The collagen α-chain helix,
another example of secondary structure, is discussed on p. 45.]

A. α-Helix

Several different polypeptide helices are found in nature, but the
α-helix is the most common. It is a rigid, right-handed spiral structure,
consisting of a tightly packed, coiled polypeptide backbone core, with
the side chains of the component ʟ-amino acids extending outward
from the central axis to avoid interfering sterically with each other
(Fig. 2.6). A very diverse group of proteins contains α-helices. For
example, the keratins are a family of closely related, rigid, fibrous proteins whose structure is nearly entirely α-helical. They are a major
component of tissues such as hair and skin. In contrast to keratin,
myoglobin, whose structure is also highly α-helical, is a globular, flexible molecule (see p. 26) found in muscles.

1. **Hydrogen bonds:** An α-helix is stabilized by extensive hydrogen
   bonding between the peptide bond carbonyl oxygens and amide
   hydrogens that are part of the polypeptide backbone (see Fig. 2.6).
   The hydrogen bonds extend up and are parallel to the spiral from
   the carbonyl oxygen of one peptide bond to the –NH group of a
   peptide linkage four residues ahead in the polypeptide. This insures
   that all but the first and last peptide bond components are linked to
   each other through intrachain hydrogen bonds. Hydrogen bonds are
   individually weak, but they collectively serve to stabilize the helix.

2. **Amino acids per turn:** Each turn of an α-helix contains 3.6 amino
   acids. Thus, amino acids spaced three or four residues apart in the
   primary sequence are spatially close together when folded in the
   α-helix.

3. **Amino acids that disrupt an α-helix:** The R group of an amino
   acid determines its propensity to be in an α-helix. Proline disrupts
   an α-helix because its rigid secondary amino group is not geometri-
   cally compatible with the right-handed spiral of the α-helix. Instead,
   it inserts a kink in the chain, which interferes with the smooth, helical structure. Glycine is also a "helix breaker" because its R group
   (a hydrogen) confers high flexibility. Additionally, amino acids with
   charged or bulky R groups (such as glutamate and tryptophan,

respectively) and those with a branch at the β-carbon, the first carbon in the R group (for example, valine), have low α-helix propensity.

B. β-Sheet

The β-sheet is another form of secondary structure in which all of the peptide bond components are involved in hydrogen bonding (Fig. 2.7A). Because the surfaces of β-sheets appear "pleated," they are often called β-pleated sheets. [Note: Pleating results from successive α-carbons being slightly above or below the plane of the sheet.] Illustrations of protein structure often show β-strands as broad arrows (Fig. 2.7B).

1. **Formation:** A β-sheet is formed by two or more peptide chains (β-strands) aligned laterally and stabilized by hydrogen bonds between the carboxyl and amino groups of amino acids that either are far apart in a single polypeptide (intrachain bonds) or are in different polypeptide chains (interchain bonds). The adjacent β-strands are arranged either antiparallel to each other (with the N-termini alternating as shown in Fig. 2.7B) or parallel to each other (with the N-termini together as shown in Fig. 2.7C). On each β-strand, the R groups of adjacent amino acids extend in opposite directions, above and below the plane of the β-sheet. [Note: β-sheets are not flat and have a right-handed curl (twist) when viewed along the polypeptide backbone.]

2. **Comparing α-helices and β-sheets:** In β-sheets, the β-strands are almost fully extended and the hydrogen bonds between the strands are perpendicular to the polypeptide backbone (see Fig. 2.7A). In contrast, in α-helices, the polypeptide is coiled and the hydrogen bonds are parallel to the backbone (see Fig. 2.6).

> The orientation of the R groups of the amino acid residues in both the α-helix and the β-sheet can result in formation of polar and nonpolar sides in these secondary structures, thereby making them amphipathic.

C. β-Bends (reverse turns, β-turns)

β-Bends reverse the direction of a polypeptide chain, helping it form a compact, globular shape. They are usually found on the surface of protein molecules and often include charged residues. [Note: β-Bends were given this name because they often connect successive strands of antiparallel β-sheets.] β-Bends are generally composed of four amino acids, one of which may be proline, the amino acid that causes a kink in the polypeptide chain. Glycine, the amino acid with the smallest R group, is also frequently found in β-bends. β-Bends are stabilized by the formation of hydrogen bonds between the first and last residues in the bend.

D. Nonrepetitive secondary structure

Approximately one half of an average globular protein is organized into repetitive structures, such as the α-helix and β-sheet. The remainder

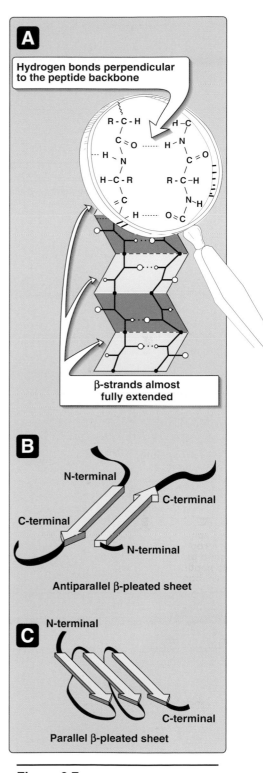

A

Hydrogen bonds perpendicular to the peptide backbone

R-C-H   H-C
C=O ···· H-N
H-N   C=O
H-C-R   R-C-H
C   N-H
H ···· O=C

β-strands almost fully extended

B

N-terminal

C-terminal

C-terminal

N-terminal

Antiparallel β-pleated sheet

C

N-terminal

C-terminal

Parallel β-pleated sheet

Figure 2.7
A. Structure of a β-sheet. B. An antiparallel β-sheet with the β-strands represented as broad arrows. C. A parallel β-sheet formed from a single polypeptide chain folding back on itself.

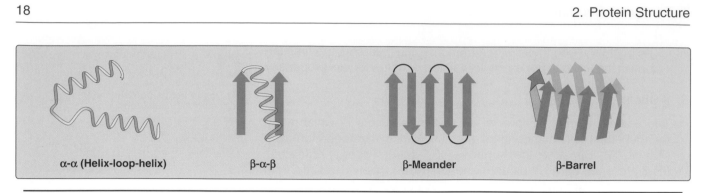

α-α (Helix-loop-helix)   **β-α-β**   **β-Meander**   **β-Barrel**

Figure 2.8
Common structural motifs involving α-helices and β-sheets. The names describe their schematic appearance.

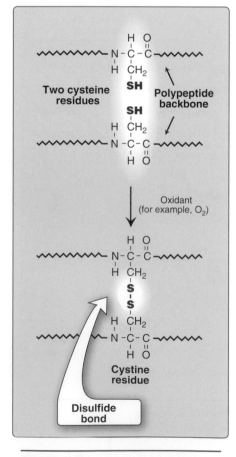

Figure 2.9
Formation of a disulfide bond by the oxidation of two cysteine residues, producing one cystine residue.
O_2 = oxygen.

of the polypeptide chain is described as having a loop or coil conformation. These nonrepetitive secondary structures are not random but rather simply have a less regular structure than those described above. [Note: The term "random coil" refers to the disordered structure obtained when proteins are denatured (see p. 20).]

E. Supersecondary structures (motifs)

Globular proteins are constructed by combining secondary structural elements (that is, α-helices, β-sheets, and coils), producing specific geometric patterns, or motifs. These form primarily the core (interior) region of the molecule. They are connected by loop regions (for example, β-bends) at the surface of the protein. Supersecondary structures are usually produced by the close packing of side chains from adjacent secondary structural elements. For example, α-helices and β-sheets that are adjacent in the amino acid sequence are also usually (but not always) adjacent in the final, folded protein. Some of the more common motifs are illustrated in Figure 2.8.

> Motifs may be associated with particular functions. Proteins that bind to DNA contain a limited number of motifs. The helix–loop–helix motif is an example found in a number of proteins that function as transcription factors (see p. 438).

IV. TERTIARY STRUCTURE

The primary structure of a polypeptide chain determines its tertiary structure. "Tertiary" refers both to the folding of domains (the basic units of structure and function; see A. below) and to the final arrangement of domains in the polypeptide. The tertiary structure of globular proteins in aqueous solution is compact, with a high density (close packing) of the atoms in the core of the molecule. Hydrophobic side chains are buried in the interior, whereas hydrophilic groups are generally found on the surface of the molecule.

A. Domains

Domains are the fundamental functional and three-dimensional structural units of polypeptides. Polypeptide chains that are >200 amino acids in length generally consist of two or more domains. The core of a domain is built from combinations of supersecondary structural elements (motifs). Folding of the peptide chain within a domain usually occurs independently of folding in other domains. Therefore, each domain has the characteristics of a small, compact globular protein that is structurally independent of the other domains in the polypeptide chain.

B. Stabilizing interactions

The unique three-dimensional structure of each polypeptide is determined by its amino acid sequence. Interactions between the amino acid side chains guide the folding of the polypeptide to form a compact structure. The following four types of interactions cooperate in stabilizing the tertiary structures of globular proteins.

1. **Disulfide bonds:** A disulfide bond (–S–S–) is a covalent linkage formed from the sulfhydryl group (–SH) of each of two cysteine residues to produce a cystine residue (Fig. 2.9). The two cysteines may be separated from each other by many amino acids in the primary sequence of a polypeptide or may even be located on two different polypeptides. The folding of the polypeptide(s) brings the cysteine residues into proximity and permits covalent bonding of their side chains. A disulfide bond contributes to the stability of the three-dimensional shape of the protein molecule and prevents it from becoming denatured in the extracellular environment. For example, many disulfide bonds are found in proteins such as immunoglobulins that are secreted by cells. [Note: *Protein disulfide isomerase* breaks and reforms disulfide bonds during folding.]

2. **Hydrophobic interactions:** Amino acids with nonpolar side chains tend to be located in the interior of the polypeptide molecule, where they associate with other hydrophobic amino acids (Fig. 2.10). In contrast, amino acids with polar or charged side chains tend to be located on the surface of the molecule in contact with the polar solvent. [Note: Recall that proteins located in nonpolar (lipid) environments, such as a membrane, exhibit the reverse arrangement (see Fig. 1.4, p. 4).] In each case, a segregation of R groups occurs that is energetically most favorable.

3. **Hydrogen bonds:** Amino acid side chains containing oxygen- or nitrogen-bound hydrogen, such as in the alcohol groups of serine and threonine, can form hydrogen bonds with electron-rich atoms, such as the oxygen of a carboxyl group or carbonyl group of a peptide bond (Fig. 2.11; see also Fig. 1.6, p. 4). Formation of hydrogen bonds between polar groups on the surface of proteins and the aqueous solvent enhances the solubility of the protein.

4. **Ionic interactions:** Negatively charged groups, such as the carboxylate group (–COO$^-$) in the side chain of aspartate or glutamate, can interact with positively charged groups such as the amino group (–NH$_3^+$) in the side chain of lysine (see Fig. 2.11).

C. Protein folding

Interactions between the side chains of amino acids determine how a linear polypeptide chain folds into the intricate three-dimensional

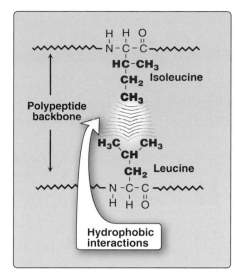

Figure 2.10
Hydrophobic interactions between amino acids with nonpolar side chains.

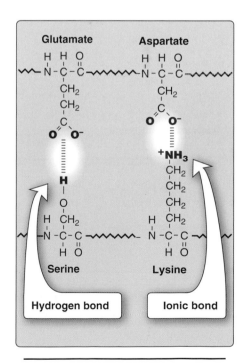

Figure 2.11
Interactions of side chains of amino acids through hydrogen bonds and ionic bonds (salt bridges).

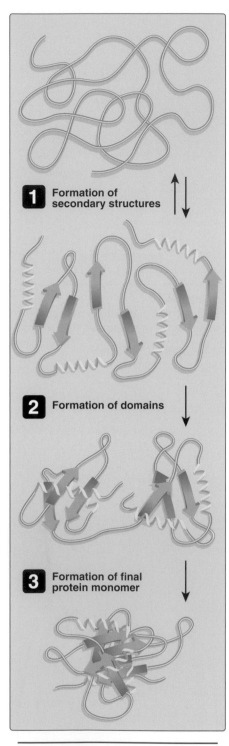

1 Formation of
secondary structures

2 Formation of domains

3 Formation of final
protein monomer

Figure 2.12
Steps in protein folding (simplified).

shape of the functional protein. Protein folding, which occurs within the cell in seconds to minutes, involves nonrandom, ordered pathways. As a peptide folds, secondary structures form, driven by the hydrophobic effect (that is, hydrophobic groups come together as water is released). These small structures combine to form larger structures. Additional events stabilize secondary structure and initiate formation of tertiary structure. In the last stage, the peptide achieves its fully folded, native (functional) form characterized by a low-energy state (Fig. 2.12). [Note: Some biologically active proteins or segments thereof lack a stable tertiary structure. They are referred to as intrinsically disordered proteins.]

D. Protein denaturation

Denaturation results in the unfolding and disorganization of a protein's secondary and tertiary structures without the hydrolysis of peptide bonds. Denaturing agents include heat, urea, organic solvents, strong acids or bases, detergents, and ions of heavy metals such as lead. Denaturation may, under ideal conditions, be reversible, such that the protein refolds into its original native structure when the denaturing agent is removed. However, most proteins remain permanently disordered once denatured. Denatured proteins are often insoluble and precipitate from solution.

E. Chaperones in protein folding

The information needed for correct protein folding is contained in the primary structure of the polypeptide. However, most denatured proteins do not resume their native conformations even under favorable environmental conditions. This is because, for many proteins, folding is a facilitated process that requires a specialized group of proteins, referred to as molecular chaperones, and ATP hydrolysis. The chaperones, also known as heat shock proteins (HSP), interact with a polypeptide at various stages during the folding process. Some chaperones bind hydrophobic regions of an extended polypeptide and are important in keeping the protein unfolded until its synthesis is completed (for example, Hsp70). Others form cage-like macromolecular structures composed of two stacked rings. The partially folded protein enters the cage, binds the central cavity through hydrophobic interactions, folds, and is released (for example, mitochondrial Hsp60). [Note: Cage-like chaperones are sometimes referred to as chaperonins.] Chaperones, then, facilitate correct protein folding by binding to and stabilizing exposed, aggregation-prone hydrophobic regions in nascent (and denatured) polypeptides, preventing premature folding.

V. QUATERNARY STRUCTURE

Many proteins consist of a single polypeptide chain and are defined as monomeric proteins. However, others may consist of two or more polypeptide chains that may be structurally identical or totally unrelated. The arrangement of these polypeptide subunits is called the quaternary structure of the protein. Subunits are held together primarily by noncovalent interactions (for example, hydrogen bonds, ionic bonds, and hydrophobic interactions). Subunits either may function independently of each other or may work cooperatively, as in hemoglobin, in which the binding of oxygen to one subunit of the tetramer increases the affinity of the other subunits for oxygen (see p. 29).

> Isoforms are proteins that perform the same function but have different primary structures. They can arise from different genes or from tissue-specific processing of the product of a single gene. If the proteins function as enzymes, they are referred to as isozymes (see p. 65).

VI. PROTEIN MISFOLDING

Protein folding is a complex process that can sometimes result in improperly folded molecules. These misfolded proteins are usually tagged and degraded within the cell (see p. 247). However, this quality control system is not perfect, and intracellular or extracellular aggregates of misfolded proteins can accumulate, particularly as individuals age. Deposits of misfolded proteins are associated with a number of diseases.

A. Amyloid diseases

Misfolding of proteins may occur spontaneously or be caused by a mutation in a particular gene, which then produces an altered protein. In addition, some apparently normal proteins can, after abnormal proteolytic cleavage, take on a unique conformation that leads to the spontaneous formation of long, fibrillar protein assemblies consisting of β-pleated sheets. Accumulation of these insoluble fibrous protein aggregates, called amyloids, has been implicated in neurodegenerative disorders such as Parkinson disease and Alzheimer disease (AD). The dominant component of the amyloid plaque that accumulates in AD is amyloid β (Aβ), an extracellular peptide containing 40–42 amino acid residues. X-ray crystallography and infrared spectroscopy demonstrate a characteristic β-pleated sheet secondary structure in nonbranching fibrils. This peptide, when aggregated in a β-pleated sheet conformation, is neurotoxic and is the central pathogenic event leading to the cognitive impairment characteristic of the disease. The Aβ that is deposited in the brain in AD is derived by enzymic cleavages (by *secretases*) from the larger amyloid precursor protein, a single transmembrane protein expressed on the cell surface in the brain and other tissues (Fig. 2.13). The Aβ peptides aggregate, generating the amyloid that is found in the brain parenchyma and around blood vessels. Most cases of AD are not genetically based, although at least 5% of cases are familial. A second biologic factor involved in the development of AD is the accumulation of neurofibrillary tangles inside neurons. A key component of these tangled fibers is an abnormal form (hyperphosphorylated and insoluble) of the tau (τ) protein, which, in its healthy version, helps in the assembly of the microtubular structure. The defective τ appears to block the actions of its normal counterpart. [Note: In Parkinson disease, amyloid is formed from α-synuclein protein.]

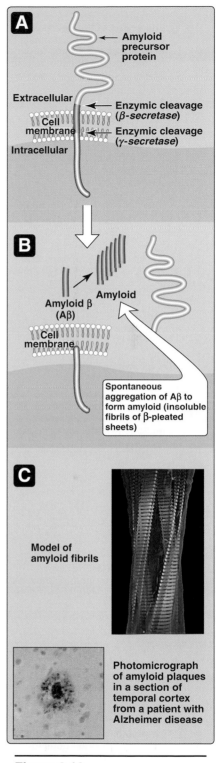

Figure 2.13
A–C. Formation of amyloid plaques found in Alzheimer disease (AD). [Note: Mutations to *presenilin*, the catalytic subunit of *γ-secretase*, are the most common cause of familial AD.]

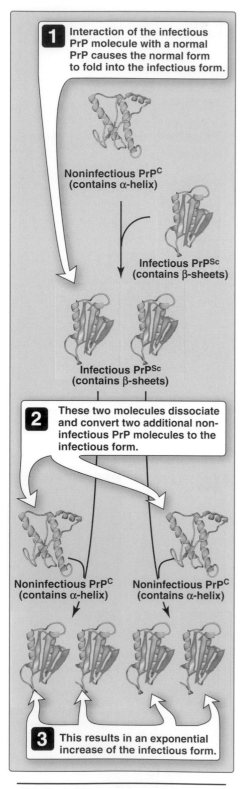

Figure 2.14
One proposed mechanism for multiplication of infectious prions. PrP = prion protein; PrP^c = prion protein cellular; PrP^{Sc} = prion protein scrapie.

B. Prion (proteinaceous infectious particle) diseases

The prion protein (PrP) is the causative agent of transmissible spongiform encephalopathies (TSE), including Creutzfeldt-Jakob disease in humans, scrapie in sheep, and bovine spongiform encephalopathy in cattle (popularly called "mad cow" disease). After an extensive series of purification procedures, scientists were surprised to find that the infectivity of the agent causing scrapie in sheep was associated with a single protein species that was not complexed with detectable nucleic acid. This infectious protein is designated PrP^{Sc} (Sc = scrapie). It is highly resistant to proteolytic degradation and tends to form insoluble aggregates of fibrils, similar to the amyloid found in some other diseases of the brain. A noninfectious form of PrP^C (C = cellular), encoded by the same gene as the infectious agent, is present in normal mammalian brains on the surface of neurons and glial cells. Thus, PrP^C is a host protein. No primary structure differences or alternate posttranslational modifications have been found between the normal and the infectious forms of the protein. The key to becoming infectious apparently lies in changes in the three-dimensional conformation of PrP^C. Research has demonstrated that a number of α-helices present in noninfectious PrP^C are replaced by β-sheets in the infectious form (Fig. 2.14). This conformational difference is presumably what confers relative resistance to proteolytic degradation of infectious prions and permits them to be distinguished from the normal PrP^C in infected tissue. The infective agent is, thus, an altered version of a normal protein, which acts as a template for converting the normal protein to the pathogenic conformation. The TSE are invariably fatal, and no treatment is currently available that can alter this outcome.

VII. CHAPTER SUMMARY

Central to understanding protein structure is the concept of the **native conformation** (Fig. 2.15), which is the functional, fully folded protein structure (for example, an active enzyme or structural protein). The unique three-dimensional structure of the native conformation is determined by its **primary structure**, that is, its amino acid sequence. Interactions between the amino acid side chains guide the folding of the polypeptide chain to form **secondary**, **tertiary**, and (sometimes) **quaternary** structures, which cooperate in stabilizing the native conformation of the protein. In addition, a specialized group of proteins named **chaperones** is required for the proper folding of many species of proteins. **Protein denaturation** results in the unfolding and disorganization of the protein's structure, which are not accompanied by hydrolysis of peptide bonds. Denaturation may be reversible or, more commonly, irreversible. Disease can occur when an apparently normal protein assumes a conformation that is cytotoxic, as in the case of **Alzheimer disease** (**AD**) and the **transmissible spongiform encephalopathies** (**TSE**), including **Creutzfeldt-Jakob disease**. In AD, normal proteins, after abnormal chemical processing, take on a unique conformational state that leads to the formation of neurotoxic **amyloid β peptide** (**Aβ**) assemblies consisting of β-pleated sheets. In TSE, the infective agent is an altered version of a normal **prion protein** that acts as a template for converting normal protein to the pathogenic conformation.

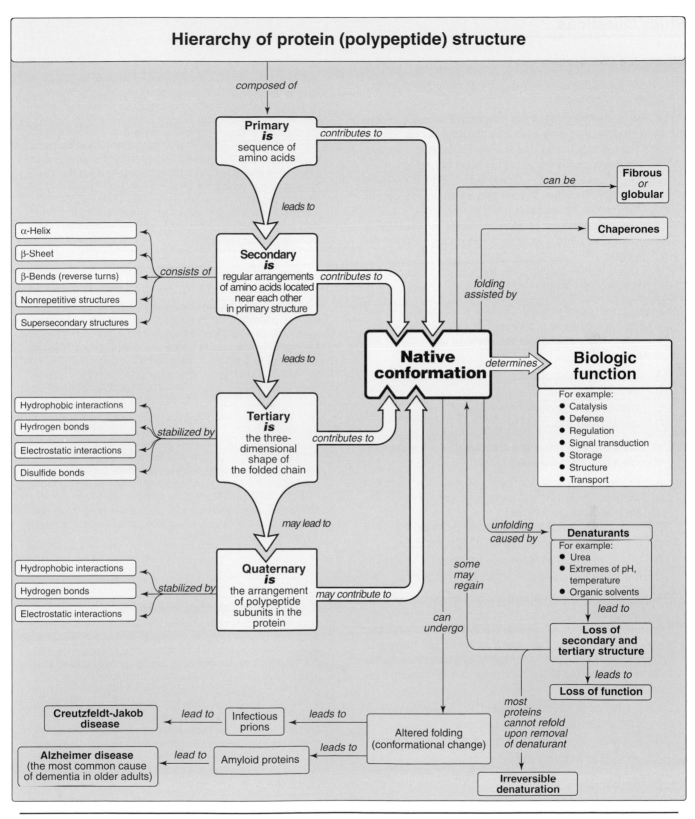

Figure 2.15
Key concept map for protein structure.

Study Questions

Choose the ONE best answer.

2.1 Which one of the following statements concerning protein structure is correct?

A. Proteins consisting of one polypeptide have quaternary structure that is stabilized by covalent bonds.

B. The peptide bonds that link amino acids in a protein most commonly occur in the cis configuration.

C. The formation of a disulfide bond in a protein requires the participating cysteine residues to be adjacent in the primary structure.

D. The denaturation of proteins leads to irreversible loss of secondary structural elements such as the α-helix.

E. The primary driving force for protein folding is the hydrophobic effect.

Correct answer = E. The hydrophobic effect, or the tendency of nonpolar entities to associate in a polar environment, is the primary driving force of protein folding. Quaternary structure requires more than one polypeptide, and, when present, it is stabilized primarily by noncovalent bonds. The peptide bond is almost always trans. The two cysteine residues participating in disulfide bond formation may be a great distance apart in the amino acid sequence of a polypeptide (or on two separate polypeptides) but are brought into close proximity by the three-dimensional folding of the polypeptide. Denaturation may be reversible or irreversible.

2.2 A particular point mutation results in disruption of the α-helical structure in a segment of the mutant protein. The most likely change in the primary structure of the mutant protein is:

A. glutamate to aspartate.

B. lysine to arginine.

C. methionine to proline.

D. valine to alanine.

Correct answer = C. Proline, because of its secondary amino group, is incompatible with an α-helix. Glutamate, aspartate, lysine, and arginine are charged amino acids, and valine is a branched amino acid. Charged and branched (bulky) amino acids may disrupt an α-helix. [Note: The flexibility of glycine's R group can also disrupt an α-helix.]

2.3 In comparing the α-helix to the β-sheet, which statement is correct only for the β-sheet?

A. Extensive hydrogen bonds between the carbonyl oxygen (C=O) and the amide hydrogen (N–H) of the peptide bond are formed.

B. It may be found in typical globular proteins.

C. It is stabilized by interchain hydrogen bonds.

D. It is an example of secondary structure.

E. It may be found in supersecondary structures.

Correct answer = C. The β-sheet is stabilized by interchain hydrogen bonds formed between separate polypeptide chains and by intrachain hydrogen bonds formed between regions of a single polypeptide. The α-helix, however, is stabilized only by intrachain hydrogen bonds. Statements A, B, D, and E are true for both of these secondary structural elements.

2.4 An 80-year-old man presented with impairment of intellectual function and alterations in behavior. His family reported progressive disorientation and memory loss over the last 6 months. There is no family history of dementia. The patient was tentatively diagnosed with Alzheimer disease (AD). Which one of the following best describes AD?

A. It is associated with β-amyloid, an abnormal protein with an altered amino acid sequence.

B. It results from accumulation of denatured proteins that have random conformations.

C. It is associated with the accumulation of amyloid precursor protein.

D. It is associated with the deposition of neurotoxic amyloid β peptide aggregates.

E. It is an environmentally produced disease not influenced by the genetics of the individual.

F. It is caused by the infectious β-sheet form of a host-cell protein.

Correct answer = D. Alzheimer disease (AD) is associated with long, fibrillar protein assemblies consisting of β-pleated sheets found in the brain and elsewhere. The disease is associated with abnormal processing of a normal protein. The accumulated altered protein occurs in a β-pleated sheet conformation that is neurotoxic. The amyloid β that is deposited in the brain in AD is derived by proteolytic cleavages from the larger amyloid precursor protein, a single transmembrane protein expressed on the cell surface in the brain and other tissues. Most cases of AD are sporadic, although at least 5% of cases are familial. Prion diseases, such as Creutzfeldt-Jakob, are caused by the infectious β-sheet form (PrP^{Sc}) of a host-cell protein (PrP^{C}).

Globular Proteins

3

I. OVERVIEW

The previous chapter described the types of secondary and tertiary structures that are the bricks and mortar of protein architecture. By arranging these fundamental structural elements in different combinations, widely diverse proteins can be constructed that are capable of various specialized functions. This chapter examines the relationship between structure and function for the clinically important globular hemeproteins. Fibrous structural proteins are discussed in Chapter 4.

II. GLOBULAR HEMEPROTEINS

Hemeproteins are a group of specialized proteins that contain heme as a tightly bound prosthetic group. (See p. 54 for a discussion of prosthetic groups.) The role of the heme group is dictated by the environment created by the three-dimensional structure of the protein. For example, the heme group of a cytochrome functions as an electron carrier that is alternately oxidized and reduced (see p. 75). In contrast, the heme group of the enzyme *catalase* is part of the active site of the enzyme that catalyzes the breakdown of hydrogen peroxide (see p. 148). In hemoglobin and myoglobin, the two most abundant hemeproteins in humans, the heme group serves to reversibly bind oxygen (O_2).

A. Heme structure

Heme is a complex of protoporphyrin IX and ferrous iron (Fe^{2+}), as shown in Figure 3.1. The iron is held in the center of the heme molecule by bonds to the four nitrogens of the porphyrin ring. The heme Fe^{2+} can form two additional bonds, one on each side of the planar porphyrin ring. In myoglobin and hemoglobin, one of these positions is coordinated to the side chain of a histidine residue of the globin molecule, whereas the other position is available to bind O_2 (Fig. 3.2). (See pp. 278 and 282, respectively, for a discussion of heme synthesis and degradation.)

B. Myoglobin structure and function

Myoglobin, a hemeprotein present in heart and skeletal muscle, functions both as an oxygen reservoir and as an oxygen carrier that increases the rate of oxygen transport within the muscle

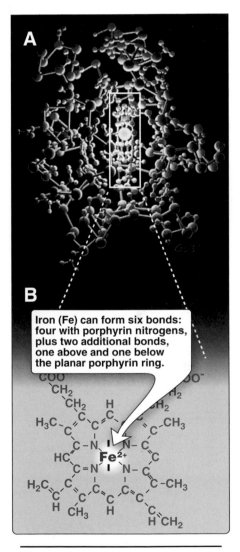

Iron (Fe) can form six bonds: four with porphyrin nitrogens, plus two additional bonds, one above and one below the planar porphyrin ring.

Figure 3.1
A. Hemeprotein (cytochrome c).
B. Structure of heme.

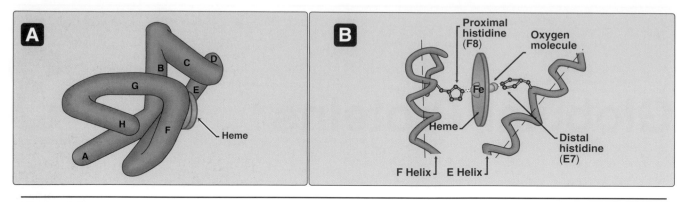

Figure 3.2
A. Model of myoglobin showing α-helices A to H. B. Schematic diagram of the oxygen-binding site of myoglobin.

cell. [Note: Surprisingly, mouse myoglobin double knockouts (see p. 502) have an apparently normal phenotype.] Myoglobin consists of a single polypeptide chain that is structurally similar to the individual polypeptide chains of the tetrameric hemoglobin molecule. This homology makes myoglobin a useful model for interpreting some of the more complex properties of hemoglobin.

1. **α-Helical content:** Myoglobin is a compact molecule, with ~80% of its polypeptide chain folded into eight stretches of α-helix. These α-helical regions, labeled A to H in Figure 3.2A, are terminated either by the presence of proline, whose five-membered ring cannot be accommodated in an α-helix (see p. 16) or by β-bends and loops stabilized by hydrogen bonds and ionic bonds (see p. 19). [Note: Ionic bonds are also termed electrostatic interactions or salt bridges.]

2. **Location of polar and nonpolar amino acid residues:** The interior of the globular myoglobin molecule is composed almost entirely of nonpolar amino acids. They are packed closely together, forming a structure stabilized by hydrophobic interactions between these clustered residues (see p. 19). In contrast, polar amino acids are located almost exclusively on the surface, where they can form hydrogen bonds, both with each other and with water.

3. **Binding of the heme group:** The heme group of the myoglobin molecule sits in a crevice, which is lined with nonpolar amino acids. Notable exceptions are two histidine residues (see Fig. 3.2B). One, the proximal histidine (F8), binds directly to the Fe^{2+} of heme. The second, or distal histidine (E7), does not directly interact with the heme group but helps stabilize the binding of O_2 to Fe^{2+}. Thus, the protein, or globin, portion of myoglobin creates a special microenvironment for the heme that permits the reversible binding of one oxygen molecule (oxygenation). The simultaneous loss of electrons by Fe^{2+} (oxidation to the ferric [Fe^{3+}] form) occurs only rarely.

C. Hemoglobin structure and function

Hemoglobin is found exclusively in red blood cells (RBC), where its main function is to transport O_2 from the lungs to the capillaries of the

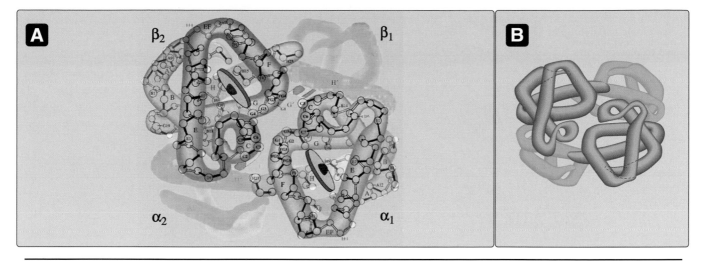

Figure 3.3
A. Structure of hemoglobin showing the polypeptide backbones. B. Simplified drawing showing the α-helices.

tissues. Hemoglobin A, the major hemoglobin in adults, is composed of four polypeptide chains (two α chains and two β chains) held together by noncovalent interactions (Fig. 3.3). Each chain (subunit) has stretches of α-helical structure and a hydrophobic heme-binding pocket similar to that described for myoglobin. However, the tetrameric hemoglobin molecule is structurally and functionally more complex than myoglobin. For example, hemoglobin can transport protons (H^+) and carbon dioxide (CO_2) from the tissues to the lungs and can carry four molecules of O_2 from the lungs to the cells of the body. Furthermore, the oxygen-binding properties of hemoglobin are regulated by interaction with allosteric effectors (see p. 29).

> Obtaining O_2 from the atmosphere solely by diffusion greatly limits the size of organisms. Circulatory systems overcome this, but transport molecules such as hemoglobin are also required because O_2 is only slightly soluble in aqueous solutions such as blood.

1. **Quaternary structure:** The hemoglobin tetramer can be envisioned as composed of two identical dimers, $(\alpha\beta)_1$ and $(\alpha\beta)_2$. The two polypeptide chains within each dimer are held tightly together primarily by hydrophobic interactions (Fig. 3.4). [Note: In this instance, hydrophobic amino acid residues are localized not only in the interior of the molecule but also in a region on the surface of each subunit. Multiple interchain hydrophobic interactions form strong associations between α-subunits and β-subunits in the dimers.] In contrast, the two dimers are held together primarily by polar bonds. The weaker interactions between the dimers allow them to move with respect to one other. This movement results in the two dimers occupying different relative positions in deoxyhemoglobin as compared with oxyhemoglobin (see Fig. 3.4).

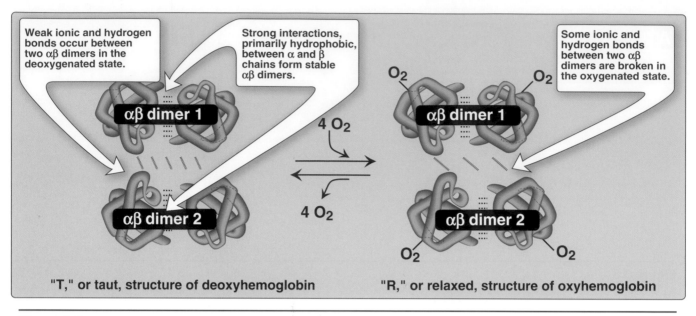

Weak ionic and hydrogen bonds occur between two αβ dimers in the deoxygenated state.

Strong interactions, primarily hydrophobic, between α and β chains form stable αβ dimers.

Some ionic and hydrogen bonds between two αβ dimers are broken in the oxygenated state.

αβ dimer 1

αβ dimer 2

4 O_2

4 O_2

O_2 O_2

αβ dimer 1

αβ dimer 2

O_2 O_2

"T," or taut, structure of deoxyhemoglobin   "R," or relaxed, structure of oxyhemoglobin

Figure 3.4
Schematic diagram showing structural changes resulting from oxygenation and deoxygenation of hemoglobin.

a. T form: The deoxy form of hemoglobin is called the "T," or taut (tense) form. In the T form, the two αβ dimers interact through a network of ionic bonds and hydrogen bonds that constrain the movement of the polypeptide chains. The T conformation is the low-oxygen-affinity form of hemoglobin.

b. R form: The binding of O_2 to hemoglobin causes the rupture of some of the polar bonds between the two αβ dimers, allowing movement. Specifically, the binding of O_2 to the heme Fe^{2+} pulls the iron into the plane of the heme (Fig. 3.5). Because the iron is also linked to the proximal histidine (F8), the resulting movement of the globin chains alters the interface between the αβ dimers. This leads to a structure called the "R," or relaxed form (see Fig. 3.4). The R conformation is the high-oxygen-affinity form of hemoglobin.

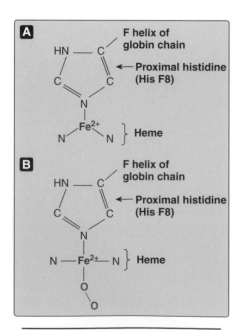

A

HN — C

F helix of globin chain

Proximal histidine (His F8)

C — C

N

Fe^{2+}

N   N

Heme

B

HN — C

F helix of globin chain

Proximal histidine (His F8)

C — C

N

N — Fe^{2+} — N

Heme

O
O

Figure 3.5
Movement of heme iron (Fe). A. Out of the plane of the heme when oxygen (O_2) is not bound. B. Into the plane of the heme upon O_2 binding.

D. Oxygen binding to myoglobin and hemoglobin

Myoglobin can bind only one molecule of O_2, because it contains only one heme group. In contrast, hemoglobin can bind four molecules of O_2, one at each of its four heme groups. The degree of saturation (Y) of these oxygen-binding sites on all myoglobin or hemoglobin molecules can vary between zero (all sites are empty) and 100% (all sites are full), as shown in Figure 3.6. [Note: Pulse oximetry is a noninvasive, indirect method of measuring the oxygen saturation of arterial blood based on differences in light absorption by oxyhemoglobin and deoxyhemoglobin.]

1. Oxygen-dissociation curve: A plot of Y measured at different partial pressures of oxygen (pO_2) is called the oxygen-dissociation curve. [Note: pO_2 may also be represented as PO_2.] The curves for myoglobin and hemoglobin show important differences (see Fig. 3.6). This graph illustrates that myoglobin has a higher oxygen affinity at all pO_2 values than does hemoglobin. The partial pressure of oxygen needed to achieve half saturation of the binding sites (P_{50}) is ~1 mm Hg for myoglobin and 26 mm Hg for hemoglobin. The higher the oxygen affinity (that is, the more tightly O_2 binds), the lower the P_{50}.

a. **Myoglobin:** The oxygen-dissociation curve for myoglobin has a hyperbolic shape (see Fig. 3.6). This reflects the fact that myoglobin reversibly binds a single molecule of O_2. Thus, oxygenated (MbO_2) and deoxygenated (Mb) myoglobin exist in a simple equilibrium:

$$Mb + O_2 \rightleftarrows MbO_2$$

The equilibrium is shifted to the right or to the left as O_2 is added to or removed from the system. [Note: Myoglobin is designed to bind O_2 released by hemoglobin at the low pO_2 found in muscle. Myoglobin, in turn, releases O_2 within the muscle cell in response to oxygen demand.]

b. **Hemoglobin:** The oxygen-dissociation curve for hemoglobin is sigmoidal in shape (see Fig. 3.6), indicating that the subunits cooperate in binding O_2. Cooperative binding of O_2 by the four subunits of hemoglobin means that the binding of an oxygen molecule at one subunit increases the oxygen affinity of the remaining subunits in the same hemoglobin tetramer (Fig. 3.7). Although it is more difficult for the first oxygen molecule to bind to hemoglobin, the subsequent binding of oxygen molecules occurs with high affinity, as shown by the steep upward curve in the region near 20–30 mm Hg (see Fig. 3.6).

E. Allosteric effectors

The ability of hemoglobin to reversibly bind O_2 is affected by the pO_2, the pH of the environment, the partial pressure of carbon dioxide (pCO_2), and the availability of 2,3-bisphosphoglycerate (2,3-BPG). These are collectively called allosteric ("other site") effectors, because their interaction at one site on the tetrameric hemoglobin molecule causes structural changes that affect the binding of O_2 to the heme iron at other sites on the molecule. [Note: The binding of O_2 to monomeric myoglobin is not influenced by allosteric effectors.]

1. **Oxygen:** The sigmoidal oxygen-dissociation curve reflects specific structural changes that are initiated at one subunit and transmitted to other subunits in the hemoglobin tetramer. The net effect of this cooperativity is that the affinity of hemoglobin for the last oxygen molecule bound is ~300 times greater than its affinity for the first oxygen molecule bound. Oxygen, then, is an allosteric effector of hemoglobin. It stabilizes the R form.

   a. **Loading and unloading oxygen:** The cooperative binding of O_2 allows hemoglobin to deliver more O_2 to the tissues in response to relatively small changes in the pO_2. This can be seen in Figure 3.6, which indicates pO_2 in the alveoli of the lung

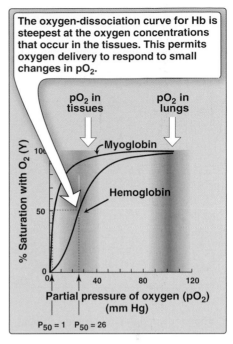

The oxygen-dissociation curve for Hb is steepest at the oxygen concentrations that occur in the tissues. This permits oxygen delivery to respond to small changes in pO_2.

Figure 3.6
Oxygen-dissociation curves for myoglobin and hemoglobin (Hb).

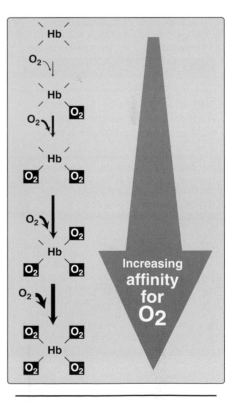

Figure 3.7
Hemoglobin (Hb) binds successive molecules of oxygen (O_2) with increasing affinity.

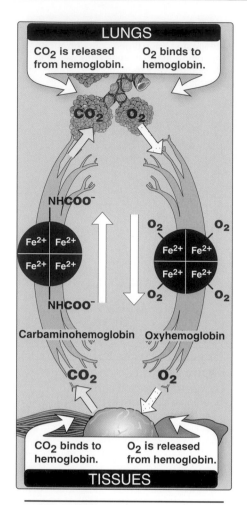

Figure 3.8
Transport of oxygen and carbon dioxide by hemoglobin. Fe = iron.

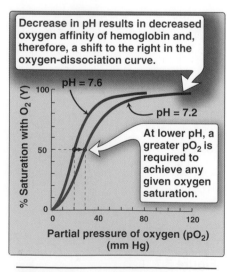

Figure 3.9
Effect of pH on the oxygen affinity of hemoglobin. Protons are allosteric effectors of hemoglobin.

and the capillaries of the tissues. For example, in the lung, oxygen concentration is high, and hemoglobin becomes virtually saturated (or "loaded") with O_2. In contrast, in the peripheral tissues, oxyhemoglobin releases (or "unloads") much of its O_2 for use in the oxidative metabolism of the tissues (Fig. 3.8).

b. **Significance of the sigmoidal oxygen-dissociation curve:** The steep slope of the oxygen-dissociation curve over the range of oxygen concentrations that occur between the lungs and the tissues permits hemoglobin to carry and deliver O_2 efficiently from sites of high to sites of low pO_2. A molecule with a hyperbolic oxygen-dissociation curve, such as myoglobin, could not achieve the same degree of O_2 release within this range of pO_2. Instead, it would have maximum affinity for O_2 throughout this oxygen pressure range and, therefore, would deliver no O_2 to the tissues.

2. **Bohr effect:** The release of O_2 from hemoglobin is enhanced when the pH is lowered (proton concentration [H^+] is increased) or when the hemoglobin is in the presence of an increased pCO_2. Both result in decreased oxygen affinity of hemoglobin and, therefore, a shift to the right in the oxygen-dissociation curve (Fig. 3.9). Both, then, stabilize the T (deoxy) form. This change in oxygen binding is called the Bohr effect. Conversely, raising the pH or lowering the concentration of CO_2 results in a greater oxygen affinity, a shift to the left in the oxygen-dissociation curve, and stabilization of the R (oxy) form.

a. **Source of the protons that lower pH:** The concentration of both H^+ and CO_2 in the capillaries of metabolically active tissues is higher than that observed in alveolar capillaries of the lungs, where CO_2 is released into the expired air. In the tissues, CO_2 is converted by zinc-containing *carbonic anhydrase* to carbonic acid:

$$CO_2 + H_2O \quad \rightleftarrows \quad H_2CO_3$$

which spontaneously loses a H^+, becoming bicarbonate (the major blood buffer):

$$H_2CO_3 \quad \rightleftarrows \quad HCO_3^- + H^+$$

The H^+ produced by this pair of reactions contributes to the lowering of pH. This differential pH gradient (that is, lungs having a higher pH and tissues a lower pH) favors the unloading of O_2 in the peripheral tissues and the loading of O_2 in the lung. Thus, the oxygen affinity of the hemoglobin molecule responds to small shifts in pH between the lungs and oxygen-consuming tissues, making hemoglobin a more efficient transporter of O_2.

b. **Mechanism of the Bohr effect:** The Bohr effect reflects the fact that the deoxy form of hemoglobin has a greater affinity for H^+ than does oxyhemoglobin. This is caused by ionizable groups such as specific histidine side chains that have a higher pK_a (see p. 6) in deoxyhemoglobin than in oxyhemoglobin. Therefore, an increase in the concentration of H^+ (resulting in a decrease in pH) causes these groups to become protonated (charged) and able to form ionic bonds (salt bridges). These bonds preferentially stabilize the deoxy form of hemoglobin, producing a decrease in oxygen affinity. [Note: Hemoglobin, then, is an important blood buffer.]

The Bohr effect can be represented schematically as:

$$HbO_2 + H^+ \rightleftharpoons HbH + O_2$$

Oxyhemoglobin   Deoxyhemoglobin

where an increase in H^+ (or a lower pO_2) shifts the equilibrium to the right (favoring deoxyhemoglobin), whereas an increase in pO_2 (or a decrease in H^+) shifts the equilibrium to the left.

3. **2,3-BPG effect on oxygen affinity:** 2,3-BPG is an important regulator of the binding of O_2 to hemoglobin. It is the most abundant organic phosphate in the RBC, where its concentration is approximately that of hemoglobin. 2,3-BPG is synthesized from an intermediate of the glycolytic pathway (Fig. 3.10; see p. 101 for a discussion of 2,3-BPG synthesis in glycolysis).

   a. **2,3-BPG binding to deoxyhemoglobin:** 2,3-BPG decreases the oxygen affinity of hemoglobin by binding to deoxyhemoglobin but not to oxyhemoglobin. This preferential binding stabilizes the T conformation of deoxyhemoglobin. The effect of binding 2,3-BPG can be represented schematically as:

   $$HbO_2 + 2,3\text{-BPG} \rightleftharpoons Hb - 2,3\text{-BPG} + O_2$$

   Oxyhemoglobin   Deoxyhemoglobin

   b. **2,3-BPG binding site:** One molecule of 2,3-BPG binds to a pocket, formed by the two β-globin chains, in the center of the deoxyhemoglobin tetramer (Fig. 3.11). This pocket contains several positively charged amino acids that form ionic bonds with the negatively charged phosphate groups of 2,3-BPG. [Note: Replacement of one of these amino acids can result in hemoglobin variants with abnormally high oxygen affinity that may be compensated for by increased RBC production (erythrocytosis).] Oxygenation of hemoglobin narrows the pocket and causes 2,3-BPG to be released.

   c. **Oxygen-dissociation curve shift:** Hemoglobin from which 2,3-BPG has been removed has high oxygen affinity. However, as seen in the RBC, the presence of 2,3-BPG significantly reduces the oxygen affinity of hemoglobin, shifting the oxygen-dissociation curve to the right (Fig. 3.12). This reduced affinity enables hemoglobin to release O_2 efficiently at the partial pressures found in the tissues.

   d. **2,3-BPG levels in chronic hypoxia or anemia:** The concentration of 2,3-BPG in the RBC increases in response to chronic hypoxia, such as that observed in chronic obstructive pulmonary disease (COPD) like emphysema, or at high altitudes, where circulating hemoglobin may have difficulty receiving sufficient O_2. Intracellular levels of 2,3-BPG are also elevated in chronic anemia, in which fewer than normal RBC are available to supply the

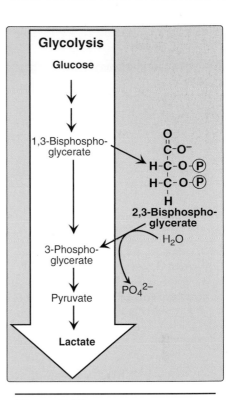

Figure 3.10
Synthesis of 2,3-bisphosphoglycerate. [Note: Ⓟ is a phosphoryl group, PO_3^{2-}.] In older literature, 2, 3-bisphosphoglycerate (2,3-BPG) may be referred to as 2,3-diphosphoglycerate (2,3-DPG).

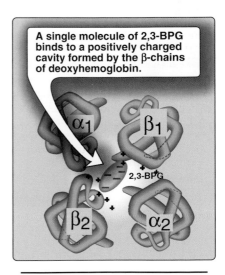

Figure 3.11
Binding of 2,3-bisphosphoglycerate (2,3-BPG) by deoxyhemoglobin.

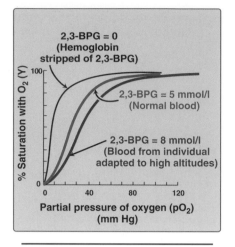

Figure 3.12
Allosteric effect of 2,3-bisphospho-glycerate (2,3-BPG) on the oxygen affinity of hemoglobin.

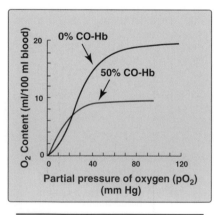

Figure 3.13
Effect of carbon monoxide (CO) on the oxygen affinity of hemoglobin. CO competes with O_2 for binding the heme iron. CO-Hb = carboxyhemoglobin (carbon monoxyhemoglobin).

body's oxygen needs. Elevated 2,3-BPG levels lower the oxygen affinity of hemoglobin, permitting greater unloading of O_2 in the capillaries of tissues (see Fig. 3.12).

e. **2,3-BPG in transfused blood:** 2,3-BPG is essential for the normal oxygen transport function of hemoglobin. However, storing blood in the currently available media results in the gradual depletion of 2,3-BPG. Consequently, stored blood displays an abnormally high oxygen affinity and fails to unload its bound O_2 properly in the tissues. Thus, hemoglobin deficient in 2,3-BPG acts as an oxygen "trap" rather than as an oxygen delivery system. Transfused RBC are able to restore their depleted supplies of 2,3-BPG in 6–24 hours. However, severely ill patients may be compromised if transfused with large quantities of such 2,3-BPG–depleted blood. Stored blood, therefore, is treated with a "rejuvenation" solution that rapidly restores 2,3-BPG. [Note: Rejuvenation also restores ATP lost during storage.]

4. **CO_2 binding:** Most of the CO_2 produced in metabolism is hydrated and transported as bicarbonate ion (see Fig. 1.12 on p. 9). However, some CO_2 is carried as carbamate bound to the terminal amino groups of hemoglobin (forming carbaminohemoglobin as shown in Fig. 3.8), which can be represented schematically as follows:

$$Hb - NH_2 + CO_2 \quad \rightleftarrows \quad Hb - NH - COO^- + H^+$$

The binding of CO_2 stabilizes the T, or deoxy, form of hemoglobin, resulting in a decrease in its oxygen affinity (see p. 28) and a right shift in the oxygen-dissociation curve. In the lungs, CO_2 dissociates from the hemoglobin and is released in the breath.

5. **CO binding:** Carbon monoxide (CO) binds tightly (but reversibly) to the hemoglobin iron, forming carboxyhemoglobin. When CO binds to one or more of the four heme sites, hemoglobin shifts to the R conformation, causing the remaining heme sites to bind O_2 with high affinity. This shifts the oxygen-dissociation curve to the left and changes the normal sigmoidal shape toward a hyperbola. As a result, the affected hemoglobin is unable to release O_2 to the tissues (Fig. 3.13). [Note: The affinity of hemoglobin for CO is 220 times greater than for O_2. Consequently, even minute concentrations of CO in the environment can produce toxic concentrations of carboxyhemoglobin in the blood. For example, increased levels of CO are found in the blood of tobacco smokers. CO toxicity appears to result from a combination of tissue hypoxia and direct CO-mediated damage at the cellular level.] CO poisoning is treated with 100% O_2 at high pressure (hyperbaric oxygen therapy), which facilitates the dissociation of CO from the hemoglobin. [Note: CO inhibits Complex IV of the electron transport chain (see p. 76).] In addition to O_2, CO_2, and CO, nitric oxide gas (NO) also is carried by hemoglobin. NO is a potent vasodilator (see p. 151). It can be taken up (salvaged) or released from RBC, thereby modulating NO availability and influencing vessel diameter.

F. Minor hemoglobins

It is important to remember that human hemoglobin A (HbA) is just one member of a functionally and structurally related family of proteins, the hemoglobins (Fig. 3.14). Each of these oxygen-carrying proteins is a tetramer, composed of two α-globin (or α-like) polypeptides and two β-globin (or β-like) polypeptides. Certain hemoglobins, such as HbF, are normally synthesized only during fetal development, whereas others, such as HbA₂, are synthesized in the adult, although at low levels compared with HbA. HbA can also become modified by the covalent addition of a hexose (see 3. below).

1. **Fetal hemoglobin:** HbF is a tetramer consisting of two α chains identical to those found in HbA, plus two γ chains ($\alpha_2\gamma_2$; see Fig. 3.14). The γ chains are members of the β-globin gene family (see p. 34).

   a. **HbF synthesis during development:** In the first month after conception, embryonic hemoglobins such as Hb Gower 1, composed of two α-like zeta (ζ) chains and two β-like epsilon (ε) chains ($\zeta_2\varepsilon_2$), are synthesized by the embryonic yolk sac. In the fifth week of gestation, the site of globin synthesis shifts, first to the liver and then to the marrow, and the primary product is HbF. HbF is the major hemoglobin found in the fetus and newborn, accounting for ~60% of the total hemoglobin in the RBC during the last months of fetal life (Fig. 3.15). HbA synthesis starts in the bone marrow at about the eighth month of pregnancy and gradually replaces HbF. Figure 3.15 shows the relative production of each type of hemoglobin chain during fetal and postnatal life. [Note: HbF represents <2% of the hemoglobin in most adults and is concentrated in RBC known as F cells.]

   b. **2,3-BPG binding to HbF:** Under physiologic conditions, HbF has a higher oxygen affinity than does HbA as a result of HbF only weakly binding 2,3-BPG. [Note: The γ-globin chains of HbF lack some of the positively charged amino acids that are responsible for binding 2,3-BPG in the β-globin chains.] Because 2,3-BPG serves to reduce the oxygen affinity of hemoglobin, the weaker interaction between 2,3-BPG and HbF results in a higher oxygen affinity for HbF relative to HbA. In contrast, if both HbA and HbF are stripped of their 2,3-BPG, they then have a similar oxygen affinity. The higher oxygen affinity of HbF facilitates the transfer of O_2 from the maternal circulation across the placenta to the RBC of the fetus.

2. **Hemoglobin A₂:** HbA₂ is a minor component of normal adult hemoglobin, first appearing shortly before birth and, ultimately, constituting ~2% of the total hemoglobin. It is composed of two α-globin chains and two δ-globin chains ($\alpha_2\delta_2$; see Fig. 3.14).

3. **Hemoglobin A₁c:** Under physiologic conditions, HbA is slowly glycated (nonenzymically condensed with a hexose), the extent of glycation being dependent on the plasma concentration of the hexose. The most abundant form of glycated hemoglobin is

Form	Chain composition	Fraction of total hemoglobin
HbA	$\alpha_2\beta_2$	90%
HbA₂	$\alpha_2\delta_2$	2%–3%
HbF	$\alpha_2\gamma_2$	<2%
HbA₁c	$\alpha_2\beta_2$-glucose	4%–6%

Figure 3.14
Normal adult human hemoglobins. HbA₁c is a subtype of HbA (or, HbA₁). [Note: The α chains in these hemoglobins are identical.] Hb = hemoglobin.

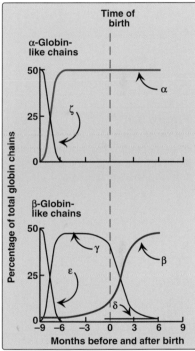

Figure 3.15
Developmental changes in globin production.

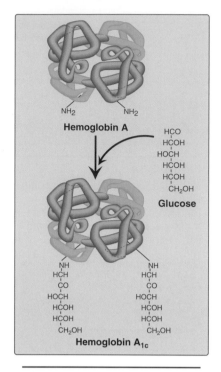

Figure 3.16
Nonenzymatic addition of glucose to hemoglobin. The nonenzymatic addition of a sugar to a protein is referred to as glycation.

HbA$_{1c}$. It has glucose residues attached predominantly to the amino groups of the N-terminal valines of the β-globin chains (Fig. 3.16). Increased amounts of HbA$_{1c}$ are found in RBC of patients with diabetes mellitus, because their HbA has contact with higher glucose concentrations during the 120-day lifetime of these cells. (See p. 340 for a discussion of the use of HbA$_{1c}$ levels in assessing average blood glucose levels in patients with diabetes.)

III. GLOBIN GENE ORGANIZATION

To understand diseases resulting from genetic alterations in the structure or synthesis of hemoglobin, it is necessary to grasp how the hemoglobin genes, which direct the synthesis of the different globin chains, are structurally organized into gene families and also how they are expressed.

A. α-Gene family

The genes coding for the α-globin and β-globin subunits of the hemoglobin chains occur in two separate gene clusters (or families) located on two different chromosomes (Fig. 3.17). The α-gene cluster on chromosome 16 contains two genes for the α-globin chains. It also contains the ζ gene that is expressed early in development as an α-globin-like component of embryonic hemoglobin. [Note: Globin gene families also contain globin-like genes that are not expressed, that is, their genetic information is not used to produce globin chains. These are called pseudogenes.]

B. β-Gene family

A single gene for the β-globin chain is located on chromosome 11 (see Fig. 3.17). There are an additional four β-globin-like genes: the ε gene (which, like the ζ gene, is expressed early in embryonic development), two γ genes (Gγ and Aγ that are expressed in HbF), and the δ gene that codes for the globin chain found in the minor adult hemoglobin HbA$_2$.

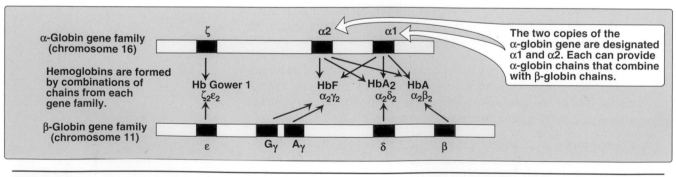

Figure 3.17
Organization of the globin gene families. Hb = hemoglobin.

C. Steps in globin chain synthesis

Expression of a globin gene begins in the nucleus of RBC precursors, where the DNA sequence encoding the gene is transcribed. The ribonucleic acid (RNA) produced by transcription is actually a precursor of the messenger RNA (mRNA) that is used as a template for the synthesis of a globin chain. Before it can serve this function, two noncoding stretches of RNA (introns) must be removed from the mRNA precursor sequence and the remaining three fragments (exons) joined in a linear manner. The resulting mature mRNA enters the cytosol, where its genetic information is translated, producing a globin chain. (A summary of this process is shown in Figure 3.18. A more detailed description of gene expression is presented in Unit VII, Chapters 30–32.)

IV. HEMOGLOBINOPATHIES

Hemoglobinopathies are defined as a group of genetic disorders caused by production of a structurally abnormal hemoglobin molecule, synthesis of insufficient quantities of normal hemoglobin, or, rarely, both. Sickle cell anemia (HbS), hemoglobin C disease (HbC), hemoglobin SC disease (HbS + HbC = HbSC), and the thalassemias are representative hemoglobinopathies that can have severe clinical consequences. The first three conditions result from production of hemoglobin with an altered amino acid sequence (qualitative hemoglobinopathy), whereas the thalassemias are caused by decreased production of normal hemoglobin (quantitative hemoglobinopathy).

A. Sickle cell anemia (hemoglobin S disease)

Sickle cell anemia, the most common of the RBC sickling diseases, is a genetic disorder caused by a single nucleotide substitution (a point mutation, see p. 449) in the gene for β-globin. It is the most common inherited blood disorder in the United States, affecting 50,000 Americans. It occurs primarily in the African American population, affecting 1 in 500 newborn African American infants. Sickle cell anemia is an autosomal-recessive disorder. It occurs in individuals who have inherited two mutant genes (one from each parent) that code for synthesis of the β chains of the globin molecules. [Note: The mutant β-globin chain is designated β^S, and the resulting hemoglobin, $\alpha_2\beta^S_2$, is referred to as HbS.] An infant does not begin showing symptoms of the disease until sufficient HbF has been replaced by HbS so that sickling can occur (see p. 36). Sickle cell anemia is characterized by lifelong episodes of pain ("crises"), chronic hemolytic anemia with associated hyperbilirubinemia (see p. 284), and increased susceptibility to infections, usually beginning in infancy. [Note: The lifetime of a RBC in sickle cell anemia is <20 days, compared with 120 days for normal RBC, hence, the anemia.] Other symptoms include acute chest syndrome, stroke, splenic and renal dysfunction, and bone changes due to marrow hyperplasia. Life expectancy is reduced. Heterozygotes, representing 1 in 12 African Americans, have one normal and one sickle

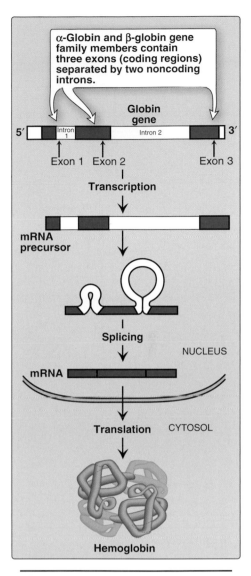

α-Globin and β-globin gene family members contain three exons (coding regions) separated by two noncoding introns.

Globin gene

5′ Intron 1   Intron 2   3′

Exon 1 Exon 2   Exon 3

Transcription

mRNA precursor

Splicing

NUCLEUS

mRNA

Translation   CYTOSOL

Hemoglobin

Figure 3.18
Synthesis of globin chains. mRNA = messenger ribonucleic acid.

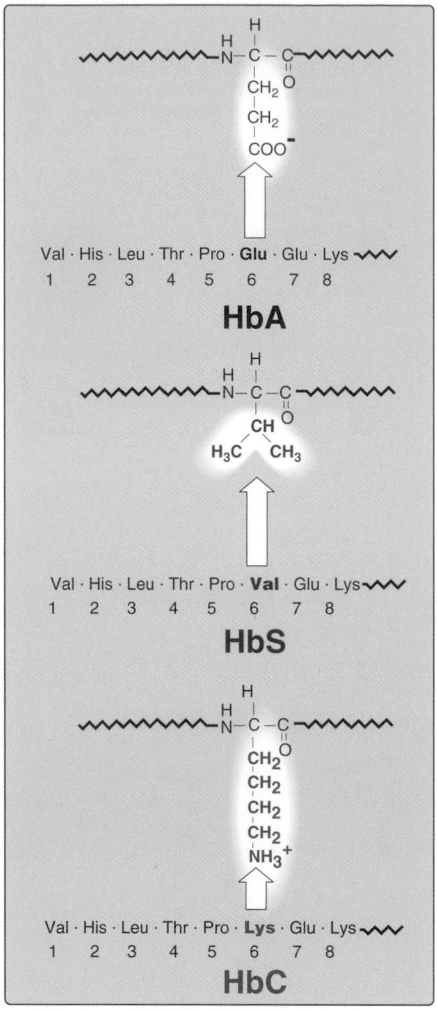

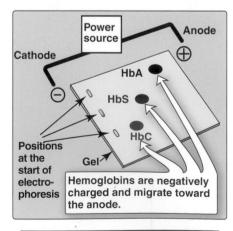

Figure 3.19
Amino acid substitutions in hemoglobin S (HbS) and hemoglobin C (HbC).

Figure 3.20
Diagram of hemoglobins (HbA), (HbS), and (HbC) after electrophoresis.

cell gene. The blood cells of such heterozygotes contain both HbS and HbA, and these individuals have sickle cell trait. They usually do not show clinical symptoms (but may under conditions of extreme physical exertion with dehydration) and can have a normal life span.

1. **Amino acid substitution in HbS β chains:** A molecule of HbS contains two normal α-globin chains and two mutant β-globin chains (β^S), in which glutamate at position six has been replaced with valine (Fig. 3.19). Therefore, during electrophoresis at alkaline pH, HbS migrates more slowly toward the anode (positive electrode) than does HbA (Fig. 3.20). This altered mobility of HbS is a result of the absence of the negatively charged glutamate residues in the two β chains, thereby rendering HbS less negative than HbA. [Note: Electrophoresis of hemoglobin obtained from lysed RBC is routinely used in the diagnosis of sickle cell trait and sickle cell anemia (or, sickle cell disease). DNA analysis also is used (see p. 493).]

2. **Sickling and tissue anoxia:** The replacement of the charged glutamate with the nonpolar valine forms a protrusion on the β chain that fits into a complementary site on the β chain of another hemoglobin molecule in the cell (Fig. 3.21). At low oxygen tension, deoxyhemoglobin S polymerizes inside the RBC, forming a network of insoluble fibrous polymers that stiffen and distort the cell, producing rigid, misshapen RBC. Such sickled cells frequently block the flow of blood in the narrow capillaries. This interruption in the supply of O_2 leads to localized anoxia (oxygen deprivation) in the tissue, causing pain and eventually ischemic death (infarction) of cells in the vicinity of the blockage. The anoxia also leads to an increase in deoxygenated HbS. [Note: The mean diameter of RBC is 7.5 μm, whereas that of the microvasculature is 3–4 μm. Compared to normal RBC, sickled cells have a decreased ability to deform and an increased tendency to adhere to vessel walls. This makes moving through small vessels difficult, thereby causing microvascular occlusion.]

3. **Variables that increase sickling:** The extent of sickling and, therefore, the severity of disease are enhanced by any variable that increases the proportion of HbS in the deoxy state (that is, reduces the oxygen affinity of HbS). These variables include decreased pO_2, increased pCO_2, decreased pH, dehydration, and an increased concentration of 2,3-BPG in RBC.

4. **Treatment:** Therapy involves adequate hydration, analgesics, aggressive antibiotic therapy if infection is present, and transfusions in patients at high risk for fatal occlusion of blood vessels. Intermittent transfusions with packed RBC reduce the risk of stroke, but the benefits must be weighed against the complications of transfusion, which include iron overload that can result in hemosiderosis (see p. 404), bloodborne infections, and immunologic complications. Hydroxyurea (hydroxycarbamide), an antitumor drug, is therapeutically useful because it increases circulating levels of HbF, which decreases RBC sickling. This

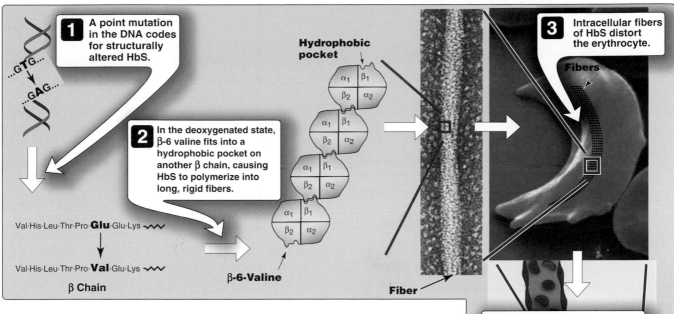

1 A point mutation in the DNA codes for structurally altered HbS.

...GTG...

...GAG...

2 In the deoxygenated state, β-6 valine fits into a hydrophobic pocket on another β chain, causing HbS to polymerize into long, rigid fibers.

Val·His·Leu·Thr·Pro·**Glu**·Glu·Lys ⌇⌇⌇

Val·His·Leu·Thr·Pro·**Val**·Glu·Lys ⌇⌇⌇

β Chain

Hydrophobic pocket

β-6-Valine

Fiber

3 Intracellular fibers of HbS distort the erythrocyte.

Fibers

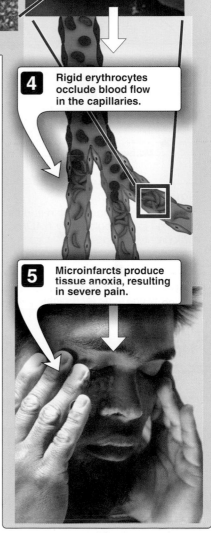

4 Rigid erythrocytes occlude blood flow in the capillaries.

5 Microinfarcts produce tissue anoxia, resulting in severe pain.

leads to decreased frequency of painful crises and reduces mortality. Stem cell transplantation is possible. [Note: The morbidity and mortality associated with sickle cell anemia has led to its inclusion in newborn screening panels to allow prophylactic antibiotic therapy to begin soon after the birth of an affected child.]

5. **Possible selective advantage of the heterozygous state:** The high frequency of the β^S mutation among black Africans, despite its damaging effects in the homozygous state, suggests that a selective advantage exists for heterozygous individuals. For example, heterozygotes for the sickle cell gene are less susceptible to the severe malaria caused by the parasite <u>Plasmodium</u> <u>falciparum</u>. This organism spends an obligatory part of its life cycle in the RBC. One theory is that because these cells in individuals heterozygous for HbS, like those in homozygotes, have a shorter life span than normal, the parasite cannot complete the intracellular stage of its development. This may provide a selective advantage to heterozygotes living in regions where malaria is a major cause of death. For example, in Africa, the geographic distribution of sickle cell anemia is similar to that of malaria.

B. Hemoglobin C disease

Like HbS, HbC is a hemoglobin variant that has a single amino acid substitution in the sixth position of the β-globin chain (see Fig. 3.19). In HbC, however, a lysine is substituted for the glutamate (as compared with a valine substitution in HbS). [Note: This substitution causes HbC to move more slowly toward the anode than HbA or HbS does (see Fig. 3.20).] Rare patients homozygous for HbC generally have a relatively mild, chronic hemolytic anemia. They do not suffer from infarctive crises, and no specific therapy is required.

Figure 3.21
Molecular and cellular events leading to sickle cell crisis. HbS = hemoglobin S.

C. Hemoglobin SC disease

HbSC disease is another of the RBC sickling diseases. In this disease, some β-globin chains have the sickle cell mutation, whereas other β-globin chains carry the mutation found in HbC disease. [Note: Patients with HbSC disease are doubly heterozygous. They are called compound heterozygotes because both of their β-globin genes are abnormal, although different from each other.] Hemoglobin levels tend to be higher in HbSC disease than in sickle cell anemia and may even be at the low end of the normal range. The clinical course of adults with HbSC anemia differs from that of sickle cell anemia in that symptoms such as painful crises are less frequent and less severe. However, there is significant clinical variability.

D. Methemoglobinemias

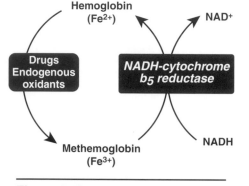

Oxidation of the heme iron in hemoglobin from Fe^{2+} to Fe^{3+} produces methemoglobin, which cannot bind O_2. This oxidation may be acquired and caused by the action of certain drugs, such as nitrates, or endogenous products such as reactive oxygen species (see p. 148). The oxidation may also result from congenital defects, for example, a deficiency of *NADH-cytochrome b_5 reductase* (also called *NADH-methemoglobin reductase*), the enzyme responsible for the conversion of methemoglobin (Fe^{3+}) to hemoglobin (Fe^{2+}), leads to the accumulation of methemoglobin (Fig. 3.22). [Note: The RBC of newborns have approximately half the capacity of those of adults to reduce methemoglobin.] Additionally, rare mutations in the α- or β-globin chain can cause the production of HbM, an abnormal hemoglobin that is resistant to the *reductase*. The methemoglobinemias are characterized by "chocolate cyanosis" (a blue coloration of the skin and mucous membranes and brown-colored blood) as a result of the dark-colored methemoglobin. Symptoms are related to the degree of tissue hypoxia and include anxiety, headache, and dyspnea. In rare cases, coma and death can occur. Treatment is with methylene blue, which is oxidized as Fe^{3+} is reduced.

Figure 3.22
Formation of methemoglobin and its reduction to hemoglobin by *NADH-cytochrome b_5 reductase.*

E. Thalassemias

The thalassemias are hereditary hemolytic diseases in which an imbalance occurs in the synthesis of globin chains. As a group, they are the most common single-gene disorders in humans. Normally, synthesis of the α- and β-globin chains is coordinated, so that each α-globin chain has a β-globin chain partner. This leads to the formation of $α_2β_2$ (HbA). In the thalassemias, the synthesis of either the α- or the β-globin chain is defective, and hemoglobin concentration is reduced. A thalassemia can be caused by a variety of mutations, including entire gene deletions, or substitutions or deletions of one of many nucleotides in the DNA. [Note: Each thalassemia can be classified as either a disorder in which no globin chains are produced ($α^0$- or $β^0$-thalassemia), or one in which some chains are synthesized but at a reduced level ($α^+$- or $β^+$-thalassemia).]

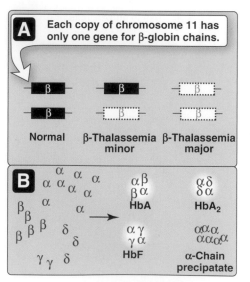

Figure 3.23
A. β-Globin gene mutations in the β-thalassemias. B. Hemoglobin (Hb) tetramers formed in β-thalassemias.

1. **β-Thalassemias:** In these disorders, synthesis of β-globin chains is decreased or absent, typically as a result of point mutations that affect the production of functional mRNA. However, α-globin

chain synthesis is normal. Excess α-globin chains cannot form stable tetramers and so precipitate, causing the premature death of cells initially destined to become mature RBC. Increase in $\alpha_2\delta_2$ (HbA$_2$) and $\alpha_2\gamma_2$ (HbF) also occurs. There are only two copies of the β-globin gene in each cell (one on each chromosome 11). Therefore, individuals with β-globin gene defects have either β-thalassemia trait (β-thalassemia minor) if they have only one defective β-globin gene or β-thalassemia major (Cooley anemia) if both genes are defective (Fig. 3.23). Because the β-globin gene is not expressed until late in prenatal development, the physical manifestations of β-thalassemias appear only several months after birth. Those individuals with β-thalassemia minor make some β chains and usually do not require specific treatment. However, those infants born with β-thalassemia major are seemingly healthy at birth but become severely anemic, usually during the first or second year of life, due to ineffective erythropoiesis. Skeletal changes as a result of extramedullary hematopoiesis also are seen. These patients require regular transfusions of blood. [Note: Although this treatment is lifesaving, the cumulative effect of the transfusions is iron overload. Use of iron chelation therapy has improved morbidity and mortality.] The only curative option available is hematopoietic stem cell transplantation.

2. **α-Thalassemias:** In these disorders, synthesis of α-globin chains is decreased or absent, typically as a result of deletional mutations. Because each individual's genome contains four copies of the α-globin gene (two on each chromosome 16), there are several levels of α-globin chain deficiencies (Fig. 3.24). If one of the four genes is defective, the individual is termed a "silent" carrier of α-thalassemia, because no physical manifestations of the disease occur. If two α-globin genes are defective, the individual is designated as having α-thalassemia trait. If three α-globin genes are defective, the individual has hemoglobin H (β_4) disease, a hemolytic anemia of variable severity. If all four α-globin genes are defective, hemoglobin Bart (γ_4) disease with hydrops fetalis and fetal death results, because α-globin chains are required for the synthesis of HbF. [Note: Heterozygote advantage against malaria is seen in both α- and β-thalassemias.]

V. CHAPTER SUMMARY

Hemoglobin A (**HbA**), the major hemoglobin in adults, is composed of four polypeptide chains (two α chains and two β chains, $\alpha_2\beta_2$) held together by noncovalent interactions (Fig. 3.25). The subunits occupy different relative positions in deoxyhemoglobin compared with oxyhemoglobin. The **deoxy form** of Hb is called the "**T**," or **taut** (**tense**), **conformation**. It has a constrained structure that limits the movement of the polypeptide chains. The T form is the **low-oxygen-affinity form** of Hb. The binding of oxygen (O$_2$) to the heme iron causes rupture of some of the ionic and hydrogen bonds and movement of the dimers. This leads to a structure called the "**R**," or **relaxed**, **conformation**. The R form is the **high-oxygen-affinity form** of Hb. The **oxygen-dissociation curve** for Hb is **sigmoidal** in shape (in contrast to

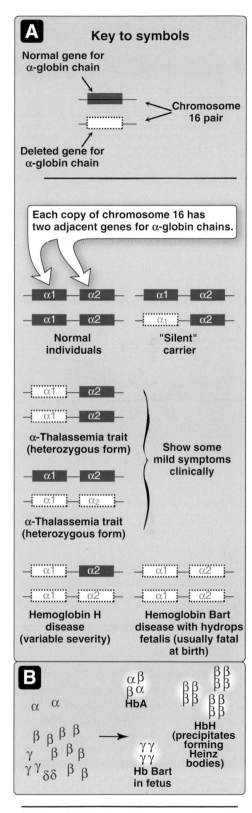

Figure 3.24
A. α-Globin gene deletions in the α-thalassemias. B. Hemoglobin (Hb) tetramers formed in α-thalassemias.

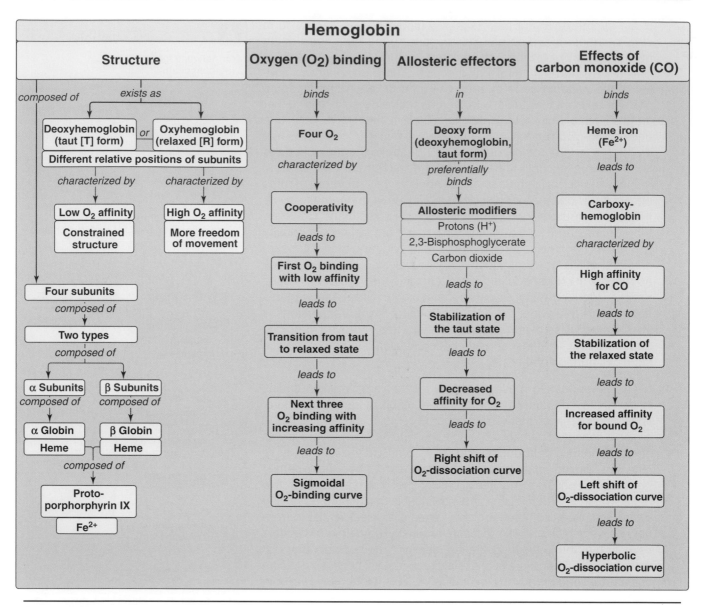

Figure 3.25
Key concept map for hemoglobin structure and function. Fe^{2+} = ferrous iron.

that of **myoglobin**, which is **hyperbolic**), indicating that the subunits cooperate in binding O_2. The binding of an oxygen molecule at one heme group increases the oxygen affinity of the remaining heme groups in the same Hb molecule (**cooperativity**). Hb's ability to bind O_2 reversibly is affected by the partial pressure of oxygen (**pO_2**), the **pH** of the environment, the partial pressure of carbon dioxide (**pCO_2**), and the availability of **2,3-bisphosphoglycerate (2,3-BPG)**. For example, the release of O_2 from Hb is enhanced when the pH is lowered or the pCO_2 is increased (the **Bohr effect**), such as in **exercising muscle**, and the oxygen-dissociation curve of Hb is shifted to the right. To cope long-term with the effects of **chronic hypoxia** or **anemia**, the concentration of **2,3-BPG** in **red blood cells** increases. **2,3-BPG** binds to the Hb and decreases its oxygen affinity. It therefore also shifts the oxygen-dissociation curve to the right. **Fetal hemoglobin (HbF)** binds 2,3-BPG less tightly than does HbA and has a higher oxygen affinity. **Carbon monoxide (CO)** binds tightly (but reversibly) to the Hb iron, forming **carboxyhemoglobin**. **Hemoglobinopathies** are disorders primarily caused either by production of a structurally abnormal Hb molecule as in **sickle cell anemia** or synthesis of insufficient quantities of normal Hb subunits as in the **thalassemias** (Fig. 3.26).

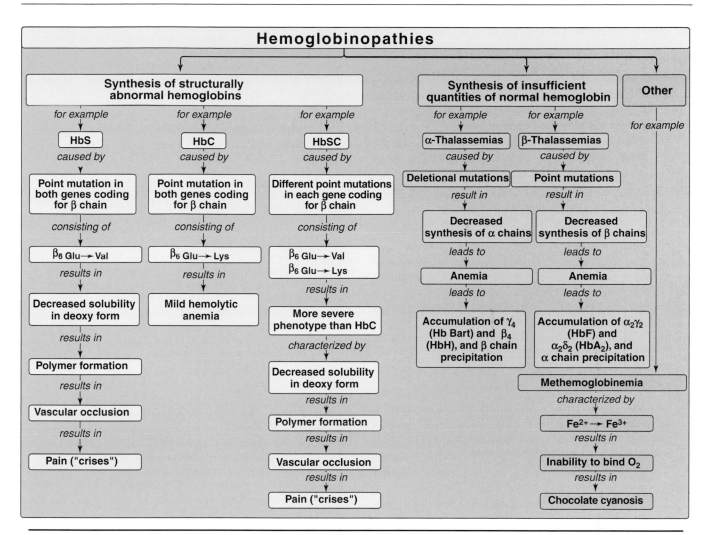

Figure 3.26
Key concept map for hemoglobinopathies. Hb = hemoglobin; Fe = iron; O_2 = oxygen.

Study Questions

Choose the ONE best answer.

3.1 Which one of the following statements concerning the hemoglobins is correct?

A. HbA is the most abundant hemoglobin in normal adults.

B. Fetal blood has a lower affinity for oxygen than does adult blood because HbF has an increased affinity for 2,3-bisphosphoglycerate.

C. The globin chain composition of HbF is $\alpha_2\delta_2$.

D. HbA_{1c} differs from HbA by a single, genetically determined amino acid substitution.

E. HbA_2 appears early in fetal life.

Correct answer = A. HbA accounts for over 90% of the hemoglobin in a normal adult. If HbA_{1c} is included, the percentage rises to ~97%. Because 2,3-bisphosphoglycerate (2,3-BPG) reduces the affinity of hemoglobin for oxygen, the weaker interaction between 2,3-BPG and HbF results in a higher oxygen affinity for HbF relative to HbA. HbF consists of $\alpha_2\gamma_2$. HbA_{1c} is a glycated form of HbA, formed nonenzymically in red blood cells. HbA_2 is a minor component of normal adult hemoglobin, first appearing shortly before birth and rising to adult levels (~2% of the total hemoglobin) by age 6 months.

3.2 Which one of the following statements concerning the ability of acidosis to precipitate a crisis in sickle cell anemia is correct?

A. Acidosis decreases the solubility of HbS.
B. Acidosis increases the oxygen affinity of hemoglobin.
C. Acidosis favors the conversion of hemoglobin from the taut to the relaxed conformation.
D. Acidosis shifts the oxygen-dissociation curve to the left.
E. Acidosis decreases the ability of 2,3-bisphosphoglycerate to bind to hemoglobin.

Correct answer = A. HbS is significantly less soluble in the deoxygenated form, compared with oxyhemoglobin S. Decreased pH (acidosis) causes the oxygen-dissociation curve to shift to the right, indicating decreased oxygen affinity (increased delivery). This favors the formation of the deoxy, or taut, form of hemoglobin and can precipitate a sickle cell crisis. The binding of 2,3-bisphosphoglycerate is increased, because it binds only to the deoxy form of hemoglobin.

3.3 Which one of the following statements concerning the binding of oxygen by hemoglobin is correct?

A. The Bohr effect results in a lower oxygen affinity at higher pH values.
B. Carbon dioxide increases the oxygen affinity of hemoglobin by binding to the C-terminal groups of the polypeptide chains.
C. The oxygen affinity of hemoglobin increases as the percentage saturation increases.
D. The hemoglobin tetramer binds four molecules of 2,3-bisphosphoglycerate.
E. Oxyhemoglobin and deoxyhemoglobin have the same affinity for protons.

Correct answer = C. The binding of oxygen at one heme group increases the oxygen affinity of the remaining heme groups in the same molecule. A rise in pH results in increased oxygen affinity. Carbon dioxide decreases oxygen affinity because it lowers the pH. Moreover, binding of carbon dioxide to the N-termini stabilizes the taut, deoxy form. Hemoglobin binds one molecule of 2,3-bisphosphoglycerate. Deoxyhemoglobin has a greater affinity for protons than does oxyhemoglobin.

3.4 β-Lysine 82 in HbA is important for the binding of 2,3-bisphosphoglycerate. In Hb Helsinki, this amino acid has been replaced by methionine. Which of the following should be true concerning Hb Helsinki?

A. It should be stabilized in the taut, rather than the relaxed, form.
B. It should have increased oxygen affinity and, consequently, decreased oxygen delivery to tissues.
C. Its oxygen-dissociation curve should be shifted to the right relative to HbA.
D. It results in anemia.

Correct answer = B. Substitution of lysine by methionine decreases the ability of negatively charged phosphate groups in 2,3-bisphosphoglycerate (2,3-BPG) to bind the β subunits of hemoglobin. Because 2,3-BPG decreases the oxygen affinity of hemoglobin, a reduction in 2,3-BPG should result in increased oxygen affinity and decreased oxygen (O_2) delivery to tissues. The relaxed form is the high-oxygen-affinity form of hemoglobin. Increased oxygen affinity (decreased delivery) results in a left shift in the oxygen-dissociation curve. Decreased delivery of O_2 is compensated for by increased RBC production.

3.5 A 67-year-old man presented to the emergency department with a 1-week history of angina and shortness of breath. He complained that his face and extremities had taken on a blue color. His medical history included chronic stable angina treated with isosorbide dinitrate and nitroglycerin. Blood obtained for analysis was brown. Which one of the following is the most likely diagnosis?

A. Carboxyhemoglobinemia
B. Hemoglobin SC disease
C. Methemoglobinemia
D. Sickle cell anemia
E. β-Thalassemia

Correct answer = C. Oxidation of the ferrous (Fe^{2+}) iron to the ferric (Fe^{3+}) state in the heme prosthetic group of hemoglobin forms methemoglobin. This may be caused by the action of certain drugs such as nitrates. The methemoglobinemias are characterized by chocolate cyanosis (a blue coloration of the skin and mucous membranes and chocolate-colored blood) as a result of the dark-colored methemoglobin. Symptoms are related to tissue hypoxia and include anxiety, headache, and dyspnea. In rare cases, coma and death can occur. [Note: Benzocaine, an aromatic amine used as a topical anesthetic, is a cause of acquired methemoglobinemia.]

3.6 Why is hemoglobin C disease a nonsickling disease?

In HbC, the polar glutamate is replaced by polar lysine rather than by nonpolar valine as in HbS.

3.7 What would be true about the extent of red blood cell sickling in individuals with HbS and hereditary persistence of HbF?

It would be decreased because HbF reduces HbS concentration. It also inhibits polymerization of deoxy HbS.

Fibrous Proteins

4

I. OVERVIEW

Collagen and elastin are examples of common, well-characterized fibrous proteins of the extracellular matrix (ECM) that serve structural functions in the body. For example, collagen and elastin are found as components of skin, connective tissue, blood vessel walls, and the sclera and cornea of the eye. Each fibrous protein exhibits special mechanical properties, resulting from its unique structure, which is obtained by combining specific amino acids into regular, secondary structural elements. This is in contrast to globular proteins (discussed in Chapter 3), whose shapes are the result of complex interactions between secondary, tertiary, and, sometimes, quaternary structural elements.

II. COLLAGEN

Collagen is the most abundant protein in the human body. A typical collagen molecule is a long, rigid structure in which three polypeptides (referred to as α chains) are wound around one another in a rope-like triple helix (Fig. 4.1). Although these molecules are found throughout the body, their types and organization are dictated by the structural role collagen plays in a particular organ. In some tissues, collagen may be dispersed as a gel that gives support to the structure, as in the ECM or the vitreous humor of the eye. In other tissues, collagen may be bundled in tight, parallel fibers that provide great strength, as in tendons. In the cornea of the eye, collagen is stacked so as to transmit light with a minimum of scattering. Collagen of bone occurs as fibers arranged at an angle to each other so as to resist mechanical shear from any direction.

A. Types

The collagen superfamily of proteins includes >25 collagen types as well as additional proteins that have collagen-like domains. The three polypeptide α chains are held together by interchain hydrogen bonds. Variations in the amino acid sequence of the α chains result in structural components that are about the same size (~1,000 amino acids long) but with slightly different properties. These α chains are combined to form the various types of collagen found in the tissues. For example, the most common collagen, type I, contains two chains called α1 and one chain called α2 (α1₂α2), whereas type II collagen contains

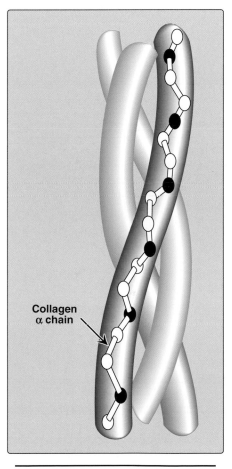

Figure 4.1
Triple-stranded helix of collagen formed from three α chains. [Note: The α chains themselves are helical in structure.]

TYPE	TISSUE DISTRIBUTION
	Fibril-forming
I	**Skin, bone, tendon, blood vessels, cornea**
II	**Cartilage, intervertebral disk, vitreous body**
III	**Blood vessels, skin, muscle**
	Network-forming
IV	**Basement membrane**
VIII	**Corneal and vascular endothelium**
	Fibril-associated*
IX	**Cartilage**
XII	**Tendon, ligaments, some other tissues**

Figure 4.2
The most abundant types of collagen.
[Note: *Fibril-associated collagens
with interrupted triple helices are
known as FACIT.]

three α1 chains (α1₃). The collagens can be organized into three groups, based on their location and functions in the body (Fig. 4.2).

1. **Fibril-forming collagens:** Types I, II, and III are the fibrillar collagens and have the rope-like structure described above for a typical collagen molecule. In the electron microscope, these linear polymers of fibrils have characteristic banding patterns, reflecting the regular staggered packing of the individual collagen molecules in the fibril (Fig. 4.3). Type I collagen fibers (composed of collagen fibrils) are found in supporting elements of high tensile strength (for example, tendons and corneas), whereas fibers formed from type II collagen molecules are restricted to cartilaginous structures. The fibers derived from type III collagen are prevalent in more distensible tissues such as blood vessels.

2. **Network-forming collagens:** Types IV and VIII form a three-dimensional mesh, rather than distinct fibrils (Fig. 4.4). For example, type IV molecules assemble into a sheet or meshwork that constitutes a major part of basement membranes.

> Basement membranes are thin, sheet-like structures that provide mechanical support for adjacent cells and function as a semipermeable filtration barrier to macromolecules in organs such as the kidney and the lung.

3. **Fibril-associated collagens:** Types IX and XII bind to the surface of collagen fibrils, linking these fibrils to one another and to other components in the ECM (see Fig. 4.2).

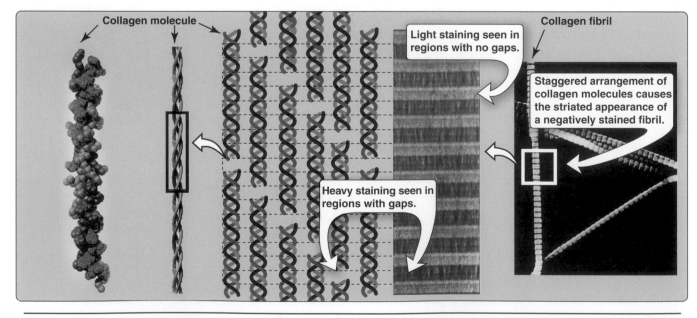

Figure 4.3
Collagen fibrils at right have a characteristic banding pattern, reflecting the regularly staggered packing of the individual collagen molecules in the fibril.

B. Structure

Unlike most globular proteins that are folded into compact structures, collagen, a fibrous protein, has an elongated, triple-helical structure that is stabilized by interchain hydrogen bonds.

1. **Amino acid sequence:** Collagen is rich in proline and glycine, both of which are important in the formation of the triple-stranded helix. Proline facilitates the formation of the helical conformation of each α chain because its ring structure causes "kinks" in the peptide chain. [Note: The presence of proline dictates that the helical conformation of the α chain cannot be an α helix (see p. 16).] Glycine, the smallest amino acid, is found in every third position of the polypeptide chain. It fits into the restricted spaces where the three chains of the helix come together. The glycine residues are part of a repeating sequence, –Gly–X–Y–, where X is frequently proline, and Y is often hydroxyproline (but can be hydroxylysine, Fig. 4.5). Thus, most of the α chain can be regarded as a polytripeptide whose sequence can be represented as (–Gly–Pro–Hyp–)$_{333}$.

2. **Hydroxyproline and hydroxylysine:** Collagen contains hydroxyproline and hydroxylysine, which are nonstandard amino acids (see p. 1) not present in most other proteins. They result from the hydroxylation of some of the proline and lysine residues after their incorporation into polypeptide chains (Fig. 4.6). Therefore, the hydroxylation is a posttranslational modification (see p. 460). [Note: Generation of hydroxyproline maximizes formation of interchain hydrogen bonds that stabilize the triple-helical structure.]

3. **Glycosylation:** The hydroxyl group of the hydroxylysine residues of collagen may be enzymatically glycosylated. Most commonly, glucose and galactose are sequentially attached to the polypeptide chain prior to triple-helix formation (Fig. 4.7).

C. Biosynthesis

The polypeptide precursors of the collagen molecule are synthesized in fibroblasts (or in the related osteoblasts of bone and chondroblasts of cartilage). They are enzymically modified and form the triple helix, which gets secreted into the ECM. After additional enzymic modification, the mature extracellular collagen fibrils aggregate and become cross-linked to form collagen fibers.

1. **Pro-α chain formation:** Collagen is one of many proteins that normally function outside of cells. Like most proteins produced for export, the newly synthesized polypeptide precursors of α chains (prepro-α chains) contain a special amino acid sequence at their amino (N)-terminal ends. This sequence acts as a signal that, in the absence of additional signals, targets the polypeptide being synthesized for secretion from the cell. The signal sequence facilitates the binding of ribosomes to the rough endoplasmic reticulum (RER) and directs the passage of the prepro-α chain into the lumen of the RER. The signal sequence is rapidly cleaved in the lumen to yield a precursor of collagen called a pro-α chain (see Fig. 4.7).

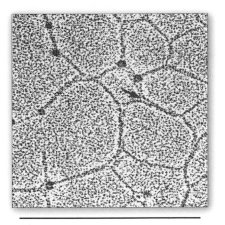

Figure 4.4
Electron micrograph of a polygonal network formed by association of collagen type IV monomers.

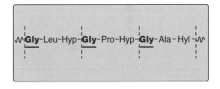

Figure 4.5
Amino acid sequence of a portion of the α1 chain of collagen. Hyp = hydroxyproline; Hyl = hydroxylysine.

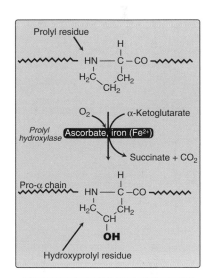

Figure 4.6
Hydroxylation of proline residues in pro-α chains of collagen by *prolyl hydroxylase.* [Note: Fe^{2+} (*hydroxylase* cofactor) is protected from oxidation to Fe^{3+} by ascorbate (vitamin C).]

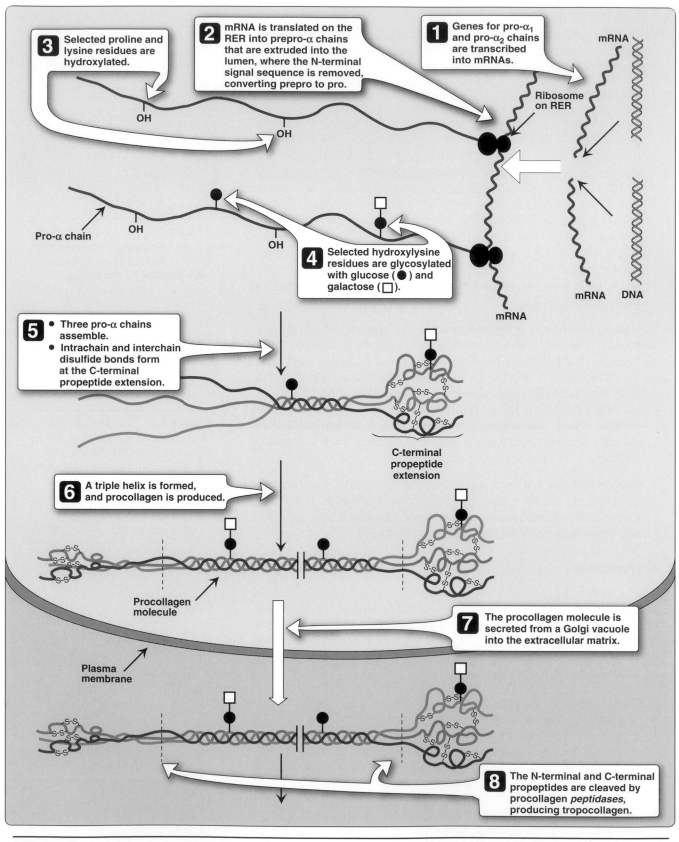

Figure 4.7
Synthesis of collagen. RER = rough endoplasmic reticulum; mRNA = messenger RNA. (continued on the next page)

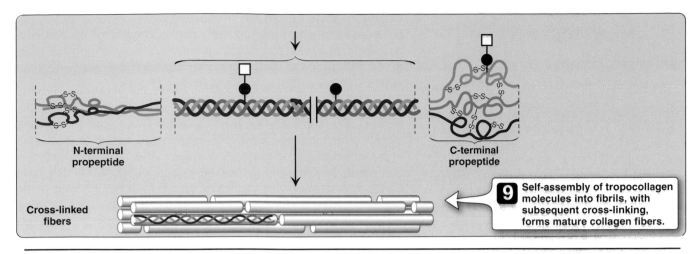

Figure 4.7
Synthesis of collagen. (continued from the previous page)

2. **Hydroxylation:** The pro-α chains are processed by a number of enzymic steps within the lumen of the RER while the polypeptides are still being synthesized (see Fig. 4.7). Proline and lysine residues found in the Y-position of the –Gly–X–Y– sequence can be hydroxylated to form hydroxyproline and hydroxylysine residues. These hydroxylation reactions require molecular oxygen, ferrous iron (Fe^{2+}), and the reducing agent vitamin C (ascorbic acid, see p. 381), without which the hydroxylating enzymes, *prolyl hydroxylase* and *lysyl hydroxylase*, are unable to function (see Fig. 4.6). In the case of ascorbic acid deficiency (and, therefore, a lack of proline and lysine hydroxylation), interchain H-bond formation is impaired, as is formation of a stable triple helix. Additionally, collagen fibrils cannot be cross-linked (see 7. below), greatly decreasing the tensile strength of the assembled fiber. The resulting deficiency disease is known as scurvy. Patients with scurvy often show ecchymoses (bruise-like discolorations) on the limbs as a result of subcutaneous extravasation (leakage) of blood due to capillary fragility (Fig. 4.8).

3. **Glycosylation:** Some hydroxylysine residues are modified by glycosylation with glucose or glucosyl-galactose (see Fig. 4.7).

4. **Assembly and secretion:** After hydroxylation and glycosylation, three pro-α chains form procollagen, a precursor of collagen that has a central region of triple helix flanked by the nonhelical N- and carboxyl (C)-terminal extensions called propeptides (see Fig. 4.7). The formation of procollagen begins with formation of interchain disulfide bonds between the C-terminal extensions of the pro-α chains. This brings the three α chains into an alignment favorable for triple helix formation. The procollagen molecules move through the Golgi apparatus, where they are packaged in secretory vesicles. The vesicles fuse with the cell membrane, causing the release of procollagen molecules into the extracellular space.

5. **Extracellular cleavage of procollagen molecules:** After their release, the triple-helical procollagen molecules are cleaved by *N-* and *C-procollagen peptidases*, which remove the terminal propeptides, producing tropocollagen molecules.

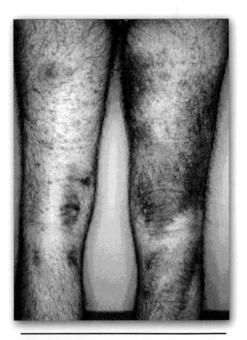

Figure 4.8
The legs of a 46-year-old man with scurvy.

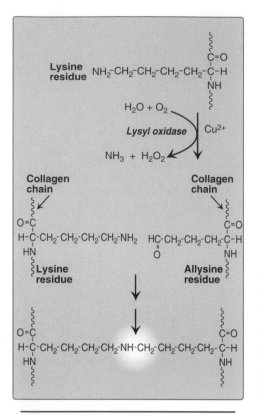

Figure 4.9
Formation of cross-links in collagen. [Note: *Lysyl oxidase* is irreversibly inhibited by a toxin present in seeds from <u>Lathyrus</u> <u>odoratus</u> (sweet pea), leading to a condition known as lathyrism that is characterized by skeletal and vascular problems.] Cu^{2+} = copper; NH_3 = ammonia; H_2O_2 = hydrogen peroxide.

6. **Collagen fibril formation:** Tropocollagen molecules spontaneously associate to form collagen fibrils. They form an ordered, parallel array, with adjacent collagen molecules arranged in a staggered pattern, each overlapping its neighbor by a length approximately three quarters of a molecule (see Fig. 4.7).

7. **Cross-link formation:** The fibrillar array of collagen molecules serves as a substrate for *lysyl oxidase*. This copper-containing extracellular enzyme oxidatively deaminates some of the lysine and hydroxylysine residues in collagen. The reactive aldehydes that result (allysine and hydroxyallysine) can spontaneously condense with lysine or hydroxylysine residues in neighboring collagen molecules to form covalent cross-links and, thus, mature collagen fibers (Fig. 4.9). [Note: Cross-links can form between two allysine residues.]

> *Lysyl oxidase* is one of several copper-containing enzymes. Others include *ceruloplasmin* (see p. 404), *cytochrome c oxidase* (see p. 76), *dopamine hydroxylase* (see p. 286), *superoxide dismutase* (see p. 148), and *tyrosinase* (see p. 273). Disruption in copper homeostasis causes copper deficiency (X-linked Menkes syndrome) or overload (Wilson disease) (see p. 402).

D. Degradation

Normal collagens are highly stable molecules, having half-lives as long as several years. However, connective tissue is dynamic and is constantly being remodeled, often in response to growth or injury of the tissue. Breakdown of collagen fibers is dependent on the proteolytic action of *collagenases*, which are part of a large family of matrix *metalloproteinases*. For type I collagen, the cleavage site is specific, generating three-quarter and one-quarter length fragments. These fragments are further degraded by other matrix *proteinases*.

E. Collagenopathies

Defects in any one of the many steps in collagen fiber synthesis can result in a genetic disease involving an inability of collagen to form fibers properly and, therefore, an inability to provide tissues with the needed tensile strength normally provided by collagen. More than 1,000 mutations have been identified in 23 genes coding for 13 of the collagen types. The following are examples of diseases (collagenopathies) that are the result of defective collagen synthesis.

1. **Ehlers-Danlos syndrome:** Ehlers-Danlos syndrome (EDS) is a heterogeneous group of connective tissue disorders that result from heritable defects in the metabolism of fibrillar collagen molecules. EDS can be caused by a deficiency of collagen-processing enzymes (for example, *lysyl hydroxylase* or *N-procollagen peptidase*) or from mutations in the amino acid sequences of collagen types I, III, and V. The classic form of EDS, caused by defects in type V collagen, is characterized by skin extensibility and fragility and joint hypermobility (Fig. 4.10). The vascular form, due to defects in type III collagen, is the most serious form of EDS because it is

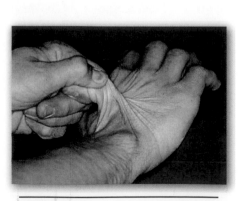

Figure 4.10
Stretchy skin of classic Ehlers-Danlos syndrome.

associated with potentially lethal arterial rupture. [Note: The classic and vascular forms show autosomal-dominant inheritance.] Collagen that contains mutant chains may have altered structure, secretion, or distribution, and it frequently is degraded. [Note: Incorporation of just one mutant chain may result in degradation of the triple helix. This is known as a dominant-negative effect.]

2. **Osteogenesis imperfecta:** This syndrome, known as "brittle bone disease," is a genetic disorder of bone fragility characterized by bones that fracture easily, with minor or no trauma (Fig. 4.11). Over 80% of cases of osteogenesis imperfecta (OI) are caused by dominant mutations to the genes that encode the α1 or α2 chains in type I collagen. The most common mutations cause the replacement of glycine (in –Gly–X–Y–) by amino acids with bulky side chains. The resultant structurally abnormal α chains prevent the formation of the required triple-helical conformation. Phenotypic severity ranges from mild to lethal. Type I OI, the most common form, is characterized by mild bone fragility, hearing loss, and blue sclerae. Type II, the most severe form, is typically lethal in the perinatal period as a result of pulmonary complications. In utero fractures are seen (see Fig. 4.11). Type III is also a severe form and is characterized by multiple fractures at birth, short stature, spinal curvature leading to a humped-back (kyphotic) appearance, and blue sclerae. Dentinogenesis imperfecta, a disorder of tooth development, may be seen in OI.

III. ELASTIN

In contrast to collagen, which forms fibers that are tough and have high tensile strength, elastin is a connective tissue fibrous protein with rubber-like properties. Elastic fibers composed of elastin and glycoprotein microfibrils are found in the lungs, the walls of large arteries, and elastic ligaments. They can be stretched to several times their normal length but recoil to their original shape when the stretching force is relaxed.

A. Structure

Elastin is an insoluble protein polymer generated from a precursor, tropoelastin, which is a soluble polypeptide composed of ~700 amino acids that are primarily small and nonpolar (for example, glycine, alanine, and valine). Elastin is also rich in proline and lysine but contains scant hydroxyproline and hydroxylysine. Tropoelastin is secreted by the cell into the ECM. There, it interacts with specific glycoprotein microfibrils, such as fibrillin, which function as a scaffold onto which tropoelastin is deposited. Some of the lysyl side chains of the tropoelastin polypeptides are oxidatively deaminated by *lysyl oxidase*, forming allysine residues. Three of the allysyl side chains plus one unaltered lysyl side chain from the same or neighboring polypeptides form a desmosine cross-link (Fig. 4.12). This produces elastin, an extensively interconnected, rubbery network that can stretch and bend in any direction when stressed, giving connective tissue elasticity (Fig. 4.13). Mutations in the fibrillin-1 protein are responsible for Marfan syndrome, a connective tissue disorder characterized by impaired structural integrity in the skeleton, the eye, and the cardiovascular system. With this disease, abnormal fibrillin protein is incorporated into microfibrils along with normal fibrillin, inhibiting the

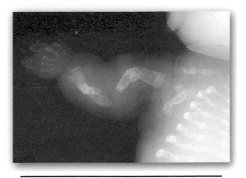

Figure 4.11
Lethal form (type II) of osteogenesis imperfecta in which the fractures appear in utero, as revealed by this radiograph of a stillborn fetus.

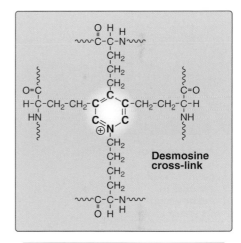

Figure 4.12
Desmosine cross-link unique to elastin.

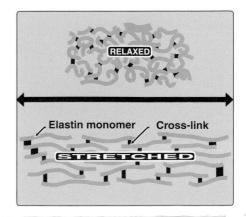

Figure 4.13
Elastin fibers in relaxed and stretched conformations.

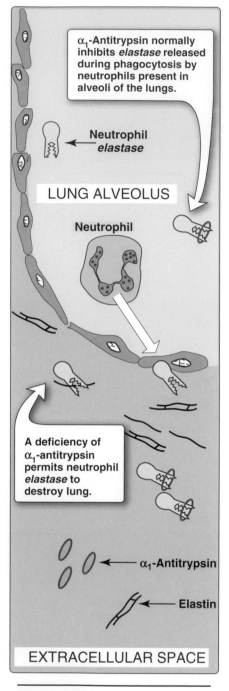

α₁-Antitrypsin normally inhibits *elastase* released during phagocytosis by neutrophils present in alveoli of the lungs.

Neutrophil *elastase*

LUNG ALVEOLUS

Neutrophil

A deficiency of α₁-antitrypsin permits neutrophil *elastase* to destroy lung.

α₁-Antitrypsin

Elastin

EXTRACELLULAR SPACE

Figure 4.14
Destruction of alveolar tissue by *elastase* released from neutrophils activated as part of the immune response to airborne pathogens.

formation of functional microfibrils. [Note: Patients with Marfan syndrome, OI, or EDS may have blue sclerae due to tissue thinning that allows underlying pigment to show through.]

B. α₁-Antitrypsin in elastin degradation

Blood and other body fluids contain a protein, α₁-antitrypsin (AAT), which inhibits a number of proteolytic enzymes (called *peptidases*, *proteases*, or *proteinases*) that hydrolyze and destroy proteins. [Note: The inhibitor was originally named AAT because it inhibits the activity of *trypsin*, a proteolytic enzyme synthesized as trypsinogen by the pancreas (see p. 248).] AAT has the important physiologic role of inhibiting neutrophil *elastase*, a powerful *protease* that is released into the extracellular space and degrades elastin of alveolar walls as well as other structural proteins in a variety of tissues (Fig. 4.14). Most of the AAT found in plasma is synthesized and secreted by the liver. Extrahepatic synthesis also occurs.

1. **α₁-Antitrypsin in the lungs:** In the normal lung, the alveoli are chronically exposed to low levels of neutrophil *elastase* released from activated and degenerating neutrophils. The proteolytic activity of *elastase* can destroy the elastin in alveolar walls if unopposed by the action of AAT, the most important inhibitor of neutrophil *elastase* (see Fig. 4.14). Because lung tissue cannot regenerate, the destruction of the connective tissue of alveolar walls caused by an imbalance between the *protease* and its inhibitor results in pulmonary disease.

2. **α₁-Antitrypsin deficiency and emphysema:** In the United States, ~2%–5% of patients with emphysema are predisposed to the disease by inherited defects in AAT. A number of different mutations in the gene for AAT are known to cause a deficiency of the protein, but one single purine base mutation (GAG to AAG, resulting in the substitution of lysine for glutamic acid at position 342 of the protein) is clinically the most widespread and severe. [Note: The mutated protein is termed the Z variant.] The mutation causes the normally monomeric AAT to misfold, polymerize, and aggregate within the RER of hepatocytes, resulting in decreased secretion of AAT by the liver. AAT deficiency is, therefore, a misfolded protein disease. Consequently, blood levels of AAT are reduced, decreasing the amount that gets to the lung. The polymer that accumulates in the liver may result in cirrhosis (scarring of the liver). In the United States, the AAT mutation is most common in Caucasians of Northern European ancestry. An individual must inherit two abnormal AAT alleles to be at risk for the development of emphysema. In a heterozygote, with one normal and one defective gene, the levels of AAT are sufficient to protect the alveoli from damage. [Note: Methionine 358 in AAT is required for the binding of the inhibitor to its target *proteases*. Smoking causes the oxidation and subsequent inactivation of the methionine, thereby rendering the inhibitor powerless to neutralize *elastase*. Smokers with AAT deficiency, therefore, have a considerably elevated rate of lung destruction and a poorer survival rate than nonsmokers with the deficiency.] The deficiency of *elastase* inhibitor can be treated by weekly augmentation therapy, that is, intravenous administration of AAT. The AAT diffuses from the blood into the lung, where it reaches therapeutic levels in the fluid surrounding the lung epithelial cells.

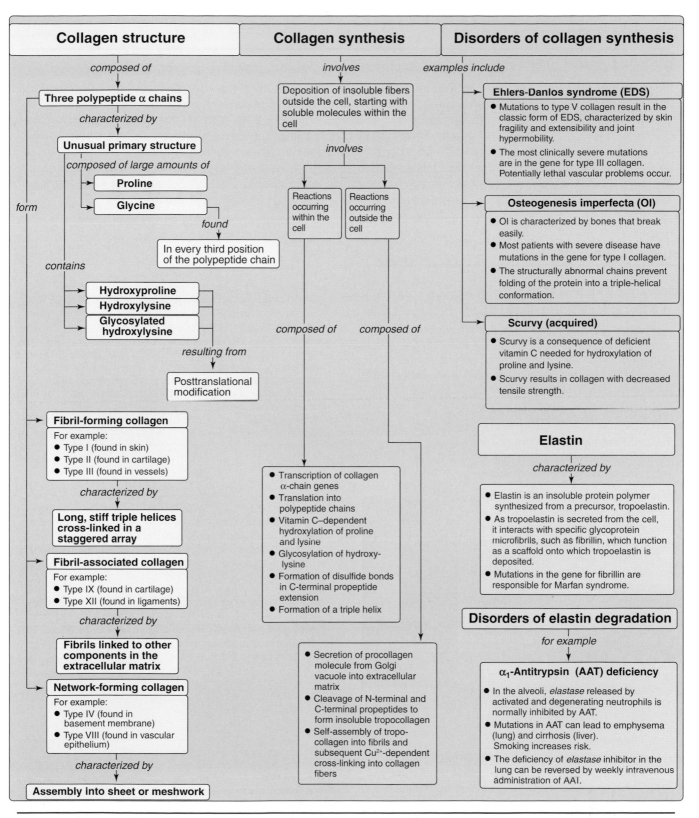

Figure 4.15
Key concept map for the fibrous proteins collagen and elastin. Cu^{2+} = copper.

IV. CHAPTER SUMMARY

Collagen and elastin are structural fibrous proteins of the extracellular matrix (Fig. 4.15). **Collagen** contains an abundance of **proline**, **lysine**, and **glycine**, the latter occurring at every third position in the primary structure. It also contains **hydroxyproline**, **hydroxylysine**, and **glycosylated hydroxylysine**, each formed by posttranslational modification. Fibrillar collagen has a long, rigid structure, in which three collagen polypeptide α chains are wound around one another in a rope-like **triple helix** stabilized by **interchain hydrogen bonds**. Diseases of fibrillar collagen synthesis affect bones, joints, skin, and blood vessels. **Elastin** is a connective tissue protein with rubber-like properties in tissues such as the lung. **α₁-Antitrypsin** (**AAT**), produced primarily by the liver, inhibits *elastase*-catalyzed degradation of elastin in the alveolar walls. A deficiency of AAT increases elastin degradation and can cause **emphysema** and, in some cases, **cirrhosis** of the liver.

Study Questions

Choose the ONE best answer.

4.1 A 30-year-old woman of Northern European ancestry presents with progressive dyspnea (shortness of breath). She denies the use of cigarettes. Family history reveals that her sister also has problems with her lungs. Which one of the following etiologies most likely explains this patient's pulmonary symptoms?

A. Deficiency in dietary vitamin C
B. Deficiency of α₁-antitrypsin
C. Deficiency of prolyl hydroxylase
D. Decreased elastase activity
E. Increased collagenase activity

Correct answer = B. α₁-Antitrypsin (AAT) deficiency is a genetic disorder that can cause pulmonary damage and emphysema even in the absence of cigarette use. A deficiency of AAT permits increased elastase activity to destroy elastin in the alveolar walls. AAT deficiency should be suspected when chronic obstructive pulmonary disease develops in a patient younger than age 45 years who does not have a history of chronic bronchitis or tobacco use or when multiple family members develop obstructive lung disease at an early age. Choices A, C, and E refer to collagen, not elastin.

4.2 A 7-month-old child "fell over" while crawling and now presents with a swollen leg. Imaging reveals a fracture of a bowed femur, secondary to minor trauma, and thin bones (see x-ray at right). Blue sclerae are also noted. At age 1 month, the infant had multiple fractures in various states of healing (right clavicle, right humerus, and right radius). A careful family history has ruled out nonaccidental trauma (child abuse) as a cause of the bone fractures. Which pairing of a defective (or deficient) molecule and the resulting pathology best fits this clinical description?

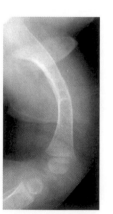

A. Elastin and emphysema
B. Fibrillin and Marfan disease
C. Type I collagen and osteogenesis imperfecta
D. Type V collagen and Ehlers-Danlos syndrome
E. Vitamin C and scurvy

Correct answer = C. The child most likely has osteogenesis imperfecta. Most cases arise from a defect in the genes encoding type I collagen. Bones in affected patients are thin, osteoporotic, often bowed, and extremely prone to fracture. Pulmonary problems are not seen in this child. Individuals with Marfan syndrome have impaired structural integrity of the skeleton, eyes, and cardiovascular system. Defects in type V collagen cause the classic form of Ehlers-Danlos syndrome characterized by skin extensibility and fragility and joint hypermobility. Scurvy caused by vitamin C deficiency is characterized by capillary fragility.

4.3 What is the differential basis of the liver and lung pathology seen in α₁-antitrypsin deficiency?

With α₁-antitrypsin (AAT) deficiency, the cirrhosis that can result is due to polymerization and retention of AAT in the liver, its site of synthesis. The alveolar damage is due to the retention-based deficiency of AAT (a serine protease inhibitor) in the lung such that elastase (a serine protease) is unopposed.

4.4 How and why is proline hydroxylated in collagen?

Proline is hydroxlyated by prolyl hydroxylase, an enzyme of the endoplasmic reticulum that requires oxygen, ferrous iron, and vitamin C. Hydroxylation increases interchain hydrogen bond formation, strengthening the triple helix of collagen. Vitamin C deficiency impairs hydroxylation.

Enzymes

I. OVERVIEW

Virtually all reactions in the body are mediated by enzymes, which are protein catalysts that increase the rate of reactions without being changed in the overall process. Among the many biologic reactions that are energetically possible, enzymes selectively channel reactants (called substrates) into useful pathways. Thus, enzymes direct all metabolic events. This chapter examines the nature of these catalytic molecules and their mechanisms of action.

II. NOMENCLATURE

Each enzyme is assigned two names. The first is its short, recommended name, convenient for everyday use. The second is the more complete systematic name, which is used when an enzyme must be identified without ambiguity.

A. Recommended name

Most commonly used enzyme names have the suffix "*-ase*" attached to the substrate of the reaction (for example, *glucosidase* and *urease*) or to a description of the action performed (for example, *lactate dehydrogenase* and *adenylyl cyclase*). [Note: Some enzymes retain their original trivial names, which give no hint of the associated enzymic reaction, for example, *trypsin* and *pepsin*.]

B. Systematic name

In the systematic naming system, enzymes are divided into six major classes (Fig. 5.1), each with numerous subgroups. For a given enzyme, the suffix *-ase* is attached to a fairly complete description of the chemical reaction catalyzed, including the names of all the substrates, for example, *lactate:nicotinamide adenine dinucleotide (NAD⁺) oxidoreductase*. [Note: Each enzyme is also assigned a classification number. *Lactate:NAD⁺ oxidoreductase* is 1.1.1.27.] The systematic names are unambiguous and informative but are frequently too cumbersome to be of general use.

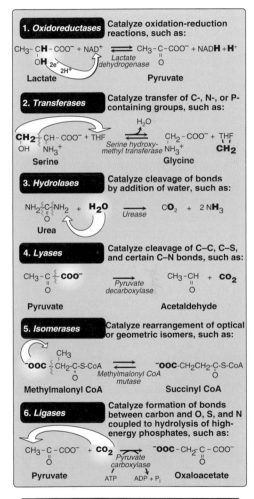

Figure 5.1

The six major classes of enzymes with examples. NAD(H) = nicotinamide adenine dinucleotide; THF = tetrahydrofolate; CoA = coenzyme A; CO_2 = carbon dioxide; NH_3 = ammonia; ADP = adenosine diphosphate; P_i = inorganic phosphate.

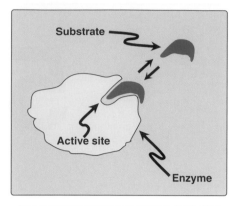

Figure 5.2
Schematic representation of an
enzyme with one active site binding a
substrate molecule.

Potentially confusing enzyme nomenclature includes *synthetase* (requires ATP), *synthase* (no ATP required), *phosphatase* (uses water to remove a phosphate group), *phosphorylase* (uses inorganic phosphate to break a bond and generate a phosphorylated product), *dehydrogenase* (NAD^+ or flavin adenine dinucleotide [FAD] is an electron acceptor in a redox reaction), *oxidase* (oxygen is the acceptor, and oxygen atoms are not incorporated into substrate), and *oxygenase* (one or both oxygen atoms are incorporated).

III. PROPERTIES

Enzymes are protein catalysts that increase the velocity of a chemical reaction and are not consumed during the reaction. [Note: Some ribonucleic acids (RNA) can catalyze reactions that affect phosphodiester and peptide bonds. RNAs with catalytic activity are called ribozymes (see p. 434) and are much less common than protein catalysts.]

A. Active site

Enzyme molecules contain a special pocket or cleft called the active site. The active site, formed by folding of the protein, contains amino acid side chains that participate in substrate binding and catalysis (Fig. 5.2). The substrate binds the enzyme noncovalently, forming an enzyme–substrate (ES) complex. Binding is thought to cause a conformational change in the enzyme (induced fit model) that allows catalysis. ES is converted to an enzyme–product (EP) complex that subsequently dissociates to enzyme and product.

B. Efficiency

Enzyme-catalyzed reactions are highly efficient, proceeding from 10^3 to 10^8 times faster than uncatalyzed reactions. The number of substrate molecules converted to product per enzyme molecule per second is called the turnover number, or k_{cat}, and typically is 10^2–10^4 s^{-1}. [Note: k_{cat} is the rate constant for the conversion of ES to E + P (see p. 58).]

C. Specificity

Enzymes are highly specific, interacting with one or a few substrates and catalyzing only one type of chemical reaction. The set of enzymes made in a cell determines which reactions occur in that cell.

D. Holoenzymes, apoenzymes, cofactors, and coenzymes

Some enzymes require nonproteins for enzymic activity. The term holoenzyme refers to the active enzyme with its nonprotein component, whereas the enzyme without its nonprotein moiety is termed an apoenzyme and is inactive. If the nonprotein moiety is a metal ion, such as zinc (Zn^{2+}) or iron (Fe^{2+}), it is called a cofactor (see Chapter 29). If it is a small organic molecule, it is termed a coenzyme. Coenzymes that only transiently associate with the enzyme are called cosubstrates. Cosubstrates dissociate from the enzyme in an altered state (NAD^+ is an example; see p. 101). If the coenzyme is permanently associated

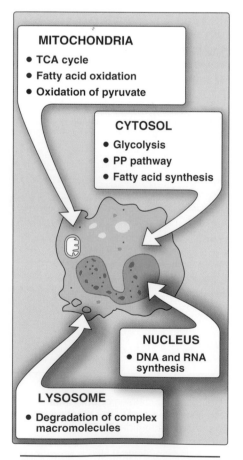

Figure 5.3
The intracellular location of some
important biochemical pathways. TCA
= tricarboxylic acid; PP = pentose
phosphate.

with the enzyme and returned to its original form, it is called a prosthetic group (FAD is an example; see p. 110). Coenzymes commonly are derived from vitamins. For example, NAD^+ contains niacin, and FAD contains riboflavin (see Chapter 28).

E. Regulation

Enzyme activity can be regulated, that is, increased or decreased, so that the rate of product formation responds to cellular need.

F. Location within the cell

Many enzymes are localized in specific organelles within the cell (Fig. 5.3). Such compartmentalization serves to isolate the reaction substrate or product from other competing reactions. This provides a favorable environment for the reaction and organizes the thousands of enzymes present in the cell into purposeful pathways.

IV. MECHANISM OF ENZYME ACTION

The mechanism of enzyme action can be viewed from two different perspectives. The first treats catalysis in terms of energy changes that occur during the reaction. That is, enzymes provide an alternate, energetically favorable reaction pathway different from the uncatalyzed reaction. The second perspective describes how the active site chemically facilitates catalysis.

A. Energy changes occurring during the reaction

Virtually all chemical reactions have an energy barrier separating the reactants and the products. This barrier, called the activation energy (E_a), is the energy difference between that of the reactants and a high-energy intermediate, the transition state (T^*), which is formed during the conversion of reactant to product. Figure 5.4 shows the changes in energy during the conversion of a molecule of reactant A to product B as it proceeds through the transition state.

$$A \rightleftarrows T^* \rightleftarrows B$$

1. **Activation energy:** The peak of energy in Figure 5.4 is the difference in free energy between the reactant and T^*, in which the high-energy, short-lived intermediate is formed during the conversion of reactant to product. Because of the high E_a, the rates of uncatalyzed chemical reactions are often slow.

2. **Rate of reaction:** For molecules to react, they must contain sufficient energy to overcome the energy barrier of the transition state. In the absence of an enzyme, only a small proportion of a population of molecules may possess enough energy to achieve the transition state between reactant and product. The rate of reaction is determined by the number of such energized molecules. In general, the lower the E_a, the more molecules have sufficient energy to pass through the transition state and, therefore, the faster the rate of the reaction.

3. **Alternate reaction pathway:** An enzyme allows a reaction to proceed rapidly under conditions prevailing in the cell by providing an alternate reaction pathway with a lower E_a (see Fig. 5.4). The enzyme does not change the free energies of the reactants

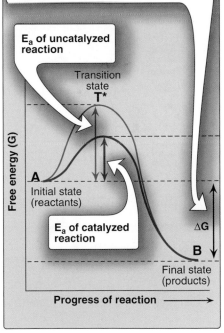

There is no difference in the free energy of the overall reaction (energy of reactants minus energy of products) between the catalyzed and uncatalyzed reactions.

E_a of uncatalyzed reaction

Transition state T^*

Free energy (G)

A
Initial state (reactants)

E_a of catalyzed reaction

ΔG

B

Final state (products)

Progress of reaction

Figure 5.4

Effect of an enzyme on the activation energy (E_a) of a reaction. ΔG = change in free energy.

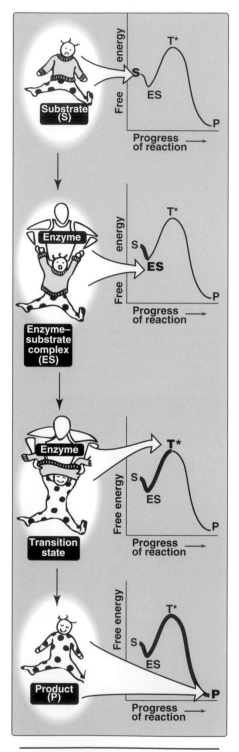

Figure 5.5
Schematic representation of energy changes accompanying formation of an enzyme–substrate complex and subsequent formation of a transition state.

(substrates) or products and, therefore, does not change the equilibrium of the reaction (see p. 70). It does, however, accelerate the rate by which equilibrium is reached.

B. Active site chemistry

The active site is not a passive receptacle for binding the substrate but, rather, is a complex molecular machine employing a diversity of chemical mechanisms to facilitate the conversion of substrate to product. A number of factors are responsible for the catalytic efficiency of enzymes, including the following examples.

1. **Transition-state stabilization:** The active site often acts as a flexible molecular template that binds the substrate and initiates its conversion to the transition state, a structure in which the bonds are not like those in the substrate or the product (see T^* at the top of the curve in Fig. 5.4). By stabilizing the transition state, the enzyme greatly increases the concentration of the reactive intermediate that can be converted to product and, thus, accelerates the reaction. [Note: The transition state cannot be isolated.]

2. **Catalysis:** The active site can provide catalytic groups that enhance the probability that the transition state is formed. In some enzymes, these groups can participate in general acid–base catalysis in which amino acid residues provide or accept protons. In other enzymes, catalysis may involve the transient formation of a covalent ES complex. [Note: The mechanism of action of *chymotrypsin*, an enzyme of protein digestion in the intestine, includes general base, general acid, and covalent catalysis. A histidine at the active site of the enzyme gains (general base) and loses (general acid) protons, mediated by the pK of histidine in proteins being close to physiologic pH. Serine at the active site forms a transient covalent bond with the substrate.]

3. **Transition-state visualization:** The enzyme-catalyzed conversion of substrate to product can be visualized as being similar to removing a sweater from an uncooperative infant (Fig. 5.5). The process has a high E_a because the only reasonable strategy for removing the garment (short of ripping it off) requires that the random flailing of the baby results in both arms being fully extended over the head, an unlikely posture. However, we can envision a parent acting as an enzyme, first coming in contact with the baby (forming ES) and then guiding the baby's arms into an extended, vertical position, analogous to the transition state. This posture (conformation) of the baby facilitates the removal of the sweater, forming the disrobed baby, which here represents product. [Note: The substrate bound to the enzyme (ES) is at a slightly lower energy than unbound substrate (S) and explains the small dip in the curve at ES.]

V. FACTORS AFFECTING REACTION VELOCITY

Enzymes can be isolated from cells and their properties studied in a test tube (that is, <u>in vitro</u>). Different enzymes show different responses to changes in substrate concentration, temperature, and pH. This section describes factors that influence the reaction velocity of enzymes. Enzymic responses to these factors give us valuable clues as to how enzymes function in living cells (that is, in vivo).

A. Substrate concentration

1. **Maximal velocity:** The rate or velocity of a reaction (v) is the number of substrate molecules converted to product per unit time. Velocity is usually expressed as μmol of product formed per minute. The rate of an enzyme-catalyzed reaction increases with substrate concentration until a maximal velocity (V_{max}) is reached (Fig. 5.6). The leveling off of the reaction rate at high substrate concentrations reflects the saturation with substrate of all available binding sites on the enzyme molecules present.

2. **Shape of the enzyme kinetics curve:** Most enzymes show Michaelis-Menten kinetics (see p. 58), in which the plot of initial reaction velocity (v_o) against substrate concentration is hyperbolic (similar in shape to that of the oxygen-dissociation curve of myoglobin; see p. 29). In contrast, allosteric enzymes do not follow Michaelis-Menten kinetics and show a sigmoidal curve (see Fig. 5.6) that is similar in shape to the oxygen-dissociation curve of hemoglobin (see p. 29).

B. Temperature

1. **Velocity increase with temperature:** The reaction velocity increases with temperature until a peak velocity is reached (Fig. 5.7). This increase is the result of the increased number of substrate molecules having sufficient energy to pass over the energy barrier and form the products of the reaction.

2. **Velocity decrease with higher temperature:** Further elevation of the temperature causes a decrease in reaction velocity as a result of temperature-induced denaturation of the enzyme (see Fig. 5.7).

> The optimum temperature for most human enzymes is between 35°C and 40°C. Human enzymes start to denature (see p. 20) at temperatures above 40°C, but thermophilic bacteria found in hot springs have optimum temperatures of 70°C.

C. pH

1. **pH effect on active site ionization:** The concentration of protons ([H⁺]) affects reaction velocity in several ways. First, the catalytic process usually requires that the enzyme and substrate have specific chemical groups in either an ionized or unionized state in order to interact. For example, catalytic activity may require that an amino group of the enzyme be in the protonated form ($-NH_3^+$). Because this group is deprotonated at alkaline pH, the rate of the reaction declines.

2. **pH effect on enzyme denaturation:** Extremes of pH can also lead to denaturation of the enzyme, because the structure of the catalytically active protein molecule depends on the ionic character of the amino acid side chains.

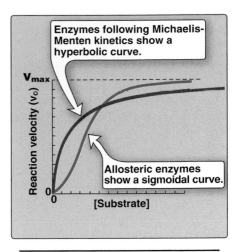

Figure 5.6
Effect of substrate concentration on reaction velocity.

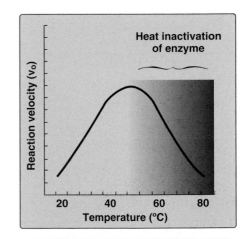

Figure 5.7
Effect of temperature on an enzyme-catalyzed reaction.

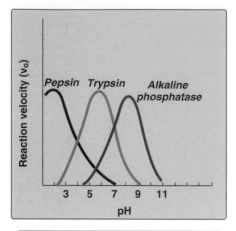

Figure 5.8
Effect of pH on enzyme-catalyzed reactions.

3. **Variable pH optimum:** The pH at which maximal enzyme activity is achieved is different for different enzymes and often reflects the $[H^+]$ at which the enzyme functions in the body. For example, *pepsin*, a digestive enzyme in the stomach, is maximally active at pH 2, whereas other enzymes, designed to work at neutral pH, are denatured by such an acidic environment (Fig. 5.8).

VI. MICHAELIS-MENTEN KINETICS

Leonor Michaelis and Maude Menten proposed a simple model that accounts for most of the features of many enzyme-catalyzed reactions. In this model, the enzyme reversibly combines with its substrate to form an ES complex that subsequently yields product, regenerating the free enzyme. The reaction model, involving one substrate molecule, is represented below:

$$E + S \underset{k_{-1}}{\overset{k_1}{\rightleftharpoons}} ES \overset{k_2}{\longrightarrow} E + P$$

where   S is the substrate.
            E is the enzyme.
            ES is the enzyme–substrate complex.
            P is the product.
            k_1, k_{-1}, and k_2 (or, k_{cat}) are rate constants.

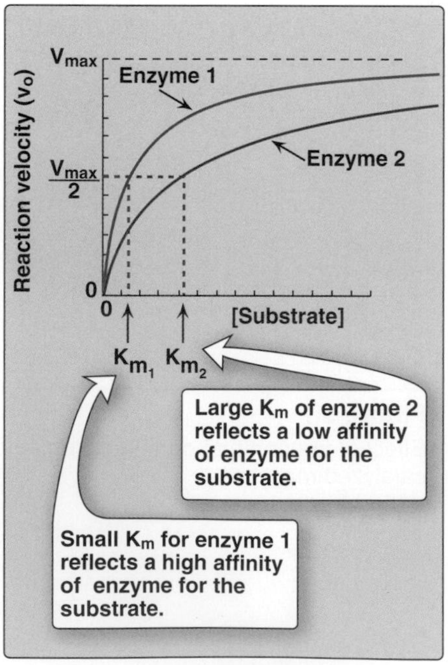

A. Michaelis-Menten equation

The Michaelis-Menten equation describes how reaction velocity varies with substrate concentration:

$$v_o = \frac{V_{max}\,[S]}{K_m + [S]}$$

where v_o = initial reaction velocity
            V_{max} = maximal velocity = $k_{cat}\,[E]_{Total}$
            K_m = Michaelis constant = $(k_{-1} + k_2)/k_1$
            $[S]$ = substrate concentration

The following assumptions are made in deriving the Michaelis-Menten rate equation.

1. **Enzyme and substrate relative concentrations:** The substrate concentration ($[S]$) is much greater than the concentration of enzyme so that the percentage of total substrate bound by the enzyme at any one time is small.

2. **Steady-state assumption:** The concentration of the ES complex does not change with time (the steady-state assumption), that is, the rate of formation of ES is equal to that of the breakdown of ES (to E + S and to E + P). In general, an intermediate in a series of reactions is said to be in steady state when its rate of synthesis is equal to its rate of degradation.

Figure 5.9
Effect of substrate concentration on reaction velocities for two enzymes: enzyme 1 with a small Michaelis constant (K_m) and enzyme 2 with a large K_m. V_{max} = maximal velocity.

Large K_m of enzyme 2 reflects a low affinity of enzyme for the substrate.

Small K_m for enzyme 1 reflects a high affinity of enzyme for the substrate.

3. **Initial velocity:** Initial reaction velocities (v_0) are used in the analysis of enzyme reactions. This means that the rate of the reaction is measured as soon as enzyme and substrate are mixed. At that time, the concentration of product is very small, and therefore, the rate of the back reaction from product to substrate can be ignored.

B. Important conclusions

1. **K_m characteristics:** K_m, the Michaelis constant, is characteristic of an enzyme and its particular substrate and reflects the affinity of the enzyme for that substrate. K_m is numerically equal to the substrate concentration at which the reaction velocity is equal to one half V_{max}. K_m does not vary with enzyme concentration.

   a. **Small K_m:** A numerically small (low) K_m reflects a high affinity of the enzyme for substrate, because a low concentration of substrate is needed to half-saturate the enzyme—that is, to reach a velocity that is one half V_{max} (Fig. 5.9).

   b. **Large K_m:** A numerically large (high) K_m reflects a low affinity of enzyme for substrate because a high concentration of substrate is needed to half-saturate the enzyme.

2. **Velocity relationship to enzyme concentration:** The rate of the reaction is directly proportional to the enzyme concentration because [S] is not limiting. For example, if the enzyme concentration is halved, the initial rates of the reaction (v_0) and that of V_{max} are reduced to half that of the original.

3. **Reaction order:** When [S] is much less (<<) than K_m, the velocity of the reaction is approximately proportional to the substrate concentration (Fig. 5.10). The rate of reaction is then said to be first order with respect to substrate. When [S] is much greater (>>) than K_m, the velocity is constant and equal to V_{max}. The rate of reaction is then independent of substrate concentration (the enzyme is saturated with substrate) and is said to be zero order with respect to substrate concentration (see Fig. 5.10).

C. Lineweaver-Burk plot

When v_0 is plotted against [S], it is not always possible to determine when V_{max} has been achieved because of the gradual upward slope of the hyperbolic curve at high substrate concentrations. However, if $1/v_0$ is plotted versus $1/[S]$, a straight line is obtained (Fig. 5.11). This plot, the Lineweaver-Burk plot (also called a double-reciprocal plot) can be used to calculate K_m and V_{max} as well as to determine the mechanism of action of enzyme inhibitors.

The equation describing the Lineweaver-Burk plot is:

$$\frac{1}{v_0} = \frac{K_m}{V_{max}\,[S]} + \frac{1}{V_{max}}$$

where the intercept on the x axis is equal to $-1/K_m$, and the intercept on the y axis is equal to $1/V_{max}$. [Note: The slope = K_m/V_{max}.]

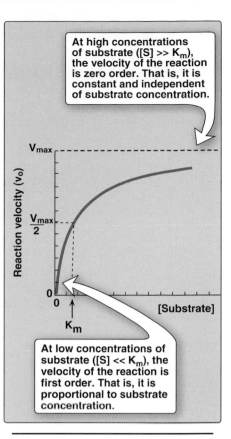

Figure 5.10
Effect of substrate concentration on reaction velocity for an enzyme-catalyzed reaction. V_{max} = maximal velocity; K_m = Michaelis constant.

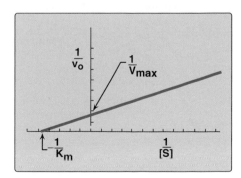

Figure 5.11
Lineweaver-Burk plot. v_0 = initial reaction velocity; V_{max} = maximal velocity; K_m = Michaelis constant; [S] = substrate concentration.

VII. ENZYME INHIBITION

Any substance that can decrease the velocity of an enzyme-catalyzed reaction is called an inhibitor. Inhibitors can be reversible or irreversible. Irreversible inhibitors bind to enzymes through covalent bonds. Lead, for example, forms covalent bonds with the sulfhydryl side chain of cysteine in proteins. *Ferrochelatase*, an enzyme involved in heme synthesis (see p. 279), is irreversibly inhibited by lead. [Note: An important group of irreversible inhibitors are the mechanism-based inhibitors that are converted by the enzyme itself to a form that covalently links to the enzyme, thereby inhibiting it. They also are referred to as "suicide" inhibitors.] Reversible inhibitors bind to enzymes through noncovalent bonds and, thus, dilution of the enzyme–inhibitor complex results in dissociation of the reversibly bound inhibitor and recovery of enzyme activity. The two most commonly encountered types of reversible inhibition are competitive and noncompetitive.

A. Competitive inhibition

This type of inhibition occurs when the inhibitor binds reversibly to the same site that the substrate would normally occupy and, therefore, competes with the substrate for that site.

1. **Effect on V_{max}:** The effect of a competitive inhibitor is reversed by increasing the concentration of substrate. At a sufficiently high [S], the reaction velocity reaches the V_{max} observed in the absence of inhibitor, that is, V_{max} is unchanged (Fig. 5.12).

2. **Effect on K_m:** A competitive inhibitor increases the apparent K_m for a given substrate. This means that, in the presence of a competitive inhibitor, more substrate is needed to achieve one half V_{max}.

3. **Effect on the Lineweaver-Burk plot:** Competitive inhibition shows a characteristic Lineweaver-Burk plot in which the plots of the

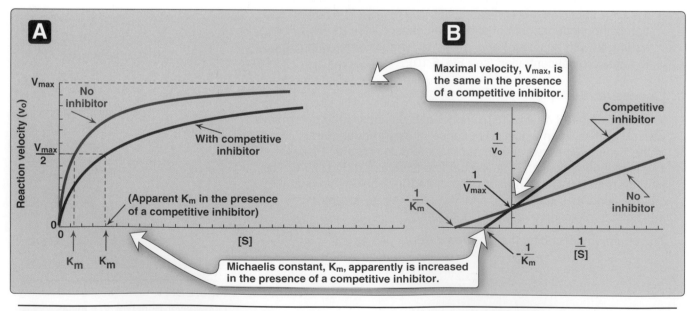

Figure 5.12
A. Effect of a competitive inhibitor on the reaction velocity versus substrate concentration ([S]) plot. B. Lineweaver-Burk plot of competitive inhibition of an enzyme. [Note: The slope increases if inhibitor concentration increases.]

inhibited and uninhibited reactions intersect on the y axis at $1/V_{max}$ (V_{max} is unchanged). The inhibited and uninhibited reactions show different x-axis intercepts, indicating that the apparent K_m is increased in the presence of the competitive inhibitor because $-1/K_m$ moves closer to zero from a negative value (see Fig. 5.12). [Note: An important group of competitive inhibitors are the transition state analogs, stable molecules that approximate the structure of the transition state, and, therefore, bind the enzyme more tightly than does the substrate.]

4. **Statin drugs as examples of competitive inhibitors:** This group of antihyperlipidemic agents competitively inhibits the rate-limiting (slowest) step in cholesterol biosynthesis. This reaction is catalyzed by *hydroxymethylglutaryl coenzyme A reductase* (*HMG CoA reductase;* see p. 221). Statins, such as atorvastatin (Lipitor) and pravastatin (Pravachol), are structural analogs of the natural substrate for this enzyme and compete effectively to inhibit *HMG CoA reductase*. By doing so, they inhibit <u>de novo</u> cholesterol synthesis, thereby lowering plasma cholesterol levels (Fig. 5.13).

B. Noncompetitive inhibition

This type of inhibition is recognized by its characteristic effect on V_{max} (Fig. 5.14). Noncompetitive inhibition occurs when the inhibitor and substrate bind at different sites on the enzyme. The noncompetitive inhibitor can bind either free enzyme or the enzyme–substrate complex, thereby preventing the reaction from occurring (Fig. 5.15).

1. **Effect on V_{max}:** Noncompetitive inhibition cannot be overcome by increasing the concentration of substrate. Therefore, noncompetitive inhibitors decrease the apparent V_{max} of the reaction.

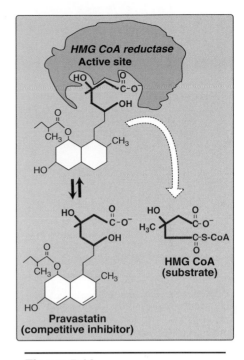

Figure 5.13
Pravastatin competes with hydroxymethylglutaryl coenzyme A (HMG CoA) for the active site of *HMG CoA reductase.*

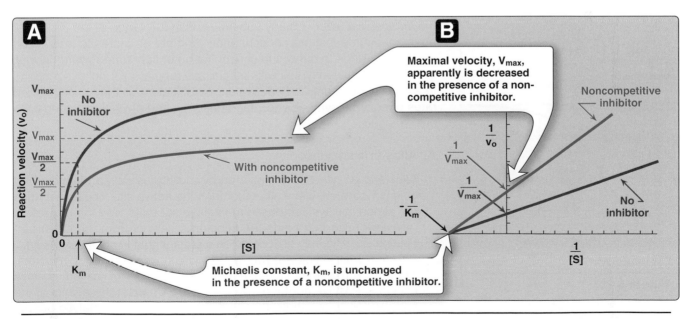

Figure 5.14
A. Effect of a noncompetitive inhibitor on the reaction velocity versus substrate concentration ([S]) plot. B. Lineweaver-Burk plot of noncompetitive inhibition of an enzyme. [Note: The slope increases if inhibitor concentration increases.]

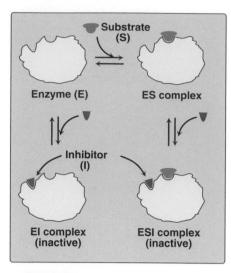

Figure 5.15
A noncompetitive inhibitor binding to both free enzyme and enzyme–substrate (ES) complex.

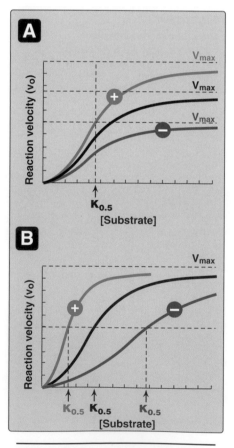

Figure 5.16
Effects of negative ⊖ or positive ⊕ effectors on an allosteric enzyme.
A. Maximal velocity (V_{max}) is altered.
B. The substrate concentration that gives half maximal velocity ($K_{0.5}$) is altered.

2. **Effect on K_m:** Noncompetitive inhibitors do not interfere with the binding of substrate to enzyme. Therefore, the enzyme shows the same K_m in the presence or absence of the noncompetitive inhibitor, that is, K_m is unchanged.

3. **Effect on Lineweaver-Burk plot:** Noncompetitive inhibition is readily differentiated from competitive inhibition by plotting $1/v_o$ versus $1/[S]$ and noting that the apparent V_{max} decreases in the presence of a noncompetitive inhibitor, whereas K_m is unchanged (see Fig. 5.14). [Note: Oxypurinol, a metabolite of the prodrug allopurinol, is a noncompetitive inhibitor of *xanthine oxidase*, an enzyme of purine degradation (see p. 301).]

C. Enzyme inhibitors as drugs

At least half of the ten most commonly prescribed drugs in the United States act as enzyme inhibitors. For example, the widely prescribed β-lactam antibiotics, such as penicillin and amoxicillin, act by inhibiting enzymes involved in bacterial cell wall synthesis. Drugs may also act by inhibiting extracellular reactions. This is illustrated by *angiotensin-converting enzyme* (*ACE*) inhibitors. They lower blood pressure by blocking plasma *ACE* that cleaves angiotensin I to form the potent vasoconstrictor, angiotensin II. These drugs, which include captopril, enalapril, and lisinopril, cause vasodilation and, therefore, a reduction in blood pressure. Aspirin, a nonprescription drug, irreversibly inhibits prostaglandin and thromboxane synthesis by inhibiting *cyclooxygenase* (see p. 214).

VIII. ENZYME REGULATION

The regulation of the reaction velocity of enzymes is essential if an organism is to coordinate its numerous metabolic processes. The rates of most enzymes are responsive to changes in substrate concentration, because the intracellular level of many substrates is in the range of the K_m. Thus, an increase in substrate concentration prompts an increase in reaction rate, which tends to return the concentration of substrate toward normal. In addition, some enzymes with specialized regulatory functions respond to allosteric effectors and/or covalent modification or they show altered rates of enzyme synthesis (or degradation) when physiologic conditions are changed.

A. Allosteric enzymes

Allosteric enzymes are regulated by molecules called effectors that bind noncovalently at a site other than the active site. These enzymes are almost always composed of multiple subunits, and the regulatory (allosteric) site that binds the effector is distinct from the substrate-binding site and may be located on a subunit that is not itself catalytic. Effectors that inhibit enzyme activity are termed negative effectors, whereas those that increase enzyme activity are called positive effectors. Positive and negative effectors can affect the affinity of the enzyme for its substrate ($K_{0.5}$), modify the maximal catalytic activity of the enzyme (V_{max}), or both (Fig. 5.16). [Note: Allosteric enzymes frequently catalyze the committed step, often the rate-limiting step, early in a pathway.]

1. **Homotropic effectors:** When the substrate itself serves as an effector, the effect is said to be homotropic. Most often, an allosteric substrate functions as a positive effector. In such a case, the presence of a substrate molecule at one site on the enzyme enhances the catalytic properties of the other substrate-binding sites. That is, their binding sites exhibit cooperativity. These enzymes show a sigmoidal curve when v_o is plotted against substrate concentration, as shown in Figure 5.16. This contrasts with the hyperbolic curve characteristic of enzymes following Michaelis-Menten kinetics, as previously discussed. [Note: The concept of cooperativity of substrate binding is analogous to the binding of oxygen to hemoglobin (see p. 29).]

2. **Heterotropic effectors:** The effector may be different from the substrate, in which case the effect is said to be heterotropic. For example, consider the feedback inhibition shown in Figure 5.17. The enzyme that converts D to E has an allosteric site that binds the end product, G. If the concentration of G increases (for example, because it is not used as rapidly as it is synthesized), the first irreversible step unique to the pathway is typically inhibited. Feedback inhibition provides the cell with appropriate amounts of a product it needs by regulating the flow of substrate molecules through the pathway that synthesizes that product. Heterotropic effectors are commonly encountered. For example, the glycolytic enzyme *phosphofructokinase-1* is allosterically inhibited by citrate, which is not a substrate for the enzyme (see p. 99).

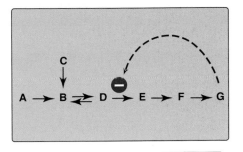

Figure 5.17
Feedback inhibition of a metabolic pathway.

B. Covalent modification

Many enzymes are regulated by covalent modification, most often by the addition or removal of phosphate groups from specific serine, threonine, or tyrosine residues of the enzyme. Protein phosphorylation is recognized as one of the primary ways in which cellular processes are regulated.

1. **Phosphorylation and dephosphorylation:** Phosphorylation reactions are catalyzed by a family of enzymes called *protein kinases* that use ATP as the phosphate donor. Phosphate groups are cleaved from phosphorylated enzymes by the action of *phosphoprotein phosphatases* (Fig. 5.18).

2. **Enzyme response to phosphorylation:** Depending on the specific enzyme, the phosphorylated form may be more or less active than the unphosphorylated enzyme. For example, hormone-mediated phosphorylation of *glycogen phosphorylase* (an enzyme that degrades glycogen) increases activity, whereas phosphorylation of *glycogen synthase* (an enzyme that synthesizes glycogen) decreases activity (see p. 132).

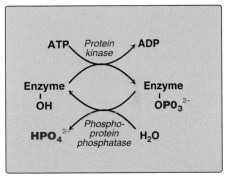

Figure 5.18
Covalent modification by the addition and removal of phosphate groups. [Note: HPO_4^{2-} may be represented as P_i and PO_3^{2-} as Ⓟ.] ADP = adenosine diphosphate.

C. Enzyme synthesis

The regulatory mechanisms described above modify the activity of existing enzyme molecules. However, cells can also regulate the amount of enzyme present by altering the rate of enzyme degradation or, more typically, the rate of enzyme synthesis. The increase (induction) or

REGULATOR EVENT	TYPICAL EFFECTOR	RESULTS	TIME REQUIRED FOR CHANGE
Substrate availability	Substrate	Change in velocity (v_o)	Immediate
Product inhibition	Reaction product	Change in V_{max} and/or K_m	Immediate
Allosteric control	Pathway end product	Change in V_{max} and/or $K_{0.5}$	Immediate
Covalent modification	Another enzyme	Change in V_{max} and/or K_m	Immediate to minutes
Synthesis or degradation of enzyme	Hormone or metabolite	Change in the amount of enzyme	Hours to days

Figure 5.19
Mechanisms for regulating enzyme activity. [Note: Inhibition by pathway end product is also referred to as feedback inhibition.]

decrease (repression) of enzyme synthesis leads to an alteration in the total population of active sites. Enzymes subject to regulation of synthesis are often those that are needed at only one stage of development or under selected physiologic conditions. For example, elevated levels of insulin as a result of high blood glucose levels cause an increase in the synthesis of key enzymes involved in glucose metabolism (see p. 105). In contrast, enzymes that are in constant use are usually not regulated by altering the rate of enzyme synthesis. Alterations in enzyme levels as a result of induction or repression of protein synthesis are slow (hours to days), compared with allosterically or covalently regulated changes in enzyme activity, which occur in seconds to minutes. Figure 5.19 summarizes the common ways that enzyme activity is regulated.

IX. ENZYMES IN CLINICAL DIAGNOSIS

Plasma enzymes can be classified into two major groups. First, a relatively small group of enzymes are actively secreted into the blood by certain cell types. For example, the liver secretes zymogens (inactive precursors) of the enzymes involved in blood coagulation. Second, a large number of enzyme species are released from cells during normal cell turnover. These enzymes almost always function intracellularly and have no physiologic use in the plasma. In healthy individuals, the levels of these enzymes are fairly constant and represent a steady state in which the rate of release from damaged cells into the plasma is balanced by an equal rate of removal from the plasma. Increased plasma levels of these enzymes may indicate tissue damage (Fig. 5.20).

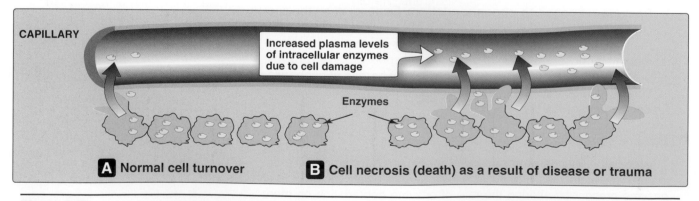

Figure 5.20
Release of enzymes from normal (A) and diseased or traumatized (B) cells.

Plasma is the fluid, noncellular part of blood. Laboratory assays of enzyme activity most often use serum, which is obtained by centrifugation of whole blood after it has been allowed to coagulate. Plasma is a physiologic fluid, whereas serum is prepared in the laboratory.

A. Plasma enzyme levels in disease states

Many diseases that cause tissue damage result in an increased release of intracellular enzymes into the plasma. The activities of many of these enzymes are routinely determined for diagnostic purposes in diseases of the heart, liver, skeletal muscle, and other tissues. The level of specific enzyme activity in the plasma frequently correlates with the extent of tissue damage. Therefore, determining the degree of elevation of a particular enzyme activity in the plasma is often useful in evaluating the prognosis for the patient.

B. Plasma enzymes as diagnostic tools

Some enzymes show relatively high activity in only one or a few tissues. Therefore, the presence of increased levels of these enzymes in plasma reflects damage to the corresponding tissue. For example, the enzyme *alanine aminotransferase* (*ALT*; see p. 251) is abundant in the liver. The appearance of elevated levels of *ALT* in plasma signals possible damage to hepatic tissue. [Note: Measurement of *ALT* is part of the liver function test panel.] Increases in plasma levels of enzymes with a wide tissue distribution provide a less specific indication of the site of cellular injury and limits their diagnostic value.

C. Isoenzymes and heart disease

Isoenzymes (also called isozymes) are enzymes that catalyze the same reaction. However, they do not necessarily have the same physical properties because of genetically determined differences in amino acid sequence. For this reason, isoenzymes may contain different numbers of charged amino acids, which allows electrophoresis (the movement of charged particles in an electric field) to separate them (Fig. 5.21). Different organs commonly contain characteristic proportions of different isoenzymes. The pattern of isoenzymes found in the plasma may, therefore, serve as a means of identifying the site of tissue damage. For example, the plasma levels of *creatine kinase* (*CK*) are commonly determined in the diagnosis of myocardial infarction (MI). They are particularly useful when the electrocardiogram (ECG) is difficult to interpret such as when there have been previous episodes of heart disease.

1. **Isoenzyme quaternary structure:** Many isoenzymes contain different subunits in various combinations. For example, *CK* occurs as three isoenzymes. Each isoenzyme is a dimer composed of two polypeptides (called B and M subunits) associated in one of three combinations: *CK1* = BB, *CK2* = MB, and *CK3* = MM. Each *CK* isoenzyme shows a characteristic electrophoretic mobility (see Fig. 5.21). [Note: Virtually all *CK* in the brain is the BB isoform, whereas it is MM in skeletal muscle. In cardiac muscle, about one third is MB with the rest as MM.]

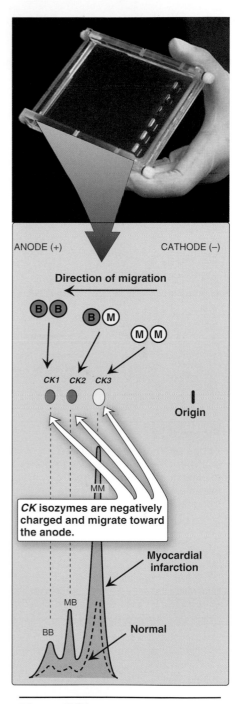

Figure 5.21
Subunit composition, electrophoretic mobility, and enzyme activity of *creatine kinase* (*CK*) isoenzymes.

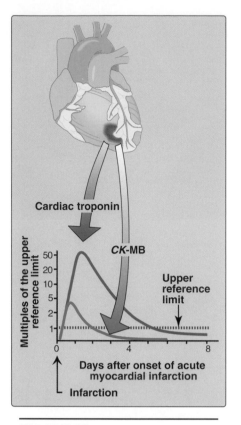

Figure 5.22
Appearance of *creatine kinase* isozyme *CK*-MB and cardiac troponin in plasma after an myocardial infarction. [Note: Either cardiac troponin T or I may be measured.]

2. **Diagnosis of myocardial infarction:** Measurement of blood levels of proteins with cardiac specificity (biomarkers) is used in the diagnosis of MI. Myocardial muscle is the only tissue that contains >5% of the total *CK* activity as the *CK2* (MB) isoenzyme. Appearance of this hybrid isoenzyme in plasma is virtually specific for infarction of the myocardium. Following an acute MI, *CK2* appears in plasma within 4–8 hours following onset of chest pain, reaches a peak of activity at ~24 hours, and returns to baseline after 48–72 hours (Fig. 5.22). Troponins T (TnT) and I (TnI) are regulatory proteins involved in muscle contractility. Cardiac-specific isoforms (cTn) are released into the plasma in response to cardiac damage. They are highly sensitive and specific for damage to cardiac tissue. cTn appear in plasma within 4–6 hours after an MI, peak in 24–36 hours, and remain elevated for 3–10 days. Elevated cTn, in combination with the clinical presentation and characteristic changes in the ECG, are currently considered the "gold standard" in the diagnosis of an MI.

X. CHAPTER SUMMARY

Enzymes are **protein catalysts** that increase the velocity of a chemical reaction by lowering the energy of the **transition state** (Fig. 5.23). They are not consumed during the reaction. Enzyme molecules contain a special cleft called the **active site**, which contains amino acid side chains that participate in substrate binding and catalysis. The active site binds the substrate, forming an **enzyme–substrate (ES) complex**. Binding is thought to cause a conformational change in the enzyme (induced fit) that allows catalysis. ES is converted to enzyme and product. An enzyme allows a reaction to proceed rapidly under conditions prevailing in the cell by providing an **alternate reaction pathway** with a **lower activation energy** (E_a). Because the enzyme does not change the free energies of the reactants or products, it does not change the equilibrium of the reaction. Most enzymes show **Michaelis-Menten kinetics**, and a plot of the **initial reaction velocity** (v_o) against **substrate concentration** (**[S]**) has a **hyperbolic** shape similar to the oxygen-dissociation curve of myoglobin. A **Lineweaver-Burk** plot of 1/v and 1/[S] allows determination of V_{max} (maximal velocity) and K_m (Michaelis constant, which reflects affinity for substrate). Any substance that can decrease the velocity of an enzyme-catalyzed reaction is called an **inhibitor**. The two most common types of reversible inhibition are **competitive** (which **increases** the **apparent K_m**) and **noncompetitive** (which **decreases** the **apparent V_{max}**). In contrast, the **multisubunit allosteric enzymes** show a **sigmoidal curve** similar in shape to the oxygen-dissociation curve of hemoglobin. They typically catalyze the **committed step** of a pathway. **Allosteric enzymes** are regulated by molecules called **effectors** that bind noncovalently at a site other than the active site. Effectors can be either **positive** (increase enzyme activity) or **negative** (decrease enzyme activity). An allosteric effector can alter the affinity of the enzyme for its substrate ($K_{0.5}$), the maximal catalytic activity of the enzyme (V_{max}), or both. Enzymes can also be regulated by **covalent modification** and by changes in the rate of synthesis or degradation. Enzymes have diagnostic and therapeutic value in medicine.

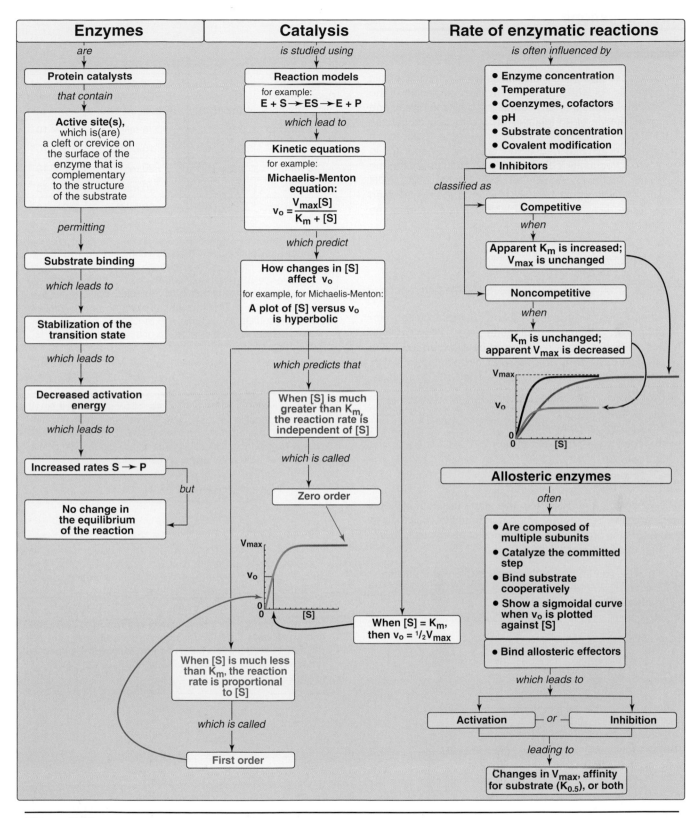

Figure 5.23
Key concept map for the enzymes. S = substrate; [S] = substrate concentration; P = product; E = enzyme; v_o = initial velocity; V_{max} = maximal velocity; K_m = Michaelis constant; $K_{0.5}$ = substrate concentration that gives half maximal velocity.

Study Questions

Choose the ONE best answer.

5.1 In cases of ethylene glycol poisoning and its characteristic metabolic acidosis, treatment involves correction of the acidosis, removal of any remaining ethylene glycol, and administration of an inhibitor of alcohol dehydrogenase (ADH), the enzyme that oxidizes ethylene glycol to the organic acids that cause the acidosis. Ethanol (grain alcohol) frequently is the inhibitor given to treat ethylene glycol poisoning. Results of experiments using ADH with and without ethanol are shown to the right. Based on these data, what type of inhibition is caused by the ethanol?

A. Competitive
B. Feedback
C. Irreversible
D. Noncompetitive

Substrate Concentration with Ethanol	Rate of Reaction (mol/L/s)	Substrate Concentration without Ethanol	Rate of Reaction (mol/L/s)
5 mM	3.0×10^{-7}	5 mM	8.0×10^{-7}
10 mM	5.0×10^{-7}	10 mM	1.2×10^{-6}
20 mM	1.0×10^{-6}	20 mM	1.8×10^{-6}
40 mM	1.6×10^{-6}	40 mM	1.9×10^{-6}
80 mM	2.0×10^{-6}	80 mM	2.0×10^{-6}

Correct answer = A. A competitive inhibitor increases the apparent K_m for a given substrate. This means that, in the presence of a competitive inhibitor, more substrate is needed to achieve one half V_{max}. The effect of a competitive inhibitor is reversed by increasing substrate concentration ([S]). At a sufficiently high [S], the reaction velocity reaches the V_{max} observed in the absence of inhibitor.

5.2 Alcohol dehydrogenase (ADH) requires oxidized nicotinamide adenine dinucleotide (NAD$^+$) for catalytic activity. In the reaction catalyzed by ADH, an alcohol is oxidized to an aldehyde as NAD$^+$ is reduced to NADH and dissociates from the enzyme. The NAD$^+$ is functioning as a/an:

A. apoenzyme.
B. coenzyme–cosubstrate.
C. coenzyme–prosthetic group.
D. cofactor.
E. heterotropic effector.

Correct answer = B. A Coenzymes–cosubstrates are small organic molecules that associate transiently with an enzyme and leave the enzyme in a changed form. Coenzyme–prosthetic groups are small organic molecules that associate permanently with an enzyme and are returned to their original form on the enzyme. Cofactors are metal ions. Heterotropic effectors are not substrates.

For Questions 5.3 and 5.4, use the graph below that shows the changes in free energy when a reactant is converted to a product in the presence and absence of an enzyme. Select the letter that best represents:

5.3 the activation energy of the catalyzed forward reaction.

5.4 the free energy of the reaction.

Correct answers = B; D. Enzymes (protein catalysts) provide an alternate reaction pathway with a lower activation energy. However, they do not change the free energy of the reactant or product. A is the activation energy of the uncatalyzed reaction. C is the activation energy of the catalyzed reverse reaction.

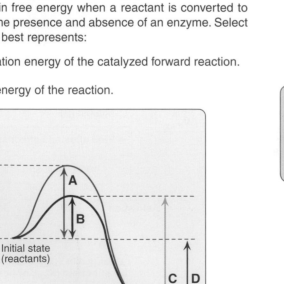

Bioenergetics and Oxidative Phosphorylation

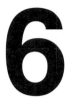

I. OVERVIEW

Bioenergetics describes the transfer and utilization of energy in biologic systems. It concerns the initial and final energy states of the reaction components, not the reaction mechanism or how much time it takes for the chemical change to occur. Bioenergetics makes use of a few basic ideas from the field of thermodynamics, particularly the concept of free energy. Because changes in free energy provide a measure of the energetic feasibility of a chemical reaction, they allow prediction of whether a reaction or process can take place. In short, bioenergetics predicts if a process is possible, whereas kinetics measures the reaction rate (see p. 54).

II. FREE ENERGY

The direction and extent to which a chemical reaction proceeds are determined by the degree to which two factors change during the reaction. These are enthalpy (ΔH, a measure of the change [Δ] in heat content of the reactants and products) and entropy (ΔS, a measure of the change in randomness or disorder of the reactants and products), as shown in Figure 6.1. Neither of these thermodynamic quantities by itself is sufficient to determine whether a chemical reaction will proceed spontaneously in the direction it is written. However, when combined mathematically (see Fig. 6.1), enthalpy and entropy can be used to define a third quantity, free energy (G), which predicts the direction in which a reaction will spontaneously proceed.

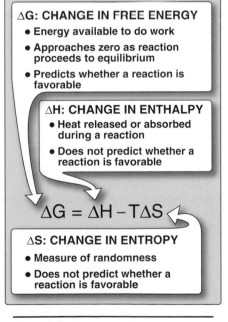

ΔG: CHANGE IN FREE ENERGY
- Energy available to do work
- Approaches zero as reaction proceeds to equilibrium
- Predicts whether a reaction is favorable

ΔH: CHANGE IN ENTHALPY
- Heat released or absorbed during a reaction
- Does not predict whether a reaction is favorable

$$\Delta G = \Delta H - T\Delta S$$

ΔS: CHANGE IN ENTROPY
- Measure of randomness
- Does not predict whether a reaction is favorable

Figure 6.1

Relationship between changes in free energy (G), enthalpy (H), and entropy (S). T is the absolute temperature in Kelvin (K), where K = °C + 273.

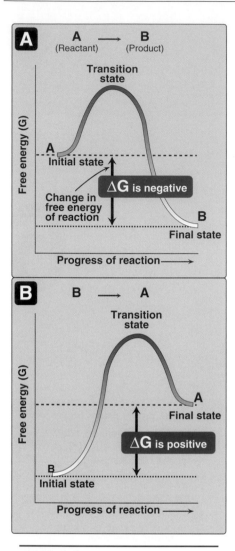

Figure 6.2
Change in free energy (ΔG) during a
reaction. A. The product has a lower
free energy (G) than the reactant.
B. The product has a higher free
energy than the reactant.

III. FREE ENERGY CHANGE

The change in free energy is represented in two ways, ΔG and ΔG^0.
The first, ΔG (without the superscript "0"), represents the change
in free energy and, thus, the direction of a reaction at any specified
concentration of products and reactants. ΔG, then, is a variable. This
contrasts with the standard free energy change, ΔG^0 (with the superscript "0"), which is the energy change when reactants and products
are at a concentration of 1 mol/l. [Note: The concentration of protons
(H^+) is assumed to be 10^{-7} mol/l (that is, pH = 7). This may be shown
by a prime sign ('), for example, $\Delta G^{0'}$.] Although ΔG^0, a constant,
represents energy changes at these nonphysiologic concentrations
of reactants and products, it is nonetheless useful in comparing the
energy changes of different reactions. Furthermore, ΔG^0 can readily be determined from measurement of the equilibrium constant
(see p. 71). [Note: This section outlines the uses of ΔG, and ΔG^0 is
described in D. below.]

A. ΔG and reaction direction

The sign of ΔG can be used to predict the direction of a reaction at
constant temperature and pressure. Consider the reaction:

$$A \rightleftarrows B$$

1. **Negative ΔG:** If ΔG is negative, then there is a net loss of energy,
   and the reaction goes spontaneously as written (that is, A is converted into B) as shown in Figure 6.2A. The reaction is said to be
   exergonic.

2. **Positive ΔG:** If ΔG is positive, then there is a net gain of energy,
   and the reaction does not go spontaneously from B to A (Fig. 6.2B).
   Energy must be added to the system to make the reaction go from
   B to A. The reaction is said to be endergonic.

3. **Zero ΔG:** If $\Delta G = 0$, then the reaction is in equilibrium. [Note:
   When a reaction is proceeding spontaneously (that is, ΔG is negative), the reaction continues until ΔG reaches zero and equilibrium
   is established.]

B. ΔG of the forward and back reactions

The free energy of the forward reaction (A → B) is equal in magnitude
but opposite in sign to that of the back reaction (B → A). For example,
if ΔG of the forward reaction is –5 kcal/mol, then that of the back reaction is +5 kcal/mol. [Note: ΔG can also be expressed in kilojoules per
mole or kJ/mol (1 kcal = 4.2 kJ).]

C. ΔG and reactant and product concentrations

The ΔG of the reaction A → B depends on the concentration of the
reactant and product. At constant temperature and pressure, the following relationship can be derived:

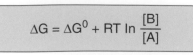

$$\Delta G = \Delta G^0 + RT \ln \frac{[B]}{[A]}$$

where ΔG^0 is the standard free energy change (see D. below)
R is the gas constant (1.987 cal/mol K)
T is the absolute temperature (K)
[A] and [B] are the actual concentrations of the reactant and product
ln represents the natural logarithm.

A reaction with a positive ΔG^0 can proceed in the forward direction if the ratio of products to reactants ([B]/[A]) is sufficiently small (that is, the ratio of reactants to products is large) to make ΔG negative. For example, consider the reaction:

Glucose 6-phosphate $\rightleftarrows$ fructose 6-phosphate

Figure 6.3A shows reaction conditions in which the concentration of reactant, glucose 6-phosphate, is high compared with the concentration of product, fructose 6-phosphate. This means that the ratio of the product to reactant is small, and RT ln([fructose 6-phosphate]/[glucose 6-phosphate]) is large and negative, causing ΔG to be negative despite ΔG^0 being positive. Thus, the reaction can proceed in the forward direction.

D. Standard free energy change

The standard free energy change, ΔG^0, is so called because it is equal to the free energy change, ΔG, under standard conditions (that is, when reactants and products are at 1 mol/l concentrations; Fig. 6.3B). Under these conditions, the natural logarithm of the ratio of products to reactants is zero (ln1 = 0), and, therefore, the equation shown at the bottom of the previous page becomes:

$$\Delta G = \Delta G^0 + 0$$

1. **ΔG^0 and reaction direction:** Under standard conditions, ΔG^0 can be used to predict the direction a reaction proceeds because, under these conditions, ΔG^0 is equal to ΔG. However, ΔG^0 cannot predict the direction of a reaction under physiologic conditions because it is composed solely of constants (R, T, and K_{eq} [see 2. below]) and is not, therefore, altered by changes in product or substrate concentrations.

2. **Relationship between ΔG^0 and K_{eq}:** In a reaction A $\rightleftarrows$ B, a point of equilibrium is reached at which no further net chemical change takes place (that is, when A is being converted to B as fast as B is being converted to A). In this state, the ratio of [B] to [A] is constant, regardless of the actual concentrations of the two compounds:

$$K_{eq} = \frac{[B]_{eq}}{[A]_{eq}}$$

where K_{eq} is the equilibrium constant, and $[A]_{eq}$ and $[B]_{eq}$ are the concentrations of A and B at equilibrium. If the reaction A $\rightleftarrows$ B is allowed to go to equilibrium at constant temperature and pressure, then, at equilibrium, the overall ΔG is zero (Fig. 6.3C). Therefore,

$$\Delta G = 0 = \Delta G^0 + RT \ln \frac{[B]_{eq}}{[A]_{eq}}$$

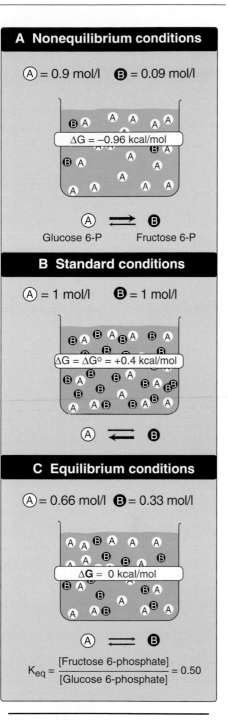

A Nonequilibrium conditions

(A) = 0.9 mol/l   (B) = 0.09 mol/l

$\Delta G = -0.96$ kcal/mol

(A) $\rightleftarrows$ (B)
Glucose 6-P   Fructose 6-P

B Standard conditions

(A) = 1 mol/l   (B) = 1 mol/l

$\Delta G = \Delta G^o = +0.4$ kcal/mol

(A) $\rightleftarrows$ (B)

C Equilibrium conditions

(A) = 0.66 mol/l (B) = 0.33 mol/l

$\Delta G = 0$ kcal/mol

(A) $\rightleftarrows$ (B)

$$K_{eq} = \frac{[\text{Fructose 6-phosphate}]}{[\text{Glucose 6-phosphate}]} = 0.50$$

Figure 6.3
Free energy change (ΔG) of a reaction depends on the concentration of reactant (A) and product (B). For the conversion of glucose 6-phosphate to fructose 6-phosphate, ΔG is negative when the ratio of reactant (A) to product (B) is large (top, panel A), is positive under standard conditions (middle, panel B), and is zero at equilibrium (bottom, panel C). ΔG^0 = standard free energy change.

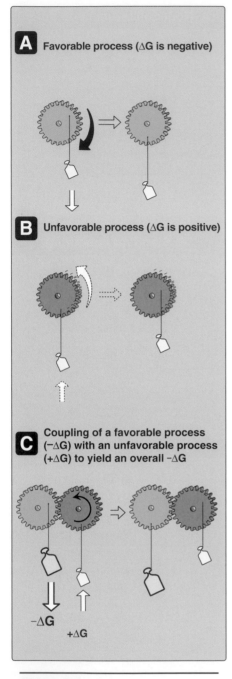

A Favorable process (ΔG is negative)

B Unfavorable process (ΔG is positive)

C Coupling of a favorable process ($-\Delta G$) with an unfavorable process ($+\Delta G$) to yield an overall $-\Delta G$

$-\Delta G$

$+\Delta G$

Figure 6.4
Mechanical model of the coupling of favorable and unfavorable processes. A. Gear with weight attached spontaneously turns in the direction that achieves the lowest energy state. B. The reverse movement is energetically unfavorable (not spontaneous). C. The energetically favorable movement can drive the unfavorable one. ΔG = change in free energy.

where the actual concentrations of A and B are equal to the equilibrium concentrations of reactant and product ($[A]_{eq}$ and $[B]_{eq}$), and their ratio is equal to the K_{eq}. Thus,

$$\Delta G^0 = -RT \ln K_{eq}$$

This equation allows some simple predictions:

If $K_{eq} = 1$, then $\Delta G^0 = 0$ $A \rightleftharpoons B$

If $K_{eq} > 1$, then $\Delta G^0 < 0$ $A \rightleftharpoons B$

If $K_{eq} < 1$, then $\Delta G^0 > 0$ $A \rightleftharpoons B$

3. **ΔG^0s of two consecutive reactions:** The ΔG^0s are additive in any sequence of consecutive reactions, as are the ΔGs. For example:

Glucose + ATP	$\rightarrow$ glucose 6-phosphate + ADP	$\Delta G^0 = -4,000$ cal/mol
Glucose 6-phosphate	$\rightarrow$ fructose 6-phosphate	$\Delta G^0 = +400$ cal/mol
Glucose + ATP	$\rightarrow$ fructose 6-phosphate + ADP	$\Delta G^0 = -3,600$ cal/mol

4. **ΔGs of a pathway:** The additive property of ΔG is very important in biochemical pathways through which substrates (reactants) must pass in a particular direction (for example, $A \rightarrow B \rightarrow C \rightarrow D \rightarrow \ldots$). As long as the sum of the ΔGs of the individual reactions is negative, the pathway can proceed as written, even if some of the individual reactions of the pathway have a positive ΔG. However, the actual rates of the reactions depend on the lowering of activation energies (E_a) by the enzymes that catalyze the reactions (see p. 55).

IV. ATP: AN ENERGY CARRIER

Reactions or processes that have a large positive ΔG, such as moving ions against a concentration gradient across a cell membrane, are made possible by coupling the endergonic movement of ions with a second, spontaneous process with a large negative ΔG such as the exergonic hydrolysis of ATP (see p. 87). [Note: In the absence of enzymes, ATP is a stable molecule because its hydrolysis has a high E_a.] Figure 6.4 shows a mechanical model of energy coupling. The simplest example of energy coupling in biologic reactions occurs when the energy-requiring and the energy-yielding reactions share a common intermediate.

A. Common intermediates

Two chemical reactions have a common intermediate when they occur sequentially in that the product of the first reaction is a substrate for the second. For example, given the reactions

$$A + B \rightarrow C + D$$

$$D + X \rightarrow Y + Z$$

D is the common intermediate and can serve as a carrier of chemical energy between the two reactions. [Note: The intermediate may be linked to an enzyme.] Many coupled reactions use ATP to generate a common intermediate. These reactions may involve the transfer of a phosphate group from ATP to another molecule. Other reactions involve the transfer of phosphate from an energy-rich intermediate to adenosine diphosphate (ADP), forming ATP.

B. Energy carried by ATP

ATP consists of a molecule of adenosine (adenine + ribose) to which three phosphate groups are attached (Fig. 6.5). Removal of one phosphate produces ADP, and removal of two phosphates produces adenosine monophosphate (AMP). For ATP, the ΔG^0 of hydrolysis is approximately -7.3 kcal/mol for each of the two terminal phosphate groups. Because of this large negative ΔG^0 of hydrolysis, ATP is called a high-energy phosphate compound. [Note: Adenine nucleotides are interconverted ($2\ ADP \rightleftarrows ATP + AMP$) by *adenylate kinase*.]

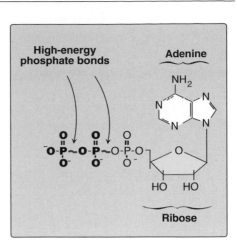

Figure 6.5
Adenosine triphosphate (ATP).

V. ELECTRON TRANSPORT CHAIN

Energy-rich molecules, such as glucose, are metabolized by a series of oxidation reactions ultimately yielding carbon dioxide and water (H_2O), as shown in Figure 6.6. The metabolic intermediates of these reactions donate electrons to specific coenzymes, nicotinamide adenine dinucleotide (NAD^+) and flavin adenine dinucleotide (FAD), to form the energy-rich reduced forms, NADH and $FADH_2$. These reduced coenzymes can, in turn, each donate a pair of electrons to a specialized set of electron carriers, collectively called the electron transport chain (ETC), described in this section. As electrons are passed down the ETC, they lose much of their free energy. This energy is used to move H^+ across the inner mitochondrial membrane, creating a H^+ gradient that drives the production of ATP from ADP and inorganic phosphate (P_i), described on p. 77. The coupling of electron transport with ATP synthesis is called oxidative phosphorylation, sometimes denoted as OXPHOS. It proceeds continuously in all tissues that contain mitochondria. [Note: The free energy not trapped as ATP is used to drive ancillary reactions such as transport of calcium ions into mitochondria and to generate heat.]

A. Mitochondrial electron transport chain

The ETC (except for cytochrome c, see p. 75) is located in the inner mitochondrial membrane and is the final common pathway by which electrons derived from different fuels of the body flow to oxygen (O_2), reducing it to H_2O (see Fig. 6.6).

1. **Mitochondrial membranes:** The mitochondrion contains an outer and an inner membrane separated by the intermembrane space. Although the outer membrane contains special channels (formed by the protein porin), making it freely permeable to most ions and small molecules, the inner membrane is a specialized structure that is impermeable to most small ions, including H^+, and small molecules such as ATP, ADP, pyruvate, and other metabolites important to mitochondrial function (Fig. 6.7). Specialized carriers or transport systems are required to move ions or molecules across this

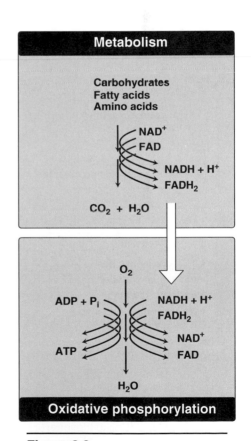

Figure 6.6
The metabolic breakdown of energy-yielding molecules. NAD(H) = nicotinamide adenine dinucleotide; $FAD(H_2)$ = flavin adenine dinucleotide; ADP = adenosine diphosphate; P_i = inorganic phosphate; CO_2 = carbon dioxide.

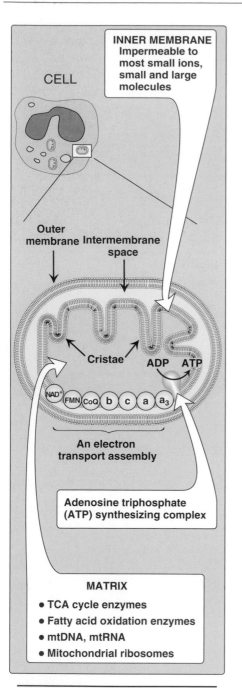

Figure 6.7
Structure of a mitochondrion showing schematic representation of the electron transport chain and the ATP synthesizing complex on the inner membrane. [Note: Unlike the inner membrane, the outer membrane is highly permeable, and the milieu of the intermembrane space is like that of the cytosol.] mt = mitochondrial; RNA = ribonucleic acid; ADP = adenosine diphosphate; TCA = tricarboxylic acid.

membrane. The inner mitochondrial membrane is unusually rich in proteins, over half of which are directly involved in oxidative phosphorylation. It also contains convolutions, called cristae, which greatly increase its surface area.

2. **Mitochondrial matrix:** The gel-like solution of the matrix (interior) of mitochondria is also rich in proteins. These include the enzymes responsible for the oxidation of pyruvate, amino acids, and fatty acids (by β-oxidation) as well as those of the tricarboxylic acid (TCA) cycle. The synthesis of glucose, urea, and heme occurs partially in the matrix of mitochondria. In addition, the matrix contains NAD^+ and FAD (the oxidized forms of the two coenzymes that are required as electron acceptors), and ADP and P_i, which are used to produce ATP. [Note: The matrix also contains mitochondrial deoxyribonucleic acid (mtDNA), ribonucleic acid (mtRNA), and ribosomes.]

B. **Organization**

The inner mitochondrial membrane contains four separate protein complexes, called Complexes I, II, III, and IV that each contain part of the ETC (Fig. 6.8). These complexes accept or donate electrons to the relatively mobile electron carrier coenzyme Q (CoQ) and cytochrome c. Each carrier in the ETC can receive electrons from an electron donor and can subsequently donate electrons to the next acceptor in the chain. The electrons ultimately combine with O_2 and H^+ to form H_2O. This requirement for O_2 makes the electron transport process the respiratory chain, which accounts for the greatest portion of the body's use of O_2.

C. **Reactions**

With the exception of CoQ, which is a lipid-soluble quinone, all members of the ETC are proteins. These may function as enzymes as is the case with the flavin-containing *dehydrogenases*, may contain iron as part of an iron-sulfur (Fe-S) center, may contain iron as part of the porphyrin prosthetic group of heme as in the cytochromes, or may contain copper (Cu) as does the cytochrome a + a_3 complex.

1. **NADH formation:** NAD^+ is reduced to NADH by *dehydrogenases* that remove two hydrogen atoms from their substrate. [Note: For examples of these reactions, see the discussion of the *dehydrogenases* of the TCA cycle, p. 112.] Both electrons but only one H^+ (that is, a hydride ion [$:H^-$]) are transferred to the NAD^+, forming NADH plus a free H^+.

2. **NADH dehydrogenase:** The free H^+ plus the hydride ion carried by NADH are transferred to *NADH dehydrogenase*, a protein complex (Complex I) embedded in the inner mitochondrial membrane. Complex I has a tightly bound molecule of flavin mononucleotide (FMN), a coenzyme structurally related to FAD (see Fig. 28.15, p. 384) that accepts the two hydrogen atoms (2 electrons + 2 H^+), becoming $FMNH_2$. *NADH dehydrogenase* also contains peptide subunits with Fe-S centers (Fig. 6.9). At Complex I, electrons move from NADH to FMN to the iron of the Fe-S centers and then to

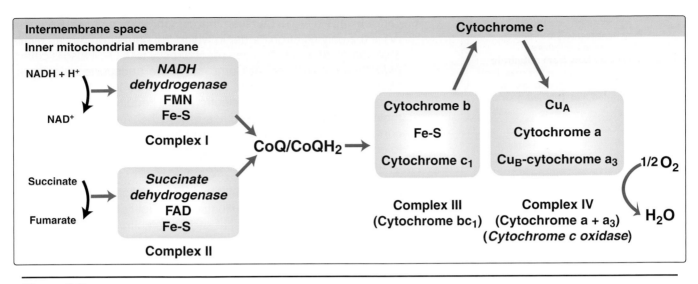

Figure 6.8
Electron transport chain. Electron flow is shown by magenta arrows. NAD(H) = nicotinamide adenine dinucleotide; FMN = flavin mononucleotide; FAD = flavin adenine dinucleotide; Fe-S = iron-sulfur; CoQ = coenzyme Q; Cu = copper.

CoQ. As electrons flow, they lose energy. This energy is used to pump four H^+ across the inner mitochondrial membrane, from the matrix to the intermembrane space.

3. **Succinate dehydrogenase:** At Complex II, electrons from the *succinate dehydrogenase*–catalyzed oxidation of succinate to fumarate move from the coenzyme, $FADH_2$, to an Fe-S protein, and then to CoQ. [Note: Because no energy is lost in this process, no H^+ are pumped at Complex II.]

4. **Coenzyme Q:** CoQ is a quinone derivative with a long, hydrophobic isoprenoid tail. It is made from an intermediate of cholesterol synthesis (see p. 221). [Note: It is also called ubiquinone because it is ubiquitous in biologic systems.] CoQ is a mobile electron carrier and can accept electrons from *NADH dehydrogenase* (Complex I), from *succinate dehydrogenase* (Complex II) and from other mitochondrial *dehydrogenases*, such as *glycerol 3-phosphate dehydrogenase* (see p. 80) and *acyl CoA dehydrogenases* (see p. 192). CoQ transfers electrons to Complex III (cytochrome bc_1). Thus, a function of CoQ is to link the flavoprotein *dehydrogenases* to the cytochromes.

5. **Cytochromes:** The remaining members of the ETC are cytochrome proteins. Each contains a heme group (a porphyrin ring plus iron). Unlike the heme groups of hemoglobin, the cytochrome iron is reversibly converted from its ferric (Fe^{3+}) to its ferrous (Fe^{2+}) form as a normal part of its function as an acceptor and donor of electrons. Electrons are passed along the chain from cytochrome bc_1 (Complex III), to cytochrome c, and then to cytochromes a + a_3 ([Complex IV] see Fig. 6.8). As electrons flow, four H^+ are pumped across the inner mitochondrial membrane at Complex III and two at Complex IV. [Note: Cytochrome c is located in the intermembrane space, loosely associated with the outer face of the inner membrane. As seen with CoQ, cytochrome c is a mobile electron carrier.]

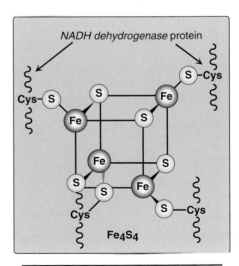

Figure 6.9
Iron-sulfur (Fe-S) center of Complex I. [Note: Complexes II and III also contain Fe-S centers.] NADH = nicotinamide adenine dinucleotide; Cys = cysteine.

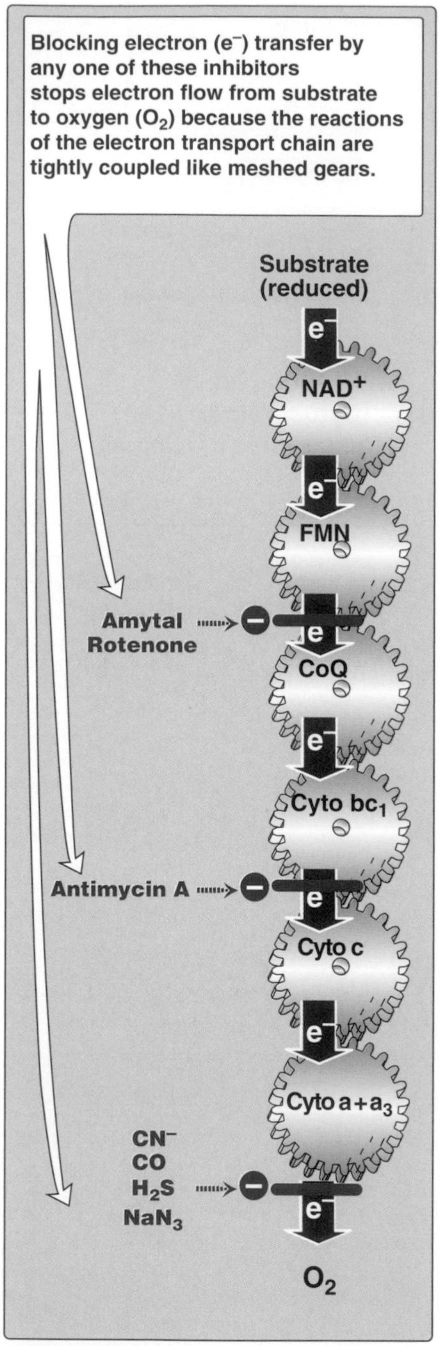

6. **Cytochrome a + a₃:** Because this cytochrome complex (Complex IV) is the only electron carrier in which the heme iron has an available coordination site that can react directly with O_2, it also is called *cytochrome c oxidase.* At Complex IV, the transported electrons, O_2, and free H^+ are brought together, and O_2 is reduced to H_2O (see Fig. 6.8). [Note: Four electrons are required to reduce one molecule of O_2 to two molecules of H_2O.] *Cytochrome c oxidase* contains Cu atoms that are required for this complicated reaction to occur. Electrons move from Cu_A to cytochrome a to cytochrome a_3 (in association with Cu_B) to O_2.

7. **Site-specific inhibitors:** Inhibitors of specific sites in the ETC have been identified and are illustrated in Figure 6.10. These respiratory inhibitors prevent the passage of electrons by binding to a component of the chain, blocking the oxidation-reduction reaction. Therefore, all electron carriers before the block are fully reduced, whereas those located after the block are oxidized. [Note: Inhibition of the ETC inhibits ATP synthesis because these processes are tightly coupled (see p. 78).]

> Leakage of electrons from the ETC produces reactive oxygen species (ROS), such as superoxide (O_2^{-}), hydrogen peroxide (H_2O_2), and hydroxyl radicals (OH·). ROS damage DNA and proteins and cause lipid peroxidation. Enzymes such as *superoxide dismutase* (*SOD*), *catalase*, and *glutathione peroxidase* are cellular defenses against ROS (see p. 148).

D. Free energy release during electron transport

The free energy released as electrons are transferred along the ETC from an electron donor (reducing agent or reductant) to an electron acceptor (oxidizing agent or oxidant) is used to pump H^+ at Complexes I, III, and IV. [Note: The electrons can be transferred as hydride ions to NAD^+; as hydrogen atoms to FMN, CoQ, and FAD; or as electrons to cytochromes.]

1. **Redox pairs:** Oxidation (loss of electrons) of one substance is always accompanied by reduction (gain of electrons) of a second. For example, Figure 6.11 shows the oxidation of NADH to NAD^+ by *NADH dehydrogenase* at Complex I, accompanied by the reduction of FMN, the prosthetic group, to $FMNH_2$. Such redox reactions can be written as the sum of two separate half reactions, one an oxidation and the other a reduction (see Fig. 6.11). NAD^+ and NADH form a redox pair, as do FMN and $FMNH_2$. Redox pairs differ in their tendency to lose electrons. This tendency is a characteristic of a particular redox pair and can be quantitatively specified by a constant, E_0 (the standard reduction potential), with units in volts.

2. **Standard reduction potential:** The E_0 of various redox pairs can be ordered from the most negative E_0 to the most positive. The more negative the E_0 of a redox pair, the greater the tendency of the reductant member of that pair to lose electrons. The more positive the E_0, the greater the tendency of the oxidant member of that

Figure 6.10
Site-specific inhibitors of electron transport shown using a mechanical model for the coupling of oxidation-reduction reactions. [Note: Normal direction of electron flow is illustrated.] NAD^+ = nicotinamide adenine dinucleotide; FMN = flavin mononucleotide; CoQ = coenzyme Q; Cyto = cytochrome; CN^- = cyanide; CO = carbon monoxide; H_2S = hydrogen sulfide; NaN_3 = sodium azide.

pair to accept electrons. Therefore, electrons flow from the pair with the more negative E_0 to that with the more positive E_0. The E_0 values for some members of the ETC are shown in Figure 6.12. [Note: The components of the chain are arranged in order of increasingly positive E_0 values.]

3. **Relationship of ΔG^0 to ΔE_0:** The ΔG^0 is related directly to the magnitude of the change in E_0:

$$\Delta G^0 = -n\,F\,\Delta E_0,$$

where   n = number of electrons transferred (1 for
a cytochrome, 2 for NADH, $FADH_2$, and CoQ)
F = Faraday constant (23.1 kcal/volt mol)
ΔE_0 = E_0 of the electron-accepting pair minus the E_0 of the electron-donating pair
ΔG^0 = change in the standard free energy

4. **ΔG^0 of ATP:** The ΔG^0 for the phosphorylation of ADP to ATP is +7.3 kcal/mol. The transport of a pair of electrons from NADH to O_2 through the ETC releases 52.6 kcal. Therefore, more than sufficient energy is available to produce three ATP from three ADP and three P_i ($3 \times 7.3 = 21.9$ kcal/mol), sometimes expressed as a P/O ratio (ATP made per O atom reduced) of 3:1. The remaining calories are used for ancillary reactions or released as heat. [Note: The P:O for $FADH_2$ is 2:1 because Complex I is bypassed.]

VI. PHOSPHORYLATION OF ADP TO ATP

The transfer of electrons down the ETC is energetically favored because NADH is a strong electron donor and O_2 is an avid electron acceptor. However, the flow of electrons does not directly result in ATP synthesis.

A. Chemiosmotic hypothesis

The chemiosmotic hypothesis (also known as the Mitchell hypothesis) explains how the free energy generated by the transport of electrons by the ETC is used to produce ATP from ADP + P_i.

1. **Proton pump:** Electron transport is coupled to ADP phosphorylation by the pumping of H^+ across the inner mitochondrial membrane, from the matrix to the intermembrane space, at Complexes I, III, and IV. For each pair of electrons transferred from NADH to O_2, 10 H^+ are pumped. This creates an electrical gradient (with more positive charges on the cytosolic side of the membrane than on the matrix side) and a pH (chemical) gradient (the cytosolic side of the membrane is at a lower pH than the matrix side), as shown in Figure 6.13. The energy (proton-motive force) generated by these gradients is sufficient to drive ATP synthesis. Thus, the H^+ gradient serves as the common intermediate that couples oxidation to phosphorylation.

2. **ATP synthase:** The multisubunit enzyme *ATP synthase* ([Complex V] Fig. 6.14) synthesizes ATP using the energy of the H^+ gradient. It contains a membrane domain (F_0) that spans the inner mitochondrial membrane and an extramembranous domain (F_1) that

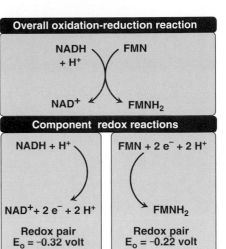

Figure 6.11
Oxidation of NADH by FMN, separated into two component half reactions. NAD(H) = nicotinamide adenine dinucleotide; FMN(H₂) = flavin mononucleotide; e⁻ = electron; H^+ = proton; E_0 = standard reduction potential.

Compounds with a large negative E_0 (located at top of the table) are strong reducing agents, or reductants (that is, they have a strong tendency to lose electrons).	

Redox pair	E_0
NAD^+/NADH	−0.32
FMN/$FMNH_2$	−0.22
Cytochrome c Fe^{3+}/Fe^{2+}	+0.22
1/2 O_2/H_2O	+0.82

Compounds at the bottom of the table are strong oxidizing agents, or oxidants (that is, they accept electrons).

Figure 6.12
Standard reduction potentials (E_0) of some reactions. NAD(H) = nicotinamide adenine dinucleotide; FMN(H₂) = flavin mononucleotide; Fe = iron.

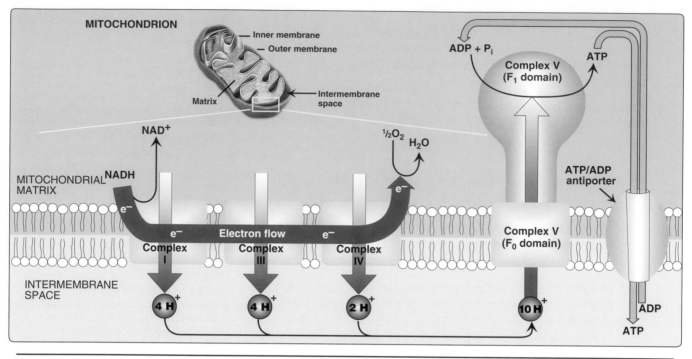

Figure 6.13

Electron transport chain shown in association with proton (H^+) pumping. Ten H^+ are pumped for each nicotinamide adenine dinucleotide (NADH) oxidized. [Note: H^+ are not pumped at Complex II.] e^- = electron; Complex V = *ATP synthase*.

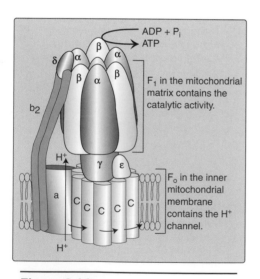

Figure 6.14

ATP synthase (F_1F_o-ATPase). [Note: The c ring of vertebrates contains eight subunits. One complete turn of the ring is driven by eight H^+ (protons) moving through the F_o domain. The resulting conformational changes in the three β subunits of the F_1 domain allow phosphorylation of three adenosine diphosphates (ADP) to three ATP.] P_i = inorganic phosphate.

appears as a sphere that protrudes into the mitochondrial matrix (see Fig. 6.13). The chemiosmotic hypothesis proposes that after H^+ have been pumped to the cytosolic side of the inner mitochondrial membrane, they reenter the matrix by passing through a H^+ channel in the F_o domain, driving rotation of the c ring of F_o and, at the same time, dissipating the pH and electrical gradients. Rotation in F_o causes conformational changes in the three β subunits of F_1 that allow them to bind ADP + P_i, phosphorylate ADP to ATP, and release ATP. One complete rotation of the c ring produces three ATP. [Note: *ATP synthase* is also called *F_1/F_o-ATPase* because the enzyme can also catalyze the hydrolysis of ATP to ADP and P_i.]

a. **Coupling in oxidative phosphorylation:** In normal mitochondria, ATP synthesis is coupled to electron transport through the H^+ gradient. Increasing (or decreasing) one process has the same effect on the other. For example, hydrolysis of ATP to ADP and P_i in energy-requiring reactions increases the availability of substrates for *ATP synthase* and, thus, increases H^+ flow through the enzyme. Electron transport and H^+ pumping by the ETC increase to maintain the H^+ gradient and allow ATP synthesis.

b. **Oligomycin:** This drug binds to the F_o (hence the letter "o") domain of *ATP synthase*, closing the H^+ channel and preventing reentry of H^+ into the matrix, thereby inhibiting phosphorylation of ADP to ATP. Because the pH and electrical gradients cannot be dissipated in the presence of this phosphorylation inhibitor, electron transport stops because of the difficulty of pumping any more H^+ against the steep gradient. This dependency of cellular respiration on the ability to phosphorylate ADP to ATP is known as respiratory control and is the consequence of the tight coupling of these processes.

c. **Uncoupling proteins:** Uncoupling proteins (UCP) occur in the inner mitochondrial membrane of mammals, including humans. These proteins form channels that allow H^+ to reenter the mitochondrial matrix without energy being captured as ATP (Fig. 6.15). The energy is released as heat, and the process is called nonshivering thermogenesis. UCP1, also called thermogenin, is responsible for heat production in the mitochondria-rich brown adipocytes of mammals. [Note: Cold causes catecholamine-dependent activation of UCP1 expression.] In brown fat, unlike the more abundant white fat, ~90% of its respiratory energy is used for thermogenesis in infants in response to cold. Thus, brown fat is involved in energy expenditure, whereas white fat is involved in energy storage. [Note: Brown fat depots have recently been shown to be present in adults.]

d. **Synthetic uncouplers:** Electron transport and phosphorylation of ADP can also be uncoupled by compounds that shuttle H^+ across the inner mitochondrial membrane, dissipating the gradient. The classic example is 2,4-dinitrophenol, a lipophilic H^+ carrier (ionophore) that readily diffuses through the mitochondrial membrane (Fig. 6.16). This uncoupler causes electron transport to proceed at a rapid rate without establishing a H^+ gradient, much as do the UCP. Again, energy is released as heat rather than being used to synthesize ATP. [Note: In high doses, aspirin and other salicylates uncouple oxidative phosphorylation. This explains the fever that accompanies toxic overdoses of these drugs.]

B. Membrane transport systems

The inner mitochondrial membrane is impermeable to most charged or hydrophilic substances. However, it contains numerous transport proteins that permit passage of certain molecules from the cytosol to the mitochondrial matrix.

1. **ATP and ADP transport:** The inner membrane requires specialized carriers to transport ADP and P_i from the cytosol (where ATP is hydrolyzed to ADP in many energy-requiring reactions) into mitochondria, where ATP can be resynthesized. An adenine nucleotide antiporter imports one ADP from the cytosol into the matrix, while exporting one ATP from the matrix into the cytosol (see Fig. 6.13). A symporter cotransports P_i and H^+ from the cytosol into the matrix.

2. **Reducing equivalent transport:** The inner mitochondrial membrane lacks an NADH transporter, and NADH produced in the cytosol (for example, in glycolysis; see p. 101) cannot directly enter the mitochondrial matrix. However, reducing equivalents of NADH are transported from the cytosol into the matrix using substrate shuttles. In the glycerol 3-phosphate shuttle

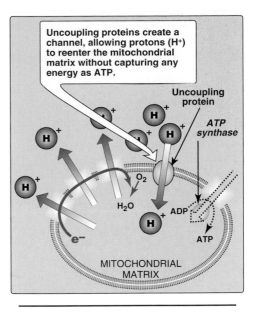

Figure 6.15
Transport of protons across the mitochondrial membrane by an uncoupling protein. ADP = adenosine diphosphate; e^- = electrons.

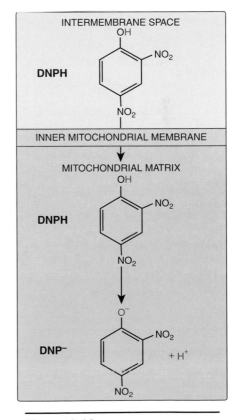

Figure 6.16
2,4-Dinitrophenol (DNP), a proton (H^+) carrier, shown in its reduced (DNPH) and oxidized (DNP$^-$) forms.

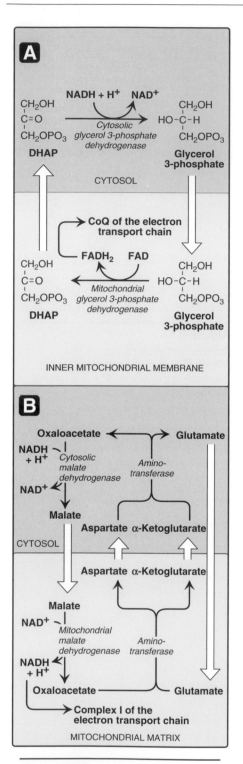

Figure 6.17
Substrate shuttles for the transport of reducing equivalents across the inner mitochondrial membrane.
A. Glycerol 3-phosphate shuttle.
B. Malate-aspartate shuttle. DHAP = dihydroxyacetone phosphate; NAD(H) = nicotinamide adenine dinucleotide; H$^+$ = proton; FAD(H$_2$) = flavin adenine dinucleotide; CoQ = coenzyme Q.

(Fig. 6.17A), two electrons are transferred from NADH to dihydroxyacetone phosphate by cytosolic *glycerol 3-phosphate dehydrogenase*. The glycerol 3-phosphate produced is oxidized by the mitochondrial isozyme as FAD is reduced to FADH$_2$. CoQ of the ETC oxidizes the FADH$_2$. Therefore, the glycerol 3-phosphate shuttle results in the synthesis of two ATP for each cytosolic NADH oxidized. This contrasts with the malate-aspartate shuttle (Fig. 6.17B), which produces NADH (rather than FADH$_2$) in the mitochondrial matrix, thereby yielding three ATP for each cytosolic NADH oxidized by *malate dehydrogenase* as oxaloacetate is reduced to malate. A transport protein moves malate into the mitochondrial matrix.

C. Inherited defects in oxidative phosphorylation

Thirteen of the ~90 polypeptides required for oxidative phosphorylation are encoded by mtDNA and synthesized in mitochondria, whereas the remaining proteins are encoded by nuclear DNA, synthesized in the cytosol, and then transported into mitochondria. Defects in oxidative phosphorylation are more likely a result of alterations in mtDNA, which has a mutation rate about 10 times greater than that of nuclear DNA. Tissues with the greatest ATP requirement (for example, the central nervous system, skeletal and heart muscle, and the liver) are most affected by defects in oxidative phosphorylation. Mutations in mtDNA are responsible for several diseases, including some cases of mitochondrial myopathies, and Leber hereditary optic neuropathy, a disease in which bilateral loss of central vision occurs as a result of neuroretinal degeneration, including damage to the optic nerve. [Note: mtDNA is maternally inherited because mitochondria from the sperm cell do not enter the fertilized egg.]

D. Mitochondria and apoptosis

The process of apoptosis (programmed cell death) may be initiated through the intrinsic (mitochondrial-mediated) pathway by the formation of pores in the outer mitochondrial membrane. These pores allow cytochrome c to leave the intermembrane space and enter the cytosol. There, cytochrome c, in association with proapoptotic factors, activates a family of proteolytic enzymes (the *caspases*), causing cleavage of key proteins and resulting in the morphologic and biochemical changes characteristic of apoptosis.

VII. CHAPTER SUMMARY

The **change** in **free energy** (**ΔG**) occurring during a reaction predicts the **direction** in which that reaction will spontaneously proceed. If ΔG is **negative** (that is, the product has a lower free energy than the substrate), then the reaction is **spontaneous** as written. If ΔG is **positive**, then the reaction is **not spontaneous**. If ΔG = **0**, then the reaction is in **equilibrium**. The ΔG of the forward reaction is equal in magnitude but opposite in sign to that of the back reaction. The ΔG are **additive** in any sequence of consecutive reactions, as are the standard free energy changes (**ΔG^0**). Therefore, reactions or processes that have a large, positive ΔG are made possible by **coupling** with those that have a large, negative ΔG such as **ATP hydrolysis**. The reduced coenzymes **nicotinamide adenine**

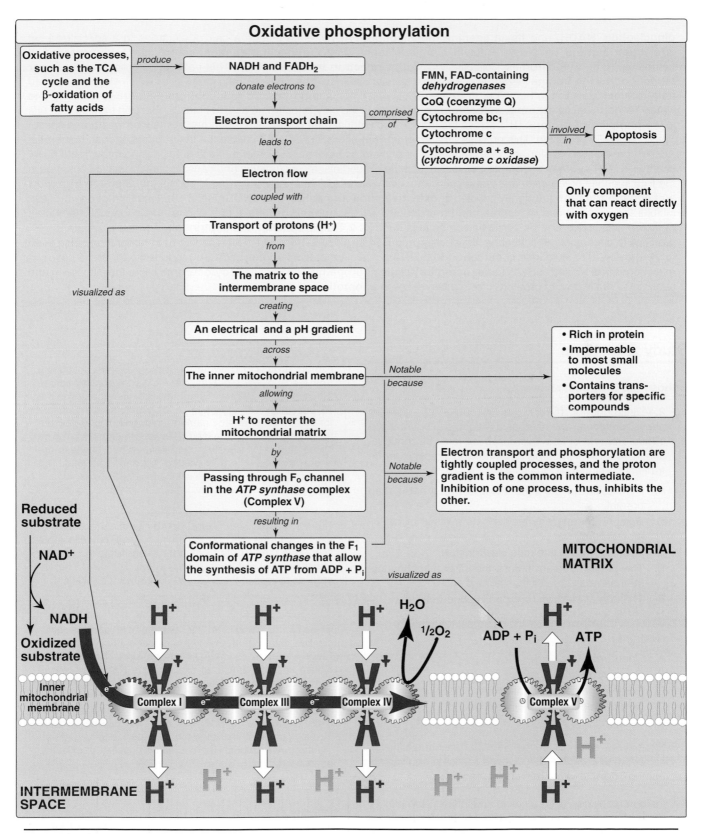

Figure 6.18
Key concept map for oxidative phosphorylation (OXPHOS). [Note: Electron (e⁻) flow and ATP synthesis are shown as sets of interlocking gears to emphasize coupling.] TCA = tricarboxylic acid; NAD(H) = nicotinamide adenine dinucleotide; FAD(H₂) = flavin adenine dinucleotide; FMN = flavin mononucleotide; ADP = adenosine diphosphate.

dinucleotide (**NADH**) and **flavin adenine dinucleotide** (**FADH₂**) each donate a pair of electrons to a specialized set of **electron carriers**, consisting of **flavin mononucleotide** (**FMN**), **iron-sulfur centers**, **coenzyme Q**, and a series of heme-containing **cytochromes**, collectively called the **electron transport chain**. This pathway is present in the **inner mitochondrial membrane** (impermeable to most substances) and is the final common pathway by which electrons derived from different fuels of the body flow to oxygen (O_2), which has a large, positive **reduction potential** (E_0), reducing it to water. The terminal cytochrome, *cytochrome c oxidase*, is the only cytochrome able to bind O_2. Electron transport results in the **pumping of protons** (H^+) across the inner mitochondrial membrane from the matrix to the intermembrane space, 10 H^+ per NADH oxidized. This process creates **electrical** and **pH gradients** across the inner mitochondrial membrane. After H^+ have been transferred to the cytosolic side of the membrane, they reenter the matrix by passing through the F_o H^+ channel in *ATP synthase* (**Complex V**), dissipating the pH and electrical gradients and causing conformational changes in the F_1 β subunits of the *synthase* that result in the synthesis of ATP from ADP + inorganic phosphate. **Electron transport** and **phosphorylation** are tightly coupled in **oxidative phosphorylation** ([**OXPHOS**] Fig. 6.18). Inhibition of one process inhibits the other. These processes can be uncoupled by **uncoupling protein-1** of the inner mitochondrial membrane of brown adipocytes and by synthetic compounds such as **2,4-dinitrophenol** and **aspirin**, all of which dissipate the H^+ gradient. In uncoupled mitochondria, the energy produced by electron transport is released as **heat** rather than being used to synthesize ATP. Mutations in **mitochondrial DNA**, which is **maternally inherited**, are responsible for some cases of mitochondrial diseases such as **Leber hereditary optic neuropathy**. The release of **cytochrome c** into the cytoplasm and subsequent activation of proteolytic *caspases* results in **apoptotic cell death**.

Study Questions

Choose the ONE best answer.

6.1 2,4-Dinitrophenol (DNP), an uncoupler of oxidative phosphorylation, was used as a weight-loss agent in the 1930s. Reports of fatal overdoses led to its discontinuation in 1939. Which of the following would most likely be true concerning individuals taking 2,4-DNP?

A. ATP levels in the mitochondria are greater than normal.

B. Body temperature is elevated as a result of hypermetabolism.

C. Cyanide has no effect on electron flow.

D. The proton gradient across the inner mitochondrial membrane is greater than normal.

E. The rate of electron transport is abnormally low.

6.2 Which of the following has the strongest tendency to gain electrons?

A. Coenzyme Q

B. Cytochrome c

C. Flavin adenine dinucleotide

D. Nicotinamide adenine dinucleotide

E. Oxygen

6.3 Explain why and how the malate-aspartate shuttle moves nicotinamide adenine dinucleotide reducing equivalents from the cytosol to the mitochondrial matrix.

6.4 Carbon monoxide (CO) binds to and inhibits Complex IV of the electron transport chain. What effect, if any, should this respiratory inhibitor have on phosphorylation of adenosine diphosphate (ADP) to ATP?

Correct answer = B. When phosphorylation is uncoupled from electron flow, a decrease in the proton gradient across the inner mitochondrial membrane and, therefore, impaired ATP synthesis are expected. In an attempt to compensate for this defect in energy capture, metabolism and electron flow to oxygen are increased. This hypermetabolism will be accompanied by elevated body temperature because the energy in fuels is largely wasted, appearing as heat. The electron transport chain will still be inhibited by cyanide.

Correct answer = E. Oxygen is the terminal acceptor of electrons in the electron transport chain (ETC). Electrons flow down the ETC to oxygen because it has the highest (most positive) reduction potential (E_0). The other choices precede oxygen in the ETC and have lower E_0 values.

There is no transporter for nicotinamide adenine dinucleotide (NADH) in the inner mitochondrial membrane. However, cytoplasmic NADH can be oxidized to NAD^+ by malate dehydrogenase as oxaloacetate (OAA) is reduced to malate. The malate is transported across the inner membrane to the matrix where the mitochondrial isozyme of malate dehydrogenase oxidizes it to OAA as mitochondrial NAD^+ is reduced to NADH. This NADH can be oxidized by Complex I of the electron transport chain, generating three ATP through the coupled processes of oxidative phosphorylation.

Inhibition of electron transport by respiratory inhibitors such as CO results in an inability to maintain the proton (H^+) gradient. Therefore, phosphorylation of ADP to ATP is inhibited, as are ancillary reactions such as calcium uptake by mitochondria, because they also require the H^+ gradient.

Introduction to Carbohydrates

7

I. OVERVIEW

Carbohydrates (saccharides) are the most abundant organic molecules in nature. They have a wide range of functions, including providing a significant fraction of the dietary calories for most organisms, acting as a storage form of energy in the body, and serving as cell membrane components that mediate some forms of intercellular communication. Carbohydrates also serve as a structural component of many organisms, including the cell walls of bacteria, the exoskeleton of insects, and the fibrous cellulose of plants. [Note: The full set of carbohydrates produced by an organism is its glycome.] The empiric formula for many of the simpler carbohydrates is $(CH_2O)_n$, where $n \geq 3$, hence the name "hydrate of carbon."

II. CLASSIFICATION AND STRUCTURE

Monosaccharides (simple sugars) can be classified according to the number of carbon atoms they contain. Examples of some monosaccharides commonly found in humans are listed in Figure 7.1. They can also be classified by the type of carbonyl group they contain. Carbohydrates with an aldehyde as their carbonyl group are called aldoses, whereas those with a keto as their carbonyl group are called ketoses (Fig. 7.2). For example, glyceraldehyde is an aldose, whereas dihydroxyacetone is a ketose. Carbohydrates that have a free carbonyl group have the suffix -ose. [Note: Ketoses have an additional "ul" in their suffix such as xylulose. There are exceptions, such as fructose, to this rule.] Monosaccharides can be linked by glycosidic bonds to create larger structures (Fig. 7.3). Disaccharides contain two monosaccharide units, oligosaccharides contain three to ten monosaccharide units, and polysaccharides contain more than ten monosaccharide units and can be hundreds of sugar units in length.

A. Isomers and epimers

Compounds that have the same chemical formula but have different structures are called isomers. For example, fructose, glucose, mannose, and galactose are all isomers of each other, having the same chemical formula, $C_6H_{12}O_6$. Carbohydrate isomers that differ in configuration around only one specific carbon atom (with the exception of the carbonyl carbon, see C. 1. below) are defined as epimers of each

GENERIC NAMES		EXAMPLES
3 Carbons:	trioses	Glyceraldehyde
4 Carbons:	tetroses	Erythrose
5 Carbons:	pentoses	Ribose
6 Carbons:	hexoses	Glucose
7 Carbons:	heptoses	Sedoheptulose
9 Carbons:	nonoses	Neuraminic acid

Figure 7.1
Examples of monosaccharides found in humans, classified according to the number of carbons they contain.

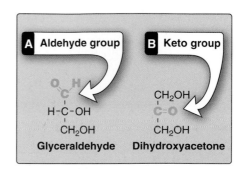

Figure 7.2
Examples of an aldose (A) and a ketose (B) sugar.

83

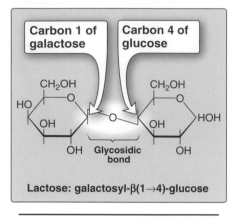

Figure 7.3
A glycosidic bond between two hexoses producing a disaccharide.

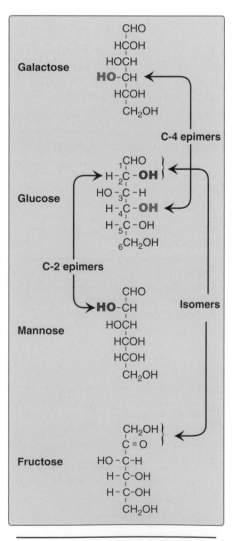

Figure 7.4
Carbon-2 (C-2) and C-4 epimers and an isomer of glucose.

other. For example, glucose and galactose are C-4 epimers because their structures differ only in the position of the −OH (hydroxyl) group at carbon 4. [Note: The carbons in sugars are numbered beginning at the end that contains the carbonyl carbon (that is, the aldehyde or keto group), as shown in Fig. 7.4.] Glucose and mannose are C-2 epimers. However, because galactose and mannose differ in the position of −OH groups at two carbons (carbons 2 and 4), they are isomers rather than epimers (see Fig. 7.4).

B. Enantiomers

A special type of isomerism is found in the pairs of structures that are mirror images of each other. These mirror images are called enantiomers, and the two members of the pair are designated as a D- and an L-sugar (Fig. 7.5). The vast majority of the sugars in humans are D-isomers. In the D-isomeric form, the −OH group on the asymmetric carbon (a carbon linked to four different atoms or groups) farthest from the carbonyl carbon is on the right, whereas in the L-isomer, it is on the left. Most enzymes are specific for either the D or the L form, but enzymes known as *isomerases* are able to interconvert D- and L-isomers.

C. Monosaccharide cyclization

Less than 1% of each of the monosaccharides with five or more carbons exists in the open-chain (acyclic) form in solution. Rather, they are predominantly found in a ring (cyclic) form, in which the aldehyde (or keto) group has reacted with a hydroxyl group on the same sugar, making the carbonyl carbon (carbon 1 for an aldose, carbon 2 for a ketose) asymmetric. This asymmetric carbon is referred to as the anomeric carbon.

1. **Anomers:** Creation of an anomeric carbon (the former carbonyl carbon) generates a new pair of isomers, the α and β configurations of the sugar (for example, α-D-glucopyranose and β-D-glucopyranose), as shown in Figure 7.6, that are anomers of each other. [Note: In the α configuration, the −OH group on the anomeric carbon projects to the same side as the ring in a modified Fischer projection formula (see Fig. 7.6A) and is trans to the CH_2OH group in a Haworth projection formula (see Fig. 7.6B). The α and β forms are not mirror images, and they are referred to as diastereomers.] Enzymes are able to distinguish between these two structures and use one or the other preferentially. For example, glycogen is synthesized from α-D-glucopyranose, whereas cellulose is synthesized from β-D-glucopyranose. The cyclic α and β anomers of a sugar in solution spontaneously (but slowly) form an equilibrium mixture, a process known as mutarotation (see Fig. 7.6). [Note: For glucose, the α form makes up 36% of the mixture.]

2. **Reducing sugars:** If the hydroxyl group on the anomeric carbon of a cyclized sugar is not linked to another compound by a glycosidic bond (see E. below), the ring can open. The sugar can act as a reducing agent and is termed a reducing sugar. Such sugars can react with chromogenic agents (for example, the Benedict reagent) causing the reagent to be reduced and colored as the aldehyde

group of the acyclic sugar is oxidized to a carboxyl group. All monosaccharides, but not all disaccharides, are reducing sugars. [Note: Fructose, a ketose, is a reducing sugar because it can be isomerized to an aldose.]

A colorimetric test can detect a reducing sugar in urine. A positive result is indicative of an underlying pathology (because sugars are not normally present in urine) and can be followed up by more specific tests to identify the reducing sugar.

D. Monosaccharide joining

Monosaccharides can be joined to form disaccharides, oligosaccharides, and polysaccharides. Important disaccharides include lactose (galactose + glucose), sucrose (glucose + fructose), and maltose (glucose + glucose). Important polysaccharides include branched glycogen (from animal sources) and starch (plant sources) and unbranched cellulose (plant sources). Each is a polymer of glucose.

E. Glycosidic bonds

The bonds that link sugars are called glycosidic bonds. They are formed by enzymes known as *glycosyltransferases* that use nucleotide sugars (activated sugars) such as uridine diphosphate glucose as substrates. Glycosidic bonds between sugars are named according to the numbers of the connected carbons and with regard to the position of the anomeric hydroxyl group of the first sugar involved in the bond. If this anomeric hydroxyl is in the α configuration, then the linkage is an α-bond. If it is in the β configuration, then the linkage is a β-bond. Lactose, for example, is synthesized by forming a glycosidic bond between carbon 1 of β-galactose and carbon 4 of glucose. Therefore, the linkage is a β(1→4) glycosidic bond (see Fig. 7.3). [Note: Because the anomeric end of the glucose residue is not involved in the glycosidic linkage, it (and, therefore, lactose) remains a reducing sugar.]

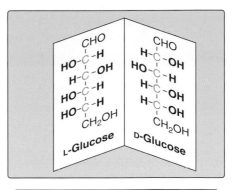

Figure 7.5
Enantiomers (mirror images) of glucose. Designation of D and L is by comparison to a triose, glyceraldehyde. [Note: The asymmetric carbons are shown in green.]

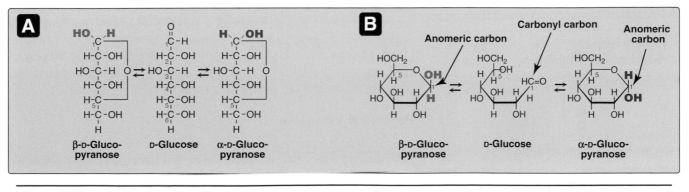

Figure 7.6
A. The interconversion (mutarotation) of the α and β anomeric forms of glucose shown as modified Fischer projection formulas. B. The interconversion shown as Haworth projection formulas. [Note: A sugar with a six-membered ring (5 C + 1 O) is termed a pyranose, whereas one with a five-membered ring (4 C + 1 O) is a furanose. Virtually all glucose in solution is in the pyranose form.]

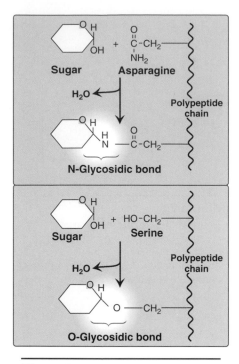

Figure 7.7
Examples of N- and O-glycosidic bonds in glycoproteins.

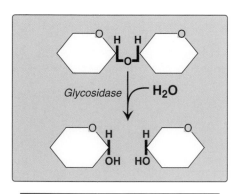

Figure 7.8
Hydrolysis of a glycosidic bond.

F. Carbohydrate linkage to noncarbohydrates

Carbohydrates can be attached by glycosidic bonds to noncarbohydrate structures, including purine and pyrimidine bases (found in nucleic acids), aromatic rings (such as those found in steroids and bilirubin), proteins (found in glycoproteins and proteoglycans), and lipids (found in glycolipids). If the group on the noncarbohydrate molecule to which the sugar is attached is an –NH$_2$ group, then the bond is called an N-glycosidic link. If the group is an –OH, then the bond is an O-glycosidic link (Fig. 7.7). [Note: All sugar-sugar glycosidic bonds are O-type linkages.]

III. DIETARY CARBOHYDRATE DIGESTION

The principal sites of dietary carbohydrate digestion are the mouth and intestinal lumen. This digestion is rapid and is catalyzed by enzymes known as *glycoside hydrolases* (*glycosidases*) that hydrolyze glycosidic bonds (Fig. 7.8). Because little monosaccharide is present in diets of mixed animal and plant origin, the enzymes are primarily *endoglycosidases* that hydrolyze polysaccharides and oligosaccharides and *disaccharidases* that hydrolyze tri- and disaccharides into their reducing sugar components. *Glycosidases* are usually specific for the structure and configuration of the glycosyl residue to be removed as well as for the type of bond to be broken. The final products of carbohydrate digestion are the monosaccharides glucose, galactose, and fructose that are absorbed by cells (enterocytes) of the small intestine.

A. Salivary α-amylase

The major dietary polysaccharides are of plant (starch, composed of amylose and amylopectin) and animal (glycogen) origin. During mastication (chewing), *salivary α-amylase* acts briefly on dietary starch and glycogen, hydrolyzing random α(1→4) bonds. [Note: There are both *α(1→4)-* and *β(1→4)-endoglucosidases* in nature, but humans do not produce the latter. Therefore, we are unable to digest cellulose, a carbohydrate of plant origin containing β(1→4) glycosidic bonds between glucose residues.] Because branched amylopectin and glycogen also contain α(1→6) bonds, which *α-amylase* cannot hydrolyze, the digest resulting from its action contains a mixture of short, branched and unbranched oligosaccharides known as dextrins (Fig. 7.9). [Note: Disaccharides are also present as they, too, are resistant to *amylase*.] Carbohydrate digestion halts temporarily in the stomach, because the high acidity inactivates *salivary α-amylase*.

B. Pancreatic α-amylase

When the acidic stomach contents reach the small intestine, they are neutralized by bicarbonate secreted by the pancreas, and *pancreatic α-amylase* continues the process of starch digestion.

C. Intestinal disaccharidases

The final digestive processes occur primarily at the mucosal lining of the duodenum and upper jejunum and include the action of several *disaccharidases* (see Fig. 7.9). For example, *isomaltase* cleaves the α(1→6) bond in isomaltose, and *maltase* cleaves the α(1→4) bond in maltose and maltotriose, each producing glucose. *Sucrase* cleaves the α(1→2) bond in sucrose, producing glucose and fructose, and *lactase* (*β-galactosidase*) cleaves the β(1→4) bond in lactose, producing galactose and glucose. [Note: The substrates for *isomaltase* are broader than its name suggests, and it hydrolyzes the majority of maltose.] Trehalose, an α(1→1) disaccharide of glucose found in mushrooms and other fungi, is cleaved by *trehalase*. These enzymes are transmembrane proteins of the brush border on the luminal (apical) surface of the enterocytes.

> *Sucrase* and *isomaltase* are enzymic activities of a single protein that is cleaved into two functional subunits, which remain associated in the cell membrane and form the *sucrase-isomaltase* (*SI*) complex. In contrast, *maltase* is one of two enzymic activities of the single membrane protein *maltase-glucoamylase* (*MGA*) that does not get cleaved. Its second enzymic activity, *glucoamylase*, cleaves α(1→4) glycosidic bonds in dextrins.

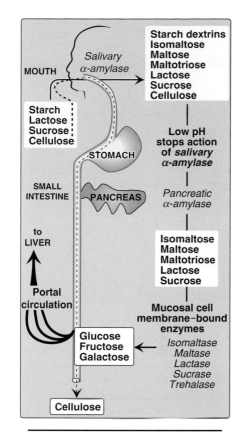

Figure 7.9
Digestion of carbohydrates. [Note: Indigestible cellulose enters the colon and is excreted.]

D. Intestinal absorption of monosaccharides

The upper jejunum absorbs the bulk of the monosaccharide products of digestion. However, different sugars have different mechanisms of absorption (Fig. 7.10). For example, galactose and glucose are taken into enterocytes by secondary active transport that requires a concurrent uptake (symport) of sodium (Na$^+$) ions. The transport protein is the sodium-dependent glucose cotransporter 1 (SGLT-1). [Note: Sugar transport is driven by the Na$^+$ gradient created by the *Na$^+$-potassium* (*K$^+$*) *ATPase* that moves Na$^+$ out of the enterocyte and K$^+$ in (see Fig. 7.10).] Fructose absorption utilizes an energy- and Na$^+$-independent monosaccharide transporter (GLUT-5). All three monosaccharides are transported from the enterocytes into the portal circulation by yet another transporter, GLUT-2. [Note: See p. 97 for a discussion of these transporters.]

E. Abnormal degradation of disaccharides

The overall process of carbohydrate digestion and absorption is so efficient in healthy individuals that ordinarily all digestible dietary carbohydrate is absorbed by the time the ingested material reaches the lower jejunum. However, because only monosaccharides are absorbed, any deficiency (genetic or acquired) in a specific *disaccharidase* activity of the intestinal mucosa causes the passage of undigested carbohydrate into the large intestine. As a consequence of the presence of this osmotically active material, water is drawn from the mucosa into the large intestine, causing osmotic diarrhea. This is reinforced by the bacterial fermentation of the remaining carbohydrate to two- and three-carbon compounds (which are also osmotically active) plus large volumes of carbon dioxide and hydrogen gas (H$_2$), causing abdominal cramps, diarrhea, and flatulence.

1. **Digestive enzyme deficiencies:** Genetic deficiencies of the individual *disaccharidases* result in disaccharide intolerance.

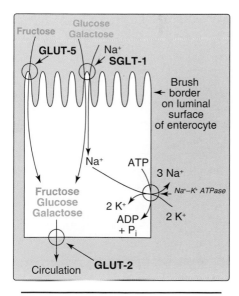

Figure 7.10
Absorption by enterocytes of the monosaccharide products of carbohydrate digestion. GLUT = glucose transporter; SGLT-1 = sodium (Na$^+$)-dependent glucose cotransporter. K$^+$ = potassium.

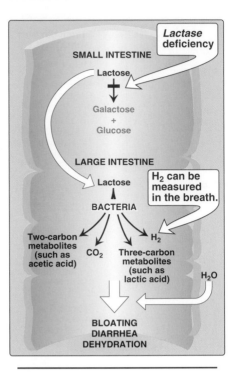

Figure 7.11
Abnormal lactose metabolism.
CO_2 = carbon dioxide; H_2 = hydrogen
gas.

Alterations in disaccharide degradation can also be caused by a variety of intestinal diseases, malnutrition, and drugs that injure the mucosa of the small intestine. For example, brush border enzymes are rapidly lost in normal individuals with severe diarrhea, causing a temporary, acquired enzyme deficiency. Therefore, patients suffering or recovering from such a disorder cannot drink or eat significant amounts of dairy products or sucrose without exacerbating the diarrhea.

2. **Lactose intolerance:** Over 60% of the world's adults are lactose intolerant (Fig. 7.11). This is particularly manifested in certain populations. For example, up to 90% of adults of African or Asian descent are *lactase* deficient. Consequently, they are less able to metabolize lactose than are individuals of Northern European origin. The age-dependent loss of *lactase* activity starting at approximately age 2 years represents a reduction in the amount of enzyme produced. It is thought to be caused by small variations in the DNA sequence of a region on chromosome 2 that controls expression of the gene for *lactase*, also on chromosome 2. Treatment for this disorder is to reduce consumption of milk; eat yogurts and some cheeses (bacterial action and aging process decrease lactose content) as well as green vegetables, such as broccoli, to ensure adequate calcium intake; use *lactase*-treated products; or take *lactase* in pill form prior to eating. [Note: Because the loss of *lactase* is the norm for most of the world's adults, use of the terms adult-type hypolactasia or *lactase* nonpersistence rather than lactose intolerance is becoming more common.] Rare cases of congenital *lactase* deficiency are known.

3. **Congenital sucrase-isomaltase deficiency:** This autosomal-recessive disorder results in an intolerance of ingested sucrose. Congenital *SI* deficiency has a prevalence of 1:5,000 in individuals of European descent and appears to be much more common (up to 1:20) in the Inuit people of Greenland and Canada. Treatment includes the dietary restriction of sucrose and enzyme replacement therapy.

4. **Diagnosis:** Identification of a specific enzyme deficiency can be obtained by performing oral tolerance tests with the individual disaccharides. Measurement of H_2 in the breath is a reliable test for determining the amount of ingested carbohydrate not absorbed by the body, but which is metabolized instead by the intestinal flora (see Fig. 7.11).

IV. CHAPTER SUMMARY

Monosaccharides (Fig. 7.12) containing an aldehyde group are called **aldoses**, and those with a keto group are called **ketoses**. **Disaccharides**, **oligosaccharides**, and **polysaccharides** consist of monosaccharides linked by **glycosidic bonds**. Compounds with the same chemical formula but different structures are called **isomers**. Two monosaccharide isomers differing in configuration around one specific carbon atom (not the carbonyl carbon) are defined as **epimers**. In **enantiomers** (mirror images), the members of the sugar pair are designated as ᴅ- and ʟ-**isomers**. When the aldehyde group on an acyclic sugar gets oxidized as a chromogenic agent gets reduced, that sugar is a **reducing sugar**. When a sugar cyclizes, an **anomeric carbon** is created from the carbonyl carbon of the aldehyde or keto group. The sugar can have two configurations, forming α or β **anomers**. A sugar can have its anomeric carbon linked to an –NH₂ or an –OH group on another structure through **N-** and **O-glycosidic bonds**, respectively. *Salivary α-amylase* initiates digestion of **dietary polysaccharides** (for example, starch or glycogen), producing oligosaccharides. *Pancreatic α-amylase* continues the process. The final digestive processes occur at the **mucosal lining** of the **small intestine**. Several *disaccharidases* (for example, *lactase* [*β-galactosidase*], *sucrase*, *isomaltase*, and *maltase*) produce monosaccharides (glucose, galactose, and fructose). These enzymes are **transmembrane proteins** of the luminal **brush border** of **intestinal mucosal cells (enterocytes)**. Absorption of the monosaccharides requires specific **transporters**. If carbohydrate degradation is deficient (as a result of heredity, disease, or drugs that injure the intestinal mucosa), undigested carbohydrate will pass into the large intestine, where it can cause **osmotic diarrhea**. Bacterial fermentation of the material produces large volumes of carbon dioxide and hydrogen gas, causing abdominal cramps, diarrhea, and flatulence. **Lactose intolerance**, primarily caused by the age-dependent loss of *lactase* (**adult-type hypolactasia**), is by far the most common of these deficiencies.

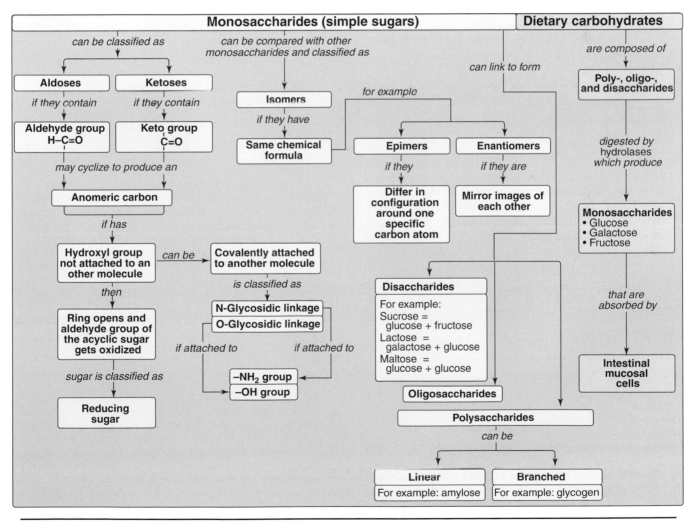

Figure 7.12

Key concept map for the classification and structure of monosaccharides and the digestion of dietary carbohydrates.

Study Questions

Choose the ONE best answer.

7.1 Which of the following statements best describes glucose?

   A. It is a C-4 epimer of galactose.

   B. It is a ketose and usually exists as a furanose ring in solution.

   C. It is produced from dietary starch by the action of α-amylase.

   D. It is utilized in biological systems only in the L-isomeric form.

7.2 A young man entered his physician's office complaining of bloating and diarrhea. His eyes were sunken, and the physician noted additional signs of dehydration. The patient's temperature was normal. He explained that the episode had occurred following a birthday party at which he had participated in an ice cream–eating contest. The patient reported prior episodes of a similar nature following ingestion of a significant amount of dairy products. This clinical picture is most probably due to a deficiency in the activity of:

   A. isomaltase.

   B. lactase.

   C. pancreatic α-amylase.

   D. salivary α-amylase.

   E. sucrase.

7.3 Routine examination of the urine of an asymptomatic pediatric patient showed a positive reaction with Clinitest (a copper reduction method of detecting reducing sugars) but a negative reaction with the glucose oxidase test for detecting glucose. Using these data, show on the chart below which of the sugars could (YES) or could not (NO) be present in the urine of this individual.

SUGAR	YES	NO
Fructose		
Galactose		
Glucose		
Lactose		
Sucrose		
Xylulose		

7.4 Why are α-glucosidase inhibitors that are taken with meals, such as acarbose and miglitol, used in the treatment of diabetes? What effect should these drugs have on the digestion of lactose?

Correct answer = A. Because glucose and galactose differ only in configuration around carbon 4, they are C-4 epimers that are interconvertible by the action of an epimerase. Glucose is an aldose sugar that typically exists as a pyranose ring in solution. Fructose, however, is a ketose with a furanose ring. α-Amylase does not produce monosaccharides. The D-isomeric form of carbohydrates is the form typically found in biologic systems, in contrast to amino acids that typically are found in the L-isomeric form.

Correct answer = B. The physical symptoms suggest a deficiency in an enzyme responsible for carbohydrate degradation. The symptoms observed following the ingestion of dairy products suggest that the patient is deficient in lactase as a result of the age-dependent reduction in expression of the enzyme.

Each of the listed sugars, except for sucrose and glucose, could be present in the urine of this individual. Clinitest is a nonspecific test that produces a change in color if urine is positive for reducing substances such as reducing sugars (fructose, galactose, glucose, lactose, xylulose). Because sucrose is not a reducing sugar, it is not detected by Clinitest. The glucose oxidase test will detect only glucose, and it cannot detect other sugars. The negative glucose oxidase test coupled with a positive reducing sugar test means that glucose cannot be the reducing sugar in the patient's urine.

α-Glucosidase inhibitors slow the production of glucose from dietary carbohydrates, thereby reducing the postprandial rise in blood glucose and facilitating better blood glucose control in diabetic patients. These drugs have no effect on lactose digestion because the disaccharide lactose contains a β-glycosidic bond, not an α-glycosidic bond.

Introduction to Metabolism and Glycolysis

8

I. METABOLISM OVERVIEW

In Chapter 5, individual enzymic reactions were analyzed in an effort to explain the mechanisms of catalysis. However, in cells, these reactions rarely occur in isolation. Instead, they are organized into multistep sequences called pathways, such as that of glycolysis (Fig. 8.1). In a pathway, the product of one reaction serves as the substrate of the subsequent reaction. Most pathways can be classified as either catabolic (degradative) or anabolic (synthetic). Catabolic pathways break down complex molecules, such as proteins, polysaccharides, and lipids, to a few simple molecules (for example, carbon dioxide, ammonia, and water). Anabolic pathways form complex end products from simple precursors, for example, the synthesis of the polysaccharide glycogen from glucose. [Note: Pathways that regenerate a component are called cycles.] Different pathways can intersect, forming an integrated and purposeful network of chemical reactions. Metabolism is the sum of all the chemical changes occurring in a cell, a tissue, or the body. The next several chapters focus on the central metabolic pathways that are involved in synthesizing and degrading carbohydrates, lipids, and amino acids.

A. Metabolic map

Metabolism is best understood by examining its component pathways. Each pathway is composed of multienzyme sequences, and each enzyme, in turn, may exhibit important catalytic or regulatory features. A metabolic map containing the important central pathways of energy metabolism is presented in Figure 8.2. This "big picture" view of metabolism is useful in tracing connections between pathways, visualizing the purposeful movement of metabolic intermediates (metabolites), and depicting the effect on the flow of intermediates if a pathway is blocked (for example, by a drug or an inherited deficiency of an enzyme). [Note: The metabolome is the full complement of metabolites in an organism.] Throughout the next three units of this book, each pathway under discussion will be repeatedly featured as part of the major metabolic map shown in Figure 8.2.

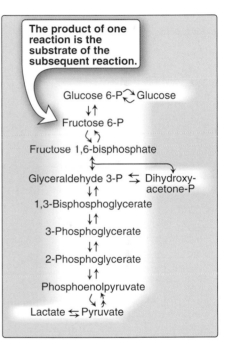

Figure 8.1
Glycolysis, an example of a metabolic pathway. [Note: Pyruvate to phosphoenolpyruvate requires two reactions.] Curved reaction arrows indicate forward and reverse reactions that are catalyzed by different enzymes. P = phosphate.

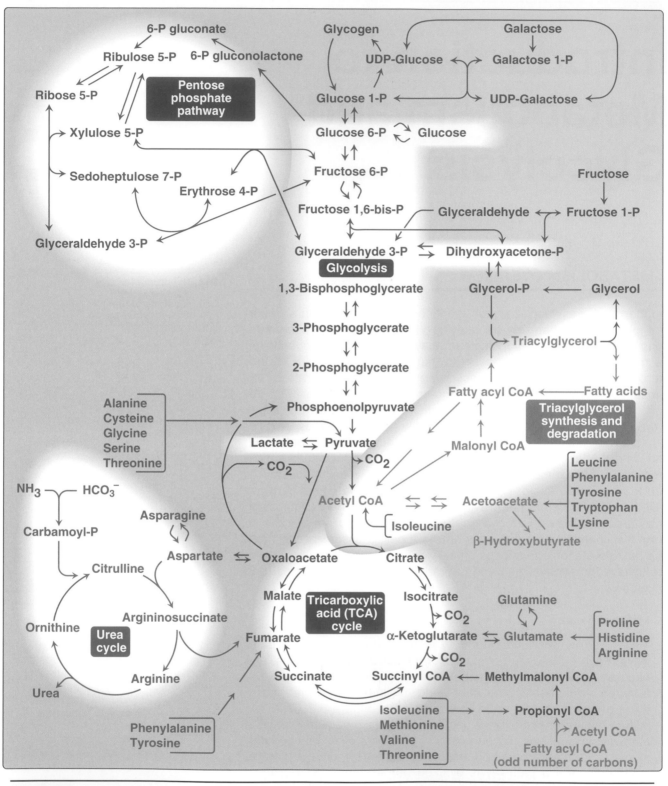

Figure 8.2

Important reactions of intermediary metabolism. Several important pathways to be discussed in later chapters are highlighted. Curved reaction arrows (⤵) indicate forward and reverse reactions that are catalyzed by different enzymes. The straight arrows (⇄) indicate forward and reverse reactions that are catalyzed by the same enzyme. **Blue text** = intermediates of carbohydrate metabolism; **brown text** = intermediates of lipid metabolism; **green text** = intermediates of protein metabolism. UDP = uridine diphosphate; P = phosphate; CoA = coenzyme A; CO_2 = carbon dioxide; HCO_3^- = bicarbonate; NH_3 = ammonia.

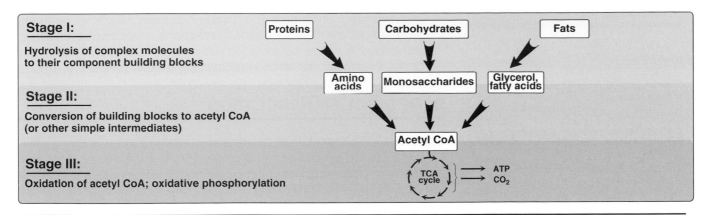

Figure 8.3
Three stages of catabolism. CoA = coenzyme A; TCA = tricarboxylic acid; CO_2 = carbon dioxide.

B. Catabolic pathways

Catabolic reactions serve to capture chemical energy in the form of ATP from the degradation of energy-rich fuel molecules. ATP generation by degradation of complex molecules occurs in three stages, as shown in Figure 8.3. [Note: Catabolic pathways are typically oxidative and require oxidized coenzymes such as nicotinamide adenine dinucleotide (NAD^+).] Catabolism also allows molecules in the diet (or nutrient molecules stored in cells) to be converted into basic building blocks needed for the synthesis of complex molecules. Catabolism, then, is a convergent process (that is, a wide variety of molecules are transformed into a few common end products).

1. **Hydrolysis of complex molecules:** In the first stage, complex molecules are broken down into their component building blocks. For example, proteins are degraded to amino acids, polysaccharides to monosaccharides, and fats (triacylglycerols) to free fatty acids and glycerol.

2. **Conversion of building blocks to simple intermediates:** In the second stage, these diverse building blocks are further degraded to acetyl coenzyme A (CoA) and a few other simple molecules. Some energy is captured as ATP, but the amount is small compared with the energy produced during the third stage of catabolism.

3. **Oxidation of acetyl coenzyme A:** The tricarboxylic acid (TCA) cycle (see p. 109) is the final common pathway in the oxidation of fuel molecules that produce acetyl CoA. Oxidation of acetyl CoA generates large amounts of ATP via oxidative phosphorylation as electrons flow from NADH and flavin adenine dinucleotide ($FADH_2$) to oxygen ([O_2] see p. 73).

C. Anabolic pathways

In contrast to catabolism, anabolism is a divergent process in which a few biosynthetic precursors (such as amino acids) form a wide variety of polymeric, or complex, products (such as proteins [Fig. 8.4]). Anabolic reactions require energy (are endergonic), which is generally provided by the hydrolysis of ATP to adenosine diphosphate (ADP)

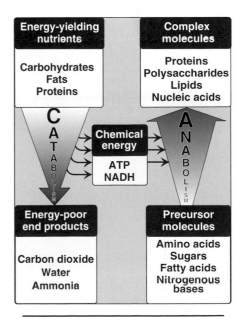

Figure 8.4
Comparison of catabolic and anabolic pathways. NADH = nicotinamide adenine dinucleotide.

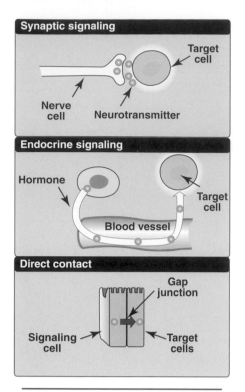

Figure 8.5
Some commonly used mechanisms for transmission of regulatory signals between cells.

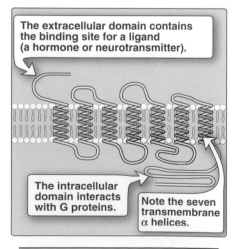

Figure 8.6
Structure of a typical G protein–coupled receptor of the plasma membrane.

and inorganic phosphate (P_i). [Note: Catabolic reactions generate energy (are exergonic).] Anabolic reactions often involve chemical reductions in which the reducing power is most frequently provided by the electron donor NADPH (phosphorylated NADH, see p. 147).

II. METABOLISM REGULATION

The pathways of metabolism must be coordinated so that the production of energy or the synthesis of end products meets the needs of the cell. Furthermore, individual cells function as part of a community of interacting tissues, not in isolation. Thus, a sophisticated communication system has evolved to coordinate the functions of the body. Regulatory signals that inform an individual cell of the metabolic state of the body as a whole include hormones, neurotransmitters, and the availability of nutrients. These, in turn, influence signals generated within the cell (Fig. 8.5).

A. Intracellular communication

The rate of a metabolic pathway can respond to regulatory signals that arise from within the cell. For example, the rate may be influenced by the availability of substrates, product inhibition, or alterations in the levels of allosteric activators or inhibitors. These intracellular signals typically elicit rapid responses and are important for the moment-to-moment regulation of metabolism.

B. Intercellular communication

The ability to respond to intercellular signals is essential for the development and survival of organisms. Signaling between cells provides for long-range integration of metabolism and usually results in a response, such as a change in gene expression, that is slower than is seen with intracellular signals. Communication between cells can be mediated, for example, by surface-to-surface contact and, in some tissues, by formation of gap junctions, allowing direct communication between the cytoplasms of adjacent cells. However, for energy metabolism, the most important route of communication is chemical signaling between cells by blood-borne hormones or by neurotransmitters.

C. Second messenger systems

Hormones and neurotransmitters can be thought of as signals and their receptors as signal detectors. Receptors respond to a bound ligand by initiating a series of reactions that ultimately result in specific intracellular responses. Second messenger molecules, so named because they intervene between the original extracellular messenger (the neurotransmitter or hormone) and the ultimate intracellular effect, are part of the cascade of events that converts (transduces) ligand binding into a response. Two of the most widely recognized second messenger systems are the calcium/phosphatidylinositol system (see p. 205) and the *adenylyl cyclase* (*adenylate cyclase*) system, which is particularly important in regulating the pathways of intermediary metabolism. Both involve the binding of ligands, such as epinephrine or glucagon, to specific G protein–coupled receptors (GPCR) on the cell (plasma) membrane. GPCR are characterized by an extracellular ligand-binding domain, seven transmembrane α helices, and an intracellular domain that interacts with trimeric G proteins (Fig. 8.6).

[Note: Insulin, another key regulator of metabolism, binds a membrane tyrosine kinase receptor (see p. 311) and not a GPCR.]

D. Adenylyl cyclase

The recognition of a chemical signal by some GPCR, such as the β- and α2-adrenergic receptors, triggers either an increase or a decrease in the activity of *adenylyl cyclase* (*AC*). This is a membrane-bound enzyme that converts ATP to 3′,5′-adenosine monophosphate (cyclic AMP, or cAMP). The chemical signals are most often hormones or neurotransmitters, each of which binds to a unique type of GPCR. Therefore, tissues that respond to more than one signal must have several different GPCR, each of which can be linked to *AC*.

1. **Guanosine triphosphate–dependent regulatory proteins:** The effect of the activated, occupied GPCR on second messenger formation is indirect, mediated by specialized trimeric proteins (α, β, and γ subunits) of the cell membrane. These proteins, referred to as G proteins because the α subunit binds guanosine di- or triphosphates (GDP or GTP), form a link in the chain of communication between the receptor and *AC*. In the inactive form of a G protein, the α subunit is bound to GDP (Fig. 8.7). Ligand binding causes a conformational change in the receptor, triggering replacement of this GDP with GTP. The GTP-bound form of the α subunit dissociates from the βγ subunits and moves to *AC*, affecting enzyme activity. Many molecules of active Gα protein are formed by one activated receptor. [Note: The ability of a hormone or neurotransmitter to stimulate or inhibit *AC* depends on the type of Gα protein that is linked to the receptor. One type, designated Gs, stimulates *AC* (see Fig. 8.7), whereas another type, designated Gi, inhibits the enzyme (not shown).] The actions of the Gα–GTP complex are short-lived because Gα has an inherent *GTPase* activity, resulting in the rapid hydrolysis of GTP to GDP. This causes inactivation of Gα, its dissociation from *AC*, and its reassociation with the βγ dimer.

> Toxins from <u>Vibrio</u> <u>cholerae</u> (cholera) and <u>Bordetella</u> <u>pertussis</u> (whooping cough) cause inappropriate activation of *AC* through covalent modification (ADP-ribosylation) of different G proteins. With cholera, the *GTPase* activity of Gαs is inhibited in intestinal cells. With whooping cough, Gαi is inactivated in respiratory tract cells.

2. **Protein kinases:** The next step in the cAMP second messenger system is the activation of a family of enzymes called *cAMP-dependent protein kinases* such as *protein kinase A* (*PKA*), as shown in Figure 8.8. cAMP activates *PKA* by binding to its two regulatory subunits, causing the release of its two catalytically active subunits. These subunits transfer phosphate from ATP to specific serine or threonine residues of protein substrates. The phosphorylated proteins may act directly on the cell's ion channels or, if enzymes, may become activated or inhibited. [Note: Several types of *protein kinases* are not cAMP dependent, for example, *protein kinase C*, described on p. 205.]

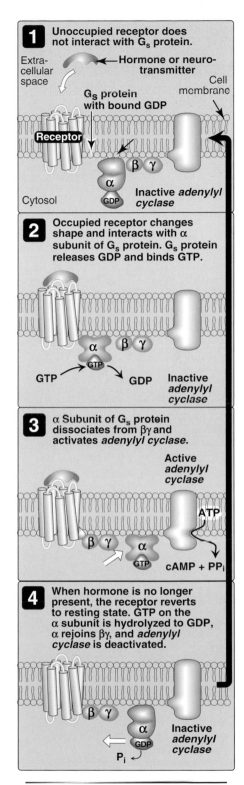

1 Unoccupied receptor does not interact with Gs protein.

Extracellular space — Hormone or neurotransmitter

Gs protein with bound GDP

Cell membrane

Receptor

Cytosol

Inactive *adenylyl cyclase*

2 Occupied receptor changes shape and interacts with α subunit of Gs protein. Gs protein releases GDP and binds GTP.

GTP → GDP

Inactive *adenylyl cyclase*

3 α Subunit of Gs protein dissociates from βγ and activates *adenylyl cyclase*.

Active *adenylyl cyclase*

ATP

cAMP + PPi

4 When hormone is no longer present, the receptor reverts to resting state. GTP on the α subunit is hydrolyzed to GDP, α rejoins βγ, and *adenylyl cyclase* is deactivated.

Inactive *adenylyl cyclase*

Pi

Figure 8.7
The recognition of chemical signals by certain membrane receptors triggers an increase (or, less often, a decrease) in the activity of *adenylyl cyclase*. GDP and GTP = guanosine di- and triphosphates; cAMP = cyclic adenosine monophosphate.

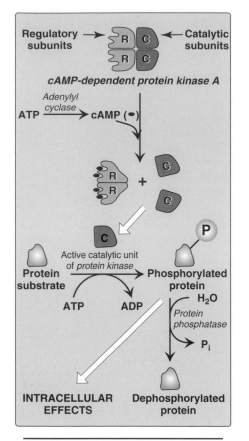

Figure 8.8
Actions of cyclic adenosine monophosphate (cAMP). P = phosphate;
ADP = adenosine diphosphate;
P_i = inorganic phosphate.

3. **Protein phosphatases:** The phosphate groups added to proteins by *protein kinases* are removed by *protein phosphatases*,
enzymes that hydrolytically cleave phosphate esters (see Fig. 8.8).
This insures that changes in protein activity induced by phosphorylation are not permanent.

4. **cAMP hydrolysis:** cAMP is rapidly hydrolyzed to 5′-AMP by *cAMP
phosphodiesterase* that cleaves the cyclic 3′,5′-phosphodiester bond.
5′-AMP is not an intracellular signaling molecule. Therefore, the effects
of neurotransmitter- or hormone-mediated increases of cAMP are rapidly terminated if the extracellular signal is removed. [Note: *cAMP phosphodiesterase* is inhibited by caffeine, a methylxanthine derivative.]

III. GLYCOLYSIS OVERVIEW

The glycolytic pathway is used by all tissues for the oxidation of glucose
to provide energy (as ATP) and intermediates for other metabolic pathways. Glycolysis is at the hub of carbohydrate metabolism because virtually all sugars, whether arising from the diet or from catabolic reactions in
the body, can ultimately be converted to glucose (Fig. 8.9A). Pyruvate is
the end product of glycolysis in cells with mitochondria and an adequate
supply of O_2. This series of ten reactions is called aerobic glycolysis
because O_2 is required to reoxidize the NADH formed during the oxidation of glyceraldehyde 3-phosphate (Fig. 8.9B). Aerobic glycolysis sets
the stage for the oxidative decarboxylation of pyruvate to acetyl CoA, a
major fuel of the TCA cycle. Alternatively, pyruvate is reduced to lactate
as NADH is oxidized to NAD^+ (Fig. 8.9C). This conversion of glucose to
lactate is called anaerobic glycolysis because it can occur without the
participation of O_2. Anaerobic glycolysis allows the production of ATP in
tissues that lack mitochondria (for example, red blood cells [RBC] and
parts of the eye) or in cells deprived of sufficient O_2 (hypoxia).

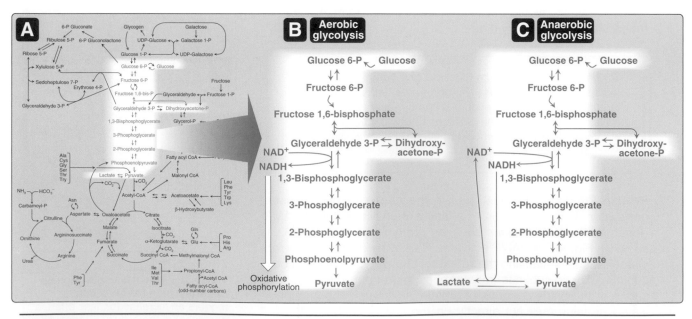

Figure 8.9
A. Glycolysis shown as one of the essential pathways of energy metabolism. B. Reactions of aerobic glycolysis.
C. Reactions of anaerobic glycolysis. NAD(H) = nicotinamide adenine dinucleotide; P = phosphate.

IV. GLUCOSE TRANSPORT INTO CELLS

Glucose cannot diffuse directly into cells but enters by one of two transport systems: a sodium (Na^+)- and ATP-independent transport system or a Na^+- and ATP-dependent cotransport system.

A. Sodium- and ATP-independent transport system

This passive system is mediated by a family of 14 glucose transporter (GLUT) isoforms found in cell membranes. They are designated GLUT-1 to GLUT-14. These monomeric protein transporters exist in the membrane in two conformational states (Fig. 8.10). Extracellular glucose binds to the transporter, which then alters its conformation, transporting glucose across the cell membrane via facilitated diffusion. Because GLUT transport one molecule at a time, they are uniporters.

1. **Tissue specificity:** GLUT display a tissue-specific pattern of expression. For example, GLUT-3 is the primary isoform in neurons. GLUT-1 is abundant in RBC and the blood–brain barrier but is low in adult muscle, whereas GLUT-4 is abundant in muscle and adipose tissue. [Note: The number of GLUT-4 transporters active in these tissues is increased by insulin. (See p. 311 for a discussion of insulin and glucose transport.)] GLUT-2 is abundant in the liver, kidneys, and pancreatic β cells. The other GLUT isoforms also have tissue-specific distributions.

2. **Specialized functions:** In facilitated diffusion, transporter-mediated glucose movement is down a concentration gradient (that is, from a high concentration to a lower one, therefore requiring no energy). For example, GLUT-1, GLUT-3, and GLUT-4 are primarily involved in glucose uptake from the blood. In contrast, GLUT-2, in the liver and kidneys, can either transport glucose into these cells when blood glucose levels are high or transport glucose from these cells when blood glucose levels are low (for example, during fasting). GLUT-5 is unusual in that it is the primary transporter for fructose (not glucose) in the small intestine and the testes (see p. 87).

B. Sodium- and ATP-dependent cotransport system

This energy-requiring process transports glucose against (up) its concentration gradient (that is, from low extracellular concentrations to higher intracellular concentrations) as Na^+ is transported down its electrochemical gradient. [Note: The gradient is created by the *Na$^+$-potassium (K$^+$) ATPase* (see Fig. 7.10, p. 87).] Because this secondary active transport process requires the concurrent uptake (symport) of Na^+, the transporter is a sodium-dependent glucose cotransporter (SGLT). This type of cotransport occurs in the epithelial cells of the intestine (see p. 87), renal tubules, and choroid plexus. [Note: The choroid plexus, part of the blood–brain barrier, also contains GLUT-1.]

V. GLYCOLYSIS REACTIONS

The conversion of glucose to pyruvate occurs in two stages (Fig. 8.11). The first five reactions of glycolysis correspond to an energy-investment phase in which the phosphorylated forms of intermediates are

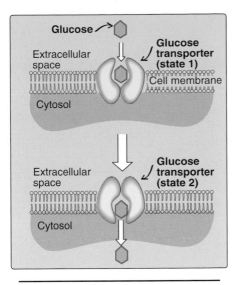

Figure 8.10
Schematic representation of the facilitated transport of glucose through a cell membrane. [Note: Glucose transporter proteins are monomeric and contain 12 transmembrane α helices.]

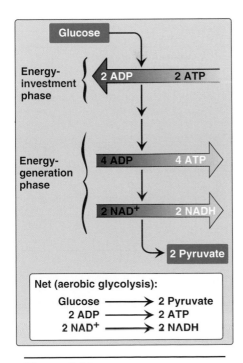

Figure 8.11
Two phases of aerobic glycolysis. NAD(H) = nicotinamide adenine dinucleotide; ADP = adenosine diphosphate.

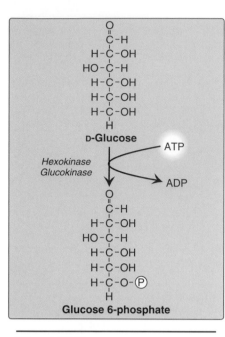

Figure 8.12
Energy-investment phase:
phosphorylation of glucose. [Note:
Kinases utilize ATP complexed with
a divalent metal ion, most typically
magnesium.] ADP = adenosine
diphosphate; Ⓟ = phosphate.

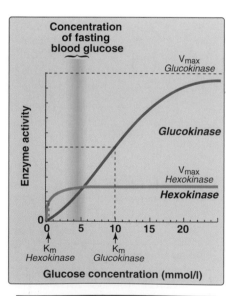

Figure 8.13
Effect of glucose concentration on the
rate of phosphorylation catalyzed by
hexokinase and *glucokinase*. K_m =
Michaelis constant; V_{max} = maximal
velocity.

synthesized at the expense of ATP. The subsequent reactions of glycolysis constitute an energy-generation phase in which a net of two molecules of ATP are formed by substrate-level phosphorylation (see p. 102) per glucose molecule metabolized.

A. Glucose phosphorylation

Phosphorylated sugar molecules do not readily penetrate cell membranes because there are no specific transmembrane carriers for these compounds and because they are too polar to diffuse through the lipid core of membranes. Therefore, the irreversible phosphorylation of glucose (Fig. 8.12) effectively traps the sugar as cytosolic glucose 6-phosphate and commits it to further metabolism in the cell. Mammals have four isozymes (I–IV) of the enzyme *hexokinase* that catalyze the phosphorylation of glucose to glucose 6-phosphate.

1. **Hexokinases I–III:** In most tissues, glucose phosphorylation is catalyzed by one of these isozymes of *hexokinase*, which is one of three regulatory enzymes of glycolysis (along with *phosphofructokinase* and *pyruvate kinase*). They are inhibited by the reaction product glucose 6-phosphate, which accumulates when further metabolism of this hexose phosphate is reduced. *Hexokinases I– III* have a low Michaelis constant (K_m) and, therefore, a high affinity (see p. 59) for glucose. This permits the efficient phosphorylation and subsequent metabolism of glucose even when tissue concentrations of glucose are low (Fig. 8.13). However, because these isozymes have a low maximal velocity ([V_{max}] see p. 57) for glucose, they do not sequester (trap) cellular phosphate in the form of phosphorylated glucose or phosphorylate more glucose than the cell can use. [Note: These isozymes have broad substrate specificity and are able to phosphorylate several hexoses in addition to glucose.]

2. **Hexokinase IV:** In liver parenchymal cells and pancreatic β cells, *glucokinase* (the *hexokinase IV* isozyme) is the predominant enzyme responsible for glucose phosphorylation. In β cells, *glucokinase* functions as a glucose sensor, determining the threshold for insulin secretion (see p. 309). [Note: *Hexokinase IV* also serves as a glucose sensor in hypothalamic neurons, playing a key role in the adrenergic response to hypoglycemia (see p. 315).] In the liver, the enzyme facilitates glucose phosphorylation during hyperglycemia. Despite the popular but misleading name *glucokinase*, the sugar specificity of the enzyme is similar to that of other *hexokinase* isozymes.

   a. **Kinetics:** *Glucokinase* differs from *hexokinases I–III* in several important properties. For example, it has a much higher K_m, requiring a higher glucose concentration for half-saturation (see Fig. 8.13). Thus, *glucokinase* functions only when the intracellular concentration of glucose in the hepatocyte is elevated such as during the brief period following consumption of a carbohydrate-rich meal, when high levels of glucose are delivered to the liver via the portal vein. *Glucokinase* has a high V_{max}, allowing the liver to effectively remove the flood of glucose delivered by the portal blood. This prevents large amounts of glucose from entering the systemic circulation following such a meal, thereby minimizing hyperglycemia during the absorptive period. [Note: GLUT-2 insures that blood glucose equilibrates rapidly across the hepatocyte membrane.]

b. **Regulation:** *Glucokinase* activity is not directly inhibited by glucose 6-phosphate as are the other *hexokinases*. Instead, it is indirectly inhibited by fructose 6-phosphate (which is in equilibrium with glucose 6-phosphate, a product of *glucokinase*) and is indirectly stimulated by glucose (a substrate of *glucokinase*). Regulation is achieved by reversible binding to the hepatic protein glucokinase regulatory protein (GKRP). In the presence of fructose 6-phosphate, *glucokinase* binds tightly to GKRP and is translocated to the nucleus, thereby rendering the enzyme inactive (Fig. 8.14). When glucose levels in the blood (and also in the hepatocyte, as a result of GLUT-2) increase, *glucokinase* is released from GKRP, and the enzyme reenters the cytosol where it phosphorylates glucose to glucose 6-phosphate. [Note: GKRP is a competitive inhibitor of glucose use by *glucokinase*.]

> ‖ *Glucokinase* functions as a glucose sensor in blood glucose homeostasis. Inactivating mutations of *glucokinase* are the cause of a rare form of diabetes, maturity onset diabetes of the young type 2 (MODY 2) that is characterized by impaired insulin secretion and hyperglycemia.

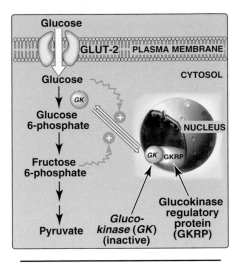

Figure 8.14
Regulation of *glucokinase* activity by glucokinase regulatory protein. GLUT = glucose transporter.

B. Glucose 6-phosphate isomerization

The isomerization of glucose 6-phosphate to fructose 6-phosphate is catalyzed by *phosphoglucose isomerase* (Fig. 8.15). The reaction is readily reversible and is not a rate-limiting or regulated step.

C. Fructose 6-phosphate phosphorylation

The irreversible phosphorylation reaction catalyzed by *phosphofructokinase-1* (*PFK-1*) is the most important control point and the rate-limiting and committed step of glycolysis (Fig. 8.16). *PFK-1* is controlled by the available concentrations of the substrates ATP and fructose 6-phosphate as well as by other regulatory molecules.

1. **Regulation by intracellular energy levels:** *PFK-1* is inhibited allosterically by elevated levels of ATP, which act as an energy-rich signal indicating an abundance of high-energy compounds. Elevated levels of citrate, an intermediate in the TCA cycle (see p. 111), also inhibit *PFK-1*. [Note: Inhibition by citrate favors the use of glucose for glycogen synthesis (see p. 126).] Conversely, *PFK-1* is activated allosterically by high concentrations of AMP, which signal that the cell's energy stores are depleted.

2. **Regulation by fructose 2,6-bisphosphate:** Fructose 2,6-bisphosphate is the most potent activator of *PFK-1* (see Fig. 8.16) and is able to activate the enzyme even when ATP levels are high. It is formed from fructose 6-phosphate by *phosphofructokinase-2*

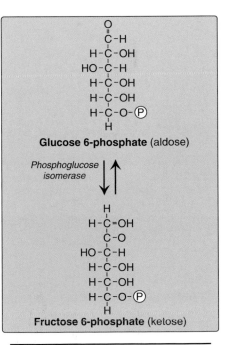

Figure 8.15
Aldose-ketose isomerization of glucose 6-phosphate to fructose 6-phosphate. Ⓟ = phosphate.

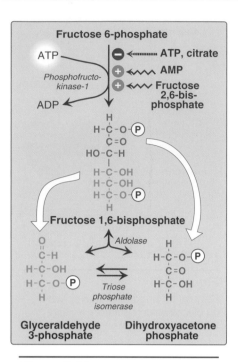

Figure 8.16
Energy-investment phase (continued): conversion of fructose 6-phosphate to triose phosphates. Ⓟ = phosphate; AMP and ADP = adenosine mono- and diphosphates.

(*PFK-2*). Unlike *PFK-1*, *PFK-2* is a bifunctional protein that has both the *kinase* activity that produces fructose 2,6-bisphosphate and the *phosphatase* activity that dephosphorylates fructose 2,6-bisphosphate to fructose 6-phosphate. In the liver isozyme, phosphorylation of *PFK-2* inactivates the *kinase* domain and activates the *phosphatase* domain (Fig. 8.17). The opposite is seen in the cardiac isozyme. Skeletal *PFK-2* is not covalently regulated. [Note: Fructose 2,6-bisphosphate is an inhibitor of *fructose 1,6-bisphosphatase*, an enzyme of gluconeogenesis (see p. 121). The reciprocal actions of fructose 2,6-bisphosphate on glycolysis (activation) and gluconeogenesis (inhibition) insure that both pathways are not fully active at the same time, preventing a futile cycle of glucose oxidation to pyruvate followed by glucose resynthesis from pyruvate.]

a. **During the well-fed state:** Decreased levels of glucagon and elevated levels of insulin (such as occur following a carbohydrate-rich meal) cause an increase in hepatic fructose 2,6-bisphosphate (*PFK-2* is dephosphorylated) and, thus, in the rate of glycolysis (see Fig. 8.17). Therefore, fructose 2,6-bisphosphate acts as an intracellular signal of glucose abundance.

b. **During fasting:** By contrast, the elevated levels of glucagon and low levels of insulin that occur during fasting (see p. 327) cause a decrease in hepatic fructose 2,6-bisphosphate (*PFK-2* is phosphorylated). This results in inhibition of glycolysis and activation of gluconeogenesis.

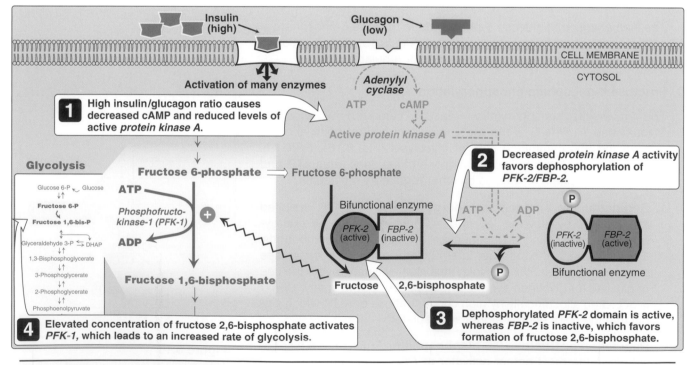

Figure 8.17
Effect of elevated insulin concentration on the intracellular concentration of fructose 2,6-bisphosphate in the liver. *PFK-2* = *phosphofructokinase-2*; *FBP-2* = *fructose 2,6-bisphosphatase*; AMP and ADP = adenosine mono- and diphosphates; cAMP = cyclic AMP; Ⓟ = phosphate.

D. Fructose 1,6-bisphosphate cleavage

Aldolase cleaves fructose 1,6-bisphosphate to dihydroxyacetone phosphate (DHAP) and glyceraldehyde 3-phosphate (see Fig. 8.16). The reaction is reversible and not regulated. [Note: *Aldolase B*, the hepatic isoform, also cleaves fructose 1-phosphate and functions in dietary fructose metabolism (see p. 138).]

E. Dihydroxyacetone phosphate isomerization

Triose phosphate isomerase interconverts DHAP and glyceraldehyde 3-phosphate (see Fig. 8.16). DHAP must be isomerized to glyceraldehyde 3-phosphate for further metabolism by the glycolytic pathway. This isomerization results in the net production of two molecules of glyceraldehyde 3-phosphate from the cleavage products of fructose 1,6-bisphosphate. [Note: DHAP is utilized in triacylglycerol synthesis (see p. 188).]

F. Glyceraldehyde 3-phosphate oxidation

The conversion of glyceraldehyde 3-phosphate to 1,3-bisphosphoglycerate (1,3-BPG) by *glyceraldehyde 3-phosphate dehydrogenase* is the first oxidation-reduction reaction of glycolysis (Fig. 8.18). [Note: Because there is a limited amount of NAD$^+$ in the cell, the NADH formed by the *dehydrogenase* reaction must be oxidized for glycolysis to continue. Two major mechanisms for oxidizing NADH to NAD$^+$ are the reduction of pyruvate to lactate by *lactate dehydrogenase* (*LDH*) (anaerobic, see p. 96) and the electron transport chain ([ETC] aerobic, see p. 74). Because NADH cannot cross the inner mitochondrial membrane, the ETC requires the malate-aspartate and glycerol 3-phosphate substrate shuttles to move NADH reducing equivalents into the mitochondrial matrix (see p. 79).]

1. **1,3-Bisphosphoglycerate synthesis:** The oxidation of the aldehyde group of glyceraldehyde 3-phosphate to a carboxyl group is coupled to the attachment of P$_i$ to the carboxyl group. This phosphate group, linked to carbon 1 of the 1,3-BPG product by a high-energy bond (see p. 73), conserves much of the free energy (see p. 69) produced by the oxidation of glyceraldehyde 3-phosphate. This high-energy phosphate drives ATP synthesis in the next reaction of glycolysis.

2. **Arsenic poisoning:** The toxicity of arsenic is due primarily to the inhibition by trivalent arsenic (arsenite) of enzymes such as the *pyruvate dehydrogenase complex* (*PDHC*), which require lipoic acid as a coenzyme (see p. 110). However, pentavalent arsenic (arsenate) can prevent net ATP and NADH production by glycolysis without inhibiting the pathway itself. It does so by competing with P$_i$ as a substrate for *glyceraldehyde 3-phosphate dehydrogenase*, forming a complex that spontaneously hydrolyzes to form 3-phosphoglycerate (see Fig. 8.18). By bypassing the synthesis of and phosphate transfer from 1,3-BPG, the cell is deprived of energy usually obtained from the glycolytic pathway. [Note: Arsenate also competes with P$_i$ binding to the F$_1$ domain of *ATP synthase* (see p. 78), resulting in formation of ADP-arsenate that is rapidly hydrolyzed.]

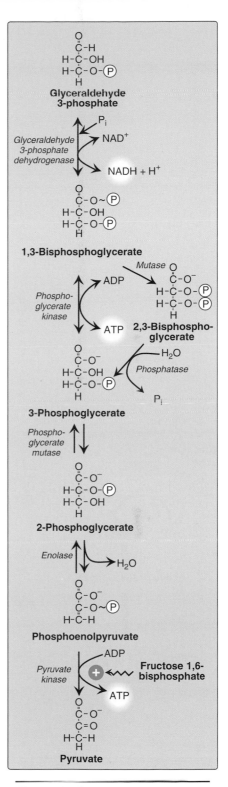

Figure 8.18
Energy-generating phase: conversion of glyceraldehyde 3-phosphate to pyruvate. NAD(H) = nicotinamide adenine dinucleotide; Ⓟ = phosphate; P$_i$ = inorganic phosphate; ~ = high-energy bond; ADP = adenosine diphosphate.

3. 2,3-Bisphosphoglycerate synthesis in RBC: Some of the 1,3-BPG is converted to 2,3-BPG by the action of *bisphosphoglycerate mutase* (see Fig. 8.18). 2,3-BPG, which is found in only trace amounts in most cells, is present at high concentration in RBC and serves to increase O$_2$ delivery (see p. 31). 2,3-BPG is hydrolyzed by a *phosphatase* to 3-phosphoglycerate, which is also an intermediate in glycolysis (see Fig. 8.18). In the RBC, glycolysis is modified by inclusion of these shunt reactions.

G. 3-Phosphoglycerate synthesis and ATP production

When 1,3-BPG is converted to 3-phosphoglycerate, the high-energy phosphate group of 1,3-BPG is used to synthesize ATP from ADP (see Fig. 8.18). This reaction is catalyzed by *phosphoglycerate kinase*, which, unlike most other *kinases*, is physiologically reversible. Because two molecules of 1,3-BPG are formed from each glucose molecule, this *kinase* reaction replaces the two ATP molecules consumed by the earlier formation of glucose 6-phosphate and fructose 1,6-bisphosphate. [Note: This reaction is an example of substrate-level phosphorylation, in which the energy needed for the production of a high-energy phosphate comes from a substrate rather than from the ETC (see J. below and p. 113 for other examples).]

H. Phosphate group shift

The shift of the phosphate group from carbon 3 to carbon 2 of phosphoglycerate by *phosphoglycerate mutase* is freely reversible.

I. 2-Phosphoglycerate dehydration

The dehydration of 2-phosphoglycerate by *enolase* redistributes the energy within the substrate, forming phosphoenolpyruvate (PEP), which contains a high-energy enol phosphate (see Fig. 8.18). The reaction is reversible, despite the high-energy nature of the product. [Note: Fluoride inhibits *enolase*, and water fluoridation reduces lactate production by mouth bacteria, decreasing dental caries (see p. 405).]

J. Pyruvate synthesis and ATP production

The conversion of PEP to pyruvate, catalyzed by *pyruvate kinase* (*PK*), is the third irreversible reaction of glycolysis. The high-energy enol phosphate in PEP is used to synthesize ATP from ADP and is another example of substrate-level phosphorylation (see Fig. 8.18).

1. Feedforward regulation: *PK* is activated by fructose 1,6-bisphosphate, the product of the *PFK-1* reaction. This feedforward (instead of the more usual feedback) regulation has the effect of linking the two *kinase* activities: increased *PFK-1* activity results in elevated levels of fructose 1,6-bisphosphate, which activates *PK*. [Note: *PK* is inhibited by ATP.]

2. Covalent regulation in the liver: Phosphorylation by *cAMP-dependent PKA* leads to inactivation of the hepatic isozyme of *PK* (Fig. 8.19). When blood glucose levels are low, elevated glucagon increases the intracellular level of cAMP, which causes the phosphorylation and inactivation of *PK* in the liver only. Therefore,

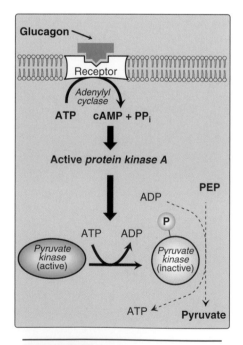

Figure 8.19
Covalent modification of hepatic *pyruvate kinase* results in inactivation of the enzyme. cAMP = cyclic adenosine monophosphate; PEP = phosphoenolpyruvate; (P) = phosphate; PP$_i$ = pyrophosphate; ADP = adenosine diphosphate.

PEP is unable to continue in glycolysis and, instead, enters the gluconeogenesis pathway. This partly explains the observed inhibition of hepatic glycolysis and stimulation of gluconeogenesis by glucagon. Dephosphorylation of *PK* by a *phosphatase* results in reactivation of the enzyme.

3. **Pyruvate kinase deficiency:** Because mature RBC lack mitochondria, they are completely dependent on glycolysis for ATP production. ATP is required to meet the metabolic needs of RBC and to fuel the ion pumps necessary for the maintenance of the flexible, biconcave shape that allows them to squeeze through narrow capillaries. The anemia observed in glycolytic enzyme deficiencies is a consequence of the reduced rate of glycolysis, leading to decreased ATP production by substrate-level phosphorylation. The resulting alterations in the RBC membrane lead to changes in cell shape and, ultimately, to phagocytosis by cells of the mononuclear phagocyte system, particularly splenic macrophages. The premature death and lysis of RBC result in mild-to-severe nonspherocytic hemolytic anemia, with the severe form requiring regular transfusions. Among patients with rare genetic defects of glycolytic enzymes, the majority has a deficiency in *PK*. [Note: Liver *PK* is encoded by the same gene as the RBC isozyme. However, liver cells show no effect because they can synthesize more *PK* and can also generate ATP by oxidative phosphorylation.] Severity depends both on the degree of enzyme deficiency (generally 5%–35% of normal levels) and on the extent to which RBC compensate by synthesizing increased levels of 2,3-BPG (see p. 31). Almost all individuals with *PK* deficiency have a mutant enzyme that shows altered kinetics or decreased stability (Fig. 8.20). Individuals heterozygous for *PK* deficiency have resistance to the most severe forms of malaria.

> The tissue-specific expression of *PK* in RBC and the liver results from the use of different start sites in transcription (see p. 473) of the gene that encodes the enzyme.

K. Pyruvate reduction to lactate

Lactate, formed from pyruvate by *LDH*, is the final product of anaerobic glycolysis in eukaryotic cells (Fig. 8.21). Reduction to lactate is the major fate for pyruvate in tissues that are poorly vascularized (for example, the lens and cornea of the eye and the kidney medulla) or in RBC that lack mitochondria.

1. **Lactate formation in muscle:** In exercising skeletal muscle, NADH production (by *glyceraldehyde 3-phosphate dehydrogenase* and by the three NAD+-linked *dehydrogenases* of the TCA cycle, see p. 113) exceeds the oxidative capacity of the ETC. This results in an elevated NADH/NAD+ ratio, favoring reduction of pyruvate to lactate by *LDH*. Therefore, during intense exercise, lactate accumulates in muscle, causing a drop in the intracellular pH, potentially resulting in cramps. Much of this lactate eventually diffuses into the bloodstream and can be used by the liver to make glucose (see p. 118).

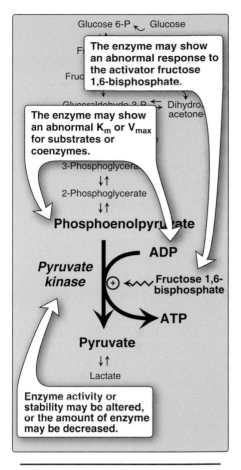

Figure 8.20
Alterations observed with various mutant forms of *pyruvate kinase*. K_m = Michaelis constant; V_{max} = maximal velocity; ADP = adenosine diphosphate.

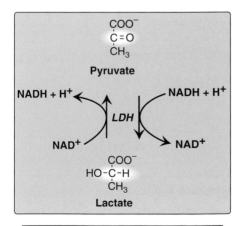

Figure 8.21
Interconversion of pyruvate and lactate by *lactate dehydrogenase* (*LDH*). NAD(H) = nicotinamide adenine dinucleotide.

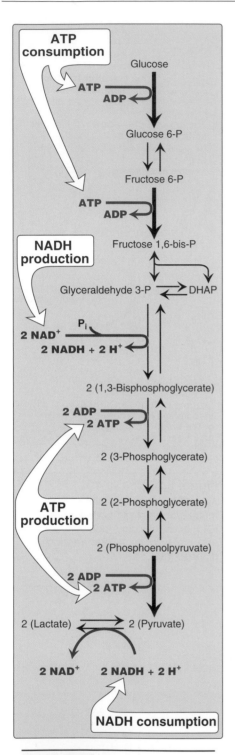

Figure 8.22
Summary of anaerobic glycolysis.
Reactions involving the production
or consumption of ATP or
nicotinamide adenine dinucleotide
(NADH) are indicated. The three
irreversible reactions of glycolysis
are shown with thick arrows.
DHAP = dihydroxyacetone phosphate;
ADP = adenosine diphosphate;
P = phosphate.

2. **Lactate utilization:** The direction of the *LDH* reaction depends on the relative intracellular concentrations of pyruvate and lactate and on the ratio of NADH/NAD$^+$. For example, in the liver and heart, this ratio is lower than in exercising muscle. Consequently, the liver and heart oxidize lactate (obtained from the blood) to pyruvate. In the liver, pyruvate is either converted to glucose by gluconeogenesis or converted to acetyl CoA that is oxidized in the TCA cycle. Heart muscle exclusively oxidizes lactate to carbon dioxide and water via the TCA cycle.

3. **Lactic acidosis:** Elevated concentrations of lactate in the plasma, termed lactic acidosis (a type of metabolic acidosis), occur when there is a collapse of the circulatory system, such as with myocardial infarction, pulmonary embolism, and uncontrolled hemorrhage, or when an individual is in shock. The failure to bring adequate amounts of O_2 to the tissues results in impaired oxidative phosphorylation and decreased ATP synthesis. To survive, the cells rely on anaerobic glycolysis for generating ATP, producing lactic acid as the end product. [Note: Production of even meager amounts of ATP may be lifesaving during the period required to reestablish adequate blood flow to the tissues.] The additional O_2 required to recover from a period when O_2 availability has been inadequate is termed the O_2 debt. [Note: The O_2 debt is often related to patient morbidity or mortality. In many clinical situations, measuring the blood levels of lactic acid allows the rapid, early detection of O_2 debt in patients and the monitoring of their recovery.]

L. Energy yield from glycolysis

Despite the production of some ATP by substrate-level phosphorylation during glycolysis, the end product, pyruvate or lactate, still contains most of the energy originally contained in glucose. The TCA cycle is required to release that energy completely (see p. 109).

1. **Anaerobic glycolysis:** A net of two molecules of ATP are generated for each molecule of glucose converted to two molecules of lactate (Fig. 8.22). There is no net production or consumption of NADH.

2. **Aerobic glycolysis:** The generation of ATP is the same as in anaerobic glycolysis (that is, a net gain of two ATP per molecule of glucose). Two molecules of NADH are also produced per molecule of glucose. Ongoing aerobic glycolysis requires the oxidation of most of this NADH by the ETC, producing three ATP for each NADH molecule entering the chain (see p. 77). [Note: NADH cannot cross the inner mitochondrial membrane, and substrate shuttles are required (see p. 79).]

VI. HORMONAL REGULATION

Regulation of the activity of the irreversible glycolytic enzymes by allosteric activation/inhibition or covalent phosphorylation/dephosphorylation is short term (that is, the effects occur over minutes or hours). Superimposed on these effects on the activity of preexisting enzyme molecules are the long-term hormonal effects on the number of new enzyme molecules. These hormonal effects can result in 10- to 20-fold increases in enzyme synthesis that typically occur over hours to days. Regular consumption of meals rich in carbohydrate or administration of insulin initiates an increase in the amount of *glucokinase*, *PFK-1*, and *PK* in the liver (Fig. 8.23). The change reflects an increase in gene transcription, resulting in increased enzyme synthesis. Increased availability of these three enzymes favors the conversion of glucose to pyruvate, a characteristic of the absorptive state (see p. 321). [Note: The transcriptional effects of insulin and carbohydrate (specifically glucose) are mediated by the transcription factors sterol regulatory element–binding protein-1c and carbohydrate response element–binding protein, respectively. These factors also regulate transcription of genes involved in fatty acid synthesis (see p. 184).] Conversely, gene expression of the three enzymes is decreased when plasma glucagon is high and insulin is low (for example, as seen in fasting or diabetes).

VII. ALTERNATE FATES OF PYRUVATE

Pyruvate can be metabolized to products other than lactate.

A. Oxidative decarboxylation to acetyl CoA

Oxidative decarboxylation of pyruvate by the *PDHC* is an important pathway in tissues with a high oxidative capacity such as cardiac muscle (Fig. 8.24). *PDHC* irreversibly converts pyruvate, the end product of aerobic glycolysis, into acetyl CoA, a TCA cycle substrate (see p. 109) and the carbon source for fatty acid synthesis (see p. 183).

B. Carboxylation to oxaloacetate

Carboxylation of pyruvate to oxaloacetate by *pyruvate carboxylase* is a biotin-dependent reaction (see Fig. 8.24). This irreversible reaction is important because it replenishes the TCA cycle intermediate and provides substrate for gluconeogenesis (see p. 118).

C. Reduction to ethanol (microorganisms)

The reduction of pyruvate to ethanol occurs by the two reactions summarized in Figure 8.24. The decarboxylation of pyruvate to acetaldehyde by thiamine-requiring *pyruvate decarboxylase* occurs in yeast and certain other microorganisms but not in humans.

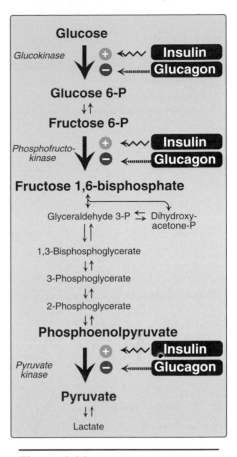

Figure 8.23
Effect of insulin and glucagon on the expression of key enzymes of glycolysis in the liver. P = phosphate.

VIII. CHAPTER SUMMARY

Most **pathways** can be classified as either **catabolic** (degrade complex molecules to a few simple products with **ATP production**) or **anabolic** (synthesize complex end products from simple precursors with **ATP hydrolysis**). The rate of a metabolic pathway can respond to **regulatory signals** such as **intracellular allosteric activators** or **inhibitors**. **Intercellular** signaling provides for the integration of metabolism. The primary route of

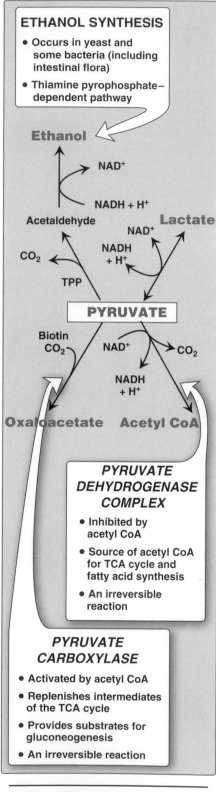

ETHANOL SYNTHESIS

- Occurs in yeast and some bacteria (including intestinal flora)
- Thiamine pyrophosphate–dependent pathway

Ethanol

NAD$^+$

NADH + H$^+$

Acetaldehyde

Lactate

NAD$^+$

NADH + H$^+$

CO_2

TPP

PYRUVATE

Biotin CO_2

NAD$^+$

CO_2

NADH + H$^+$

Oxaloacetate   Acetyl CoA

PYRUVATE DEHYDROGENASE COMPLEX

- Inhibited by acetyl CoA
- Source of acetyl CoA for TCA cycle and fatty acid synthesis
- An irreversible reaction

PYRUVATE CARBOXYLASE

- Activated by acetyl CoA
- Replenishes intermediates of the TCA cycle
- Provides substrates for gluconeogenesis
- An irreversible reaction

Figure 8.24

Summary of the metabolic fates of pyruvate. TPP = thiamine pyrophosphate. TCA = tricarboxylic acid; NAD(H) = nicotinamide adenine dinucleotide; CoA = coenzyme A; CO_2 = carbon dioxide.

this communication is **chemical signaling** (for example, by **hormones** or **neurotransmitters**). **Second messenger molecules** transduce a chemical signal (hormone or neurotransmitter binding) to appropriate intracellular responders. ***Adenylyl cyclase*** (**AC**) is a cell membrane enzyme that synthesizes **cyclic adenosine monophosphate** (**cAMP**) in response to chemical signals, such as the hormones **glucagon** and **epinephrine**. Following binding of a hormone to its **cell-surface G protein–coupled receptor**, a **guanosine triphosphate**–dependent regulatory protein (**G protein**) is activated that, in turn, activates *AC*. The cAMP produced activates ***protein kinase A***, which phosphorylates a variety of enzymes, causing their activation or deactivation. Phosphorylation is reversed by ***phosphatases***. **Aerobic glycolysis**, in which **pyruvate** is the end product, occurs in cells with mitochondria and an adequate supply of oxygen ([O$_2$], Fig. 8.25). **Anaerobic glycolysis**, in which **lactic acid** is the end product, occurs in cells that lack mitochondria and in cells deprived of sufficient O$_2$. Glucose is passively transported across membranes by 1 of 14 **glucose transporter** (**GLUT**) **isoforms**. GLUT-1 is abundant in RBC and the brain, **GLUT-4** (which is **insulin dependent**) in muscle and adipose tissue, and **GLUT-2** in the liver, kidneys, and pancreatic β cells. The oxidation of glucose to pyruvate (**glycolysis**, see Fig. 8.25) occurs through an **energy-investment** phase in which phosphorylated intermediates are synthesized at the expense of ATP and an **energy-generation** phase in which ATP is produced by **substrate-level phosphorylation**. In the energy-investment phase, glucose is phosphorylated by ***hexokinase*** (found in most tissues) or ***glucokinase*** (a *hexokinase* found in **liver cells** and **pancreatic β cells**). **Hexokinase** has a **high affinity** (**low K$_m$**) and a **low maximal velocity** (**V$_{max}$**) for glucose and is inhibited by **glucose 6-phosphate**. *Glucokinase* has a high K$_m$ and a high V$_{max}$ for glucose. It is regulated indirectly by **fructose 6-phosphate** (inhibits) and **glucose** (activates) via **glucokinase regulatory protein**. Glucose 6-phosphate is isomerized to **fructose 6-phosphate**, which is phosphorylated to **fructose 1,6-bisphosphate** by ***phosphofructokinase-1*** (**PFK-1**). This enzyme is allosterically inhibited by **ATP** and **citrate** and activated by **AMP**. **Fructose 2,6-bisphosphate**, whose synthesis by bifunctional ***phosphofructokinase-2*** (**PFK-2**) is increased in the liver by insulin and decreased by glucagon, is the most potent allosteric activator of **PFK-1**. A total of **two ATP** are used during this phase of glycolysis. Fructose 1,6-bisphosphate is cleaved to form two trioses that are further metabolized by the glycolytic pathway, forming pyruvate. During this phase, **four ATP** and **two nicotinamide adenine dinucleotide** (**NADH**) are produced per glucose molecule. The final step in pyruvate synthesis from **phosphoenolpyruvate** is catalyzed by ***pyruvate kinase*** (**PK**). This enzyme is allosterically activated by **fructose 1,6-bisphosphate**, and the hepatic isozyme is inhibited covalently by **glucagon** via the cAMP pathway. *PK* **deficiency** accounts for the majority of all inherited defects in glycolytic enzymes. Effects are restricted to **RBC** and present as mild-to-severe **chronic, nonspherocytic hemolytic anemia**. Glycolytic gene **transcription** is enhanced by insulin and glucose. In **anaerobic glycolysis**, NADH is reoxidized to NAD$^+$ by the reduction of pyruvate to lactate via ***lactate dehydrogenase***. This occurs in cells such as RBC that lack mitochondria and in tissues such as exercising muscle, where production of NADH exceeds the oxidative capacity of the respiratory chain. Elevated concentrations of lactate in the plasma (**lactic acidosis**) occur with circulatory system collapse or shock. Pyruvate also can be 1) **oxidatively decarboxylated** to acetyl CoA by ***pyruvate dehydrogenase***, 2) **carboxylated** to oxaloacetate (a TCA cycle intermediate) by ***pyruvate carboxylase***, or 3) **reduced** to ethanol by microbial ***pyruvate decarboxylase***.

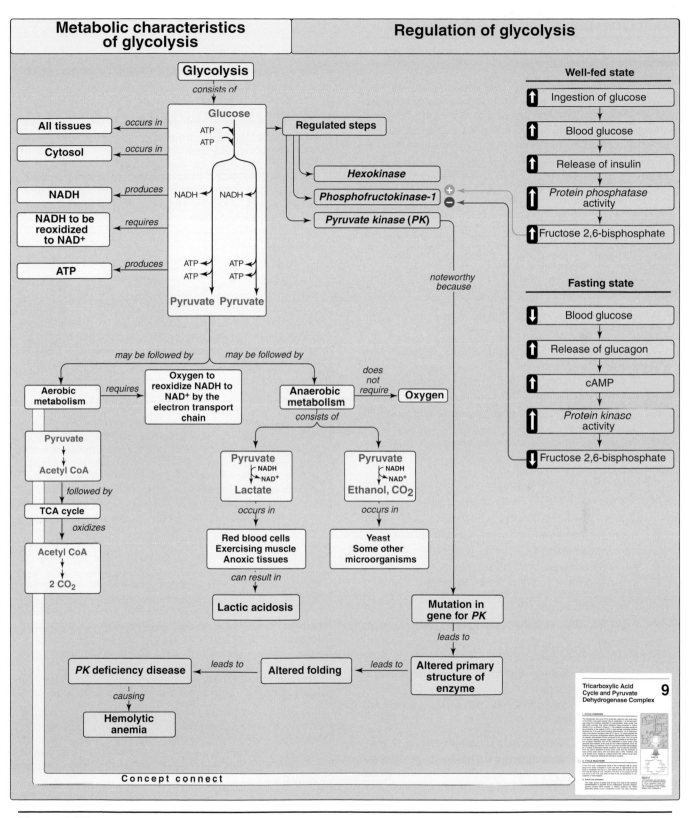

Figure 8.25

Key concept map for glycolysis. NAD(H) = nicotinamide adenine dinucleotide; cAMP = cyclic adenosine monophosphate; CoA = coenzyme A; TCA = tricarboxylic acid; CO_2 = carbon dioxide.

Study Questions

Choose the ONE best answer.

8.1 Which of the following best describes the activity level and phosphorylation state of the listed hepatic enzymes in an individual who consumed a carbohydrate-rich meal about an hour ago? PFK-1 = phosphofructokinase-1; PFK-2 = phosphofructokinase-2; Ⓟ = phosphorylated.

Choice	PFK-1		PFK-2		Pyruvate Kinase	
	Activity	Ⓟ	Activity	Ⓟ	Activity	Ⓟ
A.	Low	No	Low	No	Low	No
B.	High	Yes	Low	Yes	Low	Yes
C.	High	No	High	No	High	No
D.	High	Yes	High	Yes	High	Yes

Correct answer = C. Immediately following a meal, blood glucose levels and hepatic uptake of glucose increase. The glucose is phosphorylated to glucose 6-phosphate and used in glycolysis. In response to the rise in blood glucose, the insulin/glucagon ratio increases. As a result, the kinase domain of PFK-2 is dephosphorylated and active. Its product, fructose 2,6-bisphosphate, allosterically activates PFK-1. (PFK-1 is not covalently regulated.) Active PFK-1 produces fructose 1,6-bisphosphate that is a feedforward activator of pyruvate kinase. Hepatic pyruvate kinase is covalently regulated, and the rise in insulin favors dephosphorylation and activation.

8.2 Which of the following statements is true for anabolic pathways only?

A. Their irreversible (nonequilibrium) reactions are regulated.

B. They are called cycles if they regenerate an intermediate.

C. They are convergent and generate a few simple products.

D. They are synthetic and require energy.

E. They typically require oxidized coenzymes.

Correct answer = D. Anabolic processes are synthetic and energy requiring (endergonic). Statements A and B apply to both anabolic and catabolic processes, whereas C and E apply only to catabolic processes.

8.3 Compared with the resting state, vigorously contracting skeletal muscle shows:

A. decreased AMP/ATP ratio.

B. decreased levels of fructose 2,6-bisphosphate.

C. decreased NADH/NAD$^+$ ratio.

D. increased oxygen availability.

E. increased reduction of pyruvate to lactate.

Correct answer = E. Vigorously contracting skeletal muscle shows an increase in the reduction of pyruvate to lactate compared with resting muscle. The levels of reduced nicotinamide adenine dinucleotide (NADH) increase and exceed the oxidative capacity of the electron transport chain. Consequently, the levels of adenosine monophosphate (AMP) increase. The concentration of fructose 2,6-bisphosphate is not a key regulatory factor in skeletal muscle.

8.4 Glucose uptake by:

A. brain cells is through energy-requiring (active) transport.

B. intestinal mucosal cells requires insulin.

C. liver cells is through facilitated diffusion involving a glucose transporter.

D. most cells is through simple diffusion up a concentration gradient.

Correct answer = C. Glucose uptake in the liver, brain, muscle, and adipose tissue is down a concentration gradient, and the diffusion is facilitated by tissue-specific glucose transporters (GLUT). In adipose and muscle tissues, insulin is required for glucose uptake. Moving glucose against a concentration gradient requires energy and is seen with the sodium-dependent glucose cotransporter 1 (SGLT1) of intestinal mucosal cells.

8.5 Given that the K_m of glucokinase for glucose is 10 mM, whereas that of hexokinase is 0.1 mM, which isozyme will more closely approach V_{max} at the normal blood glucose concentration of 5 mM?

Correct answer = Hexokinase. K_m (Michaelis constant) is that substrate concentration that gives one half V_{max} (maximal velocity). When blood glucose concentration is 5 mM, hexokinase ($K_m = 0.1$ mM) will be saturated, but glucokinase ($K_m = 10$ mM) will not.

8.6 In patients with whooping cough, $G\alpha_i$ is inhibited. How does this lead to a rise in cyclic adenosine monophosphate (cAMP)?

G proteins of the $G\alpha_i$ type inhibit adenylyl cyclase (AC) when their associated G protein–coupled receptor is bound by ligand. If $G\alpha_i$ is inhibited by pertussis toxin, AC production of cAMP is inappropriately activated.

Tricarboxylic Acid Cycle and Pyruvate Dehydrogenase Complex

9

I. CYCLE OVERVIEW

The tricarboxylic acid cycle ([TCA cycle] also called the citric acid cycle, or the Krebs cycle) plays several roles in metabolism. It is the final pathway where the oxidative catabolism of carbohydrates, amino acids, and fatty acids converge, their carbon skeletons being converted to carbon dioxide (CO_2), as shown in Figure 9.1. This oxidation provides energy for the production of the majority of ATP in most animals, including humans. Because the TCA cycle occurs totally in mitochondria, it is in close proximity to the electron transport chain ([ETC] see p. 73), which oxidizes the reduced coenzymes nicotinamide adenine dinucleotide (NADH) and flavin adenine dinucleotide ($FADH_2$) produced by the cycle. The TCA cycle is an aerobic pathway, because oxygen (O_2) is required as the final electron acceptor. Reactions such as the catabolism of some amino acids generate intermediates of the cycle and are called anaplerotic (from the Greek for "filling up") reactions. The TCA cycle also provides intermediates for a number of important anabolic reactions, such as glucose formation from the carbon skeletons of some amino acids and the synthesis of some amino acids (see p. 267) and heme (see p. 278). Therefore, this cycle should not be viewed as a closed system but, instead, as an open one with compounds entering and leaving as required.

II. CYCLE REACTIONS

In the TCA cycle, oxaloacetate (OAA) is first condensed with an acetyl group from acetyl coenzyme A (CoA) and then is regenerated as the cycle is completed (see Fig. 9.1). Two carbons enter the cycle as acetyl CoA and two leave as CO_2. Therefore, the entry of one acetyl CoA into one round of the TCA cycle does not lead to the net production or consumption of intermediates.

A. Acetyl CoA production

The major source of acetyl CoA for the TCA cycle is the oxidative decarboxylation of pyruvate by the multienzyme *pyruvate dehydrogenase complex* (*PDH complex*, or *PDHC*). However, the *PDHC* (described below) is not a component of the TCA cycle. Pyruvate,

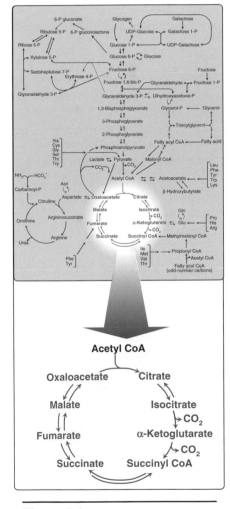

Figure 9.1
The tricarboxylic acid cycle shown as a part of the essential pathways of energy metabolism. [Note: See Fig. 8.2, p. 92 for a more detailed map of metabolism.] CO_2 = carbon dioxide; CoA = coenzyme A.

the end product of aerobic glycolysis, is transported from the cytosol into the mitochondrial matrix by the pyruvate mitochondrial carrier of the inner mitochondrial membrane. In the matrix, the *PDHC* converts pyruvate to acetyl CoA. [Note: Fatty acid oxidation is another source of acetyl CoA (see p. 192).]

1. **PDHC component enzymes:** The *PDHC* is a protein aggregate of multiple copies of three enzymes, *pyruvate decarboxylase* ([*E1*] sometimes called *pyruvate dehydrogenase*), *dihydrolipoyl transacetylase* (*E2*), and *dihydrolipoyl dehydrogenase* (*E3*). Each catalyzes a part of the overall reaction (Fig. 9.2). Their physical association links the reactions in proper sequence without the release of intermediates. In addition to the enzymes participating in the conversion of pyruvate to acetyl CoA, the *PDHC* also contains two regulatory enzymes, *pyruvate dehydrogenase kinase* (*PDH kinase*) and *pyruvate dehydrogenase phosphatase* (*PDH phosphatase*).

2. **Coenzymes:** The *PDHC* contains five coenzymes that act as carriers or oxidants for the intermediates of the reactions shown in Figure 9.2. *E1* requires thiamine pyrophosphate (TPP), *E2* requires lipoic acid and CoA, and *E3* requires FAD and NAD^+. [Note: TPP, lipoic acid, and FAD are tightly bound to the enzymes and function as coenzymes–prosthetic groups (see p. 54).]

> Deficiencies of thiamine or niacin can cause serious central nervous system problems. This is because brain cells are unable to produce sufficient ATP (via the TCA cycle) if the *PDHC* is inactive. Wernicke-Korsakoff, an encephalopathy-psychosis syndrome due to thiamine deficiency, may be seen with alcohol abuse (see p. 383).

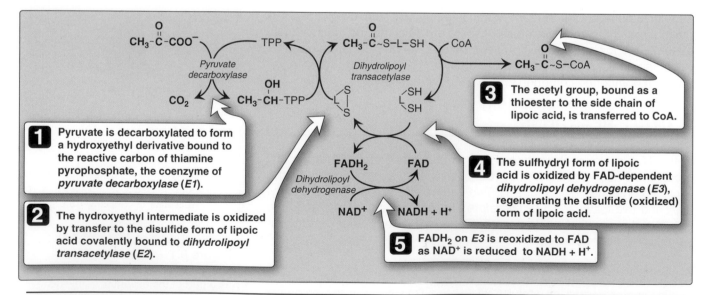

Figure 9.2
Mechanism of action of the enzymes (*E*) of the *pyruvate dehydrogenase complex*. [Note: All the coenzymes of the complex, except for lipoic acid, are derived from vitamins. TPP is from thiamine, FAD from riboflavin, NAD from niacin, and CoA from pantothenic acid.] CO_2 = carbon dioxide; TPP = thiamine pyrophosphate; L = lipoic acid; CoA = coenzyme A; FAD(H_2) and NAD(H) = flavin and nicotinamide adenine dinucleotides; ~ = high-energy bond.

3. **Regulation:** Covalent modifications by the two regulatory enzymes of the *PDHC* alternately activate and inactivate *E1*. *PDH kinase* phosphorylates and inactivates *E1*, whereas *PDH phosphatase* dephosphorylates and activates *E1* (Fig. 9.3). The *kinase* itself is allosterically activated by ATP, acetyl CoA, and NADH. Therefore, in the presence of these high-energy products, the *PDHC* is turned off. [Note: It is actually the rise in the ATP/ADP (adenosine diphosphate), NADH/NAD$^+$, or acetyl CoA/CoA ratios that affects enzymic activity.] Pyruvate is a potent inhibitor of *PDH kinase*. Therefore, if pyruvate concentrations are elevated, *E1* will be maximally active. Calcium (Ca^{2+}) is a strong activator of *PDH phosphatase*, stimulating *E1* activity. This is particularly important in skeletal muscle, where Ca^{2+} release during contraction stimulates the *PDHC* and, thus, energy production. [Note: Although covalent regulation by the *kinase* and *phosphatase* is primary, the *PDHC* is also subject to product (NADH and acetyl CoA) inhibition.]

4. **Deficiency:** A deficiency of the α subunits of the tetrameric *E1* component of the *PDHC*, although very rare, is the most common biochemical cause of congenital lactic acidosis. The deficiency results in a decreased ability to convert pyruvate to acetyl CoA, causing pyruvate to be shunted to lactate via *lactate dehydrogenase* (see p. 103). This creates particular problems for the brain, which relies on the TCA cycle for most of its energy and is particularly sensitive to acidosis. Symptoms are variable and include neurodegeneration, muscle spasticity, and, in the neonatal-onset form, early death. The gene for the α subunit is X linked, and because both males and females may be affected, the deficiency is classified as X-linked dominant. Although there is no proven treatment for *PDHC* deficiency, dietary restriction of carbohydrate and supplementation with thiamine may reduce symptoms in select patients.

> Leigh syndrome (subacute necrotizing encephalomyelopathy) is a rare, progressive, neurodegenerative disorder caused by defects in mitochondrial ATP production, primarily as a result of mutations in genes that encode proteins of the *PDHC*, the ETC, or *ATP synthase*. Both nuclear and mitochondrial DNA can be affected.

5. **Arsenic poisoning:** As previously described (see p. 101), pentavalent arsenic (arsenate) can interfere with glycolysis at the *glyceraldehyde 3-phosphate* step, thereby decreasing ATP production. However, arsenic poisoning is due primarily to inhibition of enzyme complexes that require lipoic acid as a coenzyme, including *PDH*, *α-ketoglutarate dehydrogenase* (see E. below), and *branched-chain α-keto acid dehydrogenase* (see p. 266). Arsenite (the trivalent form of arsenic) forms a stable complex with the thiol (–SH) groups of lipoic acid, making that compound unavailable to serve as a coenzyme. When it binds to lipoic acid in the *PDHC*, pyruvate (and, consequently, lactate) accumulates. As with *PDHC* deficiency, this particularly affects the brain, causing neurologic disturbances and death.

B. Citrate synthesis

The irreversible condensation of acetyl CoA and OAA to form citrate (a tricarboxylic acid) is catalyzed by *citrate synthase*, the initiating enzyme of the TCA cycle (Fig. 9.4). This aldol condensation has a

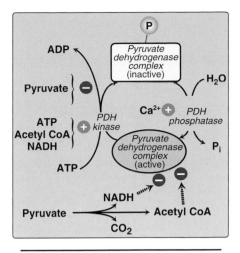

Figure 9.3
Regulation of *pyruvate dehydrogenase* (*PDH*) *complex*. (P) = phosphate [⟼ denotes product inhibition.]

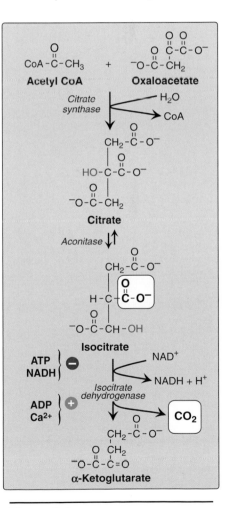

Figure 9.4
Formation of α-ketoglutarate from acetyl coenzyme A (CoA) and oxaloacetate. NAD(H) = nicotinamide adenine dinucleotide; CO_2 = carbon dioxide.

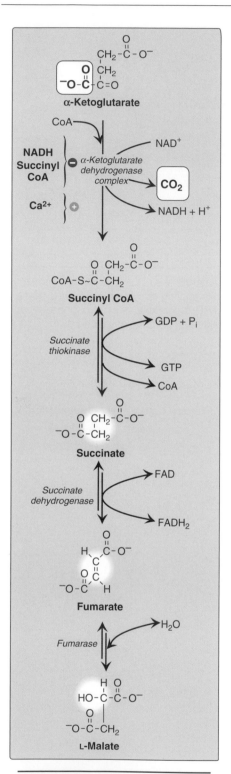

Figure 9.5
Formation of malate from
α-ketoglutarate. FAD(H₂) and
NAD(H) = flavin and nicotinamide
adenine dinucleotides; GDP
and GTP = guanosine di- and
triphosphates; ~ = high-energy
bond; CoA = coenzyme A.

highly negative change in standard free energy ([ΔG^0] see p. 70),
which strongly favors citrate formation. The enzyme is inhibited by
citrate (product inhibition). Substrate availability is another means of
regulation for *citrate synthase*. The binding of OAA greatly increases
the enzyme's affinity for acetyl CoA. [Note: Citrate, in addition to being
an intermediate in the TCA cycle, is a source of acetyl CoA for the
cytosolic synthesis of fatty acids (see p. 183) and cholesterol (see
p. 220). Citrate also inhibits *phosphofructokinase-1* (*PFK-1*), the
rate-limiting enzyme of glycolysis (see p. 99), and activates *acetyl
CoA carboxylase* (the rate-limiting enzyme of fatty acid synthesis,
see p. 183).]

C. Citrate isomerization

Citrate is isomerized to isocitrate through hydroxyl group migration
catalyzed by *aconitase* (*aconitate hydratase*), an iron-sulfur protein
(see Fig. 9.4). [Note: *Aconitase* is inhibited by fluoroacetate, a plant
toxin that is used as a pesticide. Fluoroacetate is converted to fluo-
roacetyl CoA that condenses with OAA to form fluorocitrate, a potent
inhibitor of *aconitase*.]

D. Oxidative decarboxylation of isocitrate

Isocitrate dehydrogenase catalyzes the irreversible oxidative decarboxylation of isocitrate to α-ketoglutarate, yielding the first of three
NADH molecules produced by the cycle and the first release of CO_2
(see Fig. 9.4). This is one of the rate-limiting steps of the TCA cycle.
The enzyme is allosterically activated by ADP (a low-energy signal)
and Ca^{2+} and is inhibited by ATP and NADH, levels of which are elevated when the cell has abundant energy stores.

E. Oxidative decarboxylation of α-ketoglutarate

The irreversible conversion of α-ketoglutarate to succinyl CoA is
catalyzed by the *α-ketoglutarate dehydrogenase complex*, a protein
aggregate of multiple copies of three enzymes (Fig. 9.5). The mechanism of this oxidative decarboxylation is very similar to that used
for the conversion of pyruvate to acetyl CoA by the *PDHC*. The reaction releases the second CO_2 and produces the second NADH of
the cycle. The coenzymes required are TPP, lipoic acid, FAD, NAD⁺,
and CoA. Each functions as part of the catalytic mechanism in a
way analogous to that described for the *PDHC* (see p. 110). The
large negative ΔG^0 of the reaction favors formation of succinyl CoA,
a high-energy thioester similar to acetyl CoA. The *α-ketoglutarate
dehydrogenase complex* is inhibited by its products, NADH and
succinyl CoA, and activated by Ca^{2+}. However, it is not regulated
by phosphorylation/dephosphorylation reactions as described for
the *PDHC*. [Note: α-Ketoglutarate is also produced by the oxidative
deamination (see p. 252) and transamination of the amino acid glutamate (see p. 250).]

F. Succinyl coenzyme A cleavage

Succinate thiokinase (also called *succinyl CoA synthetase*, named
for the reverse reaction) cleaves the high-energy thioester bond of

succinyl CoA (see Fig. 9.5). This reaction is coupled to phosphory-lation of guanosine diphosphate (GDP) to guanosine triphosphate (GTP). GTP and ATP are energetically interconvertible by the *nucleoside diphosphate kinase* reaction:

$$GTP + ADP \rightleftharpoons GDP + ATP$$

The generation of GTP by *succinate thiokinase* is another example of substrate-level phosphorylation (see p. 102). [Note: Succinyl CoA is also produced from propionyl CoA derived from the metabolism of fatty acids with an odd number of carbon atoms (see p. 193) and from the metabolism of several amino acids (see pp. 265–266). It can be converted to pyruvate for gluconeogenesis (see p. 118) or used in heme synthesis (see p. 278).]

G. Succinate oxidation

Succinate is oxidized to fumarate by *succinate dehydrogenase*, as its coenzyme FAD is reduced to $FADH_2$ (see Fig. 9.5). *Succinate dehydrogenase* is the only enzyme of the TCA cycle that is embedded in the inner mitochondrial membrane. As such, it functions as Complex II of the ETC (see p. 75). [Note: FAD, rather than NAD^+, is the electron acceptor because the reducing power of succinate is not sufficient to reduce NAD^+.]

H. Fumarate hydration

Fumarate is hydrated to malate in a freely reversible reaction cata-lyzed by *fumarase* (*fumarate hydratase*, see Fig. 9.5). [Note: Fumarate is also produced by the urea cycle (see p. 255), in purine synthesis (see Fig. 22.7 on p. 294), and during catabolism of the amino acids phenylalanine and tyrosine (see p. 263).]

I. Malate oxidation

Malate is oxidized to OAA by *malate dehydrogenase* (Fig. 9.6). This reaction produces the third and final NADH of the cycle. The ΔG^0 of the reaction is positive, but the reaction is driven in the direction of OAA by the highly exergonic *citrate synthase* reaction. [Note: OAA is also produced by the transamination of the amino acid aspartic acid (see p. 250).]

III. ENERGY PRODUCED BY THE CYCLE

Four pairs of electrons are transferred during one turn of the TCA cycle: three pairs reducing three NAD^+ to NADH and one pair reducing FAD to $FADH_2$. Oxidation of one NADH by the ETC leads to formation of three ATP, whereas oxidation of $FADH_2$ produces two ATP (see p. 77). The total yield of ATP from the oxidation of one acetyl CoA is shown in Figure 9.7. Figure 9.8 summarizes the reactions of the TCA cycle. [Note: The cycle does not involve the net consumption or production of intermediates. Two carbons entering as acetyl CoA are balanced by two CO_2 exiting.]

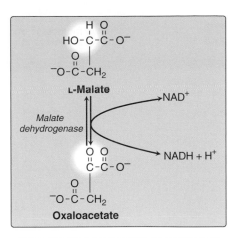

Figure 9.6
Formation (regeneration) of oxaloacetate from malate. NAD(H) = nicotinamide adenine dinucleotide.

Energy-producing reaction	Number of ATP produced
3 NADH $\longrightarrow$ 3 NAD^+	9
$FADH_2 \longrightarrow$ FAD	2
GDP + $P_i \longrightarrow$ GTP	1
	12 ATP/acetyl CoA oxidized

Figure 9.7
Number of ATP molecules produced from the oxidation of one molecule of acetyl coenzyme A (CoA) using both substrate-level and oxidative phosphorylation. NAD(H) and $FAD(H_2)$ = nicotinamide and flavin adenine dinucleotides; GDP and GTP = guanosine di- and triphosphates; P_i = inorganic phosphate.

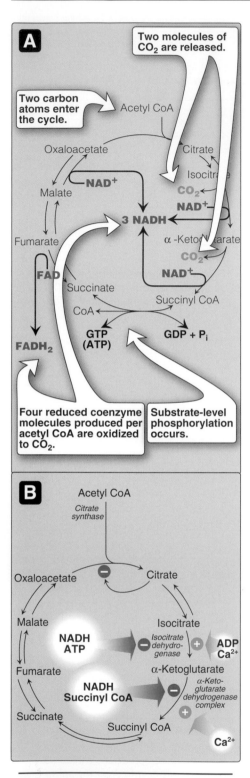

Figure 9.8
A. Production of reduced coenzymes, ATP, and carbon dioxide (CO_2) in the tricarboxylic acid cycle. [Note: Guanosine triphosphate (GTP) and ATP are interconverted by *nucleoside diphosphate kinase*.] B. Inhibitors and activators of the cycle.

IV. CYCLE REGULATION

In contrast to glycolysis, which is regulated primarily by *PFK-1*, the TCA cycle is controlled by the regulation of several enzymes (see Fig. 9.8). The most important of these regulated enzymes are those that catalyze reactions with highly negative ΔG^0: *citrate synthase*, *isocitrate dehydrogenase*, and the *α-ketoglutarate dehydrogenase complex*. Reducing equivalents needed for oxidative phosphorylation are generated by the *PDHC* and the TCA cycle, and both processes are upregulated in response to a decrease in the ATP/ADP ratio.

V. CHAPTER SUMMARY

Pyruvate is oxidatively decarboxylated by the ***pyruvate dehydrogenase complex*** (***PDHC***), producing **acetyl coenzyme A** (**CoA**), which is the major fuel for the **tricarboxylic acid** (**TCA**) **cycle** (Fig. 9.9). The multienzyme *PDHC* requires five coenzymes: **thiamine pyrophosphate**, **lipoic acid**, **flavin adenine dinucleotide** (**FAD**), **nicotinamide adenine dinucleotide** (**NAD⁺**), and **CoA**. The *PDHC* is regulated by covalent modification of *E1* (***pyruvate decarboxylase***) by ***PDH kinase*** and ***PDH phosphatase***: Phosphorylation inhibits *E1*. *PDH kinase* is allosterically activated by ATP, acetyl CoA, and NADH and inhibited by pyruvate. The *phosphatase* is activated by calcium (Ca^{2+}). ***E1 deficiency*** is the most common biochemical cause of **congenital lactic acidosis**. The brain is particularly affected in this **X-linked dominant** disorder. **Arsenic poisoning** causes inactivation of the *PDHC* by binding to lipoic acid. In the TCA cycle, **citrate** is synthesized from **oxaloacetate** (**OAA**) and **acetyl CoA** by *citrate synthase*, which is inhibited by product. Citrate is isomerized to **isocitrate** by *aconitase* (*aconitate hydratase*). Isocitrate is oxidatively decarboxylated by *isocitrate dehydrogenase* to α-ketoglutarate, producing **carbon dioxide** (**CO₂**) and **NADH**. The enzyme is inhibited by ATP and NADH and activated by adenosine diphosphate (ADP) and Ca^{2+}. α-Ketoglutarate is oxidatively decarboxylated to **succinyl CoA** by the ***α-ketoglutarate dehydrogenase complex***, producing CO_2 and NADH. The enzyme is very similar to the *PDHC* and uses the same coenzymes. The *α-ketoglutarate dehydrogenase complex* is activated by Ca^{2+} and inhibited by NADH and succinyl CoA but is not covalently regulated. Succinyl CoA is cleaved by *succinate thiokinase* (also called *succinyl CoA synthetase*), producing **succinate** and guanosine triphosphate (**GTP**). This is an example of **substrate-level phosphorylation**. Succinate is oxidized to **fumarate** by *succinate dehydrogenase*, producing **FADH₂**. Fumarate is hydrated to **malate** by *fumarase* (*fumarate hydratase*), and malate is oxidized to OAA by *malate dehydrogenase*, producing **NADH**. **Three NADH** and **one FADH₂** are produced by one round of the TCA cycle. The generation of acetyl CoA by the oxidation of pyruvate via the *PDHC* also produces an NADH. Oxidation of the NADH and FADH₂ by the ETC yields 14 ATP. The terminal phosphate of the GTP produced by substrate-level phosphorylation in the TCA cycle can be transferred to ADP by *nucleoside diphosphate kinase*, yielding another ATP. Therefore, a total of 15 ATP are produced from the complete mitochondrial oxidation of pyruvate to CO_2.

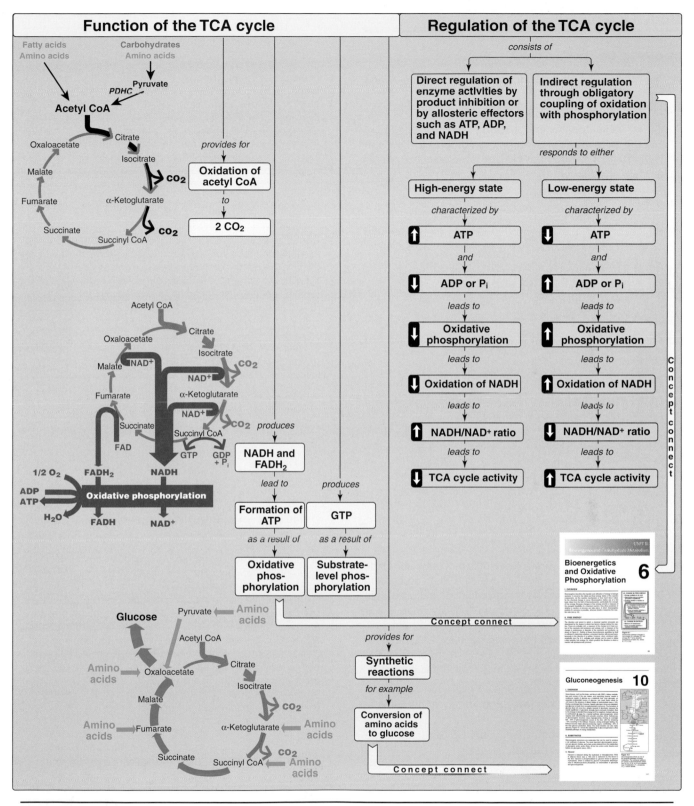

Figure 9.9
Key concept map for the tricarboxylic acid (TCA) cycle. *PDHC = pyruvate dehydrogenase complex*; CoA = coenzyme A; CO_2 = carbon dioxide; NAD(H) = nicotinamide adenine dinucleotide; FAD(H$_2$) = flavin adenine dinucleotide; GDP and GTP = guanosine di- and triphosphates; ADP = adenosine diphosphate; P$_i$ = inorganic phosphate.

Study Questions

Choose the ONE best answer.

9.1 The conversion of pyruvate to acetyl coenzyme A and carbon dioxide:

    A. involves the participation of lipoic acid.

    B. is activated when pyruvate decarboxylase of the pyruvate dehydrogenase complex (PDHC) is phosphorylated by PDH kinase in the presence of ATP.

    C. is reversible.

    D. occurs in the cytosol.

    E. requires the coenzyme biotin.

Correct answer = A. Lipoic acid is an intermediate acceptor of the acetyl group formed in the reaction. [Note: Lipoic acid linked to a lysine residue in E2 functions as a "swinging arm" that allows interaction with E1 and E3.] The PDHC catalyzes an irreversible reaction that is inhibited when the decarboxylase component (E1) is phosphorylated. The PDHC is located in the mitochondrial matrix. Biotin is utilized by carboxylases, not decarboxylases.

9.2 Which one of the following conditions decreases the oxidation of acetyl coenzyme A by the citric acid cycle?

    A. A high availability of calcium

    B. A high acetyl CoA/CoA ratio

    C. A low ATP/ADP ratio

    D. A low NAD^+/NADH ratio

Correct answer = D. A low NAD^+/NADH (oxidized to reduced nicotinamide adenine dinucleotide) ratio limits the rates of the NAD^+-requiring dehydrogenases. High availability of calcium and substrate (acetyl coenzyme A) and a low ATP/ADP (adenosine tri- to diphosphate) ratio stimulate the cycle.

9.3 The following is the sum of three steps in the citric acid cycle.

$$A + B + FAD + H_2O \rightarrow C + FADH_2 + NADH$$

Choose the lettered answer that corresponds to the missing "A," "B," and "C" in the equation.

	Reactant A	Reactant B	Product C
A.	Succinyl CoA	GDP	Succinate
B.	Succinate	NAD^+	Oxaloacetate
C.	Fumarate	NAD^+	Oxaloacetate
D.	Succinate	NAD^+	Malate
E.	Fumarate	GTP	Malate

Correct answer = B. Succinate + NAD^+ + FAD + H_2O → oxaloacetate + NADH + $FADH_2$.

9.4 A 1-month-old male shows neurologic problems and lactic acidosis. Enzyme assay for pyruvate dehydrogenase complex (PDHC) activity on extracts of cultured skin fibroblasts showed 5% of normal activity with a low concentration of thiamine pyrophosphate (TPP) but 80% of normal activity when the assay contained a thousand-fold higher concentration of TPP. Which one of the following statements concerning this patient is correct?

    A. Administration of thiamine is expected to reduce his serum lactate level and improve his clinical symptoms.

    B. A high-carbohydrate diet would be expected to be beneficial for this patient.

    C. Citrate production from aerobic glycolysis is expected to be increased.

    D. PDH kinase, a regulatory enzyme of the PDHC, is expected to be active.

Correct answer = A. The patient appears to have a thiamine-responsive PDHC deficiency. The pyruvate decarboxylase (E1) component of the PDHC fails to bind thiamine pyrophosphate at low concentration but shows significant activity at a high concentration of the coenzyme. This mutation, which affects the K_m (Michaelis constant) of the enzyme for the coenzyme, is present in some, but not all, cases of PDHC deficiency. Because the PDHC is an integral part of carbohydrate metabolism, a diet low in carbohydrates would be expected to blunt the effects of the enzyme deficiency. Aerobic glycolysis generates pyruvate, the substrate of the PDHC. Decreased activity of the complex decreases production of acetyl coenzyme A, a substrate for citrate synthase. Because PDH kinase is allosterically inhibited by pyruvate, it is inactive.

9.5 Which coenzyme–cosubstrate is used by dehydrogenases in both glycolysis and the tricarboxylic acid cycle?

Oxidized nicotinamide adenine dinucleotide (NAD^+) is used by glyceraldehyde 3-phosphate dehydrogenase of glycolysis and by isocitrate dehydrogenase, α-ketoglutarate dehydrogenase, and malate dehydrogenase of the tricarboxylic acid cycle. [Note: E3 of the pyruvate dehydrogenase complex requires oxidized flavin adenine dinucleotide (FAD) and NAD^+.]

Gluconeogenesis

10

I. OVERVIEW

Some tissues, such as the brain, red blood cells (RBC), kidney medulla, lens and cornea of the eye, testes, and exercising muscle, require a continuous supply of glucose as a metabolic fuel. Liver glycogen, an essential postprandial source of glucose, can meet these needs for <24 hours in the absence of dietary intake of carbohydrate (see p. 125). During a prolonged fast, however, hepatic glycogen stores are depleted, and glucose is made from noncarbohydrate precursors. The formation of glucose does not occur by a simple reversal of glycolysis, because the overall equilibrium of glycolysis strongly favors pyruvate formation (that is, the change in standard free energy [ΔG^0] is negative). Instead, glucose is synthesized <u>de</u> <u>novo</u> by a special pathway, gluconeogenesis, which requires both mitochondrial and cytosolic enzymes. [Note: Deficiencies of gluconeogenic enzymes cause hypoglycemia.] During an overnight fast, ~90% of gluconeogenesis occurs in the liver, with the remaining ~10% occurring in the kidneys. However, during prolonged fasting, the kidneys become major glucose-producing organs, contributing ~40% of the total glucose production. [Note: The small intestine can also make glucose.] Figure 10.1 shows the relationship of gluconeogenesis to other essential pathways of energy metabolism.

II. SUBSTRATES

Gluconeogenic precursors are molecules that can be used to produce a net synthesis of glucose. The most important gluconeogenic precursors are glycerol, lactate, and α-keto acids obtained from the metabolism of glucogenic amino acids. [Note: All but two amino acids (leucine and lysine) are glucogenic (see p. 262).]

A. Glycerol

Glycerol is released during the hydrolysis of triacylglycerols (TAG) in adipose tissue (see p. 190) and is delivered by the blood to the liver. Glycerol is phosphorylated by *glycerol kinase* to glycerol 3-phosphate, which is oxidized by *glycerol 3-phosphate dehydrogenase* to dihydroxyacetone phosphate, an intermediate of glycolysis and gluconeogenesis.

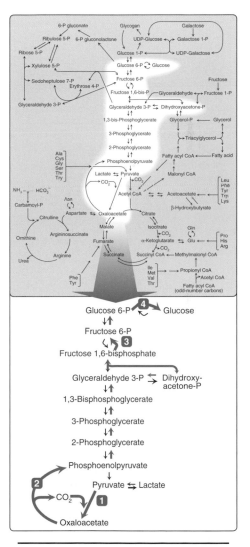

Figure 10.1
Gluconeogenesis shown as one of the essential pathways of energy metabolism. The numbered reactions are unique to gluconeogenesis. [Note: See Fig. 8.2, p. 92, for a more detailed map of metabolism.] P = phosphate; CO_2 = carbon dioxide.

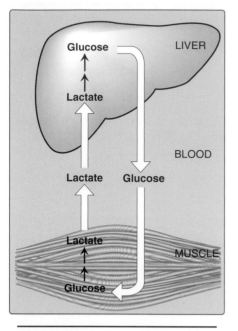

Figure 10.2
The intertissue Cori cycle links gluconeogenesis with glycolysis. [Note: Diffusion of lactate and glucose across membranes is facilitated by transport proteins.]

B. Lactate

Lactate from anaerobic glycolysis is released into the blood by exercising skeletal muscle and by cells that lack mitochondria such as RBC. In the Cori cycle, this lactate is taken up by the liver and oxidized to pyruvate that is converted to glucose, which is released back into the circulation (Fig. 10.2).

C. Amino acids

Amino acids produced by hydrolysis of tissue proteins are the major sources of glucose during a fast. Their metabolism generates α-keto acids, such as pyruvate that is converted to glucose, or α-ketoglutarate that can enter the tricarboxylic acid (TCA) cycle and form oxaloacetate (OAA), a direct precursor of phosphoenolpyruvate (PEP). [Note: Acetyl coenzyme A (CoA) and compounds that give rise only to acetyl CoA (for example, acetoacetate, lysine, and leucine) cannot give rise to a net synthesis of glucose. This is because of the irreversible nature of the *pyruvate dehydrogenase complex* (*PDHC*), which converts pyruvate to acetyl CoA (see p. 109). These compounds give rise instead to ketone bodies (see p. 195) and are termed ketogenic.]

III. REACTIONS

Seven glycolytic reactions are reversible and are used in the synthesis of glucose from lactate or pyruvate. However, three glycolytic reactions are irreversible and must be circumvented by four alternate reactions that energetically favor the synthesis of glucose. These irreversible reactions, which together are unique to gluconeogenesis, are described below.

A. Pyruvate carboxylation

The first roadblock to overcome in the synthesis of glucose from pyruvate is the irreversible conversion in glycolysis of PEP to pyruvate by *pyruvate kinase* (*PK*). In gluconeogenesis, pyruvate is carboxylated by *pyruvate carboxylase* (*PC*) to OAA, which is converted to PEP by *PEP-carboxykinase* (*PEPCK*) (Fig. 10.3).

1. **Biotin:** *PC* requires the coenzyme biotin (see p. 385) covalently bound to the ε-amino group of a lysine residue in the enzyme (see Fig. 10.3). ATP hydrolysis drives formation of an enzyme–biotin–carbon dioxide (CO_2) intermediate, which then carboxylates pyruvate to form OAA. [Note: HCO_3^- provides the CO_2.] The *PC* reaction occurs in the mitochondria of liver and kidney cells and has two purposes: to allow production of PEP, an important substrate for gluconeogenesis, and to provide OAA that can replenish the TCA cycle intermediates that may become depleted. Muscle cells also contain *PC* but use the OAA product only for the replenishment (anaplerotic) purpose and do not synthesize glucose. [Note: Pyruvate carrier protein moves pyruvate from the cytosol into mitochondria.]

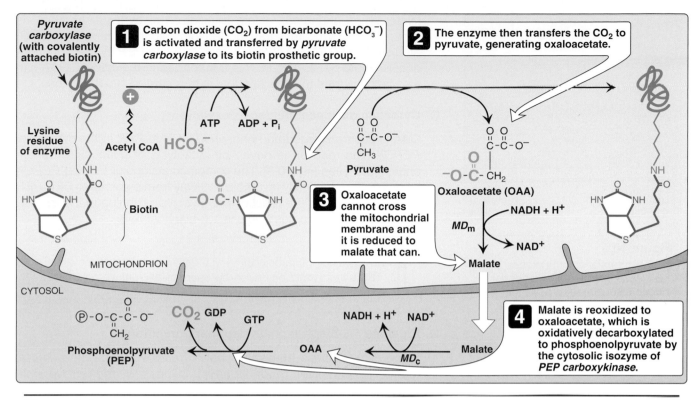

Figure 10.3
PEP synthesis in the cytosol. [Note: The process moves nicotinamide adenine dinucleotide (NADH) reducing equivalents required for gluconeogenesis out of mitochondria into the cytosol.] MD_m and MD_c = mitochondrial and cytosolic isozymes of *malate dehydrogenase*; GTP and GDP = guanosine tri- and diphosphates; ADP = adenosine diphosphate.

> *PC* is one of several *carboxylases* that require biotin. Others include *acetyl CoA carboxylase* (p. 183), *propionyl CoA carboxylase* (p. 194), and *methylcrotonyl CoA carboxylase* (p. 266).

2. **Allosteric regulation:** *PC* is allosterically activated by acetyl CoA. Elevated levels of acetyl CoA in mitochondria signal a metabolic state in which increased synthesis of OAA is required. For example, this occurs during fasting, when OAA is used for gluconeogenesis in the liver and kidneys. Conversely, at low levels of acetyl CoA, *PC* is largely inactive, and pyruvate is primarily oxidized by the *PDHC* to acetyl CoA that can be further oxidized by the TCA cycle (see p. 109).

B. Oxaloacetate transport to the cytosol

For gluconeogenesis to continue, OAA must be converted to PEP by *PEPCK*. PEP production in the cytosol requires transport of OAA out of mitochondria. However, there is no OAA transporter in the inner mitochondrial membrane, and OAA is first reduced to malate by mitochondrial *malate dehydrogenase* (*MD*). Malate is transported into the cytosol and reoxidized to OAA by cytosolic *MD* as nicotinamide adenine dinucleotide (NAD^+) is reduced to NADH (see Fig. 10.3). The NADH is used in the reduction of 1,3-bisphosphoglycerate to glyceraldehyde 3-phosphate by *glyceraldehyde 3-phosphate dehydrogenase* (see p. 101), a reaction common to glycolysis and gluconeogenesis.

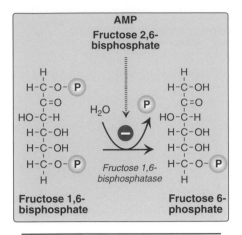

Figure 10.4
Dephosphorylation of fructose 1,6-bisphosphate. AMP = adenosine monophosphate; (P) = phosphate.

[Note: When abundant, lactate is oxidized to pyruvate as NAD^+ is reduced. The pyruvate is transported into mitochondria and carboxylated by *PC* to OAA, which can be converted to PEP by the mitochondrial isozyme of *PEPCK*. PEP is transported to the cytosol. OAA can also be converted to aspartate that is transported into the cytosol.]

C. Cytosolic oxaloacetate decarboxylation

OAA is decarboxylated and phosphorylated to PEP in the cytosol by *PEPCK*. The reaction is driven by hydrolysis of guanosine triphosphate ([GTP] see Fig. 10.3). The combined actions of *PC* and *PEPCK* provide an energetically favorable pathway from pyruvate to PEP. PEP is then acted on by the reactions of glycolysis running in the reverse direction until it becomes fructose 1,6-bisphosphate.

> The pairing of carboxylation with decarboxylation drives reactions that would otherwise be energetically unfavorable. This strategy is also used in fatty acid (FA) synthesis (see p. 184).

D. Fructose 1,6-bisphosphate dephosphorylation

Hydrolysis of fructose 1,6-bisphosphate by *fructose 1,6-bisphosphatase*, found in the liver and kidneys, bypasses the irreversible *phosphofructokinase-1* (*PFK-1*) reaction of glycolysis and provides an energetically favorable pathway for the formation of fructose 6-phosphate (Fig. 10.4). This reaction is an important regulatory site of gluconeogenesis.

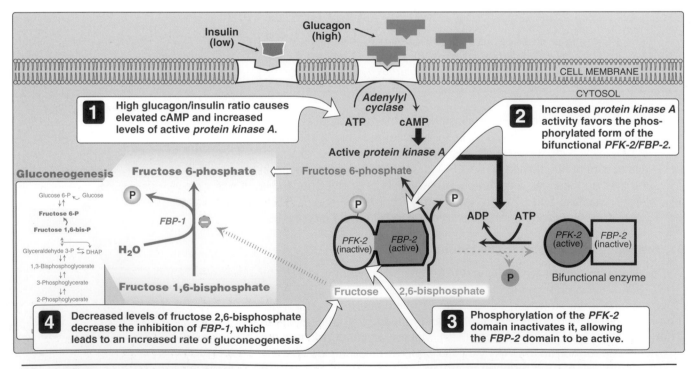

Figure 10.5
Effect of elevated glucagon on the intracellular concentration of fructose 2,6-bisphosphate in the liver. AMP and ADP = adenosine mono- and diphosphates; cAMP = cyclic AMP; *PFK-2 = phosphofructokinase-2*; *FBP-2 = fructose 2,6-bisphosphatase*; *FBP-1 = fructose 1,6-bisphosphatase*; (P) and (P) = phosphate.

1. **Regulation by intracellular energy levels:** *Fructose 1,6-bisphosphatase* is inhibited by a rise in the adenosine monophosphate (AMP)/ATP ratio, which signals a low-energy state in the cell. Conversely, low AMP and high ATP levels stimulate gluconeogenesis, an energy-requiring pathway.

2. **Regulation by fructose 2,6-bisphosphate:** *Fructose 1,6-bisphosphatase* is inhibited by fructose 2,6-bisphosphate, an allosteric effector whose concentration is influenced by the insulin/glucagon ratio. When glucagon is high, the effector is not made by hepatic *PFK-2* (see p. 99), and thus, the *phosphatase* is active (Fig. 10.5). [Note: The signals that inhibit (low energy, high fructose 2,6-bisphosphate) or activate (high energy, low fructose 2,6-bisphosphate) gluconeogenesis have the opposite effect on glycolysis, providing reciprocal control of the pathways that synthesize and oxidize glucose (see p. 100).]

E. Glucose 6-phosphate dephosphorylation

Glucose 6-phosphate hydrolysis by *glucose 6-phosphatase* bypasses the irreversible *hexokinase/glucokinase* reaction and provides an energetically favorable pathway for the formation of free glucose (Fig. 10.6). The liver is the primary organ that produces free glucose from glucose 6-phosphate. This process requires a complex of two proteins found only in gluconeogenic tissue: glucose 6-phosphate translocase, which transports glucose 6-phosphate across the endoplasmic reticular (ER) membrane, and *glucose 6-phosphatase*, which removes the phosphate, producing free glucose (see Fig. 10.6). [Note: These ER membrane proteins are also required for the final step of glycogen degradation (see p. 130). Glycogen storage diseases Ia and Ib, caused by deficiencies in the *phosphatase* and the translocase, respectively, are characterized by severe fasting hypoglycemia, because free glucose is unable to be produced from either gluconeogenesis or glycogenolysis.] Specific transporters are responsible for moving the free glucose into the cytosol and then into blood.

F. Summary of the reactions of glycolysis and gluconeogenesis

Of the 11 reactions required to convert pyruvate to free glucose, 7 are catalyzed by reversible glycolytic enzymes (Fig. 10.7). The 3 irreversible reactions (catalyzed by *hexokinase/glucokinase*, *PFK-1*, and *PK*) are circumvented by reactions catalyzed by *glucose 6-phosphatase*, *fructose 1,6-bisphosphatase*, *PC*, and *PEPCK*. In gluconeogenesis, the equilibria of the reversible glycolytic reactions are pushed toward glucose synthesis as a result of the essentially irreversible formation of PEP, fructose 6-phosphate, and glucose by the gluconeogenic enzymes. [Note: The stoichiometry of gluconeogenesis from two pyruvate molecules couples the cleavage of six high-energy phosphate bonds and the oxidation of two NADH with the formation of one glucose molecule (see Fig. 10.7).]

IV. REGULATION

The moment-to-moment regulation of gluconeogenesis is determined primarily by the circulating level of glucagon and by the availability of gluconeogenic substrates. In addition, slow adaptive changes in enzyme

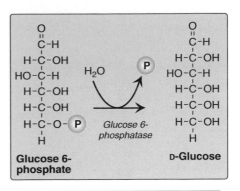

Figure 10.6
Dephosphorylation of glucose 6-phosphate allows release of free glucose from gluconeogenic tissues (primarily the liver) into blood. P = phosphate.

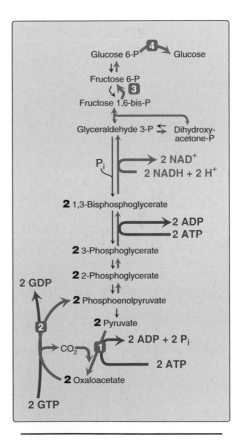

Figure 10.7
Summary of the reactions of glycolysis and gluconeogenesis, showing the energy requirements of gluconeogenesis. The numbered reactions are unique to gluconeogenesis. P = phosphate; GDP and GTP = guanosine di- and triphosphates; NAD(H) = nicotinamide adenine dinucleotide; ADP = adenosine diphosphate.

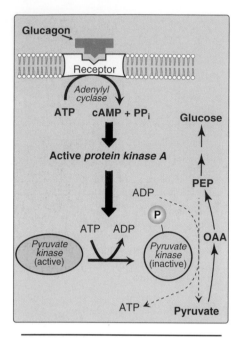

Figure 10.8
Covalent modification of *pyruvate kinase* results in inactivation of the enzyme. [Note: Only the hepatic isozyme is subject to covalent regulation.] OAA = oxaloacetate; PEP = phosphoenolpyruvate; PP_i = pyrophosphate; (P) = phosphate; AMP and ADP = adenosine mono- and diphosphates; cAMP = cyclic AMP.

amount result from an alteration in the rate of enzyme synthesis or degradation or both. [Note: Hormonal control of the glucoregulatory system is presented in Chapter 23.]

A. Glucagon

This peptide hormone from pancreatic islet α cells (see p. 313) stimulates gluconeogenesis by three mechanisms.

1. **Changes in allosteric effectors:** Glucagon lowers hepatic fructose 2,6-bisphosphate, resulting in *fructose 1,6-bisphosphatase* activation and *PFK-1* inhibition, thereby favoring gluconeogenesis over glycolysis (see Fig. 10.5). [Note: See pp. 99–100 for the role of fructose 2,6-bisphosphate in glycolysis regulation.]

2. **Covalent modification of enzyme activity:** Glucagon binds its G protein–coupled receptor (see p. 95) and, via an elevation in cyclic AMP (cAMP) level and *cAMP-dependent protein kinase A* activity, stimulates the conversion of hepatic *PK* to its inactive (phosphorylated) form. This decreases PEP conversion to pyruvate, which has the effect of diverting PEP to gluconeogenesis (Fig. 10.8).

3. **Induction of enzyme synthesis:** Glucagon increases transcription of the gene for *PEPCK* via the transcription factor cAMP response element–binding (CREB) protein, thereby increasing the availability of this enzyme as levels of its substrate rise during fasting. [Note: Cortisol (a glucocorticoid) also increases expression of the gene, whereas insulin decreases expression.]

B. Substrate availability

The availability of gluconeogenic precursors, particularly glucogenic amino acids, significantly influences the rate of glucose synthesis. Decreased insulin levels favor mobilization of amino acids from muscle protein to provide the carbon skeletons for gluconeogenesis. The ATP and NADH coenzymes required for gluconeogenesis are primarily provided by FA oxidation.

C. Allosteric activation by acetyl CoA

Allosteric activation of hepatic *PC* by acetyl CoA occurs during fasting. As a result of increased TAG hydrolysis in adipose tissue, the liver is flooded with FA (see p. 330). The rate of formation of acetyl CoA by β-oxidation of these FA exceeds the capacity of the liver to oxidize it to CO_2 and water. As a result, acetyl CoA accumulates and activates *PC*. [Note: Acetyl CoA inhibits the *PDHC* (by activating *PDH kinase*; see p. 111). Thus, this single compound can divert pyruvate toward gluconeogenesis and away from the TCA cycle (Fig. 10.9).]

D. Allosteric inhibition by AMP

Fructose 1,6-bisphosphatase is inhibited by AMP, a compound that activates *PFK-1*. This results in reciprocal regulation of glycolysis and gluconeogenesis seen previously with fructose 2,6-bisphosphate (see p. 121). [Note: Thus, elevated AMP stimulates energy-producing pathways and inhibits energy-requiring ones.]

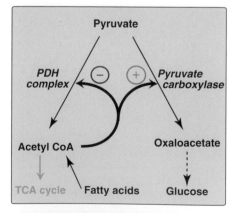

Figure 10.9
Acetyl coenzyme A (CoA) diverts pyruvate away from oxidation and toward gluconeogenesis. *PDH = pyruvate dehydrogenase*; TCA = tricarboxylic acid.

V. CHAPTER SUMMARY

Gluconeogenic precursors include **glycerol** released during triacylglycerol hydrolysis in adipose tissue, **lactate** released by cells that lack mitochondria and by exercising skeletal muscle, and **α-keto acids** (for example, **α-ketoglutarate** and **pyruvate**) derived from glucogenic amino acid metabolism (Fig. 10.10). Seven of the reactions of glycolysis are reversible and are used for gluconeogenesis in the liver and kidneys. Three reactions, catalyzed by *pyruvate kinase*, *phosphofructokinase-1*, and *glucokinase/hexokinase*, are **physiologically irreversible** and must be circumvented. **Pyruvate** is converted to **oxaloacetate** and then to **phosphoenolpyruvate** (**PEP**) by *pyruvate carboxylase* (*PC*) and *PEP-carboxykinase* (*PEPCK*). *PC* requires **biotin** and **ATP** and is allosterically activated by **acetyl coenzyme A**. *PEPCK* requires **guanosine triphosphate**. Transcription of its gene is increased by glucagon and cortisol and decreased by insulin. **Fructose 1,6-bisphosphate** is converted to **fructose 6-phosphate** by *fructose 1,6-bisphosphatase*. This enzyme is inhibited by a high **adenosine monophosphate** (**AMP**)/**ATP** ratio. It is also inhibited by **fructose 2,6-bisphosphate**, the primary allosteric activator of glycolysis. **Glucose 6-phosphate** is dephosphorylated to **glucose** by *glucose 6-phosphatase*. This enzyme of the endoplasmic reticular membrane catalyzes the final step in gluconeogenesis and in glycogen degradation. Its deficiency results in severe, fasting hypoglycemia.

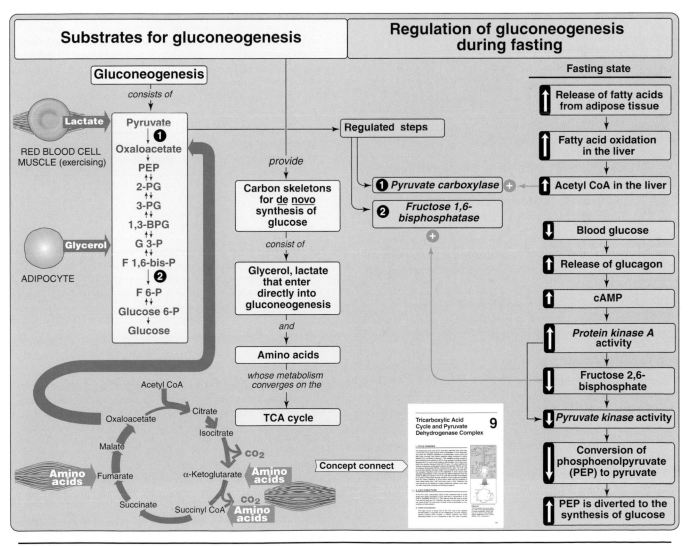

Figure 10.10

Key concept map for gluconeogenesis. TCA = tricarboxylic acid. CoA = coenzyme A; cAMP = cyclic adenosine monophosphate; P = phosphate; (B)PG = (bis)phosphoglycerate; G = glyceraldehyde; F = fructose; CO_2 = carbon dioxide.

Study Questions

Choose the ONE best answer.

10.1 Which one of the following statements concerning gluconeogenesis is correct?

    A. It is an energy-producing (exergonic) process.

    B. It is important in maintaining blood glucose during a 2-day fast.

    C. It is inhibited by a fall in the insulin/glucagon ratio.

    D. It occurs in the cytosol of muscle cells.

    E. It uses carbon skeletons provided by fatty acid degradation.

Correct answer = B. During a 2-day fast, glycogen stores are depleted, and gluconeogenesis maintains blood glucose. This is an energy-requiring (endergonic) pathway (both ATP and GTP get hydrolyzed) that occurs primarily in the liver, with the kidneys becoming major glucose producers in prolonged fasting. Gluconeogenesis uses both mitochondrial and cytosolic enzymes and is stimulated by a fall in the insulin/glucagon ratio. Fatty acid degradation yields acetyl coenzyme A (CoA), which cannot be converted to glucose. This is because there is no net gain of carbons from acetyl CoA in the tricarboxylic acid cycle, and the pyruvate dehydrogenase complex is physiologically irreversible. It is the carbon skeletons of most amino acids that are glucogenic.

10.2 Which reaction in the diagram below would be inhibited in the presence of large amounts of avidin, an egg white protein that binds and sequesters biotin?

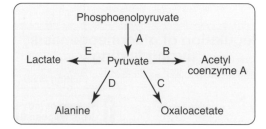

10.3 Which one of the following reactions is unique to gluconeogenesis?

    A. 1,3-Bisphosphoglycerate → 3-phosphoglycerate

    B. Lactate → pyruvate

    C. Oxaloacetate → phosphoenolpyruvate

    D. Phosphoenolpyruvate → pyruvate

Correct answer = C. Pyruvate is carboxylated to oxaloacetate by pyruvate carboxylase, a biotin-requiring enzyme. B (pyruvate dehydrogenase complex) requires thiamine pyrophosphate, lipoic acid, flavin and nicotinamide adenine dinucleotides (FAD and NAD$^+$), and coenzyme A; D (transaminase) requires pyridoxal phosphate; E (lactate dehydrogenase) requires NADH.

Correct answer = C. The other reactions are common to both gluconeogenesis and glycolysis.

10.4 Use the chart below to show the effect of adenosine monophosphate (AMP) and fructose 2,6-bisphosphate on the listed enzymes of gluconeogenesis and glycolysis.

Enzyme	Fructose 2,6-bisphosphate	AMP
Fructose 1,6-bisphosphatase		
Phosphofructokinase-1		

Both fructose 2,6-bisphosphate and adenosine monophosphate inhibit fructose 1,6-bisphosphatase of gluconeogenesis and activate phosphofructokinase-1 of glycolysis. This results in reciprocal regulation of the two pathways.

10.5 The metabolism of ethanol by alcohol dehydrogenase produces reduced nicotinamide adenine dinucleotide (NADH) from the oxidized (NAD$^+$) form. What effect is the fall in the NAD$^+$/NADH ratio expected to have on gluconeogenesis? Explain.

The increase in NADH as ethanol is oxidized decreases the availability of oxaloacetate (OAA) because the reversible oxidation of malate to OAA by malate dehydrogenase of the tricarboxylic acid cycle is driven in the reverse direction by NADH. Additionally, the reversible reduction of pyruvate to lactate by lactate dehydrogenase is driven to lactate by NADH. Thus, two important gluconeogenic substrates, OAA and pyruvate, decrease as a result of the increase in NADH during ethanol metabolism. Consequently, gluconeogenesis decreases.

10.6 Given that acetyl coenzyme A cannot be a substrate for gluconeogenesis, why is its production in fatty acid oxidation essential for gluconeogenesis?

Acetyl coenzyme A inhibits the pyruvate dehydrogenase complex and activates pyruvate carboxylase, pushing pyruvate to gluconeogenesis and away from oxidation.

Glycogen Metabolism

I. OVERVIEW

A constant source of blood glucose is an absolute requirement for human life. Glucose is the greatly preferred energy source for the brain and the required energy source for cells with few or no mitochondria such as mature red blood cells. Glucose is also essential as an energy source for exercising muscle, where it is the substrate for anaerobic glycolysis. Blood glucose can be obtained from three primary sources: the diet, glycogen degradation, and gluconeogenesis. Dietary intake of glucose and glucose precursors, such as starch (a polysaccharide), disaccharides, and monosaccharides, is sporadic and, depending on the diet, is not always a reliable source of blood glucose. In contrast, gluconeogenesis (see p. 117) can provide sustained synthesis of glucose, but it is somewhat slow in responding to a falling blood glucose level. Therefore, the body has developed mechanisms for storing a supply of glucose in a rapidly mobilized form, namely, glycogen. In the absence of a dietary source of glucose, this sugar is rapidly released into the blood from liver glycogen. Similarly, muscle glycogen is extensively degraded in exercising muscle to provide that tissue with an important energy source. When glycogen stores are depleted, specific tissues synthesize glucose de novo, using glycerol, lactate, pyruvate, and amino acids as carbon sources for gluconeogenesis (see Chapter 10). Figure 11.1 shows the reactions of glycogen synthesis and degradation as part of the essential pathways of energy metabolism.

II. STRUCTURE AND FUNCTION

The main stores of glycogen are found in skeletal muscle and liver, although most other cells store small amounts of glycogen for their own use. The function of muscle glycogen is to serve as a fuel reserve for the synthesis of ATP during muscle contraction. That of liver glycogen is to maintain the blood glucose concentration, particularly during the early stages of a fast (Fig. 11.2; also see p. 329). [Note: Liver glycogen can maintain blood glucose for <24 hours.]

A. Amounts in liver and muscle

Approximately 400 g of glycogen make up 1%–2% of the fresh weight of resting muscle, and ~100 g of glycogen make up to 10% of the fresh weight of a well-fed adult liver. What limits the production of

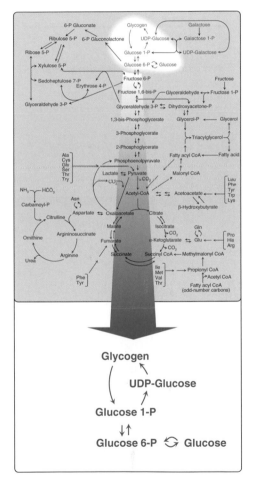

Figure 11.1
Glycogen synthesis and degradation shown as a part of the essential pathways of energy metabolism. [Note: See Fig. 8.2, p. 92, for a more detailed map of metabolism.] P = phosphate; UDP = uridine diphosphate.

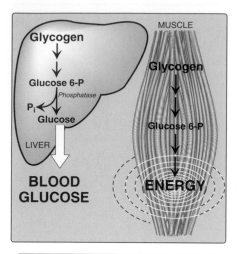

Figure 11.2

Functions of muscle and liver glycogen. [Note: The presence of *glucose 6-phosphatase* in liver allows release of glucose into blood.] P = phosphate; P_i = inorganic phosphate.

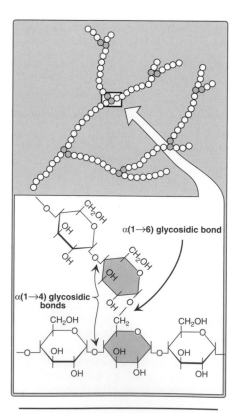

Figure 11.3

Branched structure of glycogen, showing $\alpha(1\rightarrow4)$ and $\alpha(1\rightarrow6)$ glycosidic bonds.

glycogen at these levels is not clear. However, in some glycogen storage diseases (GSD) (see Fig. 11.8), the amount of glycogen in the liver and/or muscle can be significantly higher. [Note: In the body, muscle mass is greater than liver mass. Consequently, most of the body's glycogen is found in skeletal muscle.]

B. Structure

Glycogen is a branched-chain polysaccharide made exclusively from α-D-glucose. The primary glycosidic bond is an $\alpha(1\rightarrow4)$ linkage. After an average of 8–14 glucosyl residues, there is a branch containing an $\alpha(1\rightarrow6)$ linkage (Fig. 11.3). A single glycogen molecule can contain up to 55,000 glucosyl residues. These polymers of glucose exist as large, spherical, cytoplasmic granules (particles) that also contain most of the enzymes necessary for glycogen synthesis and degradation.

C. Glycogen store fluctuation

Liver glycogen stores increase during the well-fed state (see p. 323) and are depleted during a fast (see p. 329). Muscle glycogen is not affected by short periods of fasting (a few days) and is only moderately decreased in prolonged fasting (weeks). Muscle glycogen is synthesized to replenish muscle stores after they have been depleted following strenuous exercise. [Note: Glycogen synthesis and degradation go on continuously. The difference between the rates of these two processes determines the levels of stored glycogen during specific physiologic states.]

III. SYNTHESIS (GLYCOGENESIS)

Glycogen is synthesized from molecules of α-D-glucose. The process occurs in the cytosol and requires energy supplied by ATP (for the phosphorylation of glucose) and uridine triphosphate (UTP).

A. Uridine diphosphate glucose synthesis

α-D-Glucose attached to uridine diphosphate (UDP) is the source of all the glucosyl residues that are added to the growing glycogen molecule. UDP-glucose (Fig. 11.4) is synthesized from glucose 1-phosphate and UTP by *UDP–glucose pyrophosphorylase* (Fig. 11.5). Pyrophosphate (PP_i), the second product of the reaction, is hydrolyzed to two inorganic phosphates (P_i) by *pyrophosphatase*. The hydrolysis is exergonic, insuring that the *UDP–glucose pyrophosphorylase* reaction proceeds in the direction of UDP-glucose production. [Note: Glucose 1-phosphate is generated from glucose 6-phosphate by *phosphoglucomutase*. Glucose 1,6-bisphosphate is an obligatory intermediate in this reversible reaction (Fig. 11.6).]

B. Primer requirement and synthesis

Glycogen synthase makes the $\alpha(1\rightarrow4)$ linkages in glycogen. This enzyme cannot initiate chain synthesis using free glucose as an acceptor of a molecule of glucose from UDP-glucose. Instead, it can only elongate already existing chains of glucose and, therefore, requires a primer. A fragment of glycogen can serve as a primer. In the absence of a fragment, the homodimeric protein *glycogenin* can serve as an acceptor of glucose from UDP-glucose (see Fig. 11.5). The side-chain hydroxyl group of tyrosine-194 in the protein is the site at which the initial glucosyl unit is attached. Because the reaction is catalyzed by *glycogenin* itself via autoglucosylation, *glycogenin* is an enzyme. *Glycogenin* then catalyzes the transfer of at least four molecules of glucose from UDP-glucose, producing a short, $\alpha(1\rightarrow4)$-linked glucosyl chain. This short chain serves as a primer that is able to be elongated by *glycogen synthase*, which is recruited by *glycogenin*, as described in C. below. [Note: *Glycogenin* stays associated with and forms the core of a glycogen granule.]

C. Elongation by glycogen synthase

Elongation of a glycogen chain involves the transfer of glucose from UDP-glucose to the nonreducing end of the growing chain, forming a new glycosidic bond between the anomeric hydroxyl group of carbon 1 of the activated glucose and carbon 4 of the accepting glucosyl residue (see Fig. 11.5). [Note: The nonreducing end of a carbohydrate chain is one in which the anomeric carbon of the terminal sugar is linked by a glycosidic bond to another molecule, making the terminal sugar nonreducing (see p. 84).] The enzyme responsible for making the $\alpha(1\rightarrow4)$ linkages in glycogen is *glycogen synthase*. [Note: The UDP released when the new $\alpha(1\rightarrow4)$ glycosidic bond is made can be phosphorylated to UTP by *nucleoside diphosphate kinase* (UDP + ATP $\rightleftarrows$ UTP + ADP; see p. 296).]

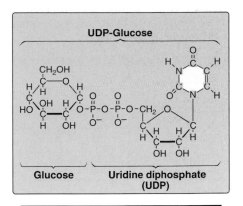

Figure 11.4
The structure of UDP-glucose, a nucleotide sugar.

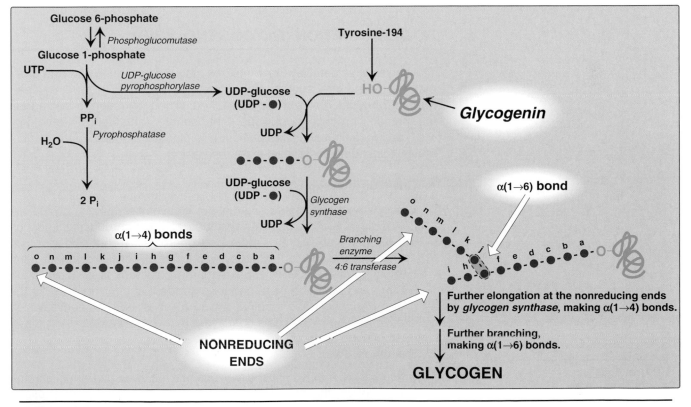

Figure 11.5
Glycogen synthesis. UDP and UTP = uridine di- and triphosphates; PP_i = pyrophosphate; P_i = inorganic phosphate.

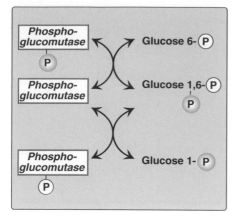

Figure 11.6
Interconversion of
glucose 6-phosphate and
glucose 1-phosphate by
phosphoglucomutase. (P) and (P) =
phosphate.

D. Branch formation

If no other synthetic enzyme acted on the chain, the resulting structure would be a linear (unbranched) chain of glucosyl residues attached by α(1→4) linkages. Such a compound is found in plant tissues and is called amylose. In contrast, glycogen has branches located, on average, eight glucosyl residues apart, resulting in a highly branched, tree-like structure (see Fig. 11.3) that is far more soluble than the unbranched amylose. Branching also increases the number of nonreducing ends to which new glucosyl residues can be added (and also, as described in IV. below, from which these residues can be removed), thereby greatly accelerating the rate at which glycogen synthesis can occur and dramatically increasing the size of the glycogen molecule.

1. **Branch synthesis:** Branches are made by the action of the branching enzyme, *amylo-α(1→4)→α(1→6)-transglycosylase*. This enzyme removes a set of six to eight glucosyl residues from the nonreducing end of the glycogen chain, breaking an α(1→4) bond to another residue on the chain, and attaches it to a nonterminal glucosyl residue by an α(1→6) linkage, thus functioning as a *4:6 transferase*. The resulting new, nonreducing end (see "i" in Fig. 11.5), as well as the old nonreducing end from which the six to eight residues were removed (see "o" in Fig. 11.5), can now be further elongated by *glycogen synthase*.

2. **Additional branch synthesis:** After elongation of these two ends has been accomplished, their terminal six to eight glucosyl residues can be removed and used to make additional branches.

IV. DEGRADATION (GLYCOGENOLYSIS)

The degradative pathway that mobilizes stored glycogen in liver and skeletal muscle is not a reversal of the synthetic reactions. Instead, a separate set of cytosolic enzymes is required. When glycogen is degraded, the primary product is glucose 1-phosphate, obtained by breaking α(1→4) glycosidic bonds. In addition, free glucose is released from each α(1→6)–linked glucosyl residue (branch point).

A. Chain shortening

Glycogen phosphorylase sequentially cleaves the α(1→4) glycosidic bonds between the glucosyl residues at the nonreducing ends of the glycogen chains by simple phosphorolysis (producing glucose 1-phosphate) until four glucosyl units remain on each chain at a branch point (Fig. 11.7). The resulting structure is called a limit dextrin, and *phosphorylase* cannot degrade it any further (Fig. 11.8). [Note: *Phosphorylase* requires pyridoxal phosphate (a derivative of vitamin B_6; see p. 382) as a coenzyme.]

B. Branch removal

Branches are removed by the two enzymic activities of a single bifunctional protein, the debranching enzyme (see Fig. 11.8). First, *oligo-α(1→4)→α(1→4)-glucantransferase* activity removes the outer three of the four glucosyl residues remaining at a branch. It next transfers

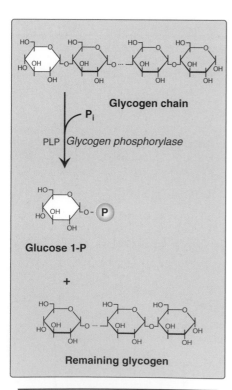

Figure 11.7
Cleavage of an α(1→4)-glycosidic
bond. PLP = pyridoxal phosphate;
P_i = inorganic phosphate; (P) =
phosphate.

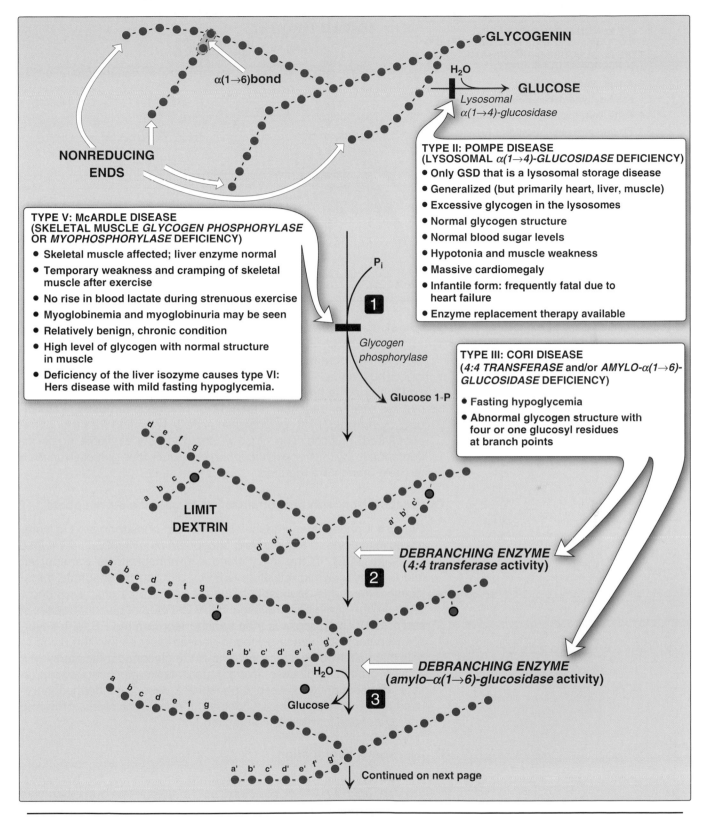

Figure 11.8

Glycogen degradation, showing some of the glycogen storage diseases (GSD). [Note: GSD type IV: Andersen disease is caused by defects in *branching enzyme*, an enzyme of synthesis, resulting in liver cirrhosis that can be fatal in early childhood.] P_i = inorganic phosphate; P = phosphate. (*Continued on next page.*)

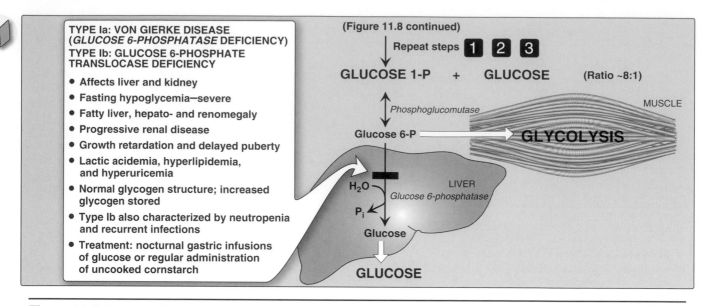

Figure 11.8 (*Continued from the previous page.*)
Glycogen degradation, showing some of the glycogen storage diseases (GSD).

them to the nonreducing end of another chain, lengthening it accordingly. Thus, an $\alpha(1\rightarrow4)$ bond is broken and an $\alpha(1\rightarrow4)$ bond is made, and the enzyme functions as a *4:4 transferase*. Next, the remaining glucose residue attached in an $\alpha(1\rightarrow6)$ linkage is removed hydrolytically by *amylo-$\alpha(1\rightarrow6)$-glucosidase* activity, releasing free (nonphosphorylated) glucose. The glucosyl chain is now available again for degradation by *glycogen phosphorylase* until four glucosyl units in the next branch are reached.

C. Glucose 1-phosphate isomerization to glucose 6-phosphate

Glucose 1-phosphate, produced by *glycogen phosphorylase*, is isomerized in the cytosol to glucose 6-phosphate by *phosphoglucomutase* (see Fig. 11.6). In the liver, glucose 6-phosphate is transported into the endoplasmic reticulum (ER) by glucose 6-phosphate translocase. There, it is dephosphorylated to glucose by *glucose 6-phosphatase* (the same enzyme used in the last step of gluconeogenesis; see p. 121). The glucose is then transported from the ER to the cytosol. Hepatocytes release glycogen-derived glucose into the blood to help maintain blood glucose levels until the gluconeogenic pathway is actively producing glucose. [Note: Muscle lacks *glucose 6-phosphatase*. Consequently, glucose 6-phosphate cannot be dephosphorylated and sent into the blood. Instead, it enters glycolysis, providing energy needed for muscle contraction.]

D. Lysosomal degradation

A small amount (1%–3%) of glycogen is degraded by the lysosomal enzyme, *acid $\alpha(1\rightarrow4)$-glucosidase* (*acid maltase*). The purpose of this autophagic pathway is unknown. However, a deficiency of this enzyme causes accumulation of glycogen in vacuoles in the lysosomes, resulting in the serious GSD type II: Pompe disease (see Fig. 11.8). [Note: Pompe disease is the only GSD that is a lysosomal storage disease.]

> Lysosomal storage diseases are genetic disorders characterized by the accumulation of abnormal amounts of carbohydrates or lipids primarily due to their decreased lysosomal degradation resulting from decreased activity or amount of lysosomal *acid hydrolases*.

V. GLYCOGENESIS AND GLYCOGENOLYSIS REGULATION

Because of the importance of maintaining blood glucose levels, the synthesis and degradation of its glycogen storage form are tightly regulated. In the liver, glycogenesis accelerates during periods when the body has been well fed, whereas glycogenolysis accelerates during periods of fasting. In skeletal muscle, glycogenolysis occurs during active exercise, and glycogenesis begins as soon as the muscle is again at rest. Regulation of synthesis and degradation is accomplished on two levels. First, *glycogen synthase* and *glycogen phosphorylase* are hormonally regulated (by covalent phosphorylation/dephosphorylation) to meet the needs of the body as a whole. Second, these same enzymes are allosterically regulated (by effector molecules) to meet the needs of a particular tissue.

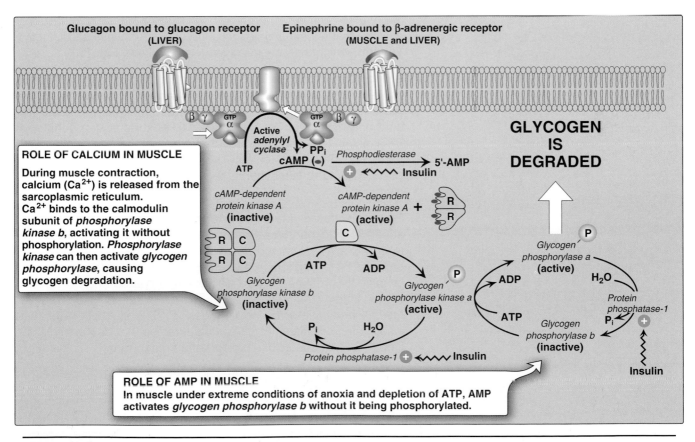

Figure 11.9
Stimulation and inhibition of glycogen degradation. AMP = adenosine monophosphate; cAMP = cyclic AMP; GTP = guanosine triphosphate; P = phosphate; PP_i = pyrophosphate; R = regulatory subunit; C = catalytic subunit.

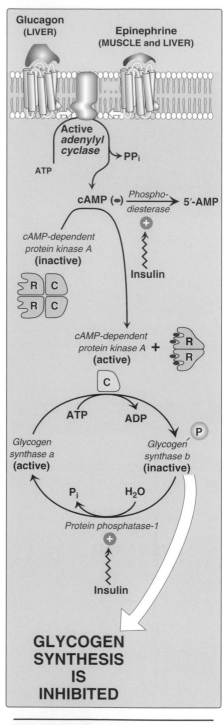

Figure 11.10
Hormonal regulation of glycogen synthesis. [Note: In contrast to *glycogen phosphorylase, glycogen synthase* is inactivated by phosphorylation.] cAMP = cyclic adenosine monophosphate; Ⓟ = phosphate; PPᵢ = pyrophosphate; R = regulatory subunit; C = catalytic subunit; ADP = adenosine diphosphate.

A. Covalent activation of glycogenolysis

The binding of hormones, such as glucagon or epinephrine, to plasma membrane G protein–coupled receptors ([GPCR] see p. 94) signals the need for glycogen to be degraded, either to elevate blood glucose levels or to provide energy for exercising muscle.

1. **Protein kinase A activation:** Binding of glucagon or epinephrine to their specific hepatocyte GPCR, or of epinephrine to a specific myocyte GPCR, results in the G protein–mediated activation of *adenylyl cyclase*. This enzyme catalyzes the synthesis of cyclic adenosine monophosphate (cAMP), which activates *cAMP-dependent protein kinase A* (*PKA*). cAMP binds the two regulatory subunits of tetrameric *PKA*, releasing two individual catalytic subunits that are active (Fig. 11.9; also see p. 95). *PKA* then phosphorylates several enzymes of glycogen metabolism, affecting their activity. [Note: When cAMP is removed, the inactive tetramer reforms.]

2. **Phosphorylase kinase activation:** *Phosphorylase kinase* exists in two forms: an inactive "b" form and an active "a" form. Active *PKA* phosphorylates the inactive "b" form of *phosphorylase kinase*, producing the active "a" form (see Fig. 11.9).

3. **Glycogen phosphorylase activation:** *Glycogen phosphorylase* also exists in a dephosphorylated, inactive "b" form and a phosphorylated, active "a" form. *Phosphorylase kinase a* is the only enzyme that phosphorylates *glycogen phosphorylase b* to its active "a" form, which then begins glycogenolysis (see Fig. 11.9).

4. **Signal amplification:** The cascade of reactions described above activates glycogenolysis. The large number of sequential steps serves to amplify the effect of the hormonal signal (that is, a few hormone molecules binding to their GPCR result in a number of *PKA* molecules being activated that can each activate many *phosphorylase kinase* molecules). This causes the production of many active *glycogen phosphorylase a* molecules that can degrade glycogen.

5. **Phosphorylated state maintenance:** The phosphate groups added to *phosphorylase kinase* and *phosphorylase* in response to cAMP are maintained because the enzyme that hydrolytically removes the phosphate, *protein phosphatase-1* (*PP1*), is inactivated by inhibitor proteins that are also phosphorylated and activated in response to cAMP (see Fig. 11.9). [Note: *PP1* is activated by a signal cascade initiated by insulin (see Fig. 27.7 on p. 311). Because insulin also activates the *phosphodiesterase* that degrades cAMP, it opposes the effects of glucagon and epinephrine.]

B. Covalent inhibition of glycogenesis

The regulated enzyme in glycogenesis, *glycogen synthase*, also exists in two forms, the active "a" form and the inactive "b" form. However, in contrast to *phosphorylase kinase* and *phosphorylase*, the active form of *glycogen synthase* is dephosphorylated, whereas the inactive form is phosphorylated at several sites on the enzyme, with the level of inactivation proportional to the degree of phosphorylation

(Fig. 11.10). Phosphorylation is catalyzed by several different *protein kinases* in response to cAMP (for example, *PKA* and *phosphorylase kinase*) or other signaling mechanisms (see C. below). *Glycogen synthase b* can be reconverted to the "a" form by *PP1*. Figure 11.11 summarizes the covalent regulation of glycogen metabolism.

C. Allosteric regulation of glycogenesis and glycogenolysis

In addition to hormonal signals, *glycogen synthase* and *glycogen phosphorylase* respond to the levels of metabolites and energy needs of the cell. Glycogenesis is stimulated when glucose and energy levels are high, whereas glycogenolysis is increased when glucose and energy levels are low. This allosteric regulation allows a rapid response to the needs of a cell and can override the effects of hormone-mediated covalent regulation. [Note: The "a" and "b" forms of the allosteric enzymes of glycogen metabolism are each in an equilibrium between the R (relaxed, more active) and T (tense, less active) conformations (see p. 28). The binding of effectors shifts the equilibrium and alters enzymic activity without directly altering the covalent modification.]

1. **Regulation in the well-fed state:** In the well-fed state, *glycogen synthase b* in both liver and muscle is allosterically activated by glucose 6-phosphate, which is present in elevated concentrations (Fig. 11.12). In contrast, *glycogen phosphorylase a* is allosterically inhibited by glucose 6-phosphate, as well as by ATP, a high-energy signal. [Note: In liver, but not muscle, free glucose is also an allosteric inhibitor of *glycogen phosphorylase a*.]

2. **Glycogenolysis activation by AMP:** Muscle *glycogen phosphorylase* (*myophosphorylase*), but not the liver isozyme, is active in the presence of the high AMP concentrations that occur under extreme conditions of anoxia and ATP depletion. AMP binds to *glycogen phosphorylase b*, causing its activation without phosphorylation (see Fig. 11.9). [Note: Recall that AMP also activates *phosphofructokinase-1* of glycolysis (see p. 99), allowing glucose from glycogenolysis to be oxidized.]

3. **Glycogenolysis activation by calcium:** Calcium (Ca^{2+}) is released into the sarcoplasm in muscle cells (myocytes) in response to neural stimulation and in the liver in response to epinephrine binding to α_1-adrenergic receptors. The Ca^{2+} binds to calmodulin (CaM), the most widely distributed member of a family of small, Ca^{2+}-binding proteins. The binding of four molecules of Ca^{2+} to CaM triggers a conformational change such that the activated Ca^{2+}–CaM complex binds to and activates protein molecules, often enzymes, that are inactive in the absence of this complex (Fig. 11.13). Thus, CaM functions as an essential subunit of many complex proteins. One such protein is the tetrameric *phosphorylase kinase*, whose "b" form is activated by the binding of Ca^{2+} to its δ subunit (CaM) without the need for the *kinase* to be phosphorylated by *PKA*. [Note: Epinephrine at β-adrenergic receptors signals through a rise in cAMP, not Ca^{2+} (see p. 131).]

   a. **Muscle phosphorylase kinase activation:** During muscle contraction, there is a rapid and urgent need for ATP. It is supplied by the degradation of muscle glycogen to glucose 6-phosphate,

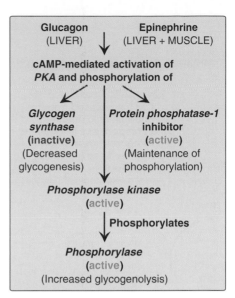

Figure 11.11
Summary of the hormone-mediated covalent regulation of glycogen metabolism. cAMP = cyclic adenosine monophosphate; *PKA* = *protein kinase A*.

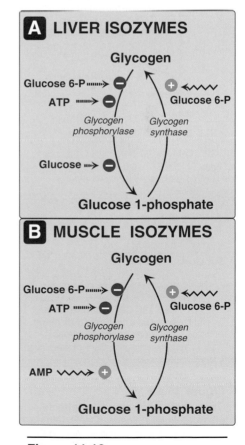

Figure 11.12
Allosteric regulation of glycogenesis and glycogenolysis in liver (A) and muscle (B). P = phosphate; AMP = adenosine monophosphate.

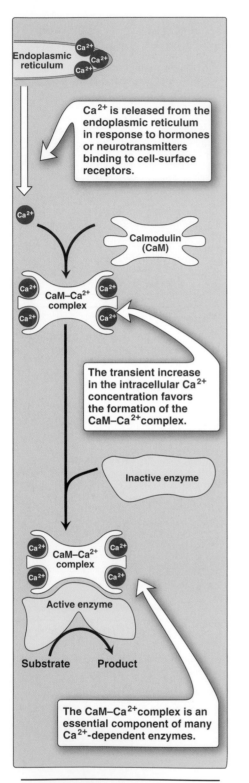

which enters glycolysis. Nerve impulses cause membrane depolarization, which promotes Ca^{2+} release from the sarcoplasmic reticulum into the sarcoplasm of myocytes. The Ca^{2+} binds the CaM subunit, and the complex activates muscle *phosphorylase kinase b* (see Fig. 11.9).

b. Liver phosphorylase kinase activation: During physiologic stress, epinephrine is released from the adrenal medulla and signals the need for blood glucose. This glucose initially comes from hepatic glycogenolysis. Binding of epinephrine to hepatocyte α_1-adrenergic GPCR activates a phospholipid-dependent cascade (see p. 205) that results in movement of Ca^{2+} from the ER into the cytoplasm. A Ca^{2+}–CaM complex forms and activates hepatic *phosphorylase kinase b*. [Note: The released Ca^{2+} also helps to activate *protein kinase C* that can phosphorylate (therefore, inactivate) *glycogen synthase a*.]

VI. GLYCOGEN STORAGE DISEASES

GSD are a group of genetic diseases caused by defects in enzymes required for glycogen degradation or, more rarely, glycogen synthesis. They result either in formation of glycogen that has an abnormal structure or in the accumulation of excessive amounts of normal glycogen in specific tissues as a result of impaired degradation. A particular enzyme may be defective in a single tissue, such as the liver (resulting in hypoglycemia) or muscle (causing muscle weakness), or the defect may be more generalized, affecting a variety of tissues, such as the heart and kidneys. Severity ranges from fatal in early childhood to mild disorders that are not life threatening. Some of the more prevalent GSD are illustrated in Figure 11.8. [Note: Only GSD II is lysosomal because glycogen metabolism occurs primarily in the cytosol.]

VII. CHAPTER SUMMARY

The main stores of **glycogen** in the body are found in **skeletal muscle**, where they serve as a fuel reserve for the synthesis of **ATP** during muscle **contraction**, and in the **liver**, where they are used to maintain the **blood glucose** concentration, particularly during the early stages of a **fast**. Glycogen is a highly **branched polymer** of α-D-**glucose**. The primary glycosidic bond is an $\alpha(1\rightarrow4)$ **linkage**. After about 8–14 glucosyl residues, there is a branch containing an $\alpha(1\rightarrow6)$ **linkage**. **Uridine diphosphate (UDP)-glucose**, the building block of glycogen, is synthesized from **glucose 1-phosphate** and UTP by *UDP–glucose pyrophosphorylase* (Fig. 11.14). **Glucose** from UDP-glucose is transferred to the **nonreducing ends** of glycogen chains by primer-requiring *glycogen synthase*, which makes the $\alpha(1\rightarrow4)$ linkages. The **primer** is made by *glycogenin*. Branches are formed by *amylo-$\alpha(1\rightarrow4)\rightarrow\alpha(1\rightarrow6)$-transglycosylase* (a *4:6 transferase*), which transfers a set of six to eight glucosyl residues from the nonreducing end of the glycogen chain (breaking an $\alpha(1\rightarrow4)$ linkage), and making an $\alpha(1\rightarrow6)$ linkage to another residue in the chain. Pyridoxal phosphate–

Figure 11.13
Calmodulin mediates many effects of intracellular calcium (Ca^{2+}). [Note: Ca^{2+} activates *phosphorylase kinase* in liver and muscles.]

requiring **glycogen phosphorylase** cleaves the α(1→4) bonds between glucosyl residues at the nonreducing ends of the glycogen chains, producing **glucose 1-phosphate**. This sequential degradation continues until four glucosyl units remain before a branch point. The resulting structure is called a **limit dextrin** that is degraded by the bifunctional **debranching enzyme**. **Oligo-α(1→4)→α(1→4)-glucantransferase** (a **4:4 transferase**) activity removes the outer three of the four glucosyl residues at a branch and transfers them to the nonreducing end of another chain, where they can be released as glucose 1-phosphate by *glycogen phosphorylase*. The remaining single glucose residue attached in an α(1→6) linkage is removed hydrolytically by the **amylo-α(1→6) glucosidase** activity of *debranching enzyme*, releasing **free glucose**. Glucose 1-phosphate is converted to **glucose 6-phosphate** by **phosphoglucomutase**. In **muscle**, glucose 6-phosphate enters glycolysis. In **liver**, the phosphate is removed by **glucose 6-phosphatase** (an enzyme of the endoplasmic reticular membrane), releasing free glucose that can be used to maintain blood glucose levels at the beginning of a fast. A deficiency of the *phosphatase* causes **glycogen storage disease Ia** (**von Gierke disease**) and results in an inability of the liver to provide free glucose to the body during a fast. It affects both glycogen degradation and gluconeogenesis. Glycogen synthesis and degradation are **reciprocally regulated** to meet whole-body needs by the same hormonal signals (namely, an **elevated insulin** level results in overall **increased glycogenesis** and **decreased glycogenolysis**, whereas an **elevated glucagon**, or **epinephrine**, level causes the opposite effects). Key enzymes are phosphorylated by a family of **protein kinases**, some of which are dependent on **cyclic adenosine monophosphate (cAMP)**, a compound increased by glucagon and epinephrine. Phosphate groups are removed by **protein phosphatase-1** (active when its inhibitor is inactive in response to elevated insulin levels). In addition to this **covalent regulation**, **glycogen synthase**, **phosphorylase kinase**, and **phosphorylase** are **allosterically regulated** to meet tissues' needs. In the well-fed state, *glycogen synthase* is activated by glucose 6-phosphate, but *glycogen phosphorylase* is inhibited by glucose 6-phosphate as well as by ATP. In the liver, free glucose also serves as an allosteric inhibitor of *glycogen phosphorylase*. The rise in **calcium** in muscle during exercise and in liver in response to epinephrine activates *phosphorylase kinase* by binding to the enzyme's **calmodulin** subunit. This allows the enzyme to activate *glycogen phosphorylase*, thereby causing glycogen degradation. **AMP** activates *glycogen phosphorylase* (**myophosphorylase**) in muscle.

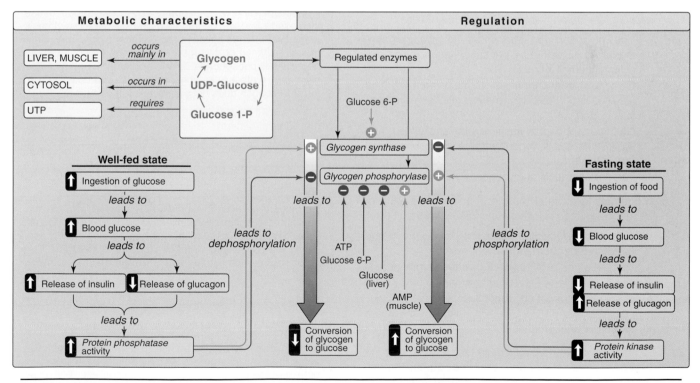

Figure 11.14

Key concept map for glycogen metabolism in the liver. [Note: *Glycogen phosphorylase* is phosphorylated by *phosphorylase kinase*, the "b" form of which can be activated by calcium.] UDP and UTP = uridine di- and triphosphates; P = phosphate; AMP = adenosine monophosphate.

Study Questions

Choose the ONE best answer.

For Questions 11.1–11.4, match the deficient enzyme to the clinical finding in selected glycogen storage diseases (GSD).

CHOICE	GSD	DEFICIENT ENZYME
A	Type Ia	Glucose 6-phosphatase
B	Type II	Acid maltase
C	Type III	4:4 Transferase
D	Type IV	4:6 Transferase
E	Type V	Myophosphorylase
F	Type VI	Liver phosphorylase

11.1 Exercise intolerance, with no rise in blood lactate during exercise

11.2 Fatal, progressive cirrhosis and glycogen with longer-than-normal outer chains

11.3 Generalized accumulation of glycogen, severe hypotonia, and death from heart failure

11.4 Severe fasting hypoglycemia, lactic acidemia, hyperuricemia, and hyperlipidemia

11.5 Epinephrine and glucagon have which one of the following effects on hepatic glycogen metabolism?

    A. Both glycogen phosphorylase and glycogen synthase are activated by phosphorylation but at significantly different rates.

    B. Glycogen phosphorylase is inactivated by the resulting rise in calcium, whereas glycogen synthase is activated.

    C. Glycogen phosphorylase is phosphorylated and active, whereas glycogen synthase is phosphorylated and inactive.

    D. The net synthesis of glycogen is increased.

11.6 In contracting skeletal muscle, a sudden elevation of the sarcoplasmic calcium concentration will result in:

    A. activation of cyclic adenosine monophosphate (cAMP)-dependent protein kinase A.

    B. conversion of cAMP to AMP by phosphodiesterase.

    C. direct activation of glycogen synthase b.

    D. direct activation of phosphorylase kinase b.

    E. inactivation of phosphorylase kinase a by the action of protein phosphatase-1.

11.7 Explain why the hypoglycemia seen with type Ia glycogen storage disease (glucose 6-phosphatase deficiency) is severe, whereas that seen with type VI (liver phosphorylase deficiency) is mild.

Correct answer = E. Myophosphorylase (the muscle isozyme of glycogen phosphorylase) deficiency (or, McArdle disease) prevents glycogen degradation in muscle, depriving muscle of glycogen-derived glucose, resulting in decreased glycolysis and its anaerobic product, lactate.

Correct answer = D. 4:6 Transferase (branching enzyme) deficiency (or, Andersen disease), a defect in glycogen synthesis, results in glycogen with fewer branches and decreased solubility.

Correct answer = B. Acid maltase [acid $\alpha(1\rightarrow4)$-glucosidase] deficiency (or, Pompe disease) prevents degradation of any glycogen brought into lysosomes. A variety of tissues are affected, with the most severe pathology resulting from heart damage.

Correct answer = A. Glucose 6-phosphatase deficiency (or, von Gierke disease) prevents the liver from releasing free glucose into the blood, causing severe fasting hypoglycemia, lactic acidemia, hyperuricemia, and hyperlipidemia.

Correct answer = C. Epinephrine and glucagon both cause increased glycogen degradation and decreased synthesis in the liver through covalent modification (phosphorylation) of key enzymes of glycogen metabolism. Glycogen phosphorylase is phosphorylated and active ("a" form), whereas glycogen synthase is phosphorylated and inactive ("b" form). Glucagon does not cause a rise in calcium.

Correct answer = D. Calcium (Ca^{2+}) released from the sarcoplasmic reticulum during exercise binds to the calmodulin subunit of phosphorylase kinase, thereby allosterically activating the dephosphorylated "b" form of this enzyme. The other choices are not caused by an elevation of cytosolic Ca^{2+}. [Note: Ca^{2+} also activates hepatic phosphorylase kinase b.]

With type Ia, the liver is unable to generate free glucose either from glycogenolysis or gluconeogenesis because both processes produce glucose 6-phosphate. With type VI, the liver is still able to produce free glucose from gluconeogenesis, but glycogenolysis is inhibited.

Monosaccharide and Disaccharide Metabolism

12

I. OVERVIEW

Glucose is the most common monosaccharide consumed by humans, and its metabolism has already been discussed. Two other monosaccharides, fructose and galactose, also occur in significant amounts in the diet (primarily in disaccharides) and make important contributions to energy metabolism. In addition, galactose is an important component of glycosylated proteins. Figure 12.1 shows the metabolism of fructose and galactose as part of the essential pathways of energy metabolism.

II. FRUCTOSE METABOLISM

About 10% of the calories in the Western diet are supplied by fructose (~55 g/day). The major source of fructose is the disaccharide sucrose, which, when cleaved in the intestine, releases equimolar amounts of fructose and glucose. Fructose is also found as a free monosaccharide in many fruits, in honey, and in high-fructose corn syrup (typically, 55% fructose and 45% glucose), which is used to sweeten soft drinks and many foods (see p. 364). Fructose transport into cells is not insulin dependent (unlike that of glucose into certain tissues; see p. 97), and, in contrast to glucose, fructose does not promote the secretion of insulin.

A. Phosphorylation

For fructose to enter the pathways of intermediary metabolism, it must first be phosphorylated (Fig. 12.2). This can be accomplished by either *hexokinase* or *fructokinase*. *Hexokinase* phosphorylates glucose in most cells of the body (see p. 98), and several additional hexoses can serve as substrates for this enzyme. However, it has a low affinity (that is, a high Michaelis constant [K_m]; see p. 59) for fructose. Therefore, unless the intracellular concentration of fructose becomes unusually high, the normal presence of saturating concentrations of glucose means that little fructose is phosphorylated by *hexokinase*. *Fructokinase* provides the primary mechanism for fructose phosphorylation (see Fig. 12.2). The enzyme has a low K_m for fructose and a high V_{max} ([maximal velocity] see p. 57). It is found in the liver (which processes most of the dietary fructose), kidneys, and the

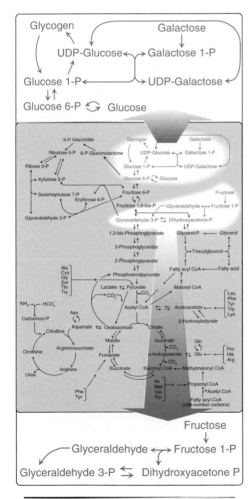

Figure 12.1

Galactose and fructose metabolism as part of the essential pathways of energy metabolism. [Note: See Fig. 8.2, p. 92, for a more detailed map of metabolism.] UDP = uridine diphosphate; P = phosphate.

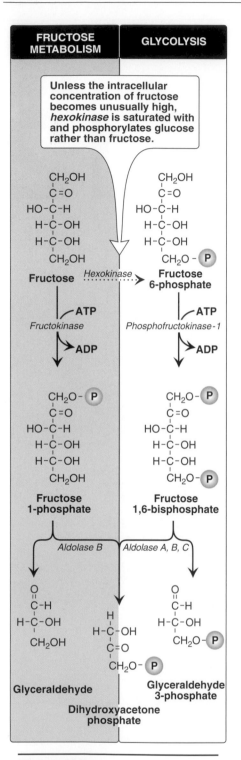

Figure 12.2
Fructose phosphorylation products
and their cleavage. **P** = phosphate;
ADP = adenosine diphosphate.

small intestine and converts fructose to fructose 1-phosphate, using ATP as the phosphate donor. [Note: These three tissues also contain *aldolase B*, discussed in section B.]

B. Fructose 1-phosphate cleavage

Fructose 1-phosphate is not phosphorylated to fructose 1,6-bisphosphate as is fructose 6-phosphate (see p. 99) but is cleaved by *aldolase B* (also called *fructose 1-phosphate aldolase*) to two trioses, dihydroxyacetone phosphate (DHAP) and glyceraldehyde. [Note: Humans express three *aldolase* isozymes (the products of three different genes): *aldolase A* in most tissues; *aldolase B* in the liver, kidneys, and small intestine; and *aldolase C* in the brain. All cleave fructose 1,6-bisphosphate produced during glycolysis to DHAP and glyceraldehyde 3-phosphate (see p. 101), but only *aldolase B* cleaves fructose 1-phosphate.] DHAP can be used in glycolysis or gluconeogenesis, whereas glyceraldehyde can be metabolized by a number of pathways, as illustrated in Figure 12.3.

C. Kinetics

The rate of fructose metabolism is more rapid than that of glucose because triose production from fructose 1-phosphate bypasses *phosphofructokinase-1,* the major rate-limiting step in glycolysis (see p. 99).

D. Disorders

A deficiency of one of the key enzymes required for the entry of fructose into metabolic pathways can result in either a benign condition as a result of *fructokinase* deficiency (essential fructosuria) or a severe disturbance of liver and kidney metabolism as a result of *aldolase B* deficiency (hereditary fructose intolerance [HFI]), which occurs in ~1:20,000 live births (see Fig. 12.3). The first symptoms of HFI appear when a baby is weaned from lactose-containing milk and begins ingesting food containing sucrose or fructose. Fructose 1-phosphate accumulates, resulting in a drop in the level of inorganic phosphate (P_i) and, therefore, of ATP production. As ATP falls, adenosine monophosphate (AMP) rises. The AMP is degraded, causing hyperuricemia (and lactic acidemia; see p. 299). The decreased availability of hepatic ATP decreases gluconeogenesis (causing hypoglycemia with vomiting) and protein synthesis (causing a decrease in blood-clotting factors and other essential proteins). Renal reabsorption of P_i is also decreased. [Note: The drop in P_i also inhibits glycogenolysis (see p. 128).] Diagnosis of HFI can be made on the basis of fructose in the urine, enzyme assay using liver cells, or by DNA-based testing (see Chapter 34). With HFI, sucrose, as well as fructose, must be removed from the diet to prevent liver failure and possible death. [Note: Individuals with HFI display an aversion to sweets and, consequently, have an absence of dental caries.]

E. Mannose conversion to fructose 6-phosphate

Mannose, the C-2 epimer of glucose (see p. 84), is an important component of glycoproteins (see p. 166). *Hexokinase* phosphorylates mannose, producing mannose 6-phosphate, which, in turn, is

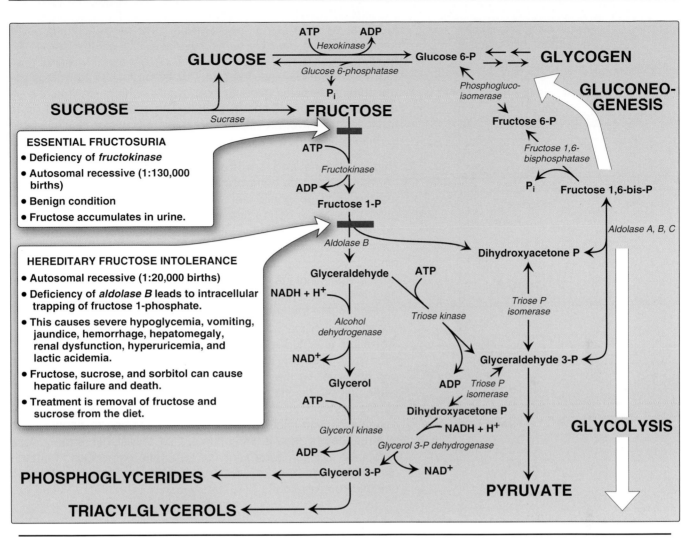

Figure 12.3
Summary of fructose metabolism. P = phosphate; P_i = inorganic phosphate; NAD(H) = nicotinamide adenine dinucleotide; ADP = adenosine diphosphate.

reversibly isomerized to fructose 6-phosphate by *phosphomannose isomerase*. [Note: Most intracellular mannose is synthesized from fructose or is preexisting mannose produced by the degradation of glycoproteins and salvaged by *hexokinase*. Dietary carbohydrates contain little mannose.]

F. Glucose conversion to fructose via sorbitol

Most sugars are rapidly phosphorylated following their entry into cells. Therefore, they are trapped within the cells, because organic phosphates cannot freely cross membranes without specific transporters. An alternate mechanism for metabolizing a monosaccharide is to convert it to a polyol (sugar alcohol) by the reduction of an aldehyde group, thereby producing an additional hydroxyl group.

1. **Sorbitol synthesis:** *Aldose reductase* reduces glucose, producing sorbitol (or, glucitol; Fig. 12.4), but the K_m is high. This enzyme is found in many tissues, including the retina, lens,

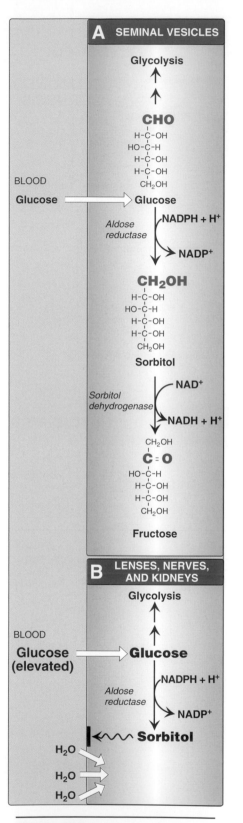

Figure 12.4
Sorbitol metabolism. NAD(H) = nicotinamide adenine dinucleotide; NADP(H) = nicotinamide adenine dinucleotide phosphate.

kidneys, peripheral nerves, ovaries, and seminal vesicles. A second enzyme, *sorbitol dehydrogenase*, can oxidize sorbitol to fructose in cells of the liver, ovaries, and seminal vesicles (see Fig. 12.4). The two-reaction pathway from glucose to fructose in the seminal vesicles benefits sperm cells, which use fructose as a major carbohydrate energy source. The pathway from sorbitol to fructose in the liver provides a mechanism by which any available sorbitol is converted into a substrate that can enter glycolysis.

2. **Hyperglycemia and sorbitol metabolism:** Because insulin is not required for the entry of glucose into cells of the retina, lens, kidneys, and peripheral nerves, large amounts of glucose may enter these cells during times of hyperglycemia (for example, in uncontrolled diabetes). Elevated intracellular glucose concentrations and an adequate supply of reduced nicotinamide adenine dinucleotide phosphate (NADPH) cause *aldose reductase* to produce a significant increase in the amount of sorbitol, which cannot pass efficiently through cell membranes and, therefore, remains trapped inside the cell (see Fig. 12.4). This is exacerbated when *sorbitol dehydrogenase* is low or absent (for example, in cells of the retina, lens, kidneys, and peripheral nerves). As a result, sorbitol accumulates in these cells, causing strong osmotic effects and cell swelling due to water influx and retention. Some of the pathologic alterations associated with diabetes can be partly attributed to this osmotic stress, including cataract formation, peripheral neuropathy, and microvascular problems leading to nephropathy and retinopathy (see p. 345). [Note: Use of NADPH in the *aldose reductase* reaction decreases the generation of reduced glutathione, an important antioxidant (see p. 148), and may be related to diabetic complications.]

III. GALACTOSE METABOLISM

The major dietary source of galactose is lactose (galactosyl β-1,4-glucose) obtained from milk and milk products. [Note: The digestion of lactose by *β-galactosidase* (*lactase*) of the intestinal mucosal cell membrane was discussed on p. 87.] Some galactose can also be obtained by lysosomal degradation of glycoproteins and glycolipids. Like fructose (and mannose), the transport of galactose into cells is not insulin dependent.

A. Phosphorylation

Like fructose, galactose must be phosphorylated before it can be further metabolized. Most tissues have a specific enzyme for this purpose, *galactokinase*, which produces galactose 1-phosphate (Fig. 12.5). As with other *kinases*, ATP is the phosphate donor.

B. Uridine diphosphate–galactose formation

Galactose 1-phosphate cannot enter the glycolytic pathway unless it is first converted to uridine diphosphate (UDP)-galactose (Fig. 12.6). This occurs in an exchange reaction, in which UDP-glucose reacts with galactose 1-phosphate, producing UDP-galactose and glucose 1-phosphate (see Fig. 12.5). The reaction is catalyzed by

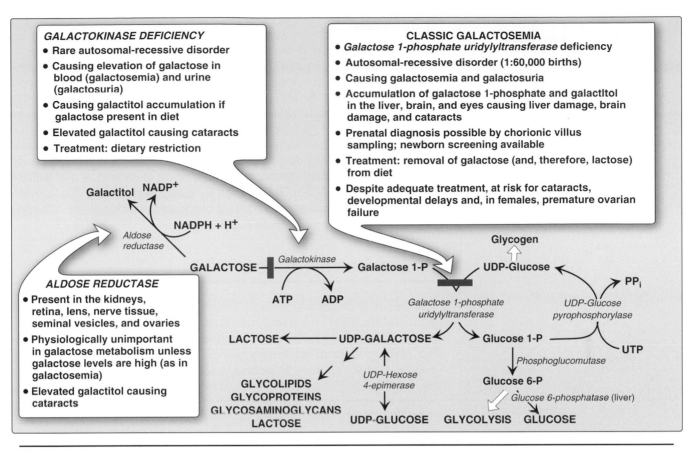

Figure 12.5

Metabolism of galactose. UDP and UTP = uridine di- and triphosphates; P = phosphate; PP$_i$ = pyrophosphate; NADP(H) = nicotinamide adenine dinucleotide phosphate; ADP = adenosine diphosphate.

galactose 1-phosphate uridylyltransferase (*GALT*). [Note: The glucose 1-phosphate product can be isomerized to glucose 6-phosphate, which can enter glycolysis or be dephosphorylated.]

C. UDP-galactose conversion to UDP-glucose

For UDP-galactose to enter the mainstream of glucose metabolism, it must first be isomerized to its C-4 epimer, UDP-glucose, by *UDP-hexose 4-epimerase*. This "new" UDP-glucose (produced from the original UDP-galactose) can participate in biosynthetic reactions (for example, glycogenesis) as well as in the *GALT* reaction. [Note: See Fig. 12.5 for a summary of the interconversions.]

D. UDP-galactose in biosynthetic reactions

UDP-galactose can serve as the donor of galactose units in a number of synthetic pathways, including synthesis of lactose (see IV. below), glycoproteins (see p. 166), glycolipids (see p. 210), and glycosaminoglycans (see p. 158). [Note: If galactose is not provided by the diet (for example, when it cannot be released from lactose owing to a lack of β-*galactosidase* in people who are lactose intolerant), all tissue requirements for UDP-galactose can be met by the action of *UDP-hexose 4-epimerase* on UDP-glucose, which is efficiently produced from glucose 1-phosphate and uridine triphosphate (see Fig. 12.5).]

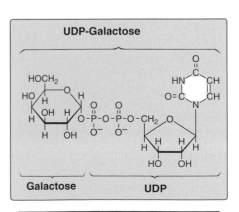

Figure 12.6

Structure of UDP-galactose. UDP = uridine diphosphate.

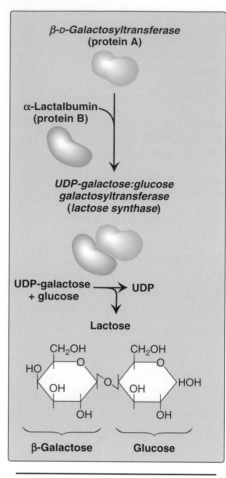

Figure 12.7
Lactose synthesis. UDP = uridine diphosphate.

E. Disorders

GALT is severely deficient in individuals with classic galactosemia (see Fig. 12.5). In this disorder, galactose 1-phosphate and, therefore, galactose accumulate. Physiologic consequences are similar to those found in HFI (see p. 138), but a broader spectrum of tissues is affected. The accumulated galactose is shunted into side pathways such as that of galactitol production. This reaction is catalyzed by *aldose reductase*, the same enzyme that reduces glucose to sorbitol (see p. 139). *GALT* deficiency is part of the newborn screening panel. Treatment of galactosemia requires removal of galactose and lactose from the diet. [Note: Deficiencies in *galactokinase* and the *epimerase* result in less severe disorders of galactose metabolism, although cataracts are common (see Fig. 12.5).]

IV. LACTOSE SYNTHESIS

Lactose is a disaccharide that consists of a molecule of β-galactose attached by a β(1→4) linkage to glucose. Therefore, lactose is galactosyl β(1→4)-glucose. Because lactose (milk sugar) is made by lactating (milk-producing) mammary glands, milk and other dairy products are the dietary sources of lactose. Lactose is synthesized in the Golgi by *lactose synthase* (*UDP-galactose:glucose galactosyltransferase*), which transfers galactose from UDP-galactose to glucose, releasing UDP (Fig. 12.7). This enzyme is composed of two proteins, A and B. Protein A is a *β-D-galactosyltransferase* and is found in a number of body tissues. In tissues other than the lactating mammary gland, this enzyme transfers galactose from UDP-galactose to N-acetyl-D-glucosamine, forming the same β(1→4) linkage found in lactose, and producing N-acetyllactosamine, a component of the structurally important N-linked glycoproteins (see p. 167). In contrast, protein B is found only in lactating mammary glands. It is α-lactalbumin, and its synthesis is stimulated by the peptide hormone prolactin. Protein B forms a complex with the enzyme, protein A, changing the specificity of that *transferase* (by decreasing the K_m for glucose) so that lactose, rather than N-acetyllactosamine, is produced (see Fig. 12.7).

V. CHAPTER SUMMARY

The major source of fructose is the disaccharide **sucrose**, which, when cleaved, releases equimolar amounts of **fructose** and **glucose** (Fig. 12.8). Transport of fructose into cells is **insulin independent**. Fructose is first phosphorylated to **fructose 1-phosphate** by *fructokinase* and then cleaved by *aldolase B* to **dihydroxyacetone phosphate** and **glyceraldehyde**. These enzymes are found in the **liver**, **kidneys**, and **small intestine**. A deficiency of *fructokinase* causes a benign condition (**essential fructosuria**), whereas a deficiency of *aldolase B* causes **hereditary fructose intolerance** (**HFI**), in which **severe hypoglycemia** and **liver failure** lead to **death** if fructose (and sucrose) is not removed from the diet. **Mannose**, an important component of **glycoproteins**, is phosphorylated by *hexokinase* to **mannose 6-phosphate**, which is reversibly isomerized to **fructose 6-phosphate** by *phosphomannose isomerase*. Glucose can be reduced to **sorbitol (glucitol)** by *aldose reductase* in many tissues, including the **lens**, **retina**, **peripheral nerves**, **kidneys**, **ovaries**, and **seminal vesicles**. In the liver, ovaries, and seminal vesicles, a second enzyme, ***sorbitol dehydrogenase***, can oxidize sorbitol to produce **fructose**. **Hyperglycemia** results in the accumulation of sorbitol in those cells lacking *sorbitol dehydrogenase*. The resulting **osmotic events** cause cell swelling and may contribute to the **cataract formation**, **peripheral neuropathy**, **nephropathy**, and **retinopathy** seen in **diabetes**. The major dietary source of **galactose** is **lactose**. The transport of galactose into cells is insulin independent. Galactose is first phosphorylated by *galactokinase* (a deficiency results in cataracts) to **galactose 1-phosphate**. This compound is converted to **uridine diphosphate (UDP)-galactose** by *galactose 1-phosphate uridylyltransferase* (***GALT***), with the nucleotide supplied by UDP-glucose. A deficiency of this enzyme causes **classic galactosemia**. Galactose 1-phosphate accumulates, and excess galactose is converted to **galactitol** by *aldose reductase*. This causes **liver damage**, **brain damage**, and **cataracts**. Treatment requires removal of galactose (and lactose) from the diet. For UDP-galactose to enter the mainstream of glucose metabolism, it must first be isomerized to UDP-glucose by ***UDP-hexose 4-epimerase***. This enzyme can also be used to produce UDP-galactose from UDP-glucose when the former is required for glycoprotein and glycolipid synthesis. **Lactose** is a disaccharide of **galactose** and **glucose**. Milk and other **dairy products** are the dietary sources of lactose. Lactose is synthesized by *lactose synthase* from **UDP-galactose** and **glucose** in the **lactating mammary gland**. The enzyme has two subunits, **protein A** (which is a *galactosyltransferase* found in most cells where it synthesizes **N-acetyllactosamine**) and **protein B** (**α-lactalbumin**, which is found only in lactating mammary glands, and whose synthesis is stimulated by the peptide hormone **prolactin**). When both subunits are present, the *transferase* produces lactose.

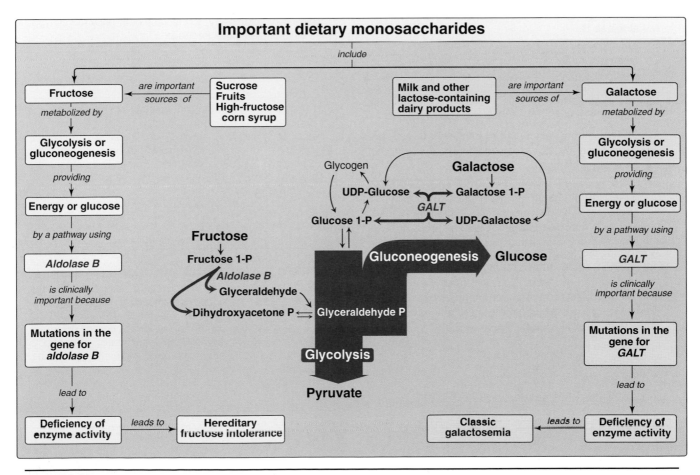

Figure 12.8

Key concept map for metabolism of fructose and galactose. *GALT = galactose 1-phosphate uridylyltransferase*; UDP = uridine diphosphate; P = phosphate.

Study Questions

Choose the ONE best answer.

12.1 A nursing female with classic galactosemia is on a galactose-free diet. She is able to produce lactose in breast milk because:

A. galactose can be produced from fructose by isomerization.

B. galactose can be produced from a glucose metabolite by epimerization.

C. hexokinase can efficiently phosphorylate galactose to galactose 1-phosphate.

D. the enzyme affected in galactosemia is activated by a hormone produced in the mammary gland.

> Correct answer = B. Uridine diphosphate (UDP)-glucose is converted to UDP-galactose by UDP-hexose 4-epimerase, thereby providing the appropriate form of galactose for lactose synthesis. Isomerization of fructose to galactose does not occur in the human body. Galactose is not converted to galactose 1-phosphate by hexokinase. A galactose-free diet provides no galactose. Galactosemia is the result of an enzyme (galactose 1-phosphate uridylyltransferase) deficiency.

12.2 A 5-month-old boy is brought to his physician because of vomiting, night sweats, and tremors. History revealed that these symptoms began after fruit juices were introduced to his diet as he was being weaned off breast milk. The physical examination was remarkable for hepatomegaly. Tests on the baby's urine were positive for reducing sugar but negative for glucose. The infant most likely suffers from a deficiency of:

A. aldolase B.

B. fructokinase.

C. galactokinase.

D. β-galactosidase.

> Correct answer = A. The symptoms suggest hereditary fructose intolerance, a deficiency in aldolase B. Deficiencies in fructokinase or galactokinase result in relatively benign conditions characterized by elevated levels of fructose or galactose in the blood and urine. Deficiency in β-galactosidase (lactase) results in a decreased ability to degrade lactose (milk sugar). Congenital lactase deficiency is quite rare and would have presented much earlier in this baby (and with different symptoms). Typical lactase deficiency (adult hypolactasia) presents at a later age.

12.3 Lactose synthesis is essential in the production of milk by mammary glands. In lactose synthesis:

A. galactose from galactose 1-phosphate is transferred to glucose by galactosyltransferase (protein A), generating lactose.

B. protein A is used exclusively in lactose synthesis.

C. α-lactalbumin (protein B) regulates the specificity of protein A by decreasing its affinity for glucose.

D. protein B expression is stimulated by prolactin.

> Correct answer = D. α-Lactalbumin (protein B) expression is increased by the hormone prolactin. Uridine diphosphate–galactose is the form used by the galactosyltransferase (protein A). Protein A is also involved in the synthesis of the amino sugar N-acetyllactosamine. Protein B decreases the Michaelis constant (K_m) and, so, increases the affinity of protein A for glucose.

12.4 A 3-month-old girl is developing cataracts. Other than not having a social smile or being able to track objects visually, all other aspects of the girl's examination are normal. Tests on the baby's urine are positive for reducing sugar but negative for glucose. Which enzyme is most likely deficient in this girl?

A. Aldolase B

B. Fructokinase

C. Galactokinase

D. Galactose 1-phosphate uridylyltransferase

> Correct answer = C. The girl is deficient in galactokinase and is unable to appropriately phosphorylate galactose. Galactose accumulates in the blood (and urine). In the lens of the eye, galactose is reduced by aldose reductase to galactitol, a sugar alcohol, which causes osmotic effects that result in cataract formation. Deficiency of galactose 1-phosphate uridylyltransferase also results in cataracts but is characterized by liver damage and neurologic effects. Fructokinase deficiency is a benign condition. Aldolase B deficiency is severe, with effects on several tissues. Cataracts are not typically seen.

Pentose Phosphate Pathway and Nicotinamide Adenine Dinucleotide Phosphate

13

I. OVERVIEW

The pentose phosphate pathway (or, hexose monophosphate shunt) occurs in the cytosol. It includes an irreversible oxidative phase, followed by a series of reversible sugar–phosphate interconversions (Fig. 13.1). In the oxidative phase, carbon 1 of a glucose 6-phosphate molecule is released as carbon dioxide (CO_2), and one pentose sugar-phosphate plus two reduced nicotinamide adenine dinucleotide phosphates (NADPH) are produced. The rate and direction of the reversible reactions are determined by the supply of and demand for intermediates of the pathway. The pentose phosphate pathway provides a major portion of the body's NADPH, which functions as a biochemical reductant. It also produces ribose 5-phosphate, required for nucleotide biosynthesis (see p. 293), and provides a mechanism for the conversion of pentose sugars to triose and hexose intermediates of glycolysis. No ATP is directly consumed or produced in the pathway.

II. IRREVERSIBLE OXIDATIVE REACTIONS

The oxidative portion of the pentose phosphate pathway consists of three irreversible reactions that lead to the formation of ribulose 5-phosphate, CO_2, and two molecules of NADPH for each molecule of glucose 6-phosphate oxidized (Fig. 13.2). This portion of the pathway is particularly important in the liver, lactating mammary glands, and adipose tissue for the NADPH-dependent biosynthesis of fatty acids (see p. 186); in the testes, ovaries, placenta, and adrenal cortex for the NADPH-dependent biosynthesis of steroid hormones (see p. 237); and in red blood cells (RBC) for the NADPH-dependent reduction of glutathione (see p. 148).

A. Glucose 6-phosphate dehydrogenation

Glucose 6-phosphate dehydrogenase (*G6PD*) catalyzes the oxidation of glucose 6-phosphate to 6-phosphogluconolactone as the coenzyme $NADP^+$ gets reduced to NADPH. This initial reaction is the committed,

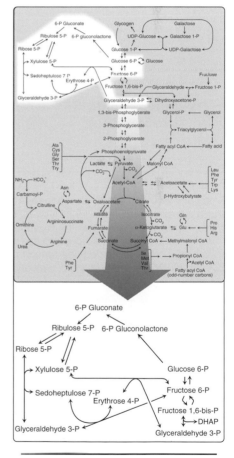

Figure 13.1
Pentose phosphate pathway shown as a component of the metabolic map. [Note: See Fig. 8.2, p. 92 for a more detailed map of metabolism.] P = phosphate; DHAP = dihydroxyacetone phosphate.

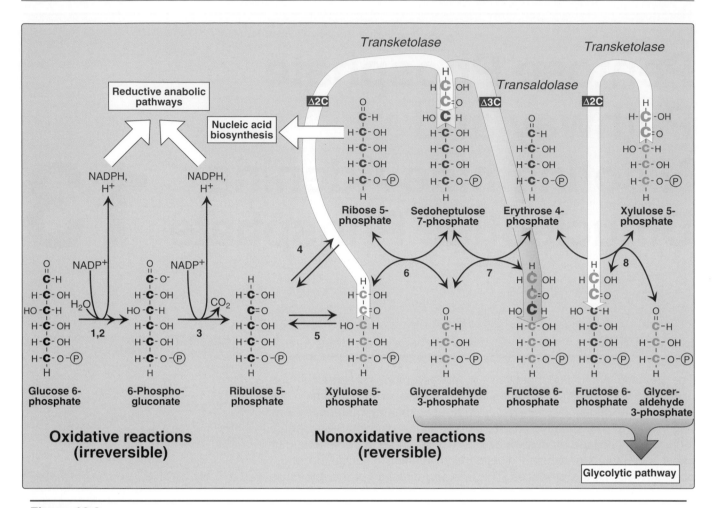

Figure 13.2
Reactions of the pentose phosphate pathway. Enzymes numbered above are: (1, 2) *glucose 6-phosphate dehydrogenase* and *6-phosphogluconolactone hydrolase*, (3) *6-phosphogluconate dehydrogenase*, (4) *ribose 5-phosphate isomerase*, (5) *phosphopentose epimerase*, (6, 8) *transketolase* (coenzyme: thiamine pyrophosphate), and (7) *transaldolase*. **Δ2C** = two carbons are transferred from a ketose donor to an aldose acceptor in *transketolase* reactions; **Δ3C** = three carbons are transferred in the *transaldolase* reaction. This can be represented as: 5C sugar + 5C sugar $\xrightarrow{\Delta 2C}$ 7C sugar + 3C sugar $\xrightarrow{\Delta 3C}$ 4C sugar + 6C sugar. NADP(H) = nicotinamide adenine dinucleotide phosphate; $\textcircled{P}$ = phosphate; CO_2 = carbon dioxide.

rate-limiting, and regulated step of the pathway. NADPH is a potent competitive inhibitor of *G6PD*, and the ratio of NADPH/NADP$^+$ is sufficiently high to substantially inhibit the enzyme under most metabolic conditions. However, with increased demand for NADPH, the ratio of NADPH/NADP$^+$ decreases, and flux through the pathway increases in response to the enhanced activity of *G6PD*. [Note: Insulin upregulates expression of the gene for *G6PD*, and flux through the pathway increases in the absorptive state (see p. 323).]

B. Ribulose 5-phosphate formation

6-Phosphogluconolactone is hydrolyzed by *6-phosphogluconolactone hydrolase* in the second step. The oxidative decarboxylation of the product, 6-phosphogluconate, is catalyzed by *6-phosphogluconate dehydrogenase*. This third irreversible step produces ribulose 5-phosphate (a pentose sugar–phosphate), CO_2 (from carbon 1 of glucose), and a second molecule of NADPH (see Fig. 13.2).

III. REVERSIBLE NONOXIDATIVE REACTIONS

The nonoxidative reactions of the pentose phosphate pathway occur in all cell types synthesizing nucleotides and nucleic acids. These reactions catalyze the interconversion of sugars containing three to seven carbons (see Fig. 13.2). These reversible reactions permit ribulose 5-phosphate (produced by the oxidative portion of the pathway) to be converted either to ribose 5-phosphate (needed for nucleotide synthesis; see p. 293) or to intermediates of glycolysis (that is, fructose 6-phosphate and glyceraldehyde 3-phosphate). For example, many cells that carry out reductive biosynthetic reactions have a greater need for NADPH than for ribose 5-phosphate. In this case, *transketolase* (which transfers two-carbon units in a thiamine pyrophosphate [TPP]-requiring reaction) and *transaldolase* (which transfers three-carbon units) convert the ribulose 5-phosphate produced as an end product of the oxidative phase to glyceraldehyde 3-phosphate and fructose 6-phosphate, which are glycolytic intermediates. In contrast, when the demand for ribose for nucleotides and nucleic acids is greater than the need for NADPH, the nonoxidative reactions can provide the ribose 5-phosphate from glyceraldehyde 3-phosphate and fructose 6-phosphate in the absence of the oxidative steps (Fig. 13.3).

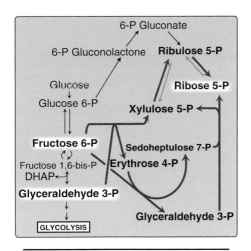

Figure 13.3
Formation of ribose 5-phosphate from intermediates of glycolysis. P = phosphate; DHAP = dihydroxyacetone phosphate.

> In addition to *transketolase*, TPP is required by the multi-enzyme complexes *pyruvate dehydrogenase* (see p. 110), *α-ketoglutarate dehydrogenase* of the tricarboxylic acid cycle (see p. 112), and *branched-chain α-keto acid dehydrogenase* of branched-chain amino acid catabolism (see p. 266).

IV. NADPH USES

The coenzyme NADPH differs from nicotinamide adenine dinucleotide (NADH) only by the presence of a phosphate group on one of the ribose units (Fig. 13.4). This seemingly small change in structure allows NADPH to interact with NADPH-specific enzymes that have unique roles in the cell. For example, in the cytosol of hepatocytes, the steady-state NADP$^+$/NADPH ratio is ~0.1, which favors the use of NADPH in reductive biosynthetic reactions. This contrasts with the high NAD$^+$/NADH ratio (~1,000), which favors an oxidative role for NAD$^+$. This section summarizes some important NADPH-specific functions in reductive biosynthesis and detoxification reactions.

A. Reductive biosynthesis

Like NADH, NADPH can be thought of as a high-energy molecule. However, the electrons of NADPH are used for reductive biosynthesis, rather than for transfer to the electron transport chain as is seen with NADH (see p. 74). Thus, in the metabolic transformations of the pentose phosphate pathway, part of the energy of glucose 6-phosphate is conserved in NADPH, a molecule with a negative reduction potential (see p. 76), that, therefore, can be used in reactions requiring an electron donor, such as fatty acid (see p. 186), cholesterol (see p. 221), and steroid hormone (see p. 237) synthesis.

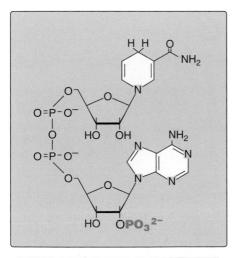

Figure 13.4
Structure of reduced nicotinamide adenine dinucleotide phosphate (NADPH).

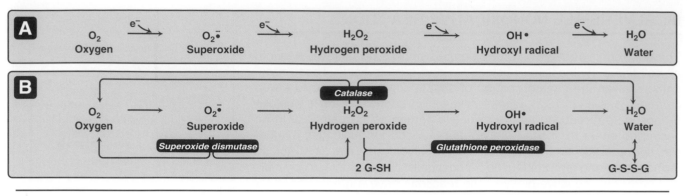

Figure 13.5

A. Formation of reactive intermediates from oxygen. e⁻ = electrons. B. Actions of antioxidant enzymes. G-SH = reduced glutathione; G-S-S-G = oxidized glutathione. [Note: See Fig. 13.6B for the regeneration of G-SH.]

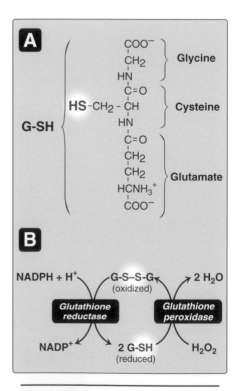

Figure 13.6

A. Structure of reduced glutathione (G-SH). [Note: Glutamate is linked to cysteine through a γ-carboxyl, rather than an α-carboxyl.] B. The roles of G-SH and reduced nicotinamide adenine dinucleotide phosphate (NADPH) in the reduction of hydrogen peroxide (H_2O_2) to water. G-S-S-G = oxidized glutathione.

B. Hydrogen peroxide reduction

Hydrogen peroxide (H_2O_2) is one of a family of reactive oxygen species (ROS) that are formed from the partial reduction of molecular oxygen ([O_2], Fig. 13.5A). These compounds are formed continuously as byproducts of aerobic metabolism, through reactions with drugs and environmental toxins, or when the level of antioxidants is diminished, all creating the condition of oxidative stress. These highly reactive oxygen intermediates can cause serious chemical damage to DNA, proteins, and unsaturated lipids and can lead to cell death. ROS have been implicated in a number of pathologic processes, including reperfusion injury, cancer, inflammatory disease, and aging. The cell has several protective mechanisms that minimize the toxic potential of these compounds. [Note: ROS can also be generated in the killing of microbes by white blood cells (WBC; see D. below).]

1. **Enzymes that catalyze antioxidant reactions:** Reduced glutathione (G-SH), a tripeptide-thiol (γ-glutamylcysteinylglycine) present in most cells, can chemically detoxify H_2O_2 (Fig. 13.5B). This reaction, catalyzed by the selenoprotein (see p. 407) *glutathione peroxidase*, forms oxidized glutathione (G-S-S-G), which no longer has protective properties. The cell regenerates G-SH in a reaction catalyzed by *glutathione reductase,* using NADPH as a source of reducing equivalents. Thus, NADPH indirectly provides electrons for the reduction of H_2O_2 (Fig. 13.6). Additional enzymes, such as *superoxide dismutase* and *catalase*, catalyze the conversion of other ROS to harmless products (see Fig. 13.5B). As a group, these enzymes serve as a defense system to guard against the toxic effects of ROS.

2. **Antioxidant chemicals:** A number of intracellular reducing agents, such as ascorbate (see p. 381), vitamin E (see p. 395), and β-carotene (see p. 386), are able to reduce and, thereby, detoxify ROS in the laboratory. Consumption of foods rich in these antioxidant compounds has been correlated with a reduced risk for certain types of cancers as well as decreased frequency of certain other chronic health problems. Therefore, it is tempting

to speculate that the effects of these compounds are, in part, an expression of their ability to quench the toxic effect of ROS. However, clinical trials with antioxidants as dietary supplements have failed to show clear beneficial effects. In the case of dietary supplementation with β-carotene, the rate of lung cancer in smokers increased rather than decreased. Thus, the health-promoting effects of dietary fruits and vegetables likely reflect a complex interaction among many naturally occurring compounds, which has not been duplicated by consumption of isolated antioxidant compounds.

C. Cytochrome P450 monooxygenase system

Monooxygenases (*mixed-function oxidases*) incorporate one atom from O_2 into a substrate (creating a hydroxyl group), with the other atom being reduced to water (H_2O). In the *cytochrome P450* (*CYP*) *monooxygenase* system, NADPH provides the reducing equivalents required by this series of reactions (Fig. 13.7). This system performs different functions in two separate locations in cells. The overall reaction catalyzed by a *CYP* enzyme is

$$R-H + O_2 + NADPH + H^+ \rightarrow R-OH + H_2O + NADP^+$$

where R may be a steroid, drug, or other chemical. [Note: *CYP* enzymes are actually a superfamily of related, heme-containing *monooxygenases* that participate in a broad variety of reactions. The P450 in the name reflects the absorbance at 450 nm by the protein.]

1. **Mitochondrial system:** An important function of the *CYP monooxygenase* system found associated with the inner mitochondrial membrane is the biosynthesis of steroid hormones. In steroidogenic tissues, such as the placenta, ovaries, testes, and adrenal cortex, it is used to hydroxylate intermediates in the conversion of cholesterol to steroid hormones, a process that makes these hydrophobic compounds more water soluble (see p. 237). The liver uses this same system in bile acid synthesis (see p. 224) and the hydroxylation of cholecalciferol to 25-hydroxycholecalciferol ([vitamin D_3] see p. 390), and the kidney uses it to hydroxylate vitamin D_3 to its biologically active 1,25-dihydroxylated form.

2. **Microsomal system:** The microsomal *CYP monooxygenase* system found associated with the membrane of the smooth endoplasmic reticulum (particularly in the liver) functions primarily in the detoxification of foreign compounds (xenobiotics). These include numerous drugs and such varied pollutants as petroleum products and pesticides. *CYP* enzymes of the microsomal system (for example, *CYP3A4*) can be used to hydroxylate these toxins (phase I). The purpose of these modifications is two-fold. First, it may itself activate or inactivate a drug and second, make a toxic compound more soluble, thereby facilitating its excretion in the urine or feces. Frequently, however, the new hydroxyl group will serve as a site for conjugation with a polar molecule, such as glucuronic acid (see p. 161), which will significantly increase the compound's solubility (phase II). [Note: Polymorphisms (see p. 491) in the genes for *CYP* enzymes can lead to differences in drug metabolism.]

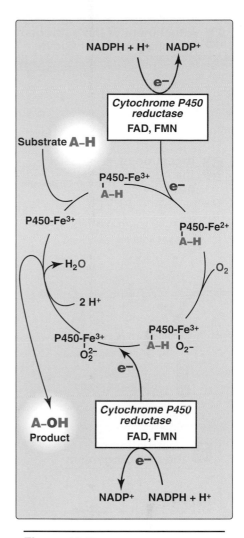

Figure 13.7
Cytochrome P450 (*CYP*) *monooxygenase* catalytic cycle (simplified). Electrons (e^-) move from nicotinamide adenine dinucleotide phosphate (NADPH) to flavin adenine dinucleotide (FAD) to flavin adenine mononucleotide (FMN) of the *reductase* and then to the heme iron (Fe) of the microsomal *CYP* enzyme. [Note: In the mitochondrial system, e^- move from FAD to an iron-sulfur protein and then to the *CYP* enzyme.]

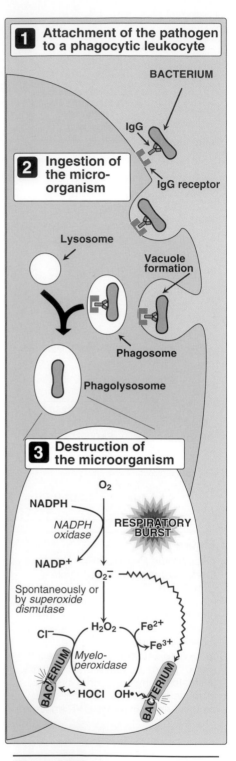

Figure 13.8

Phagocytosis and the oxygen (O_2)-dependent pathway of microbial killing. IgG = immunoglobulin G; NADP(H) = nicotinamide adenine dinucleotide phosphate; $O_2^{-\bullet}$ = superoxide; H_2O_2 = hydrogen peroxide; HOCl = hypochlorous acid; OH• = hydroxyl radical.

D. White blood cell phagocytosis and microbe killing

Phagocytosis is the ingestion by receptor-mediated endocytosis of microorganisms, foreign particles, and cellular debris by WBC (leukocytes) such as neutrophils and macrophages (monocytes). It is an important defense mechanism, particularly in bacterial infections. Neutrophils and monocytes are armed with both oxygen-independent and oxygen-dependent mechanisms for killing bacteria.

1. **Oxygen-independent:** Oxygen-independent mechanisms use pH changes in phagolysosomes and lysosomal enzymes to destroy pathogens.

2. **Oxygen-dependent:** Oxygen-dependent mechanisms include the enzymes *NADPH oxidase* and *myeloperoxidase* (*MPO*) that work together in killing bacteria (Fig. 13.8). Overall, the *MPO* system is the most potent of the bactericidal mechanisms. An invading bacterium is recognized by the immune system and attacked by antibodies that bind it to a receptor on a phagocytic cell. After internalization of the microorganism has occurred, *NADPH oxidase*, located in the leukocyte cell membrane, is activated and reduces O_2 from the surrounding tissue to superoxide ($O_2^{-\bullet}$), a free radical ROS, as NADPH is oxidized. The rapid consumption of O_2 that accompanies formation of $O_2^{-\bullet}$ is referred to as the respiratory burst. [Note: Active *NADPH oxidase* is a membrane-associated complex containing a flavocytochrome plus additional peptides that translocate from the cytoplasm upon activation of the leukocyte. Electrons move from NADPH to O_2 via flavin adenine nucleotide (FAD) and heme, generating $O_2^{-\bullet}$. Rare genetic deficiencies in *NADPH oxidase* cause chronic granulomatous disease (CGD) characterized by severe, persistent infections and the formation of granulomas (nodular areas of inflammation) that sequester the bacteria that were not destroyed.] Next, $O_2^{-\bullet}$ is converted to H_2O_2 (also a ROS), either spontaneously or catalyzed by *superoxide dismutase*. In the presence of *MPO*, a heme-containing lysosomal enzyme present within the phagolysosome, peroxide plus chloride ions are converted to hypochlorous acid ([HOCl] the major component of household bleach), which kills the bacteria. The peroxide can also be partially reduced to the hydroxyl radical (OH•), a ROS, or be fully reduced to H_2O by *catalase* or *glutathione peroxidase*. [Note: Deficiencies in *MPO* do not confer increased susceptibility to infection because peroxide from *NADPH oxidase* is bactericidal.]

E. Nitric oxide synthesis

Nitric oxide (NO) is recognized as a mediator in a broad array of biologic systems. NO is the endothelium-derived relaxing factor that causes vasodilation by relaxing vascular smooth muscle. It also acts as a neurotransmitter, prevents platelet aggregation, and plays an essential role in macrophage function. It has a very short half-life in tissues (3–10 seconds) because it reacts with O_2 and O_2^- and is converted into nitrates and nitrites including peroxynitrite (O=NOO$^-$), a reactive nitrogen species (RNS). [Note: NO is a free radical gas that is often confused with nitrous oxide (N_2O), the "laughing gas" that is used as an anesthetic and is chemically stable.]

1. **Nitric oxide synthase:** Arginine, O_2, and NADPH are substrates for cytosolic *NO synthase* ([*NOS*], Fig. 13.9). Flavin mononucleotide (FMN), FAD, heme, and tetrahydrobiopterin (see p. 268) are coenzymes, and NO and citrulline are products of the reaction. Three *NOS* isozymes, each the product of a different gene, have been identified. Two are constitutive (synthesized at a constant rate), calcium (Ca^{2+})–calmodulin (CaM)-dependent enzymes (see p. 133). They are found primarily in endothelium (*eNOS*) and neural tissue (*nNOS*) and constantly produce very low levels of NO for vasodilation and neurotransmission. An inducible, Ca^{2+}-independent enzyme (*iNOS*) can be expressed in many cells, including macrophages and neutrophils, as an early defense against pathogens. The specific inducers for *iNOS* vary with cell type and include proinflammatory cytokines, such as tumor necrosis factor-α (TNF-α) and interferon-γ (IFN-γ), and bacterial endotoxins such as lipopolysaccharide (LPS). These compounds promote synthesis of *iNOS*, which can result in large amounts of NO being produced over hours or even days.

2. **Nitric oxide and vascular endothelium:** NO is an important mediator in the control of vascular smooth muscle tone. NO is synthesized by *eNOS* in endothelial cells and diffuses to vascular smooth muscle, where it activates the cytosolic form of *guanylyl cyclase* (or, *guanylate cyclase*) to form cyclic guanosine monophosphate (cGMP). [Note: This reaction is analogous to the formation of cyclic adenosine monophosphate (cAMP) by *adenylyl cyclase* (see p. 95).] The resultant rise in cGMP causes activation of *protein kinase G*, which phosphorylates Ca^{2+} channels, causing decreased entry of Ca^{2+} into smooth muscle cells. This decreases the Ca^{2+}–CaM activation of *myosin light-chain kinase*, thereby decreasing smooth muscle contraction and favoring relaxation. Vasodilator nitrates, such as nitroglycerin, are metabolized to NO, which causes relaxation of vascular smooth muscle and, therefore, lowers blood pressure. Thus, NO can be envisioned as an endogenous nitrovasodilator. [Note: Under hypoxic conditions, nitrite (NO_2^-) can be reduced to NO, which binds to deoxyhemoglobin. The NO is released into the blood, causing vasodilation and increasing blood flow.]

3. **Nitric oxide and macrophage bactericidal activity:** In macrophages, *iNOS* activity is normally low, but synthesis of the enzyme is significantly stimulated by bacterial LPS and by release of IFN-γ and TNF-α in response to infection. Activated macrophages form $O_2^{-\bullet}$ radicals that combine with NO to form intermediates that decompose, producing the highly bactericidal OH$\bullet$ radical.

4. **Additional functions:** NO is a potent inhibitor of platelet adhesion and aggregation (by activating the cGMP pathway). It is also characterized as a neurotransmitter in the central and peripheral nervous systems.

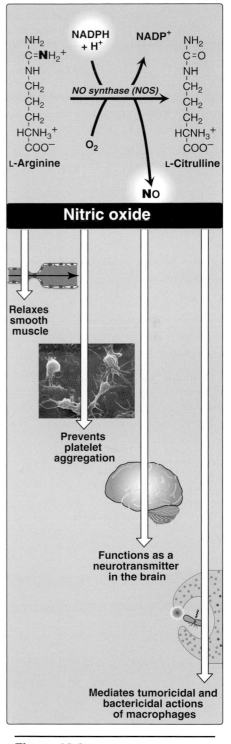

Figure 13.9
Synthesis and some actions of nitric oxide (NO). [Note: Flavin mononucleotide, flavin adenine dinucleotide, heme, and tetrahydrobiopterin are additional coenzymes required by *NOS*.] NADP(H) = nicotinamide adenine dinucleotide phosphate.

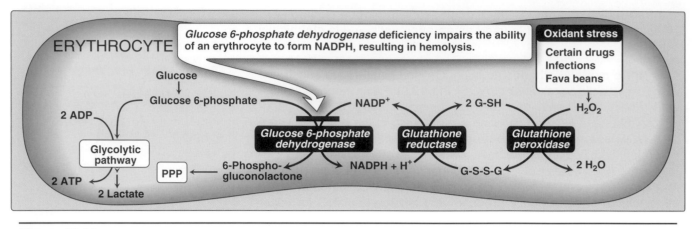

Figure 13.10
Pathways of glucose 6-phosphate metabolism in the erythrocyte. NADP(H) = nicotinamide adenine dinucleotide phosphate; G-SH = reduced glutathione; G-S-S-G = oxidized glutathione; H_2O_2 = hydrogen peroxide; PPP = pentose phosphate pathway.

V. G6PD DEFICIENCY

G6PD deficiency is a hereditary condition characterized by hemolytic anemia caused by the inability to detoxify oxidizing agents. *G6PD* deficiency is the most common disease-producing enzyme abnormality in humans, affecting >400 million individuals worldwide. This deficiency has the highest prevalence in the Middle East, tropical Africa and Asia, and parts of the Mediterranean. *G6PD* deficiency is X linked and is, in fact, a family of deficiencies caused by a number of different mutations in the gene encoding *G6PD*. Only some of the resulting protein variants cause clinical symptoms. [Note: In addition to hemolytic anemia, a clinical manifestation of *G6PD* deficiency is neonatal jaundice appearing 1–4 days after birth. The jaundice, which may be severe, typically results from increased production of unconjugated bilirubin (see p. 285).] The life span of individuals with a severe form of *G6PD* deficiency may be somewhat shortened as a result of complications arising from chronic hemolysis. This negative effect of *G6PD* deficiency has been balanced in evolution by an advantage in survival, an increased resistance to <u>Plasmodium falciparum</u> malaria. [Note: Sickle cell trait and the thalassemias also confer resistance to malaria.]

A. G6PD role in red blood cells

Diminished *G6PD* activity impairs the ability of the cell to form the NADPH that is essential for the maintenance of the G-SH pool. This results in a decrease in the detoxification of free radicals and peroxides formed within the cell (Fig. 13.10). G-SH also helps maintain the reduced states of sulfhydryl groups in proteins, including hemoglobin. Oxidation of those sulfhydryl groups leads to the formation of denatured proteins that form insoluble masses (called Heinz bodies) that attach to RBC membranes (Fig. 13.11). Additional oxidation of membrane proteins causes RBC to be rigid (less deformable), and they are removed from the circulation by macrophages in the spleen and liver. Although *G6PD* deficiency occurs in all cells of the affected individual, it is most severe in RBC, where the pentose phosphate

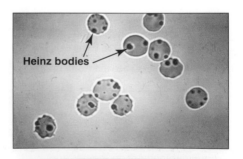

Figure 13.11
Heinz bodies in the erythrocytes of a patient with *glucose 6-phosphate dehydrogenase* deficiency.

pathway provides the only means of generating NADPH. Additionally, the RBC has no nucleus or ribosomes and cannot renew its supply of the enzyme. Thus, RBC are particularly vulnerable to enzyme variants with diminished stability. [Note: Other tissues have an alternative source of NADPH ($NADP^+$-dependent malate dehydrogenase [malic enzyme]; see p. 186) that can keep G-SH reduced.]

B. Precipitating factors in G6PD deficiency

Most individuals who have inherited one of the G6PD mutations do not show clinical manifestations (that is, they are asymptomatic). However, some patients with G6PD deficiency develop hemolytic anemia if they are treated with an oxidant drug, ingest fava beans, or contract a severe infection.

1. **Oxidant drugs:** Commonly used drugs that produce hemolytic anemia in patients with G6PD deficiency are best remembered from the mnemonic AAA: antibiotics (for example, sulfamethoxazole and chloramphenicol), antimalarials (for example, primaquine but not chloroquine or quinine), and antipyretics (for example, acetanilide but not acetaminophen).

2. **Favism:** Some forms of G6PD deficiency, for example, the Mediterranean variant, are particularly susceptible to the hemolytic effect of the fava (broad) bean, a dietary staple in the Mediterranean region. Favism, the hemolytic effect of ingesting fava beans, is not observed in all individuals with G6PD deficiency, but all patients with favism have G6PD deficiency.

3. **Infection:** Infection is the most common precipitating factor of hemolysis in G6PD deficiency. The inflammatory response to infection results in the generation of free radicals in macrophages. The radicals can diffuse into the RBC and cause oxidative damage.

C. Variant G6PD properties

Almost all G6PD variants are caused by point mutations (see p. 449) in the gene for G6PD. Some mutations do not affect enzymic activity. However, other mutations result in decreased catalytic activity, decreased stability, or an alteration of binding affinity for $NADP^+$ or glucose 6-phosphate. [Note: Active G6PD exists as a homodimer or tetramer. Mutations at the interface between subunits can affect stability.] The severity of the disease usually correlates with the amount of residual enzyme activity in the patient's RBC. For example, variants can be classified as shown in Figure 13.12. G6PD A⁻ is the prototype of the moderate (class III) form of the disease. The RBC contain an unstable but kinetically normal G6PD, with most of the enzyme activity present in the reticulocytes and younger RBC (Fig. 13.13). Therefore, the oldest RBC have the lowest level of enzyme activity and are preferentially removed in a hemolytic episode. Because hemolysis does not affect younger cells, the episodes are self-limiting. G6PD Mediterranean is the prototype of a more severe (class II) deficiency. Class I mutations (rare) are the most severe and are associated with chronic nonspherocytic hemolytic anemia, which occurs even in the absence of oxidative stress.

Class	Clinical symptoms	Residual enzyme activity
I	Very severe (chronic, nonspherocytic hemolytic anemia)	<10%
*II	Severe (acute hemolytic anemia)	<10%
*III	Moderate	10%–60%
IV	None	>60%

Figure 13.12
Classification of glucose 6-phosphate dehydrogenase (G6PD) deficiency variants. [Note: Class V variants (not shown) result in overproduction of G6PD.] * = most common.

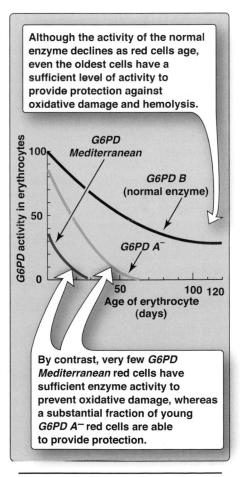

Although the activity of the normal enzyme declines as red cells age, even the oldest cells have a sufficient level of activity to provide protection against oxidative damage and hemolysis.

By contrast, very few G6PD Mediterranean red cells have sufficient enzyme activity to prevent oxidative damage, whereas a substantial fraction of young G6PD A⁻ red cells are able to provide protection.

Figure 13.13
Decline of erythrocyte glucose 6-phosphate dehydrogenase (G6PD) activity with cell age for the three most commonly encountered forms of the enzyme.

D. G6PD molecular biology

The cloning of the gene for *G6PD* and the sequencing of its DNA (see Chapter 34) have permitted the identification of mutations that cause *G6PD* deficiency. More than 400 *G6PD* variants have been identified, a finding that explains the numerous biochemical and clinical phenotypes that have been described. Most mutations that result in enzymic deficiency are missense mutations (see p. 449) in the coding region. Both *G6PD A⁻* and *G6PD Mediterranean* represent mutant enzymes that differ from the respective normal variants by a single amino acid. Large deletions or frameshift mutations have not been identified, suggesting that complete absence of *G6PD* activity is likely lethal.

VI. CHAPTER SUMMARY

The **pentose phosphate pathway** includes an irreversible oxidative phase followed by a series of reversible sugar–phosphate interconversions (Fig. 13.14). No ATP is directly consumed or produced in the pathway. The reduced nicotinamide adenine dinucleotide phosphate (NADPH)-producing **oxidative portion** of the pathway is important in providing reducing equivalents for reductive biosynthesis and detoxification reactions. In this part of the pathway, **glucose 6-phosphate** is irreversibly converted to **ribulose 5-phosphate**, and **two NADPH** are produced. The regulated step is catalyzed by **glucose 6-phosphate dehydrogenase** (**G6PD**), which is strongly inhibited by a rise in the **NADPH/NADP⁺ ratio**. **Reversible nonoxidative reactions** interconvert sugars. This part of the pathway converts ribulose 5-phosphate to **ribose 5-phosphate**, required for nucleotide and nucleic acid synthesis, or to **fructose 6-phosphate** and **glyceraldehyde 3-phosphate** (glycolytic intermediates). NADPH is a source of **reducing equivalents** in **reductive biosynthesis**, such as the production of fatty acids in liver, adipose tissue, and the mammary gland; cholesterol in the liver; and steroid hormones in the placenta, ovaries, testes, and adrenal cortex. It is also required by **red blood cells** (**RBC**) for **hydrogen peroxide reduction**. **Reduced glutathione** (**G-SH**) is used by **glutathione peroxidase** to reduce the peroxide to water. The **oxidized glutathione** (**G-S-S-G**) produced is reduced by **glutathione reductase**, using NADPH as the source of electrons. NADPH provides reducing equivalents for the **mitochondrial cytochrome P450 monooxygenase system**, which is used in **steroid hormone synthesis** in steroidogenic tissue, **bile acid synthesis** in the liver, and **vitamin D activation** in the liver and kidneys. The **microsomal system** uses NADPH to **detoxify** foreign compounds (xenobiotics), such as drugs and a variety of pollutants. NADPH provides the reducing equivalents for phagocytes in the process of eliminating invading microorganisms. **NADPH oxidase** uses molecular oxygen (O₂) and electrons from NADPH to produce **superoxide radicals**, which, in turn, can be converted to peroxide by **superoxide dismutase**. **Myeloperoxidase** catalyzes the formation of bactericidal hypochlorous acid from peroxide and chloride ions. Rare genetic defects in *NADPH oxidase* cause **chronic granulomatous disease** characterized by severe, persistent, infections and granuloma formation. NADPH is required for the synthesis of **nitric oxide** (**NO**), an important free radical gas that causes **vasodilation** by relaxing vascular smooth muscle, acts as a **neurotransmitter**, prevents **platelet aggregation**, and helps mediate **macrophage bactericidal activity**. NO is made from arginine and O₂ by three different NADPH-dependent *NO synthases* (*NOS*). The **endothelial** (*eNOS*) and **neuronal** (*nNOS*) isozymes constantly produce very low levels of NO for vasodilation and neurotransmission, respectively. The **inducible isozyme** (*iNOS*) produces large amounts of NO for defense against pathogens. *G6PD* **deficiency** impairs the ability of the cell to form the NADPH that is essential for the maintenance of the G-SH pool. The cells most affected are **RBC** because they do not have additional sources of NADPH. *G6PD* deficiency is an **X-linked disease** characterized by **hemolytic anemia** caused by the production of free radicals and peroxides following administration of **oxidant drugs**, ingestion of **fava beans**, or severe **infections**. The extent of the anemia depends on the amount of residual enzyme. Class I variants, the most severe (and least common), are associated with **chronic nonspherocytic hemolytic anemia**. Babies with *G6PD* deficiency may experience **neonatal jaundice**.

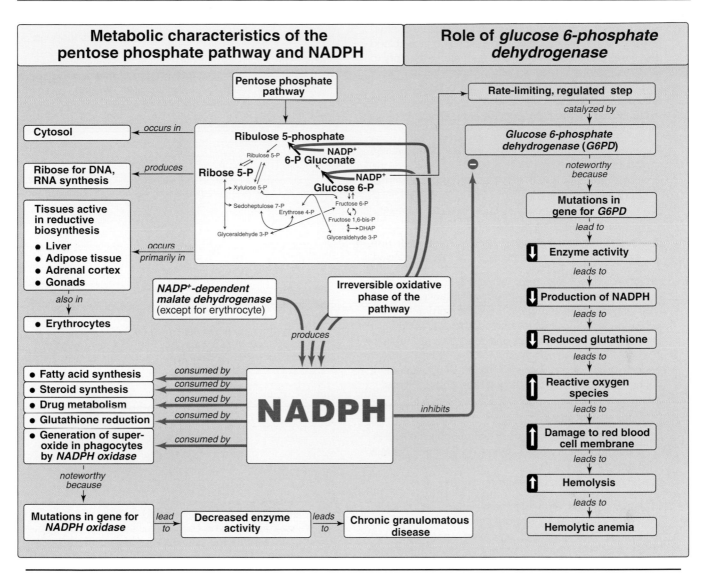

Figure 13.14
Key concept map for the pentose phosphate pathway and nicotinamide adenine dinucleotide phosphate (NADPH).

Study Questions

Choose the ONE best answer.

13.1 In preparation for a trip to an area of India where chloroquine-resistant malaria is endemic, a young man is given primaquine prophylactically. Soon thereafter, he develops a hemolytic condition due to a deficiency in glucose 6-phosphate dehydrogenase. A less-than-normal level of which of the following is a consequence of the enzyme deficiency and the underlying cause of the hemolysis?

A. Glucose 6-phosphate
B. Oxidized form of nicotinamide adenine dinucleotide
C. Reduced form of glutathione
D. Ribose 5-phosphate

Correct answer = C. Glutathione (G-SH) is essential for red cell integrity and is maintained in this reduced (functional) form by nicotinamide adenine dinucleotide phosphate (NADPH)-dependent glutathione reductase. The NADPH is from the oxidative portion of the pentose phosphate pathway. Individuals with a deficiency of the regulated enzyme of this pathway, glucose 6-phosphate dehydrogenase (G6PD), have a decreased ability to generate NADPH and, therefore, a decreased ability to keep G-SH reduced. When treated with an oxidant drug such as primaquine, some patients with G6PD deficiency develop a hemolytic anemia. Primaquine does not affect glucose 6-phosphate levels. Nicotinamide adenine dinucleotide (NAD[H]) is neither produced by the pathway nor used as a coenzyme by G-SH reductase. A decrease in ribose 5-phosphate does not cause hemolysis.

13.2 Septic shock, a state of acute circulatory failure characterized by persistent arterial hypotension (low blood pressure) and inadequate organ perfusion refractory to fluid resuscitation, results from a severe inflammatory response to bacterial infection. It has a high mortality rate and is associated with changes in the level of nitric oxide. Which statement concerning septic shock is most likely correct?

A. Activation of endothelial nitric oxide synthase causes an increase in nitric oxide.
B. High mortality is the result of the long half-life of nitric oxide.
C. Lysine, the nitrogen source for nitric oxide synthesis, is deaminated by bacteria.
D. Overproduction of nitric oxide by a calcium-independent enzyme is the cause of the hypotension.

Correct answer = D. Overproduction of short-lived (not long-lived) nitric oxide (NO) by calcium-independent, inducible nitric oxide synthase (iNOS) results in excessive vasodilation leading to hypotension. The endothelial enzyme (eNOS) is constitutive and produces low levels of NO at a consistent rate. NOS use arginine, not lysine, as the source of the nitrogen.

13.3 An individual who has recently been prescribed a drug (atorvastatin) to lower cholesterol levels is advised to limit consumption of grapefruit juice, because high intake of the juice reportedly results in an increased level of the drug in the blood, increasing the risk of side effects. Atorvastatin is a substrate for the cytochrome P450 enzyme CYP3A4, and grapefruit juice inhibits the enzyme. Which statement concerning CYP enzymes is most likely correct? They:

A. accept electrons from reduced nicotinamide adenine dinucleotide.
B. catalyze the hydroxylation of hydrophobic molecules.
C. differ from nitric oxide synthase in that they contain heme.
D. function in association with an oxidase.

Correct answer = B. The CYP enzymes hydroxylate hydrophobic compounds, making them more water soluble. Reduced nicotinamide adenine dinucleotide phosphate (NADPH) from the pentose phosphate pathway is the electron donor. Both the CYP enzymes and the nitric oxide synthase isozymes contain heme.

13.4 In male patients who are hemizygous for X-linked glucose 6-phosphate dehydrogenase deficiency, pathophysiologic consequences are more apparent in red blood cells (RBC) than in other cells such as in the liver. Which one of the following provides the most reasonable explanation for this different response?

A. Excess glucose 6-phosphate in the liver, but not in RBC, can be channeled to glycogen, thereby averting cellular damage.
B. Liver cells, in contrast to RBC, have alternative mechanisms for supplying the reduced nicotinamide adenine dinucleotide phosphate required for maintaining cell integrity.
C. Because RBC do not have mitochondria, production of ATP required to maintain cell integrity depends exclusively on the shunting of glucose 6-phosphate to the pentose phosphate pathway.
D. In RBC, in contrast to liver cells, glucose 6-phosphatase activity decreases the level of glucose 6-phosphate, resulting in cell damage.

Correct answer = B. Cellular damage is directly related to decreased ability of the cell to regenerate reduced glutathione, for which large amounts of reduced nicotinamide adenine dinucleotide phosphate (NADPH) are needed, and RBC have no means other than the pentose phosphate pathway of generating NADPH. It is decreased product (NADPH), not increased substrate (glucose 6-phosphate), that is the problem. RBC do not have glucose 6-phosphatase. The pentose phosphate pathway does not generate ATP.

13.5 An essential coenzyme for several enzymes of metabolism is derived from the vitamin thiamine. Measurement of the activity of what enzyme in red blood cells could be used to determine thiamine status in the body?

Red blood cells do not have mitochondria and, so, do not contain mitochondrial enzymes such as pyruvate dehydrogenase that require the thiamine-derived coenzyme thiamine pyrophosphate (TPP). However, they do contain the cytosolic TPP-requiring transketolase, whose activity is used clinically to assess thiamine status.

Glycosaminoglycans, Proteoglycans, and Glycoproteins

14

I. GLYCOSAMINOGLYCAN OVERVIEW

Glycosaminoglycans (GAG) are large complexes of negatively charged heteropolysaccharide chains. They are generally associated with a small amount of protein (core protein), forming proteoglycans, which typically consist of up to 95% carbohydrate. GAG have the special ability to bind large amounts of water, thereby producing the gel-like matrix that forms the basis of the body's ground substance, which, along with fibrous structural proteins such as collagen, elastin, and fibrillin-1, and adhesive proteins such as fibronectin, makes up the extracellular matrix (ECM). The hydrated GAG serve as a flexible support for the ECM, interacting with the structural and adhesive proteins, and as a molecular sieve, influencing movement of materials through the ECM. The viscous, lubricating properties of mucous secretions also result from the presence of GAG, which led to the original naming of these compounds as mucopolysaccharides.

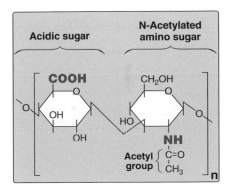

Figure 14.1
Repeating disaccharide unit of glycosaminoglycans.

II. STRUCTURE

GAG are long, unbranched, heteropolysaccharide chains composed of a repeating disaccharide unit [acidic sugar–amino sugar]$_n$ (Fig. 14.1). [Note: A single exception is keratan sulfate, which contains galactose rather than an acidic sugar.] The amino sugar is either D-glucosamine or D-galactosamine, in which the amino group is usually acetylated, thus eliminating its positive charge. The amino sugar may also be sulfated on carbon 4 or 6 or on a nonacetylated nitrogen. The acidic sugar is either D-glucuronic acid or its C-5 epimer L-iduronic acid (Fig. 14.2). These uronic sugars contain carboxyl groups that are negatively charged at physiologic pH and, together with the sulfate groups ($-SO_4^{2-}$), give GAG their strongly negative nature.

A. Structure–function relationship

Because of the high concentration of negative charges, these heteropolysaccharide chains tend to be extended in solution. They repel each other and are surrounded by a shell of water molecules. When brought together, they slide past each other, much as two magnets

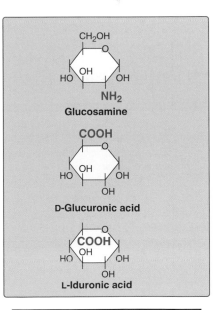

Figure 14.2
Some monosaccharide units found in glycosaminoglycans.

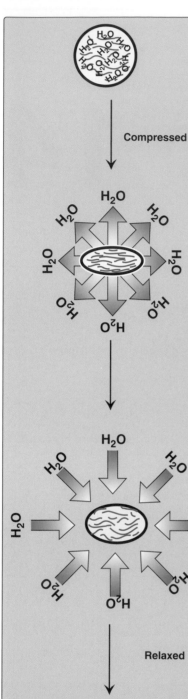

Figure 14.3
Resilience of glycosaminoglycans.

with the same polarity seem to slide past each other. This produces the slippery consistency of mucous secretions and synovial fluid. When a solution of GAG is compressed, the water is squeezed out, and the GAG are forced to occupy a smaller volume. When the compression is released, the GAG spring back to their original, hydrated volume because of the repulsion of their negative charges. This property contributes to the resilience of synovial fluid and the vitreous humor of the eye (Fig. 14.3).

B. Classification

The six major types of GAG are divided according to monomeric composition, type of glycosidic linkages, and degree and location of sulfate units. The structure of the GAG and their distribution in the body is illustrated in Figure 14.4. All GAG, except for hyaluronic acid, are sulfated and are found covalently attached to protein, forming proteoglycan monomers.

C. Proteoglycans

Proteoglycans are found in the ECM and on the outer surface of cells.

1. **Monomer structure:** A proteoglycan monomer found in cartilage consists of a core protein to which up to 100 linear chains of GAG are covalently attached. These chains, which may each be composed of up to 200 disaccharide units, extend out from the core protein and remain separated from each other because of charge repulsion. The resulting structure resembles a bottle brush (Fig. 14.5). In cartilage proteoglycans, the species of GAG include chondroitin sulfate and keratan sulfate. [Note: Proteoglycans are grouped into gene families that encode core proteins with common structural features. The aggrecan family (aggrecan, versican, neurocan, and brevican), abundant in cartilage, is an example.]

2. **GAG–protein linkage:** This covalent linkage is most commonly through a trihexoside (galactose-galactose-xylose) and a serine residue in the protein. An O-glycosidic bond (see p. 86) is formed between the xylose and the hydroxyl group of the serine (Fig. 14.6).

3. **Aggregate formation:** Many proteoglycan monomers can associate with one molecule of hyaluronic acid to form proteoglycan aggregates. The association is not covalent and occurs primarily through ionic interactions between the core protein and the hyaluronic acid. The association is stabilized by additional small proteins called link proteins (Fig. 14.7).

III. SYNTHESIS

The heteropolysaccharide chains are elongated by the sequential addition of alternating acidic and amino sugars donated primarily by their uridine diphosphate (UDP) derivatives. The reactions are catalyzed by a family of specific *glycosyltransferases*. Because GAG are produced for export from the cell, their synthesis occurs primarily in the Golgi and not in the cytosol.

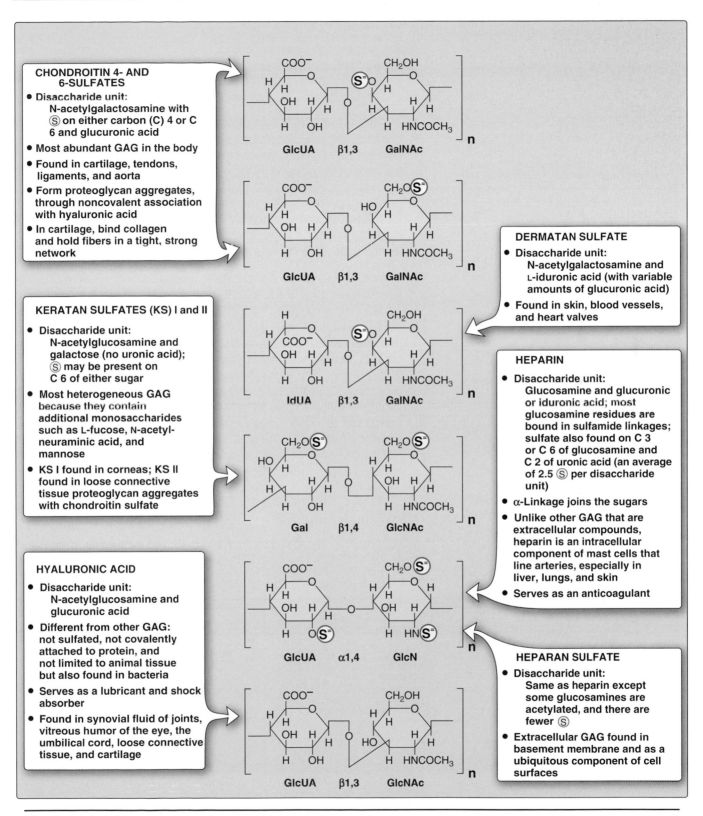

CHONDROITIN 4- AND 6-SULFATES

- Disaccharide unit: N-acetylgalactosamine with Ⓢ on either carbon (C) 4 or C 6 and glucuronic acid
- Most abundant GAG in the body
- Found in cartilage, tendons, ligaments, and aorta
- Form proteoglycan aggregates, through noncovalent association with hyaluronic acid
- In cartilage, bind collagen and hold fibers in a tight, strong network

KERATAN SULFATES (KS) I and II

- Disaccharide unit: N-acetylglucosamine and galactose (no uronic acid); Ⓢ may be present on C 6 of either sugar
- Most heterogeneous GAG because they contain additional monosaccharides such as L-fucose, N-acetyl-neuraminic acid, and mannose
- KS I found in corneas; KS II found in loose connective tissue proteoglycan aggregates with chondroitin sulfate

HYALURONIC ACID

- Disaccharide unit: N-acetylglucosamine and glucuronic acid
- Different from other GAG: not sulfated, not covalently attached to protein, and not limited to animal tissue but also found in bacteria
- Serves as a lubricant and shock absorber
- Found in synovial fluid of joints, vitreous humor of the eye, the umbilical cord, loose connective tissue, and cartilage

DERMATAN SULFATE

- Disaccharide unit: N-acetylgalactosamine and L-iduronic acid (with variable amounts of glucuronic acid)
- Found in skin, blood vessels, and heart valves

HEPARIN

- Disaccharide unit: Glucosamine and glucuronic or iduronic acid; most glucosamine residues are bound in sulfamide linkages; sulfate also found on C 3 or C 6 of glucosamine and C 2 of uronic acid (an average of 2.5 Ⓢ per disaccharide unit)
- α-Linkage joins the sugars
- Unlike other GAG that are extracellular compounds, heparin is an intracellular component of mast cells that line arteries, especially in liver, lungs, and skin
- Serves as an anticoagulant

HEPARAN SULFATE

- Disaccharide unit: Same as heparin except some glucosamines are acetylated, and there are fewer Ⓢ
- Extracellular GAG found in basement membrane and as a ubiquitous component of cell surfaces

Figure 14.4

Structure of repeating units in and distribution of glycosaminoglycans (GAG). Sulfate groups (Ⓢ) are shown in all possible positions. GlcUA and IdUA = glucuronic and iduronic acids; GalNAc = N-acetylgalactosamine; GlcNAc = N-acetylglucosamine; GlcN = glucosamine; Gal = galactose.

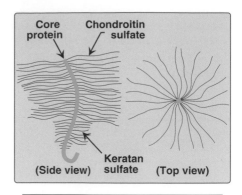

Figure 14.5
Bottle brush model of a cartilage proteoglycan monomer.

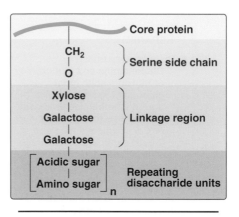

Figure 14.6
Glycosaminoglycan linkage regions.

A. Amino sugar synthesis

Amino sugars are essential components of glycoconjugates such as proteoglycans, glycoproteins, and glycolipids. The synthetic pathway of amino sugars (hexosamines) is very active in connective tissues, where as much as 20% of glucose flows through this pathway.

1. **N-Acetylglucosamine and N-acetylgalactosamine:** The monosaccharide fructose 6-phosphate is the precursor of N-acetylglucosamine (GlcNAc) and N-acetylgalactosamine (GalNAc). A hydroxyl group on the fructose is replaced by the amide nitrogen of a glutamine, and the glucosamine 6-phosphate product gets acetylated, isomerized, and activated, producing the nucleotide sugar UDP-GlcNAc (Fig. 14.8). UDP-GalNAc is generated by the epimerization of UDP-GlcNAc. It is these nucleotide sugar forms of the amino sugars that are used to elongate the carbohydrate chains.

2. **N-Acetylneuraminic acid:** NANA, a nine-carbon, acidic monosaccharide (see Fig. 17.15, p. 209), is a member of the family of sialic acids, each of which is acylated at a different site. These compounds are usually found as terminal carbohydrate residues of oligosaccharide side chains of glycoproteins, of glycolipids, or, less frequently, of GAG. N-Acetylmannosamine 6-phosphate (derived from fructose 6-phosphate) and phosphoenolpyruvate (an intermediate in glycolysis; see p. 102) are the immediate sources of the carbons and nitrogens for NANA synthesis (see Fig. 14.8). Before NANA can be added to a growing oligosaccharide, it must be activated to cytidine monophosphate (CMP)-NANA by reacting with cytidine triphosphate (CTP). *CMP-NANA synthetase* catalyzes the reaction. [Note: CMP-NANA is the only nucleotide sugar in human metabolism in which the carrier nucleotide is a monophosphate rather than a diphosphate.]

B. Acidic sugar synthesis

D-Glucuronic acid, whose structure is that of glucose with an oxidized carbon 6 ($-CH_2OH \rightarrow -COOH$), and its C-5 epimer, L-iduronic acid,

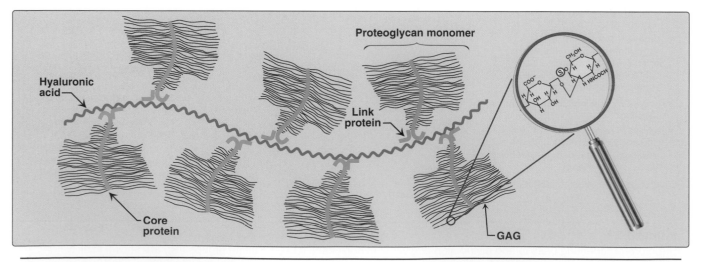

Figure 14.7
Proteoglycan aggregate. GAG = glycosaminoglycan.

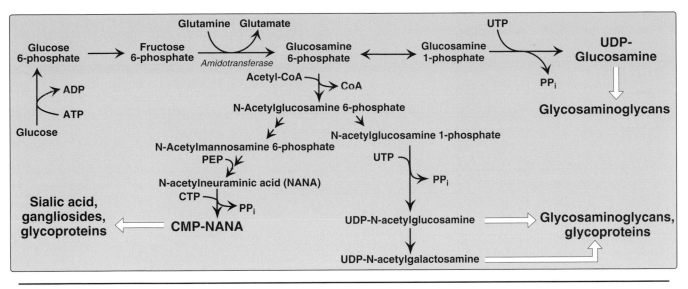

Figure 14.8
Synthesis of the amino sugars. ADP = adenosine diphosphate; UTP and UDP = uridine tri- and diphosphates; CoA = coenzyme A; PEP = phosphoenolpyruvate; CTP and CMP = cytidine tri- and monophosphates; PP_i = pyrophosphate.

are essential components of GAG. Glucuronic acid is also required for the detoxification of lipophilic compounds, such as bilirubin (see p. 282), steroids (see p. 240), and many drugs, including the statins (see p. 224), because conjugation with glucuronate (glucuronidation) increases water solubility. In plants and mammals (other than guinea pigs and primates, including humans), glucuronic acid is a precursor of ascorbic acid (vitamin C) as shown in Figure 14.9. This uronic acid pathway also provides a mechanism by which dietary D-xylulose can enter the central metabolic pathways.

1. **Glucuronic acid:** Glucuronic acid can be obtained in small amounts from the diet and from the lysosomal degradation of GAG. It also can be synthesized by the uronic acid pathway, in which glucose 1-phosphate reacts with uridine triphosphate (UTP) and is converted to UDP-glucose. Oxidation of UDP-glucose produces UDP-glucuronic acid, the form that supplies glucuronic acid for

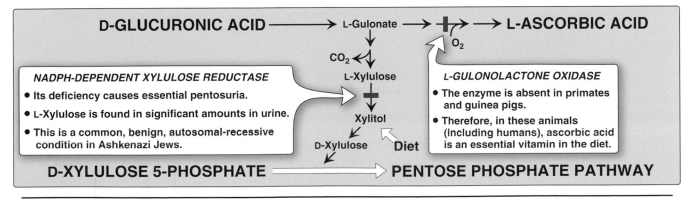

Figure 14.9
Metabolism of glucuronic acid. NADPH = reduced nicotinamide adenine dinucleotide phosphate; CO_2 = carbon dioxide.

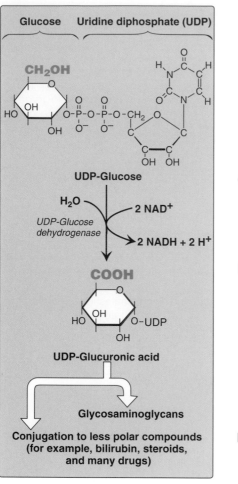

Figure 14.10
Oxidation of UDP-glucose to
UDP-glucuronic acid. NAD(H) =
nicotinamide adenine dinucleotide.

GAG synthesis and glucuronidation (Fig. 14.10). The end product of glucuronic acid metabolism in humans is D-xylulose 5-phosphate, which can enter the pentose phosphate pathway and produce the glycolytic intermediates glyceraldehyde 3-phosphate and fructose 6-phosphate (see Fig. 14.9; see also Fig. 13.2, p. 146).

2. **L-Iduronic acid:** Synthesis of L-iduronic acid occurs after D-glucuronic acid has been incorporated into the carbohydrate chain. *Uronosyl 5-epimerase* causes epimerization of the D- to the L-sugar.

C. Core protein synthesis

The core protein is made by ribosomes on the rough endoplasmic reticulum (RER), enters the RER lumen, and then moves to the Golgi, where it is glycosylated by membrane-bound *glycosyltransferases*.

D. Carbohydrate chain synthesis

Carbohydrate chain formation is initiated by synthesis of a short linker on the core protein on which carbohydrate chain synthesis will occur. The most common linker is a trihexoside formed by the transfer of a xylose from UDP-xylose to the hydroxyl group of a serine (or threonine) catalyzed by *xylosyltransferase*. Two galactose molecules are then added, completing the trihexoside. This is followed by sequential addition of alternating acidic and amino sugars (Fig. 14.11) and epimerization of some D-glucuronyl to L-iduronyl residues.

E. Sulfate group addition

Sulfation of a GAG occurs after the monosaccharide to be sulfated has been incorporated into the growing carbohydrate chain. The source of the sulfate is 3′-phosphoadenosyl-5′-phosphosulfate ([PAPS] a molecule of adenosine monophosphate with a sulfate group attached to the 5′-phosphate; see Fig. 17.16, p. 210). The sulfation reaction is catalyzed by *sulfotransferases*. Synthesis of the sulfated GAG chondroitin sulfate is shown in Figure 14.11. [Note: PAPS is also the sulfur donor in glycosphingolipid synthesis (see p. 210).]

> A defect in the sulfation of the growing GAG chains results in one of several autosomal-recessive disorders, the chondrodystrophies, which affect the proper development and maintenance of the skeletal system.

IV. DEGRADATION

GAG are degraded in lysosomes, which contain hydrolytic enzymes that are most active at a pH of ~5. Therefore, as a group, these enzymes are called *acid hydrolases*. [Note: The low pH optimum is a protective mechanism that prevents the enzymes from destroying the cell should leakage occur into the cytosol where the pH is neutral.] The half-lives of GAG vary from minutes to months and are influenced by the type of GAG and its location in the body.

A. GAG phagocytosis

Because GAG are extracellular or cell-surface compounds, they must first be engulfed by invagination of the cell membrane (phagocytosis), forming a vesicle inside of which are the GAG to be degraded. This vesicle then fuses with a lysosome, forming a single digestive vesicle in which the GAG are efficiently degraded (see p. 150 for a discussion of phagocytosis).

B. Lysosomal degradation

The lysosomal degradation of GAG requires a large number of *acid hydrolases* for complete digestion. First, the polysaccharide chains are cleaved by *endoglycosidases*, producing oligosaccharides. Further degradation of the oligosaccharides occurs sequentially from the nonreducing end (see p. 127) of each chain, the last group (sulfate or sugar) added during synthesis being the first group removed (by *sulfatases* or *exoglycosidases*). Examples of some of these enzymes and the bonds they hydrolyze are shown in Figure 14.12. [Note: *Endo-* and *exoglycosidases* are also involved in the lysosomal degradation of glycoproteins (see p. 170) and glycolipids (see p. 210). Deficiencies in these enzymes result in the accumulation of partially degraded carbohydrates, causing tissue damage.]

> Multiple *sulfatase* deficiency (Austin disease) is a rare lysosomal storage disease in which all *sulfatases* are nonfunctional because of a defect in the formation of formylglycine, an amino acid derivative required at the active site for enzymic activity to occur.

V. MUCOPOLYSACCHARIDOSES

The mucopolysaccharidoses are hereditary diseases (approximately 1:25,000 live births) caused by a deficiency of any one of the lysosomal *hydrolases* normally involved in the degradation of heparan sulfate and/ or dermatan sulfate (see Fig. 14.12). They are progressive disorders characterized by lysosomal accumulation of GAG in various tissues, causing a range of symptoms, such as skeletal and ECM deformities, and intellectual disability. All are autosomal-recessive disorders except Hunter syndrome, which is X linked. Children who are homozygous for any one of these diseases are apparently normal at birth and then gradually deteriorate. In severe deficiencies, death occurs in childhood. There currently is no cure. Incomplete lysosomal degradation of GAG results in the presence of oligosaccharides in the urine. These fragments can be used to diagnose the specific mucopolysaccharidosis by identifying the structure present on the nonreducing end of the oligosaccharide, because that residue would have been the substrate for the missing enzyme. Diagnosis is confirmed by measuring the patient's cellular level of the lysosomal *hydrolases*. Bone marrow and cord blood transplants, in which transplanted macrophages produce the enzymes that degrade GAG, have been used to treat Hurler and Hunter syndromes, with limited success. Enzyme replacement therapy is available for both syndromes but does not prevent neurologic damage.

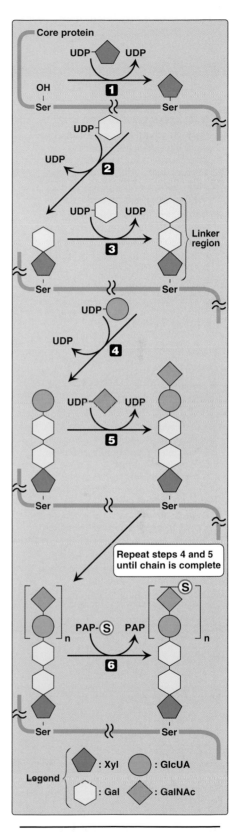

Figure 14.11
Synthesis of chondroitin sulfate. PAP-Ⓢ = 3'-phosphoadenosyl-5'-phosphosulfate; Ser = serine.

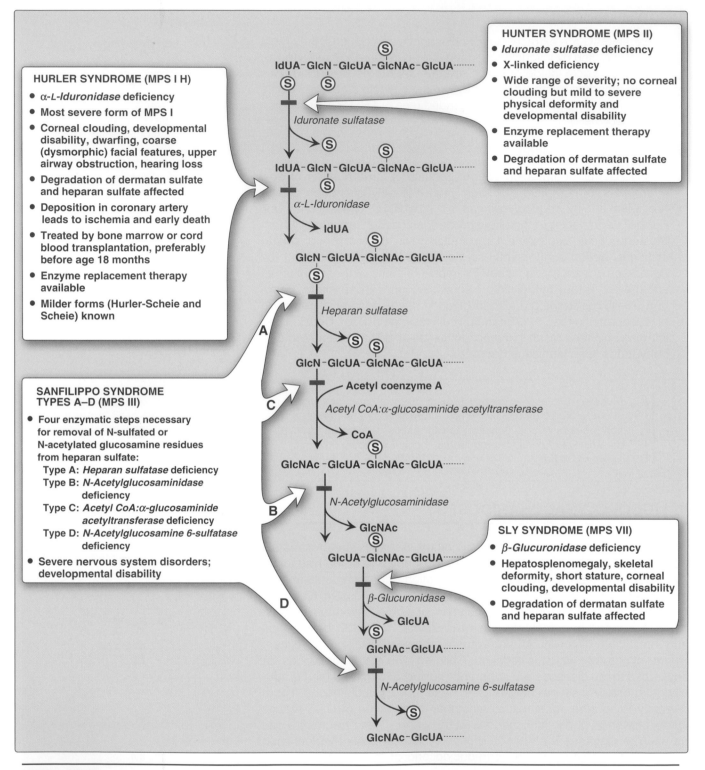

Figure 14.12

Degradation of the glycosaminoglycan heparan sulfate by lysosomal enzymes, indicating sites of enzyme deficiencies in some representative mucopolysaccharidoses (MPS). [Note: Deficiencies in *galactosamine 6-sulfatase* and *β-galactosidase* that degrade keratan sulfate result in Morquio syndrome (MPS IV), A and B, respectively. Deficiencies in *arylsulfatase B* that degrades dermatan sulfate result in Maroteaux-Lamy syndrome (MPS VI).] GlcUA and IdUA = glucuronic and iduronic acids; GalNAc = N-acetylgalactosamine; GlcNAc = N-acetylglucosamine; GlcN = glucosamine; Ⓢ = sulfate.

VI. GLYCOPROTEIN OVERVIEW

Glycoproteins are proteins to which oligosaccharides (glycans) are covalently attached. [Note: Glycosylation is the most common post-translational modification of proteins.] They differ from the proteoglycans in several important ways. Glycoproteins contain highly variable amounts of carbohydrate but typically less than that of proteoglycans. For example, the glycoprotein immunoglobulin G (IgG) contains <4% of its mass as carbohydrate, whereas the proteoglycan aggrecan contains >80%. In glycoproteins, the glycan is relatively short (usually two to ten sugar residues in length, although it can be longer); does not contain repeating disaccharide units and, consequently, is structurally diverse; is often branched instead of linear; and may or may not be negatively charged. Membrane-bound glycoproteins participate in a broad range of cellular phenomena, including cell-surface recognition (by other cells, hormones, and viruses), cell-surface antigenicity (such as the blood group antigens), and as components of the ECM and of the mucins of the gastrointestinal and urogenital tracts, where they act as protective biologic lubricants. In addition, almost all of the globular proteins present in human plasma are glycoproteins, although albumin is an exception. Figure 14.13 summarizes some glycoprotein functions.

VII. OLIGOSACCHARIDE STRUCTURE

The oligosaccharide (glycan) components of glycoproteins are generally branched heteropolymers composed primarily of D-hexoses, with the addition in some cases of neuraminic acid (a nonose) and of L-fucose, a 6-deoxyhexose.

A. Carbohydrate–protein linkage

The glycan may be attached to the protein through an N- or an O-glycosidic link (see p. 86). In the former case, the sugar chain is attached to the amide group of an asparagine side chain and, in the latter case, to the hydroxyl group of either a serine or threonine side chain. [Note: In the case of collagen, there is an O-glycosidic linkage between galactose or glucose and the hydroxyl group of hydroxylysine (see p. 47).]

B. N- and O-Linked oligosaccharides

A glycoprotein may contain only one type of glycosidic linkage (N or O linked) or may have both types within the same molecule.

1. **O-Linked:** The O-linked glycans may have one or more of a wide variety of sugars arranged in either a linear or a branched pattern. Many are found in extracellular glycoproteins or as membrane glycoprotein components. For example, O-linked oligosaccharides on the surface of red blood cells help provide the ABO blood group determinants. If the terminal sugar on the glycan is GalNAc, the blood group is A. If it is galactose, the blood group is B. If neither GalNAc nor galactose is present, the blood group is O.

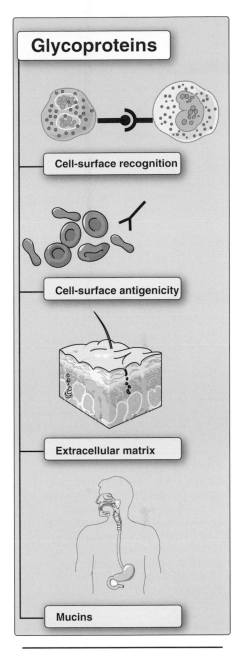

Glycoproteins

Cell-surface recognition

Cell-surface antigenicity

Extracellular matrix

Mucins

Figure 14.13
Functions of glycoproteins.

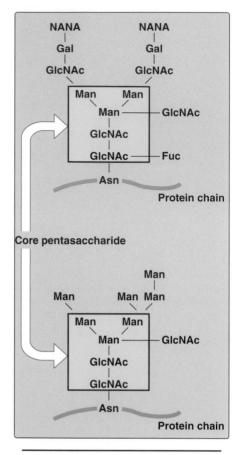

Figure 14.14
Complex (top) and high-mannose (bottom) N-linked oligosaccharides. [Note: Members of each class contain the same pentasaccharide core (shown inside the box).] NANA = N-acetylneuraminic acid; Gal = galactose; GlcNAc = N-acetylglucosamine; Man = mannose; Fuc = fucose; Asn = asparagine.

2. **N-Linked:** The N-linked glycans fall into two broad classes: complex oligosaccharides and high-mannose oligosaccharides. Both contain the same pentasaccharide core shown in Figure 14.14, but the complex oligosaccharides contain a diverse group of additional sugars, for example, GlcNAc, GalNAc, L-fucose, and NANA, whereas the high-mannose oligosaccharides contain primarily mannose.

VIII. GLYCOPROTEIN SYNTHESIS

Proteins destined to function in the cytoplasm are synthesized on free cytosolic ribosomes. However, proteins, including glycoproteins, that are destined for cellular membranes, lysosomes, or to be exported from the cell, are synthesized on ribosomes attached to the RER. These proteins contain specific signal sequences that act as molecular addresses, targeting the proteins to their proper destinations. An N-terminal hydrophobic sequence initially directs these proteins to the RER, allowing the growing polypeptide to be extruded into the lumen (see p. 459). The proteins are then transported via secretory vesicles to the Golgi, which acts as a sorting center (Fig. 14.15). In the Golgi, those glycoproteins that are to be secreted from the cell (or are targeted for lysosomes) are packaged into vesicles that fuse with the cell (or lysosomal) membrane and release their contents. Those that are destined to become components of the cell membrane are integrated into the Golgi membrane, which buds off, forming vesicles that add their membrane-bound glycoproteins to the cell membrane. [Note: Therefore, the membrane glycoproteins are oriented with the carbohydrate portion on the outside of the cell (see Fig. 14.15).]

A. Carbohydrate components

The precursors of the carbohydrate components of glycoproteins are nucleotide sugars, which include UDP-glucose, UDP-galactose, UDP-GlcNAc, and UDP-GalNAc. In addition, guanosine diphosphate (GDP)-mannose, GDP-L-fucose (which is synthesized from GDP-mannose), and CMP-NANA may donate sugars to the growing chain. [Note: When the acidic NANA is present, the oligosaccharide has a negative charge at physiologic pH.] The oligosaccharides are covalently attached to the side chains of specific amino acids in the protein, where the three-dimensional structure of the protein determines whether or not a specific amino acid is glycosylated.

B. O-Linked glycoprotein synthesis

Synthesis of the O-linked glycoproteins is very similar to that of the GAG (see p. 158). First, the protein to which sugars are to be attached is synthesized on the RER and extruded into its lumen. Glycosylation begins with the transfer of GalNAc (from UDP-GalNAc) to the hydroxyl group of a specific serine or threonine residues. The *glycosyltransferases* responsible for the stepwise synthesis (from individual sugars) of the oligosaccharides are bound to the membranes of the Golgi. They act in a specific order, without using a template as is required for DNA, ribonucleic acid (RNA), and protein synthesis (see Unit VII), but instead by recognizing the actual structure of the growing oligosaccharide as the appropriate substrate.

C. N-Linked glycoprotein synthesis

Synthesis of N-linked glycoproteins occurs in the lumen of the RER and requires the participation of the phosphorylated form of dolichol (dolichol pyrophosphate), a lipid of the RER membrane (Fig. 14.16). The initial product is processed in the RER and Golgi.

1. **Dolichol-linked oligosaccharide synthesis:** As with the O-linked glycoproteins, the protein is synthesized on the RER and enters its lumen. However, it does not become glycosylated with individual sugars. Instead, a lipid-linked oligosaccharide is first constructed. This consists of dolichol (an RER membrane lipid made from an intermediate of cholesterol synthesis; see p. 221) attached through a pyrophosphate linkage to an oligosaccharide containing GlcNAc, mannose, and glucose. The sugars to be added sequentially to the dolichol by membrane-bound *glycosyltransferases* are first GlcNAc, followed by mannose and glucose (see Fig. 14.16). The entire 14-sugar oligosaccharide is then transferred from dolichol to the amide nitrogen of an asparagine residue in the protein to be glycosylated by a *protein–oligosaccharide transferase* present in the RER. [Note: Tunicamycin inhibits N-linked glycosylation.]

Congenital disorders of glycosylation (CDG) are syndromes caused primarily by defects in the N-linked glycosylation of proteins, either oligosaccharide assembly (type I) or processing (type II).

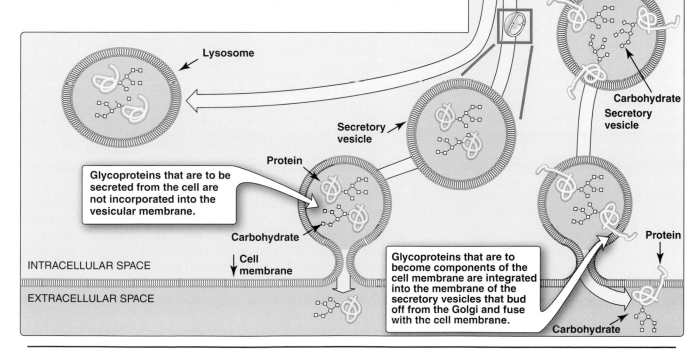

Figure 14.15

Transport of glycoproteins to and through the Golgi and their subsequent secretion or incorporation into a lysosome or the cell membrane.

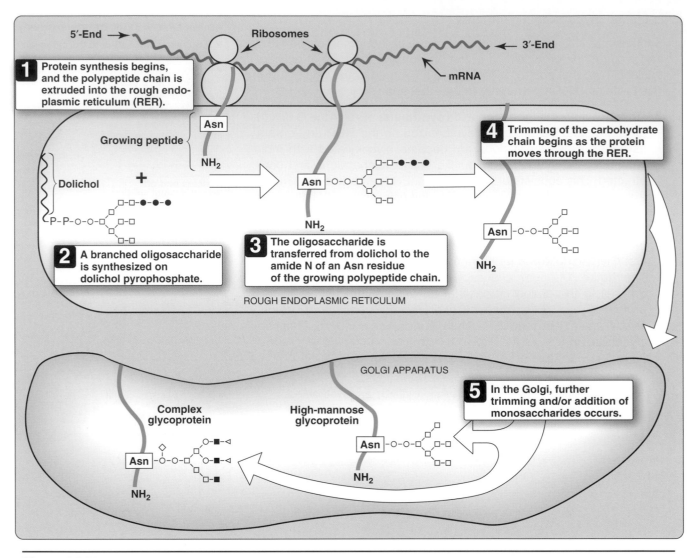

Figure 14.16
Synthesis of N-linked glycoproteins. ○ = N-acetylglucosamine; □ = mannose; ● = glucose; ■ = galactose; ◇ or ◁ = terminal group (fucose or N-acetylneuraminic acid); mRNA = messenger RNA; Asn = asparagine.

2. **N-Linked oligosaccharide processing:** After addition to the protein, the N-linked oligosaccharide is processed by the removal of specific mannosyl and glucosyl residues as the glycoprotein moves through the RER. Finally, the oligosaccharide chains are completed in the Golgi by addition of a variety of sugars (for example, GlcNAc, GalNAc, and additional mannoses and then fucose or NANA as terminal groups) to produce a complex glycoprotein. Alternatively, they are not processed further, leaving branched, mannose-containing chains in a high-mannose glycoprotein (see Fig. 14.16). The ultimate fate of N-linked glycoproteins is the same as that of the O-linked glycoproteins (for example, they can be released by the cell or become part of a cell membrane). In addition, N-linked glycoproteins can be targeted to the lysosomes. [Note: Nonenzymatic glycosylation of proteins is known as glycation (see p. 33).]

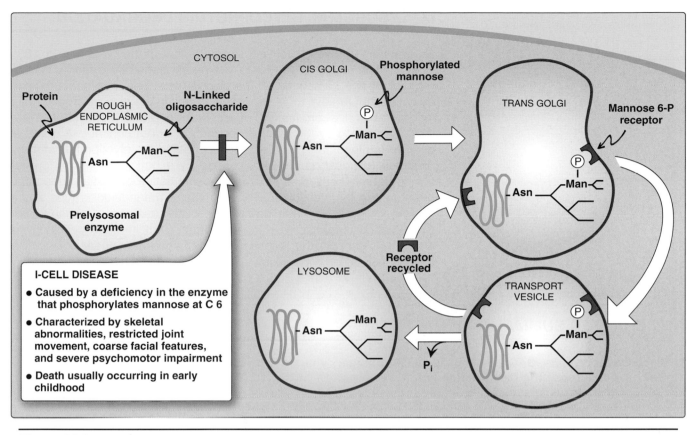

Figure 14.17
Mechanism for transport of N-linked glycoproteins to the lysosomes. Asn = asparagine; Man = mannose; $\textcircled{P}$ = phosphate; P_i = inorganic phosphate.

3. **Lysosomal enzymes:** N-Linked glycoproteins being processed in the Golgi can be phosphorylated on carbon 6 of one or more mannosyl residues. UDP-GlcNAc provides the phosphate in a reaction catalyzed by a *phosphotransferase*. Receptors, located in the Golgi membrane, bind the mannose 6-phosphate residues of these proteins, which are then packaged into vesicles and sent to the lysosomes (Fig. 14.17). I-Cell disease is a rare lysosomal storage disease in which the *phosphotransferase* is deficient. This causes the proteins to be secreted, rather than being targeted to lysosomes. Consequently, the *acid hydrolases* normally found in the lysosomal matrix are absent, resulting in an accumulation of the substrates for these missing enzymes. [Note: I-Cell disease is so named because of the large inclusion bodies seen in cells of patients with this disease.] In addition, high amounts of lysosomal enzymes are found in the patient's plasma and urine, indicating that the targeting process to lysosomes (rather than the synthetic pathway of these enzymes) is deficient. I-Cell disease is characterized by skeletal abnormalities, restricted joint movement, coarse (dysmorphic) facial features, and severe psychomotor impairment. [Note: Because I-cell disease has features in common with the mucopolysaccharidoses and sphingolipidoses (see p. 210), it is termed a mucolipidosis (type II).] Currently, there is no cure, and death from cardiopulmonary complications usually occurs in early childhood.

IX. LYSOSOMAL GLYCOPROTEIN DEGRADATION

Degradation of glycoproteins is similar to that of the GAG (see p. 163). The lysosomal *acid hydrolases* are each generally specific for the removal of one component of the glycoprotein. They are primarily exo-enzymes that remove their respective groups in the reverse order of their incorporation (last on, first off). If any one degradative enzyme is missing, degradation by the other exoenzymes cannot continue. A group of very rare autosomal-recessive diseases called the glycoprotein storage diseases (oligosaccharidoses), caused by a deficiency of any one of the degradative enzymes, results in accumulation of partially degraded structures in the lysosomes. For example, α-mannosidosis type 3 is a severe, progressive, fatal deficiency of the enzyme *α-mannosidase*. Presentation is similar to Hurler syndrome, but immune deficiency is also seen. Mannose-rich oligosaccharide fragments appear in the urine. Diagnosis is by enzyme assay.

X. CHAPTER SUMMARY

Glycosaminoglycans (GAG) are **long, negatively charged, unbranched, heteropolysaccharide chains** generally composed of a **repeating disaccharide unit** [acidic sugar–amino sugar]n (Fig. 14.18). The **amino sugar** is either ᴅ-**glucosamine** or ᴅ-**galactosamine** in which the amino group is usually acetylated, thus eliminating its positive charge. The amino sugar may also be **sulfated** on carbon 4 or 6 or on a nonacetylated nitrogen. The **acidic sugar** is either ᴅ-**glucuronic acid** or its C-5 epimer ʟ-**iduronic acid**. GAG bind large amounts of water, thereby producing the gel-like matrix that forms the basis of the body's **ground substance**. The viscous, lubricating properties of **mucous secretions** are also caused by the presence of GAG, which led to the original naming of these compounds as **mucopolysaccharides**. There are six major types of GAG, including **chondroitin 4-** and **6-sulfates**, **keratan sulfate**, **dermatan sulfate**, **heparin**, **heparan sulfate**, and **hyaluronic acid**. All GAG, except hyaluronic acid, are found covalently attached to a **core protein**, forming **proteoglycan monomers**. Many proteoglycan monomers associate with a molecule of **hyaluronic acid** to form **proteoglycan aggregates**. GAG are synthesized in the **Golgi**. The polysaccharide chains are elongated by the sequential addition of alternating acidic and amino sugars, donated by their **UDP derivatives**. ᴅ-Glucuronate may be epimerized to ʟ-iduronate. The last step in synthesis is sulfation of some of the amino sugars. The source of the sulfate is **3′-phosphoadenosyl-5′-phosphosulfate (PAPS)**. The completed proteoglycans are secreted into the **extracellular matrix (ECM)** or remain associated with the outer surface of cells. GAG are degraded by **lysosomal *acid hydrolases***. They are first broken down to oligosaccharides, which are degraded sequentially from the nonreducing end of each chain. A deficiency of any one of the *hydrolases* results in a **mucopolysaccharidosis**. These are hereditary disorders in which GAG accumulate in tissues, causing symptoms such as **skeletal** and **ECM deformities** and **intellectual disability**. Examples of these genetic diseases include **Hunter** (X-linked) and **Hurler syndromes**. **Glycoproteins** are proteins to which **oligosaccharides (glycans)** are covalently attached. They differ from the proteoglycans in that the length of the glycoprotein's carbohydrate chain is relatively short (usually two to ten sugar residues long, although it can be longer), may be branched, and does not contain serial disaccharide units. **Membrane-bound** glycoproteins participate in a broad range of cellular phenomena, including **cell-surface recognition** (by other cells, hormones, and viruses), **cell-surface antigenicity** (such as the blood group antigens), and as components of the ECM and of the **mucins** of the gastrointestinal and urogenital tracts, where they act as protective biologic lubricants. In addition, almost all of the globular proteins present in human plasma are glycoproteins. Glycoproteins are synthesized in the **rough endoplasmic reticulum (RER)** and the **Golgi**. The precursors of the carbohydrate components of glycoproteins are **nucleotide sugars**. **O-Linked glycoproteins** are synthesized in the Golgi by the sequential transfer of sugars from their nucleotide carriers to the hydroxyl group of a serine or threonine residue in the protein. **N-Linked glycoproteins** are synthesized by the transfer of a preformed oligosaccharide from its RER membrane lipid carrier, **dolichol pyrophosphate**, to the amide N of an asparagine residue in the protein. They contain varying amounts of **mannose**. A deficiency in the ***phosphotransferase*** that phosphorylates mannose residues at carbon 6 in N-linked glycoprotein enzymes destined for the lysosomes results in **I-cell disease**. Glycoproteins are degraded in lysosomes by *acid hydrolases*. A deficiency of any one of these enzymes results in a **lysosomal glycoprotein storage disease (oligosaccharidosis)**, resulting in accumulation of partially degraded structures in the lysosome.

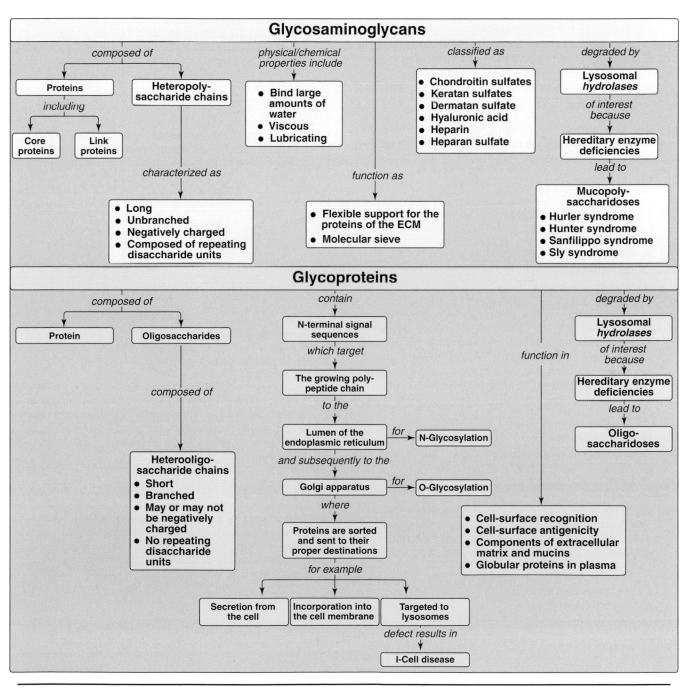

Figure 14.18
Key concept map for glycosaminoglycans and glycoproteins. ECM = extracellular matrix.

Study Questions

Choose the ONE best answer.

14.1 Mucopolysaccharidoses are hereditary lysosomal storage diseases. They are caused by:

   A. defects in the degradation of glycosaminoglycans.
   B. defects in the targeting of enzymes to lysosomes.
   C. an increased rate of synthesis of the carbohydrate component of proteoglycans.
   D. an insufficient rate of synthesis of proteolytic enzymes.
   E. the synthesis of abnormally small amounts of core proteins.
   F. the synthesis of heteropolysaccharides with an altered structure.

> Correct answer = A. The mucopolysaccharidoses are caused by deficiencies in any one of the lysosomal acid hydrolases responsible for the degradation of glycosaminoglycans (not proteins). The enzyme is correctly targeted to the lysosome, so blood levels of the enzyme do not increase, but it is nonfunctional. In these diseases, synthesis of the protein and carbohydrate components of proteoglycans is unaffected, in terms of both structure and amount.

14.2 The presence of the following compound in the urine of a patient suggests a deficiency in which one of the enzymes listed below?

$$\begin{array}{ccc} \text{Sulfate} & & \text{Sulfate} \\ | & & | \\ \text{GalNac--GlcUA--GalNAc--} \end{array}$$

   A. Galactosidase
   B. Glucuronidase
   C. Iduronidase
   D. Mannosidase
   E. Sulfatase

> Correct answer = E. Degradation of glycoproteins follows the rule: last on, first off. Because sulfation is the last step in the synthesis of this sequence, a sulfatase is required for the next step in the degradation of the compound shown.

14.3 An 8-month-old boy with coarse facial features, skeletal abnormalities, and delays in both growth and development is diagnosed with I-cell disease based on his presentation and on histologic and biochemical testing. I-Cell disease is characterized by:

   A. decreased production of cell surface O-linked glycoproteins.
   B. elevated levels of acid hydrolases in the blood.
   C. inability to N-glycosylate proteins.
   D. increased synthesis of proteoglycans.
   E. oligosaccharides in the urine.

> Correct answer = B. I-Cell disease is a lysosomal storage disease caused by deficiency of the phosphotransferase needed for synthesis of the mannose 6-phosphate signal that targets acid hydrolases to the lysosomal matrix. This results in secretion of these enzymes from the cell and accumulation of materials within the lysosome because of impaired degradation. None of the other choices relates to I-cell disease or lysosomal function. Oligosaccharides in the urine are characteristic of the muco- and polysaccharidoses but not I-cell disease (a type II mucolipidosis).

14.4 An infant with corneal clouding has dermatan sulfate and heparan sulfate in his urine. Decreased activity of which of the enzymes listed below would confirm the suspected diagnosis of Hurler syndrome?

   A. α-L-Iduronidase
   B. α-Glucuronidase
   C. Glycosyltransferase
   D. Iduronate sulfatase

> Correct answer = A. Hurler syndrome, a defect in the lysosomal degradation of glycosaminoglycans (GAG) with corneal clouding, is due to a deficiency in α-L-iduronidase. β-Glucuronidase is deficient in Sly syndrome, and iduronate sulfatase is deficient in Hunter syndrome. Glycosyltransferases are enzymes of GAG synthesis.

14.5 Distinguish between glycoproteins and proteoglycans.

> Glycoproteins are proteins to which short, branched, structurally diverse oligosaccharide chains (glycans) are attached. Proteoglycans consist of a core protein to which long, unbranched, glycosaminoglycan (GAG) chains are attached. GAG are large complexes of negatively charged heteropolysaccharides composed of repeating [acidic sugar-amino sugar]$_n$ disaccharide units.

Dietary Lipid Metabolism

15

I. OVERVIEW

Lipids are a heterogeneous group of water-insoluble (hydrophobic) organic molecules (Fig. 15.1). Because of their insolubility in aqueous solutions, body lipids are generally found compartmentalized, as in the case of membrane-associated lipids or droplets of triacylglycerol in adipocytes, or transported in blood in association with protein, as in lipoprotein particles (see p. 227) or on albumin. Lipids are a major source of energy for the body, and they also provide the hydrophobic barrier that permits partitioning of the aqueous contents of cells and subcellular structures. Lipids serve additional functions in the body (for example, some fat-soluble vitamins have regulatory or coenzyme functions, and the prostaglandins and steroid hormones play major roles in the control of the body's homeostasis). Deficiencies or imbalances of lipid metabolism can lead to some of the major clinical problems encountered by physicians, such as atherosclerosis, diabetes, and obesity.

II. DIGESTION, ABSORPTION, SECRETION, AND UTILIZATION

The average daily intake of lipids by U.S. adults is ~78 g, of which >90% is triacylglycerol ([TAG], formerly called triglyceride [TG]), that consists of three fatty acids (FA) esterified to a glycerol backbone (see Fig. 15.1). The remainder of the dietary lipids consists primarily of cholesterol, cholesteryl esters, phospholipids, and nonesterified (free) FA (FFA). The digestion of dietary lipids begins in the stomach and is completed in the small intestine. The process is summarized in Figure 15.2.

A. Digestion in the stomach

Lipid digestion in the stomach is limited. It is catalyzed by *lingual lipase* that originates from glands at the back of the tongue and *gastric lipase* that is secreted by the gastric mucosa. Both enzymes are relatively acid stable, with optimal pH values of 4 to 6. These *acid lipases*

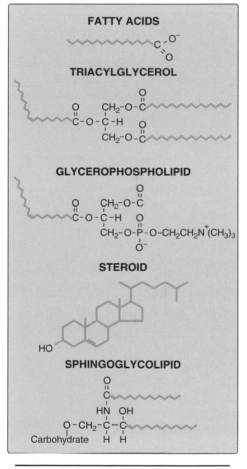

Figure 15.1
Structures of some common classes of lipids. Hydrophobic portions of the molecules are shown in orange.

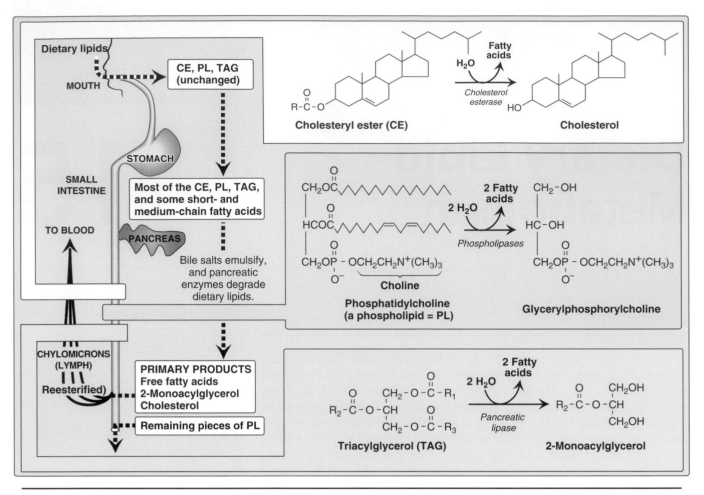

Figure 15.2
Overview of lipid digestion.

hydrolyze FA from TAG molecules, particularly those containing short- or medium-chain-length (≤12 carbons) FA such as are found in milk fat. Consequently, these *lipases* play a particularly important role in lipid digestion in infants for whom milk fat is the primary source of calories. They also become important digestive enzymes in individuals with pancreatic insufficiency such as those with cystic fibrosis (CF). *Lingual* and *gastric lipases* aid these patients in degrading TAG molecules (especially those with short- to medium-chain FA) despite a near or complete absence of *pancreatic lipase* (see Section D.1. below).

B. Cystic fibrosis

CF is the most common lethal genetic disease in Caucasians of Northern European ancestry and has a prevalence of ~1:3,300 births in the United States. CF is an autosomal-recessive disorder caused by mutations to the gene for the CF transmembrane conductance regulator (CFTR) protein that functions as a chloride channel on epithelium in the pancreas, lungs, testes, and sweat glands. Defective CFTR results in decreased secretion of chloride and increased uptake of sodium and water. In the pancreas, the depletion of water on the cell surface results in thickened mucus that clogs the pancreatic ducts, preventing pancreatic enzymes from reaching the intestine, thereby leading to pancreatic insufficiency. Treatment includes replacement of these enzymes and supplementation with fat-soluble vitamins. [Note: CF also causes chronic lung infections with progressive pulmonary disease and male infertility.]

C. Emulsification in the small intestine

The critical process of dietary lipid emulsification occurs in the duodenum. Emulsification increases the surface area of the hydrophobic lipid droplets so that the digestive enzymes, which work at the interface of the droplet and the surrounding aqueous solution, can act effectively. Emulsification is accomplished by two complementary mechanisms, namely, use of the detergent properties of the conjugated bile salts and mechanical mixing due to peristalsis. Bile salts, made in the liver and stored in the gallbladder, are amphipathic derivatives of cholesterol (see p. 224). Conjugated bile salts consist of a hydroxylated sterol ring structure with a side chain to which a molecule of glycine or taurine is covalently attached by an amide linkage (Fig. 15.3). These emulsifying agents interact with the dietary lipid droplets and the aqueous duodenal contents, thereby stabilizing the droplets as they become smaller from peristalsis and preventing them from coalescing. [Note: See p. 225 for a more complete discussion of bile salt metabolism.]

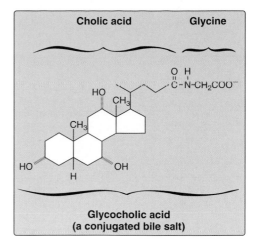

Figure 15.3
Structure of glycocholic acid.

D. Degradation by pancreatic enzymes

The dietary TAG, cholesteryl esters, and phospholipids are enzymatically degraded (digested) in the small intestine by pancreatic enzymes, whose secretion is hormonally controlled.

1. **Triacylglycerol degradation:** TAG molecules are too large to be taken up efficiently by the mucosal cells (enterocytes) of the intestinal villi. Therefore, they are hydrolyzed by an *esterase*, *pancreatic lipase*, which preferentially removes the FA at carbons 1 and 3. The primary products of hydrolysis are, thus, a mixture of 2-monoacylglycerol (2-MAG) and FFA (see Fig. 15.2). [Note: *Pancreatic lipase* is found in high concentrations in pancreatic secretions (2%–3% of the total protein present), and it is highly efficient catalytically, thus insuring that only severe pancreatic deficiency, such as that seen in CF, results in significant malabsorption of fat.] A second protein, *colipase*, also secreted by the pancreas, binds the *lipase* at a ratio of 1:1 and anchors it at the lipid–aqueous interface. *Colipase* restores activity to *lipase* in the presence of inhibitory substances like bile salts that bind the micelles. [Note: *Colipase* is secreted as the zymogen, procolipase, which is activated in the intestine by *trypsin*.] Orlistat, an antiobesity drug, inhibits *gastric* and *pancreatic lipases*, thereby decreasing fat absorption, resulting in weight loss.

2. **Cholesteryl ester degradation:** Most dietary cholesterol is present in the free (nonesterified) form, with 10%–15% present in the esterified form. Cholesteryl esters are hydrolyzed by pancreatic *cholesteryl ester hydrolase* (*cholesterol esterase*), which produces cholesterol plus FFA (see Fig. 15.2). Activity of this enzyme is greatly increased in the presence of bile salts.

3. **Phospholipid degradation:** Pancreatic juice is rich in the proenzyme of *phospholipase A_2* that, like procolipase, is activated by *trypsin* and, like *cholesteryl ester hydrolase*, requires bile salts for optimum activity. *Phospholipase A_2* removes one FA from carbon

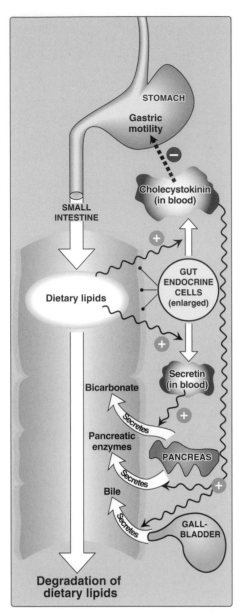

Figure 15.4
Hormonal control of lipid digestion in the small intestine. [Note: The small intestine is divided into three parts: the duodenum (upper 5%), the jejunum, and the ileum (lower 55%).]

2 of a phospholipid, leaving a lysophospholipid. For example, phosphatidylcholine (the predominant phospholipid of digestion) becomes lysophosphatidylcholine. The remaining FA at carbon 1 can be removed by *lysophospholipase*, leaving a glycerylphosphoryl base (for example, glycerylphosphorylcholine, see Fig. 15.2) that may be excreted in the feces, further degraded, or absorbed.

4. **Control:** Pancreatic secretion of the hydrolytic enzymes that degrade dietary lipids in the small intestine is hormonally controlled (Fig. 15.4). Cells in the mucosa of the lower duodenum and jejunum produce the peptide hormone cholecystokinin (CCK), in response to the presence of lipids and partially digested proteins entering these regions of the upper small intestine. CCK acts on the gallbladder (causing it to contract and release bile, a mixture of bile salts, phospholipids, and free cholesterol) and on the exocrine cells of the pancreas (causing them to release digestive enzymes). It also decreases gastric motility, resulting in a slower release of gastric contents into the small intestine (see p. 353). Other intestinal cells produce another peptide hormone, secretin, in response to the low pH of the chyme entering the intestine from the stomach. Secretin causes the pancreas to release a solution rich in bicarbonate that helps neutralize the pH of the intestinal contents, bringing them to the appropriate pH for digestive activity by pancreatic enzymes.

E. Absorption by enterocytes

FFA, free cholesterol, and 2-MAG are the primary products of lipid digestion in the jejunum. These, plus bile salts and fat-soluble vitamins (A, D, E, and K), form mixed micelles (that is, disc-shaped clusters of a mixture of amphipathic lipids that coalesce with their hydrophobic groups on the inside and their hydrophilic groups on the outside). Therefore, mixed micelles are soluble in the aqueous environment of the intestinal lumen (Fig. 15.5). These particles approach the primary site of lipid absorption, the brush border membrane of the enterocytes. This microvilli-rich apical membrane is separated from the liquid contents of the intestinal lumen by an unstirred water layer that mixes poorly with the bulk fluid. The hydrophilic surface of the micelles facilitates the transport of the hydrophobic lipids through the unstirred water layer to the brush border membrane where they are absorbed. Bile salts are absorbed in the terminal ileum, with <5% being lost in the feces. [Note: Relative to other dietary lipids, cholesterol is only poorly absorbed by the enterocytes. Drug therapy (for example, with ezetimibe) can further reduce cholesterol absorption in the small intestine.] Because short- and medium-chain FA are water soluble, they do not require the assistance of mixed micelles for absorption by the intestinal mucosa.

F. Triacylglycerol and cholesteryl ester resynthesis

The mixture of lipids absorbed by the enterocytes migrates to the smooth endoplasmic reticulum (SER) where biosynthesis of complex lipids takes place. The long-chain FA are first converted into their activated form by *fatty acyl coenzyme A (CoA) synthetase (thiokinase)*, as shown in Figure 15.6. Using the fatty acyl CoA derivatives, the 2-MAG absorbed by the enterocytes are converted to TAG through sequential reacylations by two *acyltransferases*, *acyl CoA:monoacylglycerol acyltransferase* and *acyl CoA:diacylglycerol acyltransferase*. Lysophospholipids are reacylated to form phospholipids by a family of *acyltransferases*, and cholesterol is acylated primarily by *acyl CoA:cholesterol acyltransferase* (see p. 232). [Note: Virtually all long-chain FA entering the enterocytes are used in this fashion to form TAG, phospholipids, and cholesteryl esters. Short- and medium-chain FA are not converted to their CoA derivatives and are not reesterified to 2-MAG. Instead, they are released into the portal circulation, where they are carried by serum albumin to the liver.]

G. Lipid malabsorption

Lipid malabsorption, resulting in increased lipid (including the fat-soluble vitamins and essential FA, see p. 182) in the feces, a condition known as steatorrhea, can be caused by disturbances in lipid digestion and/or absorption (Fig. 15.7). Such disturbances can result from several conditions, including CF (causing poor digestion) and short bowel syndrome (causing decreased absorption).

> The ability of short- and medium-chain FA to be taken up by enterocytes without the aid of mixed micelles has made them important in medical nutrition therapy for individuals with malabsorption disorders.

H. Secretion from enterocytes

The newly resynthesized TAG and cholesteryl esters are very hydrophobic and aggregate in an aqueous environment. Therefore, they must be packaged as particles of lipid droplets surrounded by a thin layer composed of phospholipids, nonesterified cholesterol, and a molecule of the protein apolipoprotein (apo) B-48 (see p. 228). This layer stabilizes the particle and increases its solubility, thereby preventing multiple particles from coalescing. [Note: Microsomal triglyceride transfer protein is essential for the assembly of all TAG-rich

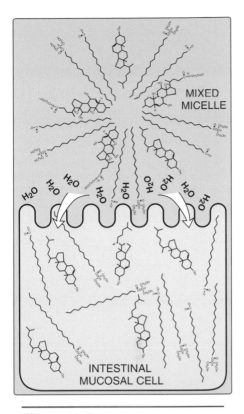

Figure 15.5
Absorption of lipids contained in a mixed micelle by an intestinal mucosal cell. The micelle itself is not absorbed. [Note: Short- and medium-chain-length fatty acids do not require incorporation into micelles.]

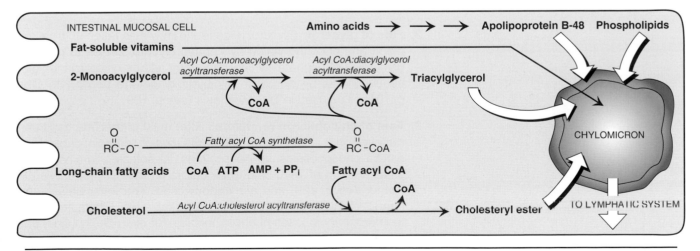

Figure 15.6
Assembly and secretion of chylomicrons by intestinal mucosal cells. [Note: Short- and medium-chain-length fatty acids do not require incorporation into chylomicrons and directly enter into the blood.] CoA = coenzyme A; AMP = adenosine monophosphate; PP$_i$ = pyrophosphate.

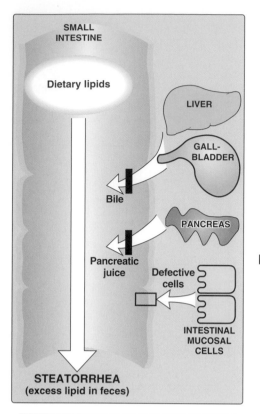

Figure 15.7
Possible causes of steatorrhea.

apo B–containing particles in the ER (see p. 228).] The lipoprotein particles are released by exocytosis from enterocytes into the lacteals (lymphatic vessels in the villi of the small intestine). The presence of these particles in the lymph after a lipid-rich meal gives it a milky appearance. This lymph is called chyle (as opposed to chyme, the name given to the semifluid mass of partially digested food that passes from the stomach to the duodenum), and the particles are named chylomicrons. Chylomicrons follow the lymphatic system to the thoracic duct and are then conveyed to the left subclavian vein, where they enter the blood. The steps in the production of chylomicrons are summarized in Figure 15.6. [Note: Once released into blood, the nascent (immature) chylomicrons pick up apolipoproteins E and C-II from high-density lipoproteins and mature. (For a more detailed description of chylomicron structure and metabolism, see p. 227.)]

I. Use by the tissues

Most of the TAG contained in chylomicrons is broken down in the capillary beds of skeletal and cardiac muscle and adipose tissue. The TAG is degraded to FFA and glycerol by *lipoprotein lipase* (*LPL*). This enzyme is synthesized and secreted primarily by adipocytes and muscle cells. Secreted *LPL* is anchored to the luminal surface of endothelial cells in the capillaries of muscle and adipose tissues. [Note: Familial chylomicronemia (type I hyperlipoproteinemia) is a rare, autosomal-recessive disorder caused by a deficiency of *LPL* or its coenzyme apo C-II (see p. 228). The result is fasting chylomicronemia and severe hypertriacylglycerolemia, which can cause pancreatitis.]

1. **Fate of free fatty acids:** The FFA derived from the hydrolysis of TAG may either directly enter adjacent muscle cells and adipocytes or be transported in the blood in association with serum albumin until they are taken up by cells. [Note: Human serum albumin is a large protein secreted by the liver. It transports a number of primarily hydrophobic compounds in the circulation, including FFA and some drugs.] Most cells can oxidize FA to produce energy (see p. 190). Adipocytes can also reesterify FFA to produce TAG molecules, which are stored until the FA are needed by the body (see p. 188).

2. **Fate of glycerol:** Glycerol released from TAG is taken up from the blood and phosphorylated by hepatic *glycerol kinase* to produce glycerol 3-phosphate, which can enter either glycolysis or gluconeogenesis by oxidation to dihydroxyacetone phosphate (see p. 101) or be used in TAG synthesis (see p. 189).

3. **Fate of chylomicron remnants:** After most of the TAG has been removed, the chylomicron remnants (which contain cholesteryl esters, phospholipids, apolipoproteins, fat-soluble vitamins, and a small amount of TAG) bind to receptors on the liver (apo E is the ligand; see p. 229) and are endocytosed. The intracellular remnants are hydrolyzed to their component parts. Cholesterol and the nitrogenous bases of phospholipids (for example, choline) can be recycled by the body. [Note: If removal of remnants by the liver is decreased because of impaired binding to their receptor, they accumulate in the plasma. This is seen in the rare type III hyperlipoproteinemia (also called familial dysbetalipoproteinemia or broad beta disease, see p. 231).]

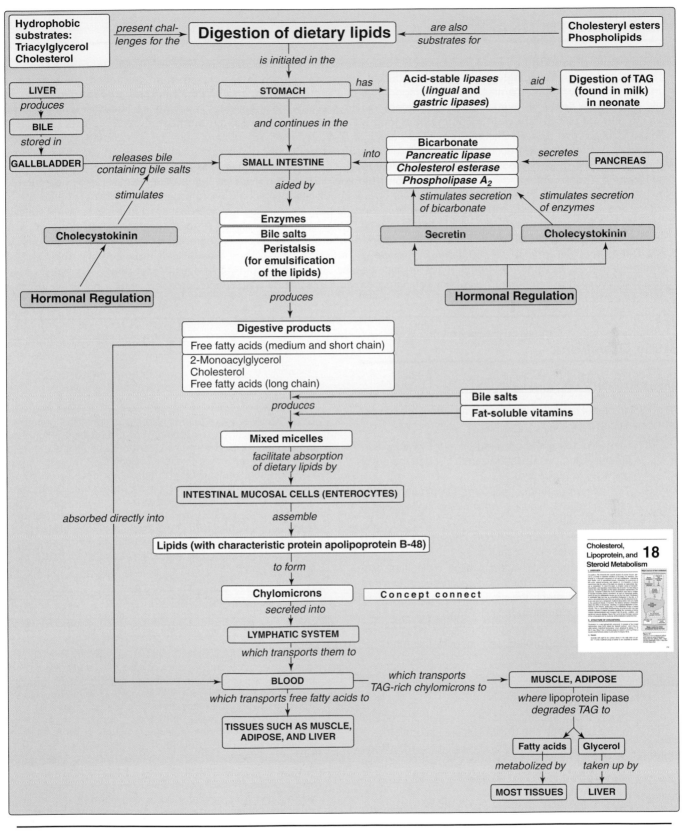

Figure 15.8
Key concept map for metabolism of dietary lipids. TAG = triacylglycerols.

III. CHAPTER SUMMARY

Dietary lipid digestion begins in the stomach and continues in the small intestine (Fig. 15.8). **Cholesteryl esters**, **phospholipids**, and **triacylglycerols** (**TAG**) containing **long-chain-length fatty acids** (**FA**) are degraded in the **small intestine** by **pancreatic enzymes**. The most important of these enzymes are *cholesterol esterase*, *phospholipase A₂*, and *pancreatic lipase*. In **cystic fibrosis**, thickened mucus prevents these enzymes reaching the intestine. In contrast, TAG in **milk fat** contain **short- to medium-chain-length FA** and are degraded in the **stomach** by *acid lipases* (*lingual lipase* and *gastric lipase*). The **hydrophobic** nature of lipids requires that dietary lipids be **emulsified** for efficient degradation. Emulsification occurs in the small intestine using **peristaltic action** (mechanical mixing) and **bile salts** (detergents). The primary products of dietary lipid degradation are **2-monoacylglycerol**, nonesterified (free) **cholesterol**, and **free FA**. These compounds, plus the **fat-soluble vitamins**, form **mixed micelles** that facilitate dietary lipid absorption by **intestinal mucosal cells** (**enterocytes**). These cells use activated long-chain FA to regenerate TAG and cholesteryl esters and also synthesize protein (**apolipoprotein [apo] B-48**), all of which are then assembled with the fat-soluble vitamins into **lipoprotein particles** called **chylomicrons**. Short- and medium-chain FA enter blood directly. Chylomicrons are first released into the **lymph** and then enter the **blood**, where their lipid core is degraded by *lipoprotein lipase* (with **apo C-II** as the coenzyme) in the **capillaries** of **muscle** and **adipose** tissues. Thus, dietary lipids are made available to the peripheral tissues. **Fat maldigestion** or malabsorption causes **steatorrhea** (lipid in the feces). A deficiency in the ability to degrade chylomicron components, or remove chylomicron remnants after TAG has been degraded, results in accumulation of these particles in blood.

Study Questions

Choose the ONE best answer.

15.1 Which one of the following statements about lipid digestion is correct?

    A. Large lipid droplets are emulsified (have their surface area increased) in the mouth through the act of chewing (mastication).

    B. The enzyme colipase facilitates the binding of bile salts to mixed micelles, maximizing the activity of pancreatic lipase.

    C. The peptide hormone secretin causes the gallbladder to contract and release bile.

    D. Patients with cystic fibrosis have difficulties with digestion because their pancreatic secretions are less able to reach the small intestine, the primary site of lipid digestion.

    E. Formation of triacylglycerol-rich chylomicrons is independent of protein synthesis in the intestinal mucosa.

Correct answer = D. Patients with cystic fibrosis, a genetic disease resulting in a deficiency of a functional chloride transporter, have thickened mucus that impedes the flow of pancreatic enzymes into the duodenum. Emulsification occurs through peristalsis, which provides mechanical mixing, and bile salts that function as detergents. Colipase restores activity to pancreatic lipase in the presence of inhibitory bile salts that bind the micelles. Cholecystokinin is the hormone that causes contraction of the gallbladder and release of stored bile, and secretin causes release of bicarbonate. Chylomicron formation requires synthesis of apolipoprotein B-48.

15.2 Which one of the following statements about lipid absorption from the intestine is correct?

    A. Dietary triacylglycerol must be completely hydrolyzed to free fatty acids and glycerol before absorption.

    B. The triacylglycerol carried by chylomicrons is degraded by lipoprotein lipase, producing fatty acids that are taken up by muscle and adipose tissues and glycerol that is taken up by the liver.

    C. Fatty acids that contain ≤12 carbon atoms are absorbed and enter the circulation primarily via the lymphatic system.

    D. Deficiencies in the ability to absorb fat result in excessive amounts of chylomicrons in the blood.

Correct answer = B. The triacylglycerols (TAG) in chylomicrons are degraded to fatty acids (FA) and glycerol by lipoprotein lipase on capillary endothelial surfaces in muscle and adipose tissue, thus providing a source of FA to these tissues for degradation or storage and providing glycerol for hepatic metabolism. In the duodenum, TAG are degraded to one 2-monoacylglycerol + two free FA that get absorbed. Medium- and short-chain FA enter directly into blood (not lymph), and they neither require micelles nor get packaged into chylomicrons. Because chylomicrons contain dietary lipids that were digested and absorbed, a defect in fat absorption would result in decreased production of chylomicrons.

Fatty Acid, Triacylglycerol, and Ketone Body Metabolism

16

I. OVERVIEW

Fatty acids exist free in the body (that is, they are nonesterified) and as fatty acyl esters in more complex molecules such as triacylglycerols (TAG). Low levels of free fatty acids (FFA) occur in all tissues, but substantial amounts can sometimes be found in the plasma, particularly during fasting. Plasma FFA (transported on serum albumin) are in route from their point of origin (TAG of adipose tissue or circulating lipoproteins) to their site of consumption (most tissues). FFA can be oxidized by many tissues, particularly liver and muscle, to provide energy and, in the liver, to provide the substrate for ketone body synthesis. Fatty acids are also structural components of membrane lipids, such as phospholipids and glycolipids (see p. 201). Fatty acids attached to certain proteins enhance the ability of those proteins to associate with membranes (see p. 206). Fatty acids are also precursors of the hormone-like prostaglandins (see p. 213). Esterified fatty acids, in the form of TAG stored in white adipose tissue (WAT), serve as the major energy reserve of the body. Alterations in fatty acid metabolism are associated with obesity and diabetes. Figure 16.1 illustrates the metabolic pathways of fatty acid synthesis and degradation and their relationship to carbohydrate metabolism.

II. FATTY ACID STRUCTURE

A fatty acid consists of a hydrophobic hydrocarbon chain with a terminal carboxyl group that has a pK_a (see p. 6) of ~4.8 (Fig. 16.2). At physiologic pH, the terminal carboxyl group (–COOH) ionizes, becoming –COO⁻. [Note: When the pH is above the pK, the deprotonated form predominates (see p. 7).] This anionic group has an affinity for water, giving the fatty acid its amphipathic nature (having both a hydrophilic and a hydrophobic region). However, for long-chain-length fatty acids (LCFA), the hydrophobic portion is predominant. These molecules are highly water insoluble and must be transported in the circulation in association with protein. More than 90% of the fatty acids found in plasma are in the form of fatty acid esters (primarily TAG, cholesteryl esters, and phospholipids) contained in

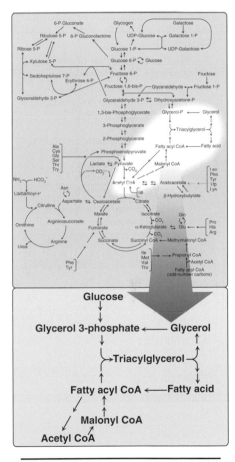

Figure 16.1
Triacylglycerol synthesis and degradation. CoA = coenzyme A.

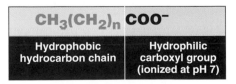

Figure 16.2
Structure of a fatty acid.

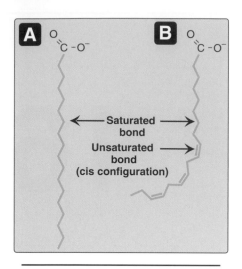

Figure 16.3
A saturated (A) and an unsaturated (B) fatty acid. Orange denotes hydrophobic portions of the molecules. [Note: Cis double bonds cause a fatty acid to kink.]

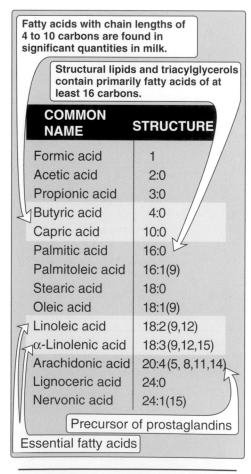

Figure 16.4
Some fatty acids of physiologic importance. [Note: A fatty acid containing 2–4 carbons is considered short; 6–12, medium; 14–20, long; and ≥22, very long.]

circulating lipoprotein particles (see p. 227). FFA are transported in the circulation in association with albumin, the most abundant protein in serum.

A. Fatty acid saturation

Fatty acid chains may contain no double bonds (that is, be saturated) or contain one or more double bonds (that is, be mono- or polyunsaturated). In humans, the majority are saturated or monounsaturated. When double bonds are present, they are nearly always in the cis rather than in the trans configuration. The introduction of a cis double bond causes the fatty acid to bend or kink at that position (Fig. 16.3). If the fatty acid has two or more double bonds, they are always spaced at three-carbon intervals. [Note: In general, addition of double bonds decreases the melting temperature (T_m) of a fatty acid, whereas increasing the chain length increases the T_m. Because membrane lipids typically contain LCFA, the presence of double bonds in some fatty acids helps maintain the fluid nature of those lipids. See p. 363 for a discussion of the dietary occurrence of cis and trans unsaturated fatty acids.]

B. Fatty acid chain length and double bond positions

The common names and structures of some fatty acids of physiologic importance are listed in Figure 16.4. In humans, fatty acids with an even number of carbon atoms (16, 18, or 20) predominate, with longer fatty acids (>22 carbons) being found in the brain. The carbon atoms are numbered, beginning with the carbonyl carbon as carbon 1. The number before the colon indicates the number of carbons in the chain, and those after the colon indicate the numbers and positions (relative to the carboxyl end) of double bonds. For example, as denoted in Figure 16.4, arachidonic acid, 20:4(5,8,11,14), is 20 carbons long and has four double bonds (between carbons 5–6, 8–9, 11–12, and 14–15). [Note: Carbon 2, the carbon to which the carboxyl group is attached, is also called the α-carbon, carbon 3 is the β-carbon, and carbon 4 is the γ-carbon. The carbon of the terminal methyl group is called the ω-carbon regardless of the chain length.] The double bonds in a fatty acid can also be referenced relative to the ω (methyl) end of the chain. Arachidonic acid is referred to as an ω-6 fatty acid because the terminal double bond is six bonds from the ω end (Fig. 16.5A). [Note: The equivalent designation of n-6 may also be used (Fig. 16.5B).] Another ω-6 fatty acid is the essential linoleic acid 18:2(9,12). In contrast, α-linolenic acid, 18:3(9,12,15), is an essential ω-3 fatty acid.

C. Essential fatty acids

Linoleic acid, the precursor of ω-6 arachidonic acid that is the substrate for prostaglandin synthesis (see p. 213), and α-linolenic acid, the precursor of ω-3 fatty acids that are important for growth and development, are dietary essentials in humans because we lack the enzymes needed to synthesize them. Plants provide us with these essential fatty acids. [Note: Arachidonic acid becomes essential if linoleic acid is deficient in the diet. See p. 362 for a discussion of the nutritional significance of ω-3 and ω-6 fatty acids.]

> Essential fatty acid deficiency (rare) can result in a dry, scaly dermatitis as a result of an inability to synthesize molecules that provide the water barrier in skin (see p. 206).

III. FATTY ACID DE NOVO SYNTHESIS

Carbohydrates and proteins obtained from the diet in excess of the body's needs for these nutrients can be converted to fatty acids. In adults, de novo fatty acid synthesis occurs primarily in the liver and lactating mammary glands and, to a lesser extent, in adipose tissue. This cytosolic process is endergonic (see p. 70) and reductive. It incorporates carbons from acetyl coenzyme A (CoA) into the growing fatty acid chain, using ATP and reduced nicotinamide adenine dinucleotide phosphate (NADPH). [Note: Dietary TAG also supply fatty acids. See p. 321 for a discussion of the metabolism of dietary nutrients in the well-fed state.]

A. Cytosolic acetyl CoA production

The first step in fatty acid synthesis is the transfer of acetate units from mitochondrial acetyl CoA to the cytosol. Mitochondrial acetyl CoA is produced by the oxidation of pyruvate (see p. 109) and by the catabolism of certain amino acids (see p. 266). However, the CoA portion of acetyl CoA cannot cross the inner mitochondrial membrane, and only the acetyl portion enters the cytosol. It does so as part of citrate produced by the condensation of acetyl CoA with oxaloacetate (OAA) by *citrate synthase* (Fig. 16.6). [Note: The transport of citrate to the cytosol occurs when the mitochondrial citrate concentration is high. This is observed when *isocitrate dehydrogenase* of the tricarboxylic acid (TCA) cycle is inhibited by the presence of large amounts of ATP, causing citrate and isocitrate to accumulate (see p. 112). Therefore, cytosolic citrate may be viewed as a high-energy signal. Because a large amount of ATP is needed for fatty acid synthesis, the increase in both ATP and citrate enhances this pathway.] In the cytosol, citrate is cleaved to OAA and acetyl CoA by *ATP citrate lyase*.

B. Acetyl CoA carboxylation to malonyl CoA

The energy for the carbon-to-carbon condensations in fatty acid synthesis is supplied by the carboxylation and then decarboxylation of acyl groups in the cytosol. The carboxylation of acetyl CoA to malonyl CoA is catalyzed by *acetyl CoA carboxylase (ACC)* (Fig. 16.7). *ACC* transfers carbon dioxide (CO_2) from bicarbonate (HCO_3^-) in an ATP-requiring reaction. The coenzyme is biotin (vitamin B_7), which is covalently bound to a lysyl residue of the *carboxylase* (see Fig. 28.16, p. 385). *ACC* carboxylates the bound biotin, which transfers the activated carboxyl group to acetyl CoA.

1. **Acetyl CoA carboxylase short-term regulation:** This carboxylation is both the rate-limiting and the regulated step in fatty acid synthesis (see Fig. 16.7). The inactive form of *ACC* is a protomer (complex of ≥2 polypeptides). The enzyme is allosterically activated by citrate, which causes protomers to polymerize, and allosterically inactivated by palmitoyl CoA (the end product of the pathway), which causes depolymerization. A second mechanism of short-term regulation is by reversible phosphorylation. *Adenosine monophosphate–activated protein kinase (AMPK)* phosphorylates and inactivates *ACC*. *AMPK* itself is activated allosterically by AMP and covalently by phosphorylation via several *kinases*. At least one of these *AMPK kinases* is activated by *cyclic AMP (cAMP)– dependent protein kinase A (PKA)*. Thus, in the presence of counterregulatory hormones, such as epinephrine and glucagon, *ACC* is

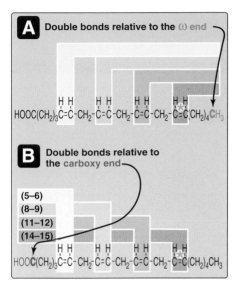

Figure 16.5
Arachidonic acid, 20:4(5,8,11,14), illustrating the position of the double bonds. A. Arachidonic acid is an ω-6 fatty acid because the first double bond from the ω end is 6 carbons from that end. B. It is also referred to as an n-6 fatty acid because the last double bond from the carboxyl end is 14 carbons from that end: 20 – 14 = 6 = n. Thus, the "ω" and "n" designations are equivalent (see *).

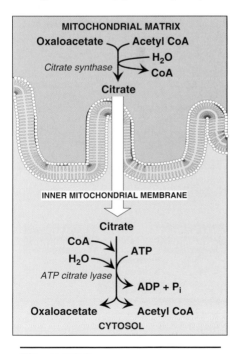

Figure 16.6
Production of cytosolic acetyl coenzyme A (CoA). [Note: Citrate is transported by the tricarboxylate transporter system.] ADP = adenosine monophosphate; P_i = inorganic phosphate.

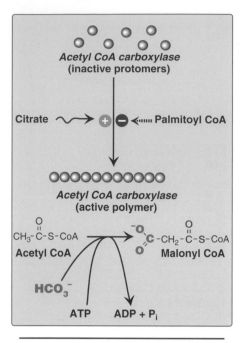

Figure 16.7
Allosteric regulation of malonyl coenzyme A (CoA) synthesis by *acetyl CoA carboxylase*. The carboxyl group contributed by bicarbonate (HCO_3^-) is shown in blue. P_i = inorganic phosphate; ADP = adenosine diphosphate.

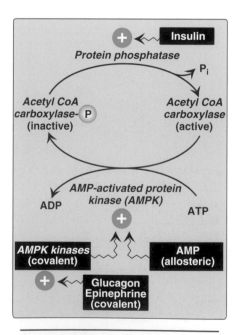

Figure 16.8
Covalent regulation of *acetyl CoA carboxylase* by *AMPK*, which itself is regulated both covalently and allosterically. CoA = coenzyme A; ADP and AMP = adenosine di- and monophosphates; (P) = phosphate; P_i = inorganic phosphate.

phosphorylated and inactive (Fig. 16.8). In the presence of insulin, *ACC* is dephosphorylated and active. [Note: This is analogous to the regulation of *glycogen synthase* (see p. 131).]

2. **Acetyl CoA carboxylase long-term regulation:** Prolonged consumption of a diet containing excess calories (particularly high-carbohydrate, low-fat diets) causes an increase in *ACC* synthesis, thereby increasing fatty acid synthesis. A low-calorie or a high-fat, low-carbohydrate diet has the opposite effect. [Note: *ACC* synthesis is upregulated by carbohydrate (specifically glucose) via the transcription factor carbohydrate response element–binding protein (ChREBP) and by insulin via the transcription factor sterol regulatory element–binding protein-1c (SREBP-1c). *Fatty acid synthase* (see C. below) is similarly regulated. The function and regulation of SREBP are described on p. 222.] Metformin, used in the treatment of type 2 diabetes, lowers plasma TAG through activation of *AMPK*, resulting in inhibition of *ACC* activity (by phosphorylation) and inhibition of *ACC* and *fatty acid synthase* expression (by decreasing SREBP-1c). Metformin lowers blood glucose by increasing *AMPK*-mediated glucose uptake by muscle.

C. Eukaryotic fatty acid synthase

The remaining series of reactions of fatty acid synthesis in eukaryotes is catalyzed by the multifunctional, homodimeric enzyme *fatty acid synthase* (*FAS*). The process involves the addition of two carbons from malonyl CoA to the carboxyl end of a series of acyl acceptors. Each *FAS* monomer is a multicatalytic polypeptide with six different enzymic domains plus a 4′-phosphopantetheine-containing acyl carrier protein (ACP) domain. 4′-Phosphopantetheine, a derivative of pantothenic acid (vitamin B_5, see p. 385), carries acyl units on its terminal thiol (–SH) group and presents them to the catalytic domains of *FAS* during fatty acid synthesis. It also is a component of CoA. [Note: In prokaryotes, *FAS* is a multienzyme complex.] The reaction numbers in brackets below refer to Figure 16.9.

[1] An acetyl group is transferred from acetyl CoA to the –SH group of the ACP. Domain: *Malonyl/acetyl CoA–ACP transacylase*.

[2] Next, this two-carbon fragment is transferred to a temporary holding site, the –SH group of a cysteine residue on the condensing enzyme domain (see [4] below).

[3] The now-vacant ACP accepts a three-carbon malonyl group from malonyl CoA. Domain: *Malonyl/acetyl CoA–ACP transacylase*.

[4] The acetyl group on the cysteine residue condenses with the malonyl group on ACP as the CO_2 originally added by *ACC* is released. The result is a four-carbon unit attached to the ACP domain. The loss of free energy from the decarboxylation drives the reaction. Domain: *3-Ketoacyl–ACP synthase*, also known as condensing enzyme.

The next three reactions convert the 3-ketoacyl group to the corresponding saturated acyl group by a pair of NADPH-requiring reductions and a dehydration step.

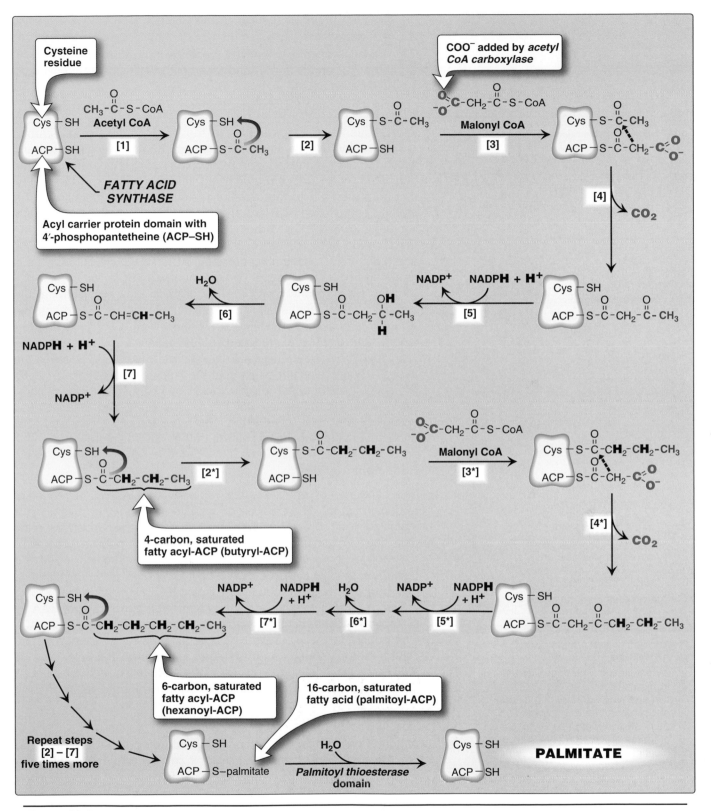

Figure 16.9

Synthesis of palmitate (16:0) by multifunctional *fatty acid synthase*. [Note: Numbers in brackets correspond to bracketed numbers in the text. A second repetition of the steps is indicated by numbers with an asterisk (*). Carbons provided directly by acetyl coenzyme A (CoA) are shown in red.] ACP = acyl carrier protein domain; CO_2 = carbon dioxide; NADP(H) = nicotinamide adenine dinucleotide phosphate.

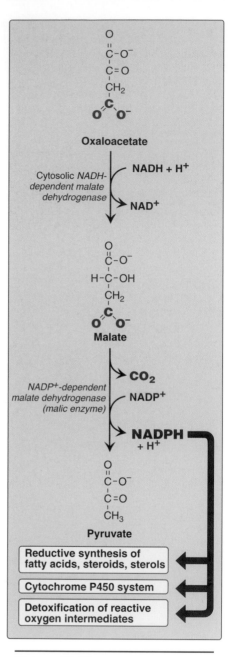

Figure 16.10
Cytosolic conversion of oxaloacetate to pyruvate with the generation of nicotinamide adenine dinucleotide phosphate (NADPH). [Note: The pentose phosphate pathway is also a source of NADPH.] NAD(H) = nicotinamide adenine dinucleotide; CO_2 = carbon dioxide.

[5] The keto group is reduced to an alcohol. Domain: *3-Ketoacyl–ACP reductase.*

[6] A molecule of water is removed, creating a trans double bond between carbons 2 and 3 (the α- and β-carbons). Domain: *3-Hydroxyacyl–ACP dehydratase.*

[7] The double bond is reduced. Domain: *Enoyl–ACP reductase.*

This sequence of steps results in the production of a four-carbon group (butyryl) whose three terminal carbons are fully saturated and which remains attached to the ACP domain. The steps are repeated (indicated by an asterisk), beginning with the transfer of the butyryl unit from the ACP to the cysteine residue [2*], the attachment of a malonyl group to the ACP [3*], and the condensation of the two groups liberating CO_2 [4*]. The carbonyl group at the β-carbon (carbon 3, the third carbon from the sulfur) is then reduced [5*], dehydrated [6*], and reduced [7*], generating hexanoyl-ACP. This cycle of reactions is repeated five more times, each time incorporating a two-carbon unit (derived from malonyl CoA) into the growing fatty acid chain at the carboxyl end. When the fatty acid reaches a length of 16 carbons, the synthetic process is terminated with palmitoyl-S-ACP. [Note: Shorter-length fatty acids are produced in the lactating mammary gland.] *Palmitoyl thioesterase*, the final catalytic activity of *FAS*, cleaves the thioester bond, releasing a fully saturated molecule of palmitate (16:0). [Note: All the carbons in palmitic acid have passed through malonyl CoA except the two donated by the original acetyl CoA (the first acyl acceptor), which are found at the methyl (ω) end of the fatty acid. This underscores the rate-limiting nature of the *ACC* reaction.]

D. Reductant sources

The synthesis of one palmitate requires 14 NADPH, a reductant (reducing agent). The pentose phosphate pathway (see p. 145) is a major supplier of the NADPH. Two NADPH are produced for each molecule of glucose 6-phosphate that enters this pathway. The cytosolic conversion of malate to pyruvate, in which malate is oxidized and decarboxylated by cytosolic *malic enzyme* (*NADP⁺-dependent malate dehydrogenase*), also produces cytosolic NADPH (and CO_2), as shown in Figure 16.10. [Note: Malate can arise from the reduction of OAA by cytosolic *NADH-dependent malate dehydrogenase* (see Fig. 16.10). One source of the cytosolic NADH required for this reaction is glycolysis (see p. 101). OAA, in turn, can arise from citrate cleavage by *ATP citrate lyase*.] A summary of the interrelationship between glucose metabolism and palmitate synthesis is shown in Figure 16.11.

E. Further elongation

Although palmitate, a 16-carbon, fully saturated LCFA (16:0), is the primary end product of *FAS* activity, it can be further elongated by the addition of two-carbon units to the carboxylate end primarily in the smooth endoplasmic reticulum (SER). Elongation requires a system of separate enzymes rather than a multifunctional enzyme. Malonyl CoA is the two-carbon donor, and NADPH supplies the electrons. The brain has additional elongation capabilities, allowing it to produce the very-long-chain fatty acids ([VLCFA] over 22 carbons) that are required for synthesis of brain lipids.

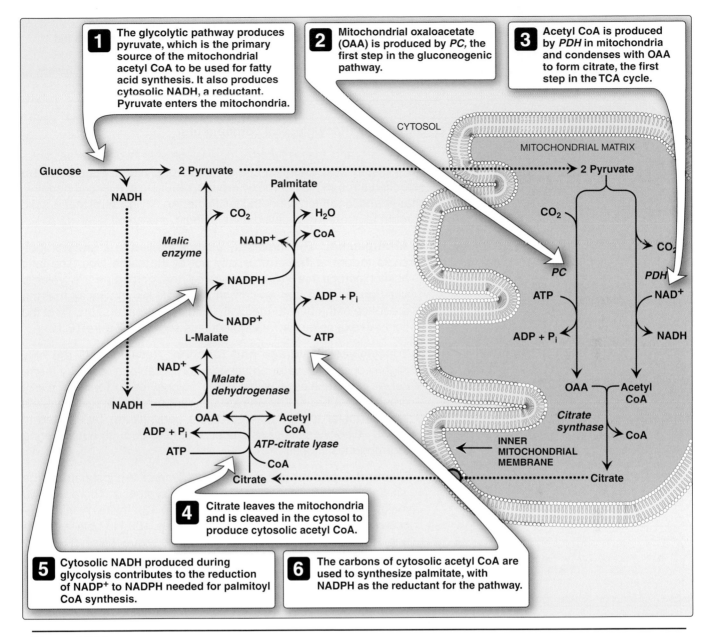

Figure 16.11
Interrelationship between glucose metabolism and palmitate synthesis. CoA = coenzyme A; NAD(H) = nicotinamide adenine nucleotide; NADP(H) = nicotinamide adenine dinucleotide phosphate; ADP = adenosine diphosphate; P$_i$ = inorganic phosphate; CO$_2$ = carbon dioxide; TCA = tricarboxylic acid; *PC = pyruvate carboxylase*; *PDH = pyruvate dehydrogenase*.

F. Chain desaturation

Enzymes (*fatty acyl CoA desaturases*) also present in the SER are responsible for desaturating LCFA (that is, adding cis double bonds). The desaturation reactions require oxygen (O$_2$), NADH, cytochrome b$_5$, and its flavin adenine dinucleotide (FAD)-linked *reductase*. The fatty acid and the NADH get oxidized as the O$_2$ gets reduced to H$_2$O. The first double bond is typically inserted between carbons 9 and 10, producing primarily oleic acid, 18:1(9), and small amounts of palmitoleic acid, 16:1(9). A variety of polyunsaturated fatty acids can be made through additional desaturation combined with elongation.

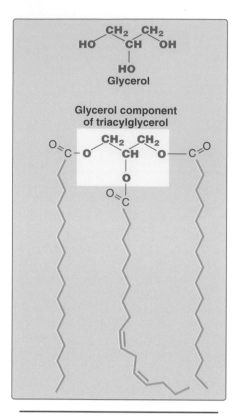

Figure 16.12
A triacylglycerol with an unsaturated fatty acid on carbon 2. Orange denotes the hydrophobic portions of the molecule.

Humans have carbon 9, 6, 5, and 4 *desaturases* but lack the ability to introduce double bonds from carbon 10 to the ω end of the chain. This is the basis for the nutritional essentiality of the polyunsaturated ω-6 linoleic acid and ω-3 linolenic acid.

G. Storage as triacylglycerol components

Mono-, di-, and triacylglycerols consist of one, two, or three molecules of fatty acid esterified to a molecule of glycerol. Fatty acids are esterified through their carboxyl groups, resulting in a loss of negative charge and formation of neutral fat. [Note: An acylglycerol that is solid at room temperature is called a fat. If liquid, it is an oil.]

1. **Arrangement:** The three fatty acids esterified to a glycerol molecule to form a TAG are usually not of the same type. The fatty acid on carbon 1 is typically saturated, that on carbon 2 is typically unsaturated, and that on carbon 3 can be either. Recall that the presence of the unsaturated fatty acid(s) decrease(s) the T_m of the lipid. An example of a TAG molecule is shown in Figure 16.12.

2. **Triacylglycerol storage and function:** Because TAG are only slightly soluble in water and cannot form stable micelles by themselves, they coalesce within white adipocytes to form large oily droplets that are nearly anhydrous. These cytosolic lipid droplets are the major energy reserve of the body. [Note: TAG stored in brown adipocytes serve as a source of heat through nonshivering thermogenesis (see p. 79).]

3. **Glycerol 3-phosphate synthesis:** Glycerol 3-phosphate is the initial acceptor of fatty acids during TAG synthesis. There are two major pathways for its production (Fig. 16.13). [Note: A third process (glyceroneogenesis) is described on p. 190.] In both liver (the primary site of TAG synthesis) and adipose tissue, glycerol 3-phosphate can be produced from glucose, first using the reactions of the glycolytic pathway to produce dihydroxyacetone phosphate ([DHAP], see p. 101). DHAP is reduced by *glycerol 3-phosphate*

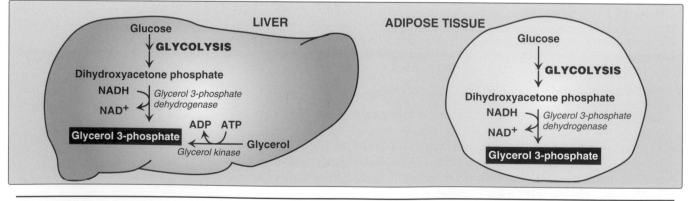

Figure 16.13
Pathways for production of glycerol 3-phosphate in liver and adipose tissue. [Note: Glycerol 3-phosphate can also be generated by glyceroneogenesis.] NAD(H) = nicotinamide adenine dinucleotide; ADP = adenosine diphosphate.

dehydrogenase to glycerol 3-phosphate. A second pathway found in the liver, but not in adipose tissue, uses *glycerol kinase* to convert free glycerol to glycerol 3-phosphate (see Fig. 16.13). [Note: The glucose transporter in adipocytes (GLUT-4) is insulin dependent (see p. 312). Thus, when plasma glucose levels are low, adipocytes have only a limited ability to synthesize glycerol phosphate and cannot produce TAG de novo.]

4. **Fatty acid activation:** A free fatty acid must be converted to its activated form (bound to CoA through a thioester link) before it can participate in metabolic processes such as TAG synthesis. This reaction, illustrated in Figure 15.6 on p. 177, is catalyzed by a family of *fatty acyl CoA synthetases* (*thiokinases*).

5. **Triacylglycerol synthesis:** This pathway from glycerol 3-phosphate involves four reactions, shown in Figure 16.14. These include the sequential addition of two fatty acids from fatty acyl CoA, the removal of phosphate, and the addition of the third fatty acid.

H. Triacylglycerol fate in liver and adipose tissue

In WAT, TAG is stored in a nearly anhydrous form as fat droplets in the cytosol of the cells. It serves as "depot fat," ready for mobilization when the body requires it for fuel. Little TAG is stored in healthy liver. Instead, most is exported, packaged with other lipids and apolipoproteins to form lipoprotein particles called very-low-density lipoproteins (VLDL). Nascent VLDL are secreted directly into the blood where they mature and function to deliver the endogenously derived lipids to the peripheral tissues. [Note: Recall from Chapter 15 that chylomicrons carry dietary (exogenously derived) lipids. Plasma lipoproteins are discussed in Chapter 18.]

IV. FAT MOBILIZATION AND FATTY ACID OXIDATION

Fatty acids stored in WAT, in the form of neutral TAG, serve as the body's major fuel storage reserve. TAG provide concentrated stores of metabolic energy because they are highly reduced and largely anhydrous. The yield from the complete oxidation of fatty acids to CO_2 and H_2O is 9 kcal/g fat (as compared to 4 kcal/g protein or carbohydrate, see Fig. 27.5 on p. 359).

A. Fatty acid release from fat

The mobilization of stored fat requires the hydrolytic release of FFA and glycerol from their TAG form. This process of lipolysis is achieved by *lipases*. It is initiated by *adipose triglyceride lipase* (*ATGL*), which generates a diacylglycerol that is the preferred substrate for *hormone-sensitive lipase* (*HSL*). The monoacylglycerol (MAG) product of *HSL* is acted upon by *MAG lipase*.

1. **Hormone-sensitive lipase regulation:** *HSL* is active when phosphorylated by *PKA*, a *cAMP-dependent protein kinase*. cAMP is produced in the adipocyte when catecholamines (such as epinephrine) bind to cell membrane β-adrenergic receptors and activate *adenylyl cyclase* (Fig. 16.15). The process is similar to that of the activation of *glycogen phosphorylase* (see Fig. 11.9, p. 131). [Note: Because *ACC* is inhibited by hormone-directed phosphorylation,

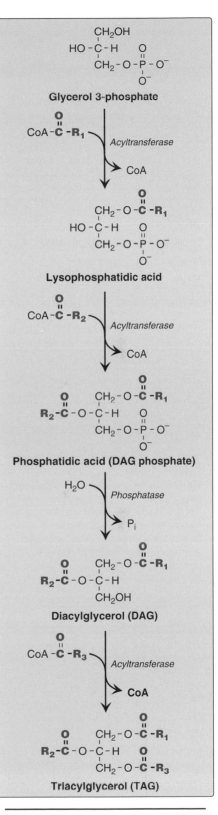

Figure 16.14
Synthesis of TAG. R1–R3 = activated fatty acids. CoA = coenzyme A; P_i = inorganic phosphate.

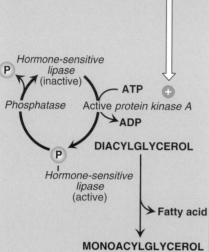

Figure 16.15
Hormonal regulation of diacylglycerol degradation in the adipocyte. [Note: Triacylglycerol is degraded to diacylglycerol by *adipose triglyceride lipase*.] cAMP = cyclic adenosine monophosphate; PP$_i$ = pyrophosphate; ADP = adenosine diphosphate; (P) = phosphate.

when the cAMP-mediated cascade is activated (see Fig. 16.8), fatty acid synthesis is turned off and TAG degradation is turned on.] In the presence of high plasma levels of insulin, *HSL* is dephosphorylated and inactivated. Insulin also suppresses expression of *ATGL*. [Note: Fat droplets are coated by a protein (perilipin) that limits access of *HSL*. Phosphorylation of perilipin by *PKA* allows translocation and binding of phosphorylated *HSL* to the droplet.]

2. **Fate of glycerol:** The glycerol released during TAG degradation cannot be metabolized by adipocytes because they lack *glycerol kinase*. Rather, glycerol is transported through the blood to the liver, which has the *kinase*. The resulting glycerol 3-phosphate can be used to form TAG in the liver or can be converted to DHAP by reversal of the *glycerol 3-phosphate dehydrogenase* reaction illustrated in Figure 16.13. DHAP can participate in glycolysis or gluconeogenesis.

3. **Fate of fatty acids:** The FFA move through the cell membrane of the adipocyte and bind to serum albumin. They are transported to tissues such as muscle, enter cells, get activated to their CoA derivatives, and are oxidized for energy in mitochondria. Regardless of their levels, plasma FFA cannot be used for fuel by red blood cells (RBC), which have no mitochondria. The brain does not use fatty acids for energy to any appreciable extent, but the reasons are less clear. [Note: Over 50% of the fatty acids released from adipose TAG are reesterified to glycerol 3-phosphate. WAT does not express *glycerol kinase*, and the glycerol 3-phosphate is produced by glyceroneogenesis, an incomplete version of gluconeogenesis: pyruvate to OAA via *pyruvate carboxylase* and OAA to phosphoenolpyruvate (PEP) via *phosphoenolpyruvate carboxykinase*. The PEP is converted (by reactions common to glycolysis and gluconeogenesis) to DHAP, which is reduced to glycerol 3-phosphate. The process decreases plasma FFA, molecules associated with insulin resistance in type 2 diabetes and obesity (see p. 343).]

B. Fatty acid β-oxidation

The major pathway for catabolism of fatty acids is a mitochondrial pathway called β-oxidation, in which two-carbon fragments are successively removed from the carboxyl end of the fatty acyl CoA, producing acetyl CoA, NADH, and FADH$_2$.

1. **Long-chain fatty acid transport into mitochondria:** After a LCFA enters a cell, it is converted in the cytosol to its CoA derivative by *long-chain fatty acyl CoA synthetase* (*thiokinase*), an enzyme of the outer mitochondrial membrane. Because β-oxidation occurs in the mitochondrial matrix, the fatty acid must be transported across the inner mitochondrial membrane that is impermeable to CoA. Therefore, a specialized carrier transports the long-chain acyl group from the cytosol into the mitochondrial matrix. This carrier is carnitine, and this rate-limiting transport process is called the carnitine shuttle (Fig. 16.16).

   a. **Translocation steps:** First, the acyl group is transferred from CoA to carnitine by *carnitine palmitoyltransferase I* (*CPT-I*), an enzyme of the outer mitochondrial membrane. [Note: *CPT-I* is

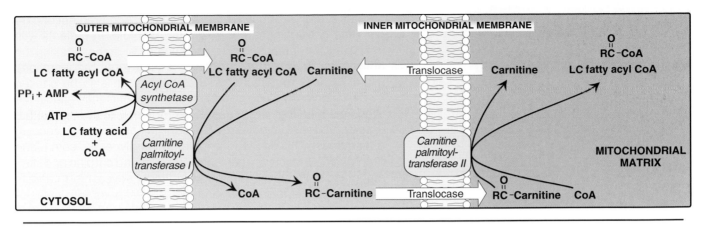

Figure 16.16
Carnitine shuttle. The net effect is that a long-chain (LC) fatty acyl coenzyme A (CoA) is transported from the outside to the inside of mitochondria. AMP = adenosine monophosphate; PP$_i$ = pyrophosphate.

also known as *CAT-I* for *carnitine acyltransferase I*.] This reaction forms an acylcarnitine and regenerates free CoA. Second, the acylcarnitine is transported into the mitochondrial matrix in exchange for free carnitine by carnitine–acylcarnitine translocase. *Carnitine palmitoyltransferase 2* (*CPT-II*, or *CAT-II*), an enzyme of the inner mitochondrial membrane, catalyzes the transfer of the acyl group from carnitine to CoA in the mitochondrial matrix, thus regenerating free carnitine.

b. Carnitine shuttle inhibitor: Malonyl CoA inhibits *CPT-I*, thus preventing the entry of long-chain acyl groups into the mitochondrial matrix. Therefore, when fatty acid synthesis is occurring in the cytosol (as indicated by the presence of malonyl CoA), the newly made palmitate cannot be transferred into mitochondria and degraded. [Note: Muscle tissue, although it does not synthesize fatty acids, contains the mitochondrial isozyme of *ACC* (*ACC2*), allowing regulation of β-oxidation. The liver contains both isozymes.] Fatty acid oxidation is also regulated by the acetyl CoA/CoA ratio: As the ratio increases, the CoA-requiring *thiolase* reaction decreases (Fig. 16.17).

c. Carnitine sources: Carnitine can be obtained from the diet, where it is found primarily in meat products. It can also be synthesized from the amino acids lysine and methionine by an enzymatic pathway found in the liver and kidneys but not in skeletal or cardiac muscle. Therefore, these latter tissues are totally dependent on uptake of carnitine provided by endogenous synthesis or the diet and distributed by the blood. [Note: Skeletal muscle contains ~97% of all carnitine in the body.]

d. Carnitine deficiencies: Such deficiencies result in decreased ability of tissues to use LCFA as a fuel. Primary carnitine deficiency is caused by defects in a membrane transporter that prevent uptake of carnitine by cardiac and skeletal muscle and the kidneys, causing carnitine to be excreted. Treatment includes carnitine supplementation. Secondary carnitine deficiency occurs primarily as a result of defects in fatty acid oxidation leading to the accumulation of acylcarnitines that are excreted in

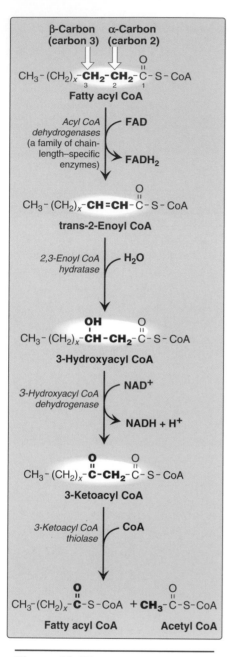

Figure 16.17
Enzymes involved in the β-oxidation
of fatty acyl coenzyme A (CoA).
[Note: *2,3-Enoyl CoA hydratase*
requires a trans double bond between
carbon 2 and carbon 3.] FAD(H₂) =
flavin adenine dinucleotide; NAD(H) =
nicotinamide adenine dinucleotide.

the urine, decreasing carnitine availability. Acquired secondary carnitine deficiency can be seen, for example, in patients with liver disease (decreased carnitine synthesis) or those taking the antiseizure drug valproic acid (decreased renal reabsorption). [Note: Defects in mitochondrial oxidation can also be caused by deficiencies in *CPT-I* and *CPT-II*. *CPT-I* deficiency affects the liver, where an inability to use LCFA for fuel greatly impairs that tissue's ability to synthesize glucose (an endergonic process) during a fast. This can lead to severe hypoglycemia, coma, and death. *CPT-II* deficiency can affect the liver and cardiac and skeletal muscle. The most common (and least severe) form affects skeletal muscle. It presents as muscle weakness with myoglobinemia following prolonged exercise. Treatment includes avoidance of fasting and adopting a diet high in carbohydrates and low in fat but supplemented with medium-chain TAG.]

2. **Shorter-chain fatty acid entry into mitochondria:** Fatty acids ≤12 carbons can cross the inner mitochondrial membrane without the aid of carnitine or the *CPT* system. Once inside the mitochondria, they are activated to their CoA derivatives by matrix enzymes and are oxidized. [Note: Medium-chain fatty acids are plentiful in human milk. Because their oxidation is not dependent on *CPT-I*, malonyl CoA is not inhibitory.]

3. **β-Oxidation reactions:** The first cycle of β-oxidation is shown in Figure 16.17. It consists of a sequence of four reactions involving the β-carbon (carbon 3) that results in shortening the fatty acid by two carbons at the carboxylate end. The steps include an oxidation that produces FADH₂, a hydration, a second oxidation that produces NADH, and a CoA-dependent thiolytic cleavage that releases a molecule of acetyl CoA. Each step is catalyzed by enzymes with chain-length specificity. [Note: For LCFA, the last three steps are catalyzed by a trifunctional protein.] These four steps are repeated for saturated fatty acids of even-numbered carbon chains (n/2) − 1 times (where n is the number of carbons), each cycle producing one acetyl CoA plus one NADH and one FADH₂. The final cycle produces two acetyl CoA. The acetyl CoA can be oxidized or used in hepatic ketogenesis (see V. below). The reduced coenzymes are oxidized by the electron transport chain, NADH by Complex I, and FADH₂ by coenzyme Q (see p. 75). [Note: Acetyl CoA is a positive allosteric effector of *pyruvate carboxylase* (see p. 119), thus linking fatty acid oxidation and gluconeogenesis.]

4. **β-Oxidation energy yield:** The energy yield from fatty acid β-oxidation is high. For example, the oxidation of a molecule of palmitoyl CoA to CO_2 and H_2O produces 8 acetyl CoA, 7 NADH, and 7 FADH₂, from which 131 ATP can be generated. However, activation of the fatty acid requires two ATP. Therefore, the net yield from palmitate is 129 ATP (Fig. 16.18). A comparison of the processes of synthesis and degradation of long-chain saturated fatty acids with an even number of carbon atoms is provided in Figure 16.19.

5. **Medium-chain fatty acyl CoA dehydrogenase deficiency:** In mitochondria, there are four *fatty acyl CoA dehydrogenase* species, each with distinct but overlapping specificity for either short-, medium-, long-, or very-long-chain fatty acids. *Medium-chain fatty acyl CoA*

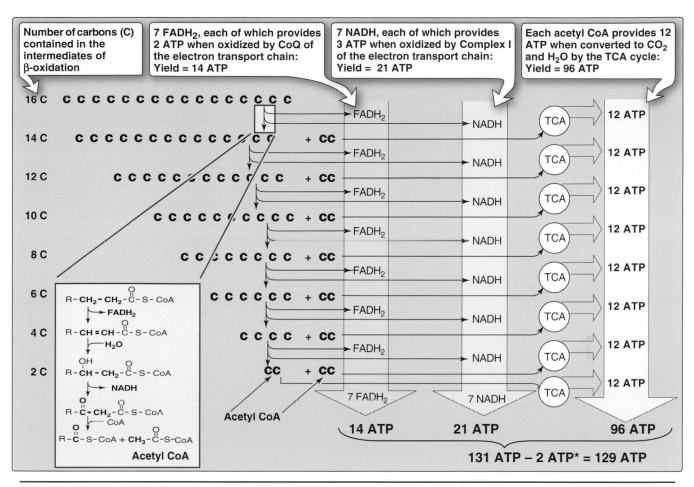

Figure 16.18
Summary of the energy yield from the oxidation of palmitoyl coenzyme A (CoA) (16 carbons). [Note: *Activation of palmitate to palmitoyl CoA requires the equivalent of 2 ATP (ATP → AMP + PP$_i$).] FADH$_2$ = flavin adenine dinucleotide; NADH = nicotinamide adenine dinucleotide; TCA = tricarboxylic acid; CoQ = coenzyme Q; CO$_2$ = carbon dioxide.

dehydrogenase (*MCAD*) deficiency, an autosomal-recessive disorder, is the most common inborn error of β-oxidation, being found in 1:14,000 births worldwide, with a higher incidence in Caucasians of Northern European descent. It results in decreased ability to oxidize fatty acids with six to ten carbons (which accumulate and can be measured in urine), severe hypoglycemia (because the tissues must increase their reliance on glucose), and hypoketonemia (because of decreased production of acetyl CoA; see p. 195). Treatment includes avoidance of fasting.

6. **Oxidation of fatty acids with an odd number of carbons:** This process proceeds by the same reaction steps as that of fatty acids with an even number of carbons, until the final three carbons are reached. This product, propionyl CoA, is metabolized by a three-step pathway (Fig. 16.20). [Note: Propionyl CoA is also produced during the metabolism of certain amino acids (see Fig. 20.11, p. 266).]

   a. **D-Methylmalonyl CoA synthesis:** First, propionyl CoA is carboxylated, forming D-methylmalonyl CoA. The enzyme *propionyl*

VARIABLE	SYNTHESIS	DEGRADATION
Greatest flux through pathway	After carbohydrate-rich meal	In starvation
Hormonal state favoring pathway	High insulin/glucagon ratio	Low insulin/glucagon ratio
Major tissue site	Primarily liver	Muscle, liver
Subcellular location	Cytosol	Primarily mitochondria
Carriers of acyl/acetyl groups between mitochondria and cytosol	Citrate (mitochondria to cytosol)	Carnitine (cytosol to mitochondria)
Phosphopantetheine-containing active carriers	Acyl carrier protein domain, coenzyme A	Coenzyme A
Oxidation/reduction coenzymes	NADPH (reduction)	NAD^+, FAD (oxidation)
Two-carbon donor/product	Malonyl CoA: donor of one acetyl group	Acetyl CoA: product of β-oxidation
Activator	Citrate	—
Inhibitor	Palmitoyl CoA (inhibits *acetyl CoA carboxylase*)	Malonyl CoA (inhibits *carnitine palmitoyltransferase-I*)
Product of pathway	Palmitate	Acetyl CoA
Repetitive four-step process	Condensation, reduction dehydration, reduction	Dehydrogenation, hydration dehydrogenation, thiolysis

Figure 16.19
Comparison of the synthesis and degradation of long-chain, even-numbered, saturated fatty acids. NADPH = nicotinamide adenine dinucleotide phosphate; NAD^+ = nicotinamide adenine dinucleotide; FAD = flavin adenine dinucleotide; CoA = coenzyme A.

CoA carboxylase has an absolute requirement for the coenzymes biotin and ATP, as do *ACC* and most other *carboxylases*.

b. **ʟ-Methylmalonyl CoA formation:** Next, the ᴅ-isomer is converted to the ʟ-form by the enzyme *methylmalonyl CoA racemase*.

c. **Succinyl CoA synthesis:** Finally, the carbons of ʟ-methylmalonyl CoA are rearranged, forming succinyl CoA, which can enter the TCA cycle (see p. 113). [Note: This is the only example of a glucogenic precursor generated from fatty acid oxidation.] The enzyme *methylmalonyl CoA mutase* requires a coenzyme form of vitamin B_{12} (deoxyadenosylcobalamin). The *mutase* reaction is one of only two reactions in the body that require vitamin B_{12} (see p. 379). [Note: In patients with vitamin B_{12} deficiency, both propionate and methylmalonate are excreted in the urine. Two types of heritable methylmalonic acidemia and aciduria have been described: one in which the *mutase* is missing or deficient (or has reduced affinity for the coenzyme) and one in which the patient is unable to convert vitamin B_{12} into its coenzyme form. Either type results in metabolic acidosis and neurologic manifestations.]

7. **Unsaturated fatty acid β-oxidation:** The oxidation of unsaturated fatty acids generates intermediates that cannot serve as substrates

for *2,3-enoyl CoA hydratase* (see Fig. 16.17). Consequently, additional enzymes are required. Oxidation of a double bond at an odd-numbered carbon, such as 18:1(9) (oleic acid), requires one additional enzyme, *3,2-enoyl CoA isomerase*, which converts the 3-cis derivative obtained after three rounds of β-oxidation to the 2-trans derivative required by the *hydratase*. Oxidation of a double bond at an even-numbered carbon, such as 18:2(9,12) (linoleic acid), requires an *NADPH-dependent 2,4-dienoyl CoA reductase* in addition to the *isomerase*. [Note: Because unsaturated fatty acids are less reduced than saturated fatty acids, fewer reducing equivalents are produced by their oxidation.]

8. **Peroxisomal β-oxidation:** VLCFA ≥22 carbons in length undergo a preliminary β-oxidation in peroxisomes, because peroxisomes and not mitochondria are the primary site of the *synthetase* that activates fatty acids of this length. The shortened fatty acid (linked to carnitine) diffuses to a mitochondrion for further oxidation. In contrast to mitochondrial β-oxidation, the initial dehydrogenation in peroxisomes is catalyzed by a FAD-containing *acyl CoA oxidase*. The $FADH_2$ produced is oxidized by O_2, which is reduced to hydrogen peroxide (H_2O_2). Therefore, no ATP is generated from this step. The H_2O_2 is reduced to H_2O by *catalase* (see p. 148). [Note: Genetic defects in the ability either to target matrix proteins to peroxisomes (resulting in Zellweger syndrome, a peroxisomal biogenesis disorder) or to transport VLCFA across the peroxisomal membrane (resulting in X-linked adrenoleukodystrophy) lead to accumulation of VLCFA in the blood and tissues.]

C. Peroxisomal α-oxidation

Branched-chain phytanic acid, a product of chlorophyll metabolism, is not a substrate for *acyl CoA dehydrogenase* because of the methyl group on its β-carbon (Fig. 16.21). Instead, it is hydroxylated at the α-carbon by *phytanoyl CoA α-hydroxylase* (*PhyH*); carbon 1 is released as CO_2; and the product, 15-carbon-long pristanal, is oxidized to pristanic acid, which is activated to its CoA derivative and undergoes β-oxidation. Refsum disease is a rare, autosomal-recessive disorder caused by a deficiency of peroxisomal *PhyH*. This results in the accumulation of phytanic acid in the plasma and tissues. The symptoms are primarily neurologic, and the treatment involves dietary restriction to halt disease progression. [Note: ω-Oxidation (at the methyl terminus) also is known and generates dicarboxylic acids. Normally a minor pathway of the SER, its upregulation is seen with conditions such as *MCAD* deficiency that limit fatty acid β-oxidation.]

V. KETONE BODIES: ALTERNATIVE FUEL FOR CELLS

Liver mitochondria have the capacity to convert acetyl CoA derived from fatty acid oxidation into ketone bodies. The compounds categorized as ketone bodies are acetoacetate, 3-hydroxybutyrate (also called β-hydroxybutyrate), and acetone (a nonmetabolized side product, Fig. 16.22). [Note: The two functional ketone bodies are organic acids.] Acetoacetate and 3-hydroxybutyrate are transported in the blood to the peripheral tissues. There they can be reconverted to acetyl CoA, which can be oxidized by the TCA cycle. Ketone bodies are important sources

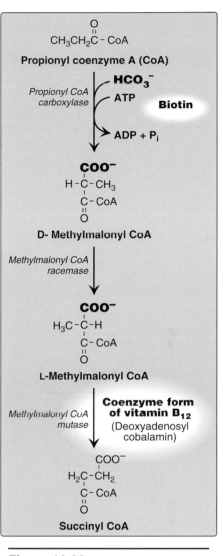

Figure 16.20
Metabolism of propionyl CoA. ADP = adenosine diphosphate; HCO_3^- = bicarbonate; P_i = inorganic phosphate.

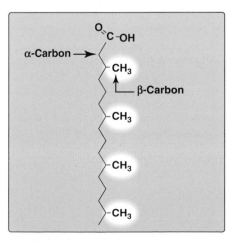

Figure 16.21
Phytanic acid, a branched-chain fatty acid 16 carbons in length.

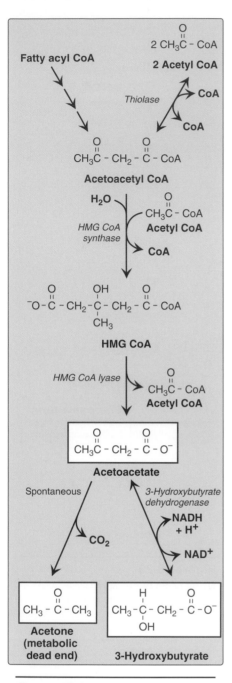

Figure 16.22
Synthesis of ketone bodies. [Note:
The release of CoA in ketogenesis
supports continued fatty acid
oxidation.] CoA = coenzyme A; HMG =
hydroxymethylglutarate; NAD(H) =
nicotinamide adenine dinucleotide;
CO_2 = carbon dioxide.

of energy for the peripheral tissues because they 1) are soluble in aqueous solution and, therefore, do not need to be incorporated into lipoproteins or carried by albumin as do the other lipids; 2) are produced in the liver during periods when the amount of acetyl CoA present exceeds the oxidative capacity of the liver; and 3) are used in proportion to their concentration in the blood by extrahepatic tissues, such as skeletal and cardiac muscle, the intestinal mucosa, and the renal cortex. Even the brain can use ketone bodies to help meet its energy needs if the blood levels rise sufficiently. Thus, ketone bodies spare glucose, which is particularly important during prolonged periods of fasting (see p. 332). [Note: Disorders of fatty acid oxidation present with the general picture of hypoketosis (because of decreased availability of acetyl CoA) and hypoglycemia (because of increased reliance on glucose for energy).]

A. Ketone body synthesis by the liver: Ketogenesis

During a fast, the liver is flooded with fatty acids mobilized from adipose tissue. The resulting elevated hepatic acetyl CoA produced by fatty acid oxidation inhibits *pyruvate dehydrogenase* (see p. 111) and activates *pyruvate carboxylase* ([*PC*] see p. 119). The OAA produced by *PC* is used by the liver for gluconeogenesis rather than for the TCA cycle. Additionally, fatty acid oxidation decreases the NAD^+/NADH ratio, and the rise in NADH shifts OAA to malate (see p. 113). The decreased availability of OAA for condensation with acetyl CoA results in the increased use of acetyl CoA for ketone body synthesis. [Note: Acetyl CoA for ketogenesis is also generated by the catabolism of ketogenic amino acids (see p. 262).]

1. **3-Hydroxy-3-methylglutaryl CoA synthesis:** The first step, formation of acetoacetyl CoA, occurs by reversal of the final *thiolase* reaction of fatty acid oxidation (see Fig. 16.17). Mitochondrial *3-hydroxy-3-methylglutaryl* (*HMG*) *CoA synthase* combines a third molecule of acetyl CoA with acetoacetyl CoA to produce HMG CoA. *HMG CoA synthase* is the rate-limiting step in the synthesis of ketone bodies and is present in significant quantities only in the liver. [Note: HMG CoA is also an intermediate in cytosolic cholesterol synthesis (see p. 220). The two pathways are separated by location in, and conditions of, the cell.]

2. **Ketone body synthesis:** HMG CoA is cleaved by *HMG CoA lyase* to produce acetoacetate and acetyl CoA, as shown in Figure 16.22. Acetoacetate can be reduced to form 3-hydroxybutyrate with NADH as the electron donor. [Note: Because ketone bodies are not linked to CoA, they can cross the inner mitochondrial membrane.] Acetoacetate can also spontaneously decarboxylate in the blood to form acetone, a volatile, biologically nonmetabolized compound that can be detected in the breath. The equilibrium between acetoacetate and 3-hydroxybutyrate is determined by the NAD^+/NADH ratio. Because this ratio is low during fatty acid oxidation, 3-hydroxybutyrate synthesis is favored.

B. Ketone body use by the peripheral tissues: Ketolysis

Although the liver constantly synthesizes low levels of ketone bodies, their production increases during fasting when ketone bodies are needed to provide energy to the peripheral tissues. 3-Hydroxybutyrate

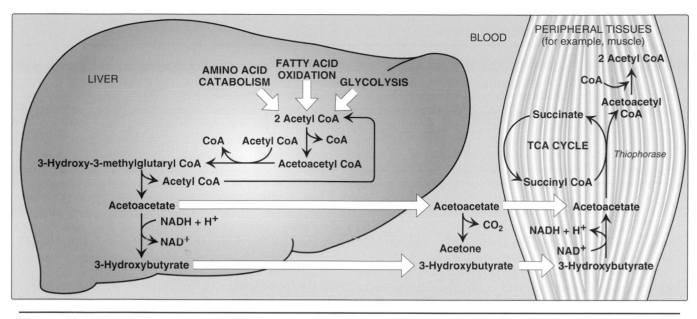

Figure 16.23
Ketone body synthesis in the liver and use in peripheral tissues. The liver and red blood cells cannot use ketone bodies.
[Note: *Thiophorase* is also known as *succinyl CoA:acetoacetate CoA transferase*.] CoA = coenzyme A; NAD(H) =
nicotinamide adenine dinucleotide; TCA = tricarboxylic acid; CO_2 = carbon dioxide.

is oxidized to acetoacetate by *3-hydroxybutyrate dehydrogenase*, producing NADH (Fig. 16.23). Acetoacetate is then provided with a CoA
molecule taken from succinyl CoA by *succinyl CoA:acetoacetate CoA
transferase* (*thiophorase*). This reaction is reversible, but the product,
acetoacetyl CoA, is actively removed by its cleavage to two acetyl CoA
by *thiolase*. This pulls the reaction forward. Extrahepatic tissues, including the brain but excluding cells lacking mitochondria (for example, RBC),
efficiently oxidize acetoacetate and 3-hydroxybutyrate in this manner.
In contrast, although the liver actively produces ketone bodies, it lacks
thiophorase and, therefore, is unable to use ketone bodies as fuel.

C. Excessive ketone body production in diabetes mellitus

When the rate of formation of ketone bodies is greater than the rate
of their use, their levels begin to rise in the blood (ketonemia) and,
eventually, in the urine (ketonuria). This is seen most often in cases
of uncontrolled type 1 diabetes mellitus (T1D), where the blood
concentration of ketone bodies may reach 90 mg/dl (versus <3 mg/dl
in normal individuals), and urinary excretion of ketone bodies may
be as high as 5,000 mg/24 hour. The elevation of the ketone body
concentration in the blood can result in acidemia. [Note: The carboxyl
group of a ketone body has a pK_a of ~4. Therefore, each ketone body
loses a proton (H^+) as it circulates in the blood, which lowers the pH.]
Also, in uncontrolled T1D, urinary loss of glucose and ketone bodies
results in dehydration. Therefore, the increased number of H^+ circulating in a decreased volume of plasma can cause a severe acidosis
(ketoacidosis, Fig. 16.24) known as diabetic ketoacidosis (DKA).] A
frequent symptom of DKA is a fruity odor on the breath, which results
from increased production of acetone. Ketoacidosis may also be seen
in cases of prolonged fasting (see p. 330) and excessive ethanol consumption (see p. 318).

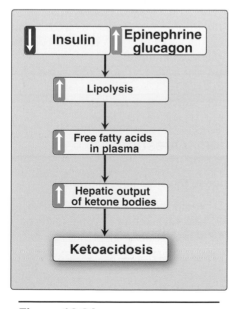

Figure 16.24
Mechanism of diabetic ketoacidosis
seen in uncontrolled type 1 diabetes.

VI. CHAPTER SUMMARY

A **fatty acid**, generally a linear hydrocarbon chain with a terminal carboxyl group, can be **saturated** or **unsaturated**. Two unsaturated fatty acids are dietary essentials: **linoleic** and **α-linolenic acids**. Fatty acids are synthesized in the **liver cytosol** following a meal containing excess carbohydrate and protein. Carbons used to synthesize fatty acids are provided by **acetyl coenzyme A** (**CoA**), energy by **ATP**, and reducing equivalents by **nicotinamide adenine dinucleotide phosphate** ([**NADPH**], Fig. 16.25) provided by the **pentose phosphate pathway** and *malic enzyme*. **Citrate** carries two-carbon acetyl units from the mitochondrial matrix to the cytosol. The regulated step in fatty acid synthesis is the carboxylation of acetyl CoA to **malonyl CoA** by biotin- and ATP-requiring *acetyl CoA carboxylase* (*ACC*). **Citrate** allosterically activates *ACC*, and **palmitoyl CoA** inhibits it. *ACC* can also be activated by **insulin** and inactivated by *adenosine monophosphate–activated protein kinase* (*AMPK*) in response to **epinephrine**, **glucagon**, or a rise in **AMP**. The remaining steps in fatty acid synthesis are catalyzed by the multifunctional enzyme, *fatty acid synthase*, which produces **palmitoyl CoA** by adding two-carbon units from malonyl CoA to a series of acyl acceptors. Fatty acids can be **elongated** and **desaturated** in the **smooth endoplasmic reticulum** (**SER**). When fatty acids are required for energy, *hormone-sensitive lipase* (**activated** by **epinephrine**, and **inhibited** by **insulin**), along with other *lipases*, degrades **triacylglycerol** (**TAG**) stored in **adipocytes**. The fatty acid products are carried by **serum albumin** to the liver and peripheral tissues, where their oxidation provides energy. The **glycerol** backbone of the degraded TAG is carried by the blood to the **liver**, where it serves as a **gluconeogenic precursor**. Fatty acid degradation (**β-oxidation**) occurs in **mitochondria**. The **carnitine shuttle** is required to transport long-chain fatty acids from the cytosol to the mitochondrial matrix. A translocase and the enzymes *carnitine palmitoyltransferases* (*CPT*) *I* and *II* are required. *CPT-I* is inhibited by **malonyl CoA**, thereby preventing simultaneous synthesis and degradation of fatty acids. Mitochondrial fatty acid β-oxidation produces **acetyl CoA**, **nicotinamide adenine dinucleotide** (**NADH**), and **flavin adenine dinucleotide** (**FADH₂**). The first step in β-oxidation is catalyzed by one of four *acyl CoA dehydrogenases*, each with chain-length specificity. *Medium-chain fatty acyl CoA dehydrogenase* (*MCAD*) **deficiency** causes a decrease in fatty acid oxidation (process stops once a medium-chain fatty acid is produced), resulting in **hypoketonemia** and severe **hypoglycemia**. Oxidation of fatty acids with an **odd number** of carbons proceeds two carbons at a time (producing acetyl CoA) until three-carbon **propionyl CoA** remains. This compound is carboxylated to **methylmalonyl CoA** (by biotin- and ATP-requiring *propionyl CoA carboxylase*), which is then converted to **succinyl CoA** (a gluconeogenic precursor) by **vitamin B₁₂**-requiring *methylmalonyl CoA mutase*. A genetic error in the *mutase* or vitamin B₁₂ deficiency causes **methylmalonic acidemia** and **aciduria**. β-Oxidation of **unsaturated** fatty acids requires additional enzymes. β-Oxidation of **very-long-chain** fatty acids and α-oxidation of **branched-chain** fatty acids occur in the **peroxisome**. Deficiencies result in **X-linked adrenoleukodystrophy** and **Refsum disease**, respectively. **ω-Oxidation**, normally a minor pathway, occurs in the SER. Liver mitochondria can convert acetyl CoA derived from fatty acid oxidation into **acetoacetate** and **3-hydroxybutyrate** (**ketone bodies**). Peripheral tissues possessing mitochondria can oxidize 3-hydroxybutyrate to acetoacetate, which can be cleaved to two acetyl CoA, thereby producing energy for the cell. Unlike fatty acids, ketone bodies are utilized by the **brain** and, therefore, are important fuels during a fast. Because the liver lacks *thiophorase* required to degrade ketone bodies, it synthesizes them specifically for the peripheral tissues. **Ketoacidosis** occurs when the rate of ketone body formation is greater than the rate of use, as is seen in cases of uncontrolled **type 1 diabetes mellitus**.

Study Questions

Choose the ONE best answer.

16.1 When oleic acid, 18:1(9), is desaturated at carbon 6 and then elongated, what is the correct representation of the product?

    A. 19:2(7,9)

    B. 20:2 (ω-6)

    C. 20:2(6,9)

    D. 20:2(8,11)

Correct answer = D. Fatty acids are elongated in the smooth endoplasmic reticulum by adding two carbons at a time to the carboxylate end (carbon 1) of the molecule. This pushes the double bonds at carbon 6 and carbon 9 farther away from carbon 1. The 20:2(8,11) product is an ω-9 (n-9) fatty acid.

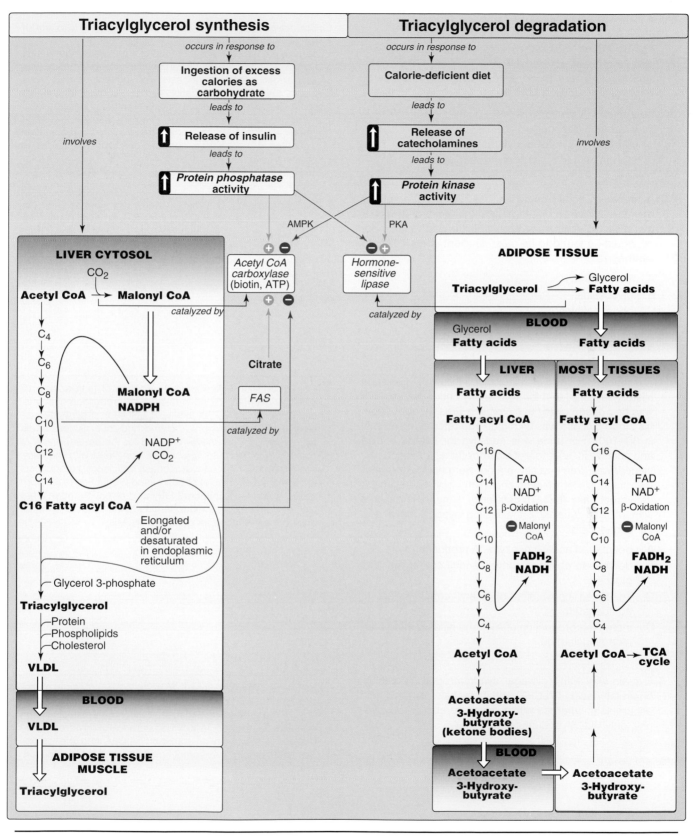

Figure 16.25

Key concept map for fatty acid and triacylglycerol metabolism. *AMPK = adenosine monophosphate–activated protein kinase; PKA = protein kinase A*; CoA = coenzyme A; NADP(H) = nicotinamide adenine dinucleotide phosphate; FAD(H$_2$) = flavin adenine dinucleotide; *FAS= fatty acid synthase*; CO$_2$ = carbon dioxide; NAD(H) = nicotinamide adenine dinucleotide; TCA = tricarboxylic acid; VLDL = very-low-density lipoprotein.

16.2 A 4-month-old child is being evaluated for fasting hypo-glycemia. Laboratory tests at admission reveal low levels of ketone bodies (hypoketonemia), free carnitine, and long-chain acylcarnitines in the blood. Free fatty acid levels in the blood were elevated. Deficiency of which of the following would best explain these findings?

A. Adipose triglyceride lipase
B. Carnitine transporter
C. Carnitine palmitoyltransferase-I
D. Long-chain fatty acid dehydrogenase

Correct answer = B. A defect in the carnitine transporter (primary carnitine deficiency) would result in low levels of carnitine in the blood (as a result of increased urinary loss) and low levels in the tissues. In the liver, this decreases fatty acid oxidation and ketogenesis. Consequently, blood levels of free fatty acids rise. Deficiencies of adipose triglyceride lipase would decrease fatty acid availability. Deficiency of carnitine palmitoyltransferase I would result in elevated blood carnitine. Defects in any of the enzymes of β-oxidation would result in secondary carnitine deficiency, with a rise in acylcarnitines.

16.3 A teenager, concerned about his weight, attempts to maintain a fat-free diet for a period of several weeks. If his ability to synthesize various lipids were examined, he would be found to be most deficient in his ability to synthesize:

A. cholesterol.
B. glycolipids.
C. phospholipids.
D. prostaglandins.
E. triacylglycerol.

Correct answer = D. Prostaglandins are synthesized from arachidonic acid. Arachidonic acid is synthesized from linoleic acid, an essential fatty acid obtained by humans from dietary lipids. The teenager would be able to synthesize all other compounds but, presumably, in somewhat decreased amounts.

16.4 A 6-month-old boy was hospitalized following a seizure. History revealed that for several days prior, his appetite was decreased owing to a stomach virus. At admission, his blood glucose was 24 mg/dl (age-referenced normal is 60–100). His urine was negative for ketone bodies and positive for a variety of dicarboxylic acids. Blood carnitine levels (free and acyl bound) were normal. A tentative diagnosis of medium-chain fatty acyl coenzyme A dehydrogenase (MCAD) deficiency is made. In patients with MCAD deficiency, the fasting hypoglycemia is a consequence of:

A. decreased acetyl coenzyme A production.
B. decreased ability to convert acetyl coenzyme A to glucose.
C. increased conversion of acetyl coenzyme A to acetoacetate.
D. increased production of ATP and nicotinamide adenine dinucleotide.

Correct answer = A. Impaired oxidation of fatty acids <12 carbons in length results in decreased production of acetyl-coenzyme A (CoA), the allosteric activator of pyruvate carboxylase, a gluconeogenic enzyme, and, thus, glucose levels fall. Acetyl CoA can never be used for the net synthesis of glucose. Acetoacetate is a ketone body, and with medium-chain fatty acyl CoA dehydrogenase deficiency, ketogenesis is decreased as a result of decreased production of the substrate, acetyl CoA. Impaired fatty acid oxidation means that less ATP and nicotinamide adenine dinucleotide are made, and both are needed for gluconeogenesis.

16.5 Explain why with Zellweger syndrome both very-long-chain fatty acids (VLCFA) and long-chain phytanic acid accumulate, whereas with X-linked adrenoleukodystrophy, only VLCFA accumulate.

Zellweger syndrome is caused by an inability to target matrix proteins to the peroxisome. Therefore, all peroxisomal activities are affected because functional peroxisomes are unable to be formed. In X-linked adrenoleukodystrophy, the defect is an inability to transport VLCFA into the peroxisome, but other peroxisomal functions, such as α-oxidation, are normal.

Phospholipid, Glycosphingolipid, and Eicosanoid Metabolism 17

I. PHOSPHOLIPID OVERVIEW

Phospholipids are polar, ionic compounds composed of an alcohol that is attached by a phosphodiester bond to either diacylglycerol (DAG) or sphingosine. Like fatty acids (FA), phospholipids are amphipathic in nature. That is, each has a hydrophilic head, which is the phosphate group plus whatever alcohol is attached to it (for example, serine, ethanolamine, and choline; highlighted in blue in Fig. 17.1A), and a long, hydrophobic tail containing FA or FA-derived hydrocarbons (shown in orange in Fig. 17.1A). Phospholipids are the predominant lipids of cell membranes. In membranes, the hydrophobic portion of a phospholipid molecule is associated with the nonpolar portions of other membrane constituents, such as glycolipids, proteins, and cholesterol. The hydrophilic (polar) head of the phospholipid extends outward, interacting with the intracellular or extracellular aqueous environment (see Fig. 17.1A). Membrane phospholipids also function as a reservoir for intracellular messengers, and, for some proteins, phospholipids serve as anchors to cell membranes. Nonmembrane phospholipids serve additional functions in the body, for example, as components of lung surfactant and essential components of bile, where their detergent properties aid cholesterol solubilization.

II. PHOSPHOLIPID STRUCTURE

There are two classes of phospholipids: those that have glycerol (from glucose) as a backbone and those that have sphingosine (from serine and palmitate). Both classes are found as structural components of membranes, and both play a role in the generation of lipid signaling molecules.

A. Glycerophospholipids

Phospholipids that contain glycerol are called glycerophospholipids (or phosphoglycerides). Glycerophospholipids constitute the major class of phospholipids and are the predominant lipids in membranes. All contain (or are derivatives of) phosphatidic acid (PA), which is DAG with a phosphate group on carbon 3 (Fig. 17.1B). PA is the simplest phosphoglyceride and is the precursor of the other members of this group.

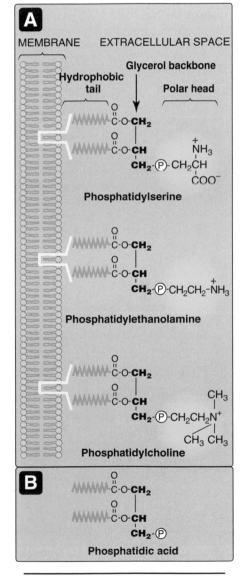

Figure 17.1
A. Structures of some glycerophospholipids. B. Phosphatidic acid. Ⓟ = phosphate (an anion).

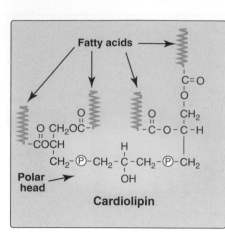

Figure 17.2
Structure of cardiolipin (diphosphatidylglycerol). $\textcircled{P}$ = phosphate.

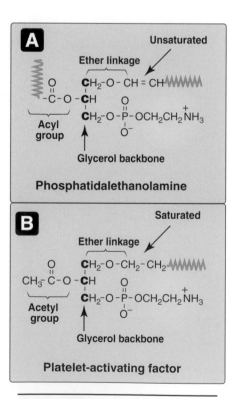

Figure 17.3
The ether glycerophospholipids.
A. The plasmalogen phosphatidalethanolamine. B. Platelet-activating factor. (∿∿∿∿∿ is a long, hydrophobic hydrocarbon chain.)

1. **From phosphatidic acid and an alcohol:** The phosphate group on PA can be esterified to a compound containing an alcohol group (see Fig. 17.1). For example:

Serine	+ PA →	phosphatidylserine (PS)
Ethanolamine	+ PA →	phosphatidylethanolamine (PE)
Choline	+ PA →	phosphatidylcholine (PC) (lecithin)
Inositol	+ PA →	phosphatidylinositol (PI)
Glycerol	+ PA →	phosphatidylglycerol (PG)

2. **Cardiolipin:** Two molecules of PA esterified through their phosphate groups to an additional molecule of glycerol form cardiolipin, or diphosphatidylglycerol (Fig. 17.2). Cardiolipin is found in membranes in bacteria and eukaryotes. In eukaryotes, cardiolipin is virtually exclusive to the inner mitochondrial membrane, where it maintains the structure and function of certain respiratory complexes of the electron transport chain. [Note: Cardiolipin is antigenic and is recognized by antibodies (Ab) raised against Treponema pallidum, the bacterium that causes syphilis. The Wasserman test for syphilis detects these Ab.]

3. **Plasmalogens:** When the FA at carbon 1 of a glycerophospholipid is replaced by an unsaturated alkyl group attached by an ether (rather than by an ester) linkage to the core glycerol molecule, an ether phosphoglyceride known as a plasmalogen is produced. For example, phosphatidalethanolamine, which is abundant in nerve tissue (Fig. 17.3A), is the plasmalogen that is similar in structure to phosphatidylethanolamine. Phosphatidalcholine (abundant in heart muscle) is the other quantitatively significant ether lipid in mammals. [Note: Plasmalogens have "al" rather than "yl" in their names.]

4. **Platelet-activating factor:** A second example of an ether glycerophospholipid is platelet-activating factor (PAF), which has a saturated alkyl group in an ether link to carbon 1 and an acetyl residue (rather than a FA) at carbon 2 of the glycerol backbone (Fig. 17.3B). PAF is synthesized and released by a variety of cell types. It binds to surface receptors, triggering potent thrombotic and acute inflammatory events. For example, PAF activates inflammatory cells and mediates hypersensitivity, acute inflammatory, and anaphylactic reactions. It causes platelets to aggregate and activate and neutrophils and alveolar macrophages to generate superoxide radicals to kill bacteria (see p. 150). It also lowers blood pressure. [Note: PAF is one of the most potent bioactive molecules known, causing effects at concentrations as low as 10^{-11} mol/l.]

B. Sphingophospholipids: Sphingomyelin

The backbone of sphingomyelin is the amino alcohol sphingosine, rather than glycerol (Fig. 17.4). A long-chain-length FA (LCFA) is attached to the amino group of sphingosine through an amide linkage, producing a ceramide, which can also serve as a precursor of glycolipids (see p. 209). The alcohol group at carbon 1 of sphingosine is esterified to phosphorylcholine, producing sphingomyelin, the only significant sphingophospholipid in humans. Sphingomyelin is an important constituent of the myelin sheath of nerve fibers. [Note: The myelin sheath is a layered, membranous structure that insulates and protects neuronal axons of the central nervous system (CNS).]

III. PHOSPHOLIPID SYNTHESIS

Glycerophospholipid synthesis involves either the donation of PA from cytidine diphosphate (CDP)-DAG to an alcohol or the donation of the phosphomonoester of the alcohol from CDP-alcohol to DAG (Fig. 17.5). In both cases, the CDP-bound structure is considered an activated intermediate, and cytidine monophosphate (CMP) is released as a side product. Therefore, a key concept in glycerophospholipid synthesis is activation, of either DAG or the alcohol to be added, by linkage with CDP. [Note: This is similar in principle to the activation of sugars by their attachment to uridine diphosphate (UDP) (see p. 126).] The FA esterified to the glycerol alcohol groups can vary widely, contributing to the heterogeneity of this group of compounds, with saturated FA typically found at carbon 1 and unsaturated ones at carbon 2. Most phospholipids are synthesized in the smooth endoplasmic reticulum (SER). From there, they are transported to the Golgi and then to membranes of organelles or the plasma membrane or are secreted from the cell by exocytosis. [Note: Ether lipid synthesis from dihydroxyacetone phosphate begins in peroxisomes.]

A. Phosphatidic acid

PA is the precursor of other glycerophospholipids. The steps in its synthesis from glycerol 3-phosphate and two fatty acyl coenzyme A (CoA) molecules were illustrated in Figure 16.14, p. 189, in which PA is shown as a precursor of triacylglycerol (TAG).

> Essentially all cells except mature erythrocytes can synthesize phospholipids, whereas TAG synthesis occurs essentially only in the liver, adipose tissue, lactating mammary glands, and intestinal mucosal cells.

B. Phosphatidylcholine and phosphatidylethanolamine

The neutral phospholipids PC and PE are the most abundant phospholipids in most eukaryotic cells. The primary route of their synthesis uses choline and ethanolamine obtained either from the diet or from the turnover of the body's phospholipids. [Note: In the liver, PC also can be synthesized from PS and PE (see 2. below).]

1. **Synthesis from preexisting choline and ethanolamine:** These synthetic pathways involve the phosphorylation of choline or ethanolamine by *kinases*, followed by conversion to the activated form, CDP-choline or CDP-ethanolamine. Finally, choline phosphate or ethanolamine phosphate is transferred from the nucleotide (leaving CMP) to a molecule of DAG (see Fig. 17.5).

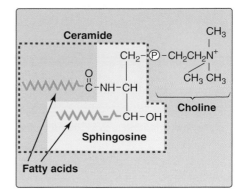

Figure 17.4
Structure of sphingomyelin, showing sphingosine (in green box) and ceramide components (in dashed box). (P) = phosphate.

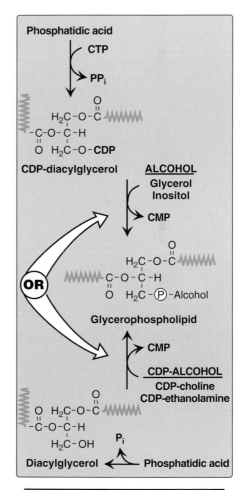

Figure 17.5
Glycerophospholipid synthesis requires activation of either diacylglycerol or an alcohol by linkage to cytidine diphosphate (CDP). CMP and CTP = cytidine mono- and triphosphates; P_i = inorganic phosphate; PP_i = pyrophosphate. (⌇⌇⌇⌇ is a fatty acid hydrocarbon chain.)

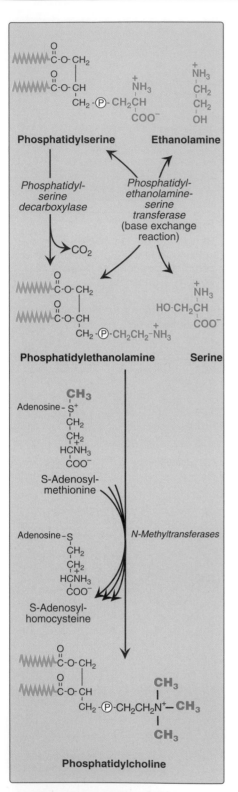

Figure 17.6

Synthesis of phosphatidylcholine from phosphatidylserine in the liver. (〰〰 is a fatty acid hydrocarbon chain.) Ⓟ = phosphate; CO_2 = carbon dioxide.

a. Significance of choline reutilization: The reutilization of choline is important because, although humans can synthesize choline de novo, the amount made is insufficient for our needs. Thus, choline is an essential dietary nutrient with an adequate intake (see p. 358) of 550 mg for men and 425 mg for women. [Note: Choline is also used for the synthesis of acetylcholine, a neurotransmitter.]

b. Phosphatidylcholine in lung surfactant: The pathway described above is the principal pathway for the synthesis of dipalmitoylphosphatidylcholine (DPPC or, dipalmitoyl lecithin). In DPPC, positions 1 and 2 on the glycerol are occupied by palmitate, a saturated LCFA. DPPC, made and secreted by type II pneumocytes, is a major lipid component of lung surfactant, which is the extracellular fluid layer lining the alveoli. Surfactant serves to decrease the surface tension of this fluid layer, reducing the pressure needed to reinflate alveoli, thereby preventing alveolar collapse (atelectasis). [Note: Surfactant is a complex mixture of lipids (90%) and proteins (10%), with DPPC being the major component for reducing surface tension.]

> Fetal lung maturity can be gauged by determining the DPPC/sphingomyelin ratio, usually written as L (for lecithin)/S, in amniotic fluid. A value ≥2 is evidence of maturity, because it reflects the shift from sphingomyelin to DPPC synthesis that occurs in pneumocytes at ~32 weeks' gestation.

c. Lung maturity: Respiratory distress syndrome (RDS) in preterm infants is associated with insufficient surfactant production and/or secretion and is a significant cause of all neonatal deaths in Western countries. Lung maturation can be accelerated by giving the mother glucocorticoids shortly before delivery to induce expression of specific genes. Postnatal administration of natural or synthetic surfactant (by intratracheal instillation) is also used. [Note: Acute RDS, seen in all age groups, is the result of alveolar damage (due to infection, injury, or aspiration) that causes fluid to accumulate in the alveoli, impeding the exchange of oxygen (O_2) and carbon dioxide (CO_2).]

2. Phosphatidylcholine synthesis from phosphatidylserine: The liver requires a mechanism for producing PC, even when free choline levels are low, because it exports significant amounts of PC in the bile and as a component of plasma lipoproteins. To provide the needed PC, PS is decarboxylated to PE by *PS decarboxylase*. PE then undergoes three methylation steps to produce PC, as illustrated in Figure 17.6. S-adenosylmethionine is the methyl group donor (see p. 264).

C. Phosphatidylserine

PS synthesis in mammalian tissues is provided by the base exchange reaction, in which the ethanolamine of PE is exchanged for free serine (see Fig. 17.6). This reaction, although reversible, is used primarily to produce the PS required for membrane synthesis. PS has a net negative charge. (See online Chapter 35 for the role of PS in clotting.)

D. Phosphatidylinositol

PI is synthesized from free inositol and CDP-DAG, as shown in Figure 17.5. PI is an unusual phospholipid in that it most frequently contains stearic acid on carbon 1 and arachidonic acid on carbon 2 of the glycerol. Therefore, PI serves as a reservoir of arachidonic acid in membranes and, thus, provides the substrate for prostaglandin (see p. 213) synthesis when required. Like PS, PI has a net negative charge. [Note: There is asymmetry in the phospholipid composition of the cell membrane. PS and PI, for example, are found primarily on the inner leaflet. Asymmetry is achieved by ATP-dependent enzymes known as "flippases" and "floppases."]

1. **Role in signal transduction across membranes:** The phosphorylation of membrane-bound PI produces polyphosphoinositides such as phosphatidylinositol 4,5-bisphosphate ([PIP$_2$]; Fig. 17.7). The cleavage of PIP$_2$ by *phospholipase C* occurs in response to the binding of various neurotransmitters, hormones, and growth factors to G protein–coupled receptors (GPCR), such as the α_1 adrenergic receptor, on the cell membrane and activation of the G$_q$ α-subunit (Fig. 17.8). The products of this cleavage, inositol 1,4,5-trisphosphate (IP$_3$) and DAG, mediate the mobilization of intracellular calcium and the activation of *protein kinase C*, which act synergistically to evoke specific cellular responses. Signal transduction across the membrane is, thus, accomplished.

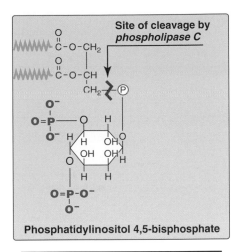

Phosphatidylinositol 4,5-bisphosphate

Figure 17.7
Structure of phosphatidylinositol 4,5-bisphosphate (PIP$_2$). Cleavage by *phospholipase C* produces inositol 1,4,5-trisphosphate (IP$_3$) and diacylglycerol. (〰〰 is a fatty acid hydrocarbon chain.) Ⓟ = phosphate.

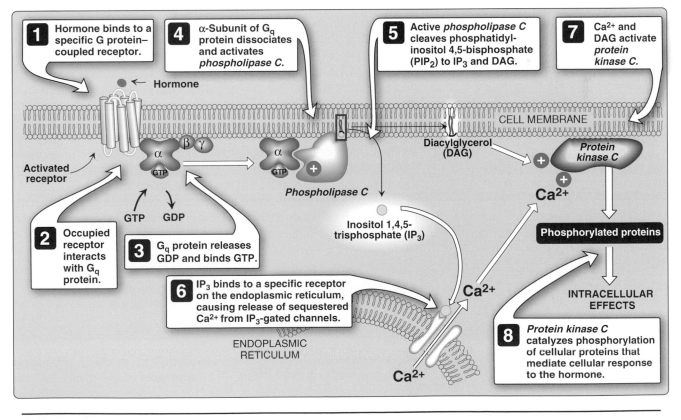

Figure 17.8
Role of inositol triphosphate and diacylglycerol in cell signaling. GDP and GTP = guanosine di- and triphosphates; Ca^{2+} = calcium.

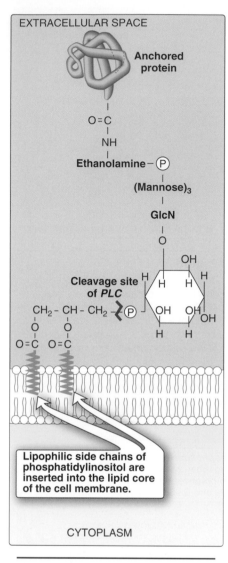

Figure 17.9
Example of a glycosyl phosphatidylinositol (GPI) membrane protein
anchor. GlcN = glucosamine; (P) =
phosphate; *PLC = phospholipase C*.

2. Role in membrane protein anchoring: Specific proteins can be covalently attached through a carbohydrate bridge to membrane-bound PI (Fig. 17.9). For example, *lipoprotein lipase*, an enzyme that degrades triacylglycerol in lipoprotein particles (see p. 228), is attached to capillary endothelial cells by a glycosyl phosphatidylinositol (GPI) anchor. [Note: GPI-linked proteins are also found in a variety of parasitic protozoans, such as trypanosomes and leishmania.] Being attached to a membrane lipid (rather than being an integral part of the membrane) allows GPI-anchored proteins increased lateral mobility on the extracellular surface of the plasma membrane. The protein can be cleaved from its anchor by the action of *phospholipase C* (see Fig. 17.9). [Note: A deficiency in the synthesis of GPI in hematopoietic cells results in the hemolytic disease paroxysmal nocturnal hemoglobinuria, because GPI-anchored proteins protect blood cells from complement-mediated lysis.]

E. Phosphatidylglycerol and cardiolipin

Phosphatidylglycerol occurs in relatively large amounts in mitochondrial membranes and is a precursor of cardiolipin (diphosphatidyglycerol). It is synthesized from CDP-DAG and glycerol 3-phosphate. Cardiolipin (see Fig. 17.2) is synthesized by the transfer of DAG 3-phosphate from CDP-DAG to a pre-existing molecule of phosphatidylglycerol.

F. Sphingomyelin

Sphingomyelin, a sphingosine-based phospholipid, is found in cell membranes and in the myelin sheath. The synthesis of sphingomyelin is shown in Figure 17.10. Briefly, palmitoyl CoA condenses with serine, as CoA and the carboxyl group (as CO_2) of serine are lost. [Note: This reaction, like the decarboxylation reactions involved in the synthesis of PE from PS and of regulators from amino acids (for example, the catecholamines from tyrosine; see p. 286), requires pyridoxal phosphate (a derivative of vitamin B_6) as a coenzyme.] The product is reduced in a nicotinamide adenine dinucleotide phosphate (NADPH)-requiring reaction to sphinganine (dihydrosphingosine). The sphinganine is acylated at the amino group with one of a variety of LCFA and then desaturated to produce a ceramide, the immediate precursor of sphingomyelin (and other sphingolipids, as described on p. 208).

> Ceramides play a key role in maintaining the skin's water-permeability barrier. Decreased ceramide levels are associated with a number of skin diseases.

Phosphorylcholine from PC is transferred to the ceramide, producing sphingomyelin and DAG. [Note: Sphingomyelin of the myelin sheath contains predominantly longer-chain FA such as lignoceric acid and nervonic acid, whereas gray matter of the brain has sphingomyelin that contains primarily stearic acid.]

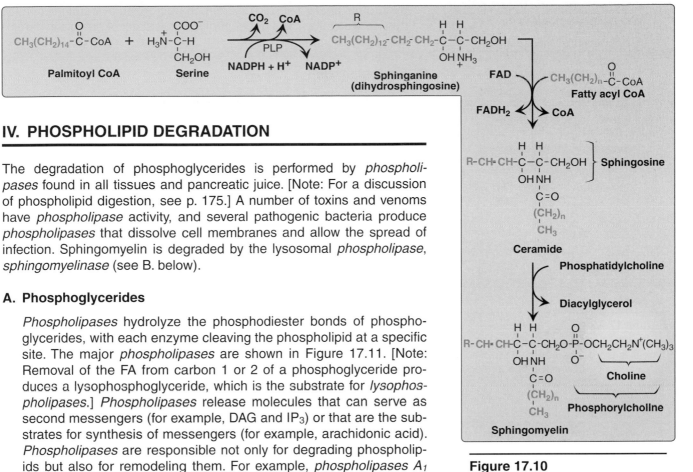

IV. PHOSPHOLIPID DEGRADATION

The degradation of phosphoglycerides is performed by *phospholipases* found in all tissues and pancreatic juice. [Note: For a discussion of phospholipid digestion, see p. 175.] A number of toxins and venoms have *phospholipase* activity, and several pathogenic bacteria produce *phospholipases* that dissolve cell membranes and allow the spread of infection. Sphingomyelin is degraded by the lysosomal *phospholipase*, *sphingomyelinase* (see B. below).

A. Phosphoglycerides

Phospholipases hydrolyze the phosphodiester bonds of phosphoglycerides, with each enzyme cleaving the phospholipid at a specific site. The major *phospholipases* are shown in Figure 17.11. [Note: Removal of the FA from carbon 1 or 2 of a phosphoglyceride produces a lysophosphoglyceride, which is the substrate for *lysophospholipases*.] *Phospholipases* release molecules that can serve as second messengers (for example, DAG and IP_3) or that are the substrates for synthesis of messengers (for example, arachidonic acid). *Phospholipases* are responsible not only for degrading phospholipids but also for remodeling them. For example, *phospholipases A_1* and A_2 remove specific FA from membrane-bound phospholipids, which can be replaced with different FA using *fatty acyl CoA transferase*. This mechanism is used as one way to create the unique lung surfactant DPCC (see p. 204) and to insure that carbon 2 of PI (and sometimes of PC) is bound to arachidonic acid. [Note: Barth

Figure 17.10

Synthesis of sphingomyelin. PLP = pyridoxal phosphate; NADP(H) = nicotinamide adenine dinucleotide phosphate; $FAD(H_2)$ = flavin adenine dinucleotide; CoA = coenzyme A.

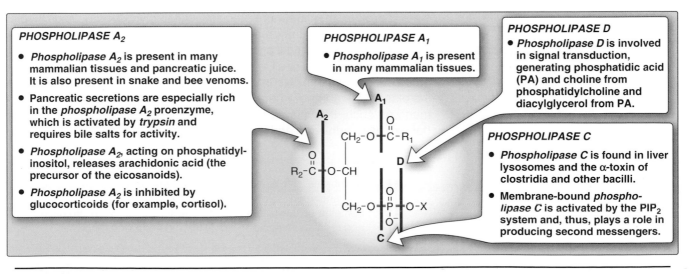

PHOSPHOLIPASE A_2

- *Phospholipase A_2* is present in many mammalian tissues and pancreatic juice. It is also present in snake and bee venoms.

- Pancreatic secretions are especially rich in the *phospholipase A_2* proenzyme, which is activated by *trypsin* and requires bile salts for activity.

- *Phospholipase A_2*, acting on phosphatidylinositol, releases arachidonic acid (the precursor of the eicosanoids).

- *Phospholipase A_2* is inhibited by glucocorticoids (for example, cortisol).

PHOSPHOLIPASE A_1

- *Phospholipase A_1* is present in many mammalian tissues.

PHOSPHOLIPASE D

- *Phospholipase D* is involved in signal transduction, generating phosphatidic acid (PA) and choline from phosphatidylcholine and diacylglycerol from PA.

PHOSPHOLIPASE C

- *Phospholipase C* is found in liver lysosomes and the α-toxin of clostridia and other bacilli.

- Membrane-bound *phospholipase C* is activated by the PIP_2 system and, thus, plays a role in producing second messengers.

Figure 17.11

Degradation of glycerophospholipids by *phospholipases*. PIP_2 = phosphatidylinositol 4,5-bisphosphate; R_1 and R_2 = fatty acids; X = an alcohol.

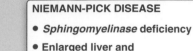

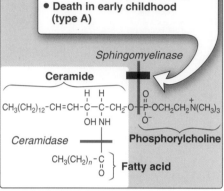

NIEMANN-PICK DISEASE

- *Sphingomyelinase* deficiency
- Enlarged liver and spleen filled with lipid
- Severe intellectual disability and neurodegeneration (type A)
- Death in early childhood (type A)

Figure 17.12
Degradation of sphingomyelin. [Note: Type B is the nonneuropathic form. It has a later age of onset and a longer survival time than type A.]

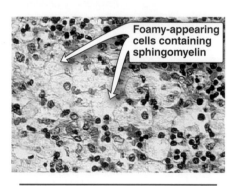

Foamy-appearing cells containing sphingomyelin

Figure 17.13
Accumulation of lipids in spleen cells from a patient with Niemann-Pick disease.

syndrome, a rare X-linked disorder characterized by cardiomyopathy, muscle weakness, and neutropenia, is the result of defects in cardiolipin remodeling.]

B. Sphingomyelin

Sphingomyelin is degraded by *sphingomyelinase*, a lysosomal enzyme that removes phosphorylcholine, leaving a ceramide. The ceramide is, in turn, cleaved by *ceramidase* into sphingosine and a free FA (Fig. 17.12). [Note: The released ceramide and sphingosine regulate signal transduction pathways, in part by influencing the activity of *protein kinase C* and, thus, the phosphorylation of its protein substrates. They also promote apoptosis.] Niemann-Pick disease (types A and B) is an autosomal-recessive disorder caused by the inability to degrade sphingomyelin due to a deficiency of *sphingomyelinase*, a type of *phospholipase C*. In the severe infantile form (type A, which shows <1% of normal enzymic activity), the liver and spleen are the primary sites of lipid deposits and are, therefore, greatly enlarged. The lipid consists primarily of the sphingomyelin that cannot be degraded (Fig. 17.13). Infants with this lysosomal storage disease experience rapid and progressive neurodegeneration as a result of deposition of sphingomyelin in the CNS, and they die in early childhood. A less severe variant (type B, which shows up to 10% of normal activity) with a later age of onset and a longer survival time causes little to no damage to neural tissue, but lungs, spleen, liver, and bone marrow are affected, resulting in a chronic form of the disease. Although Niemann-Pick disease occurs in all ethnic groups, type A occurs with greater frequency in the Ashkenazi Jewish population.

V. GLYCOLIPID OVERVIEW

Glycolipids are molecules that contain both carbohydrate and lipid components. Like the phospholipid sphingomyelin, glycolipids are derivatives of ceramides in which a LCFA is attached to the amino alcohol sphingosine. Therefore, they are more precisely called glycosphingolipids. [Note: Thus, ceramides are the precursors of both phosphorylated and glycosylated sphingolipids.] Like the phospholipids, glycosphingolipids are essential components of all membranes in the body, but they are found in greatest amounts in nerve tissue. They are located in the outer leaflet of the plasma membrane, where they interact with the extracellular environment. As such, they play a role in the regulation of cellular interactions (for example, adhesion and recognition), growth, and development.

> Membrane glycosphingolipids associate with cholesterol and GPI-anchored proteins to form lipid rafts, laterally mobile microdomains of the plasma membrane that function to organize and regulate membrane signaling and trafficking functions.

Glycosphingolipids are antigenic and are the source of ABO blood group antigens (see p. 165), various embryonic antigens specific for particular stages of fetal development, and some tumor antigens. [Note: The carbohydrate portion of a glycolipid is the antigenic determinant.] They have been coopted for use as cell surface receptors for cholera and tetanus toxins as well as for certain viruses and microbes. Genetic disorders associated with an inability to properly degrade the glycosphingolipids result in lysosomal accumulation of these compounds. [Note: Changes in the carbohydrate portion of glycosphingolipids (and glycoproteins) are characteristic of transformed cells (cells with dysregulated growth).]

VI. GLYCOSPHINGOLIPID STRUCTURE

The glycosphingolipids differ from sphingomyelin in that they do not contain phosphate, and the polar head function is provided by a monosaccharide or oligosaccharide attached directly to the ceramide by an O-glycosidic bond (Fig. 17.14). The number and type of carbohydrate moieties present determine the type of glycosphingolipid.

A. Neutral glycosphingolipids

The simplest neutral glycosphingolipids are the cerebrosides. These are ceramide monosaccharides that contain either a molecule of galactose (forming ceramide-galactose or galactocerebroside, the most common cerebroside found in myelin, as shown in Fig. 17.14) or glucose (forming ceramide-glucose or glucocerebroside, an intermediate in the synthesis and degradation of the more complex glycosphingolipids). [Note: Members of a group of galacto- or glucocerebrosides may also differ from each other in the type of FA attached to the sphingosine.] As their name implies, cerebrosides are found predominantly in the brain and peripheral nerves, with high concentrations in the myelin sheath. Ceramide oligosaccharides (or globosides) are produced by attaching additional monosaccharides to a glucocerebroside, for example, ceramide-glucose-galactose (also known as lactosylceramide). The additional monosaccharides can include substituted sugars such as N-acetylgalactosamine.

B. Acidic glycosphingolipids

Acidic glycosphingolipids are negatively charged at physiologic pH. The negative charge is provided by N-acetylneuraminic acid ([NANA], a sialic acid, as shown in Fig. 17.15) in gangliosides or by sulfate groups in sulfatides.

1. **Gangliosides:** These are the most complex glycosphingolipids and are found primarily in the ganglion cells of the CNS, particularly at the nerve endings. They are derivatives of ceramide oligosaccharides and contain one or more molecules of NANA (from CMP-NANA). The notation for these compounds is G (for ganglioside) plus a subscript M, D, T, or Q to indicate whether there is one (mono), two (di), three (tri), or four (quatro) molecules of NANA in the ganglioside, respectively. Additional numbers and letters in the subscript designate the monomeric sequence of the carbohydrate attached to the ceramide. (See Fig. 17.15 for the structure of G_{M2}.) Gangliosides are of medical interest because several lipid storage disorders involve the accumulation of NANA-containing glycosphingolipids in cells (see Fig. 17.20, p. 212).

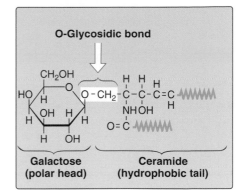

Figure 17.14
Structure of a neutral glycosphingolipid, galactocerebroside. (〰〰 is a hydrophobic hydrocarbon chain.)

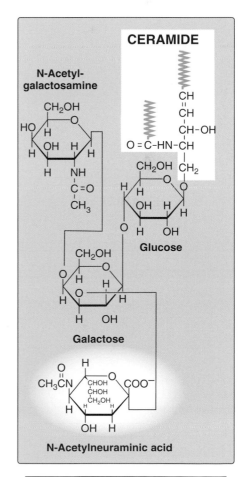

Figure 17.15
Structure of the ganglioside G_{M2}. (〰〰 is a hydrophobic hydrocarbon chain.)

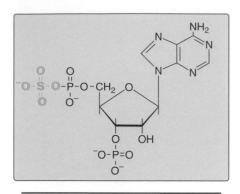

Figure 17.16
Structure of 3′-phosphoadenosine-5′-phosphosulfate.

2. Sulfatides: These sulfoglycosphingolipids are sulfated galactocerebrosides that are negatively charged at physiologic pH. Sulfatides are found predominantly in the brain and kidneys.

VII. GLYCOSPHINGOLIPID SYNTHESIS AND DEGRADATION

Synthesis of glycosphingolipids occurs primarily in the Golgi by sequential addition of glycosyl monomers transferred from UDP-sugar donors to the acceptor molecule. The mechanism is similar to that used in glycoprotein synthesis (see p. 166).

A. Enzymes involved in synthesis

The enzymes involved in the synthesis of glycosphingolipids are *glycosyltransferases* that are specific for the type and location of the glycosidic bond formed. [Note: These enzymes can recognize both glycosphingolipids and glycoproteins as substrates.]

B. Sulfate group addition

A sulfate group from the sulfate carrier 3′-phosphoadenosine-5′-phosphosulfate ([PAPS], Fig. 17.16) is added by a *sulfotransferase* to the 3′-hydroxyl group of the galactose in a galactocerebroside, forming the sulfatide galactocerebroside 3-sulfate (Fig. 17.17). [Note: PAPS is also the sulfur donor in glycosaminoglycan synthesis (see p. 162) and steroid hormone catabolism (see p. 240).] An overview of the synthesis of sphingolipids is shown in Figure 17.18.

C. Glycosphingolipid degradation

Glycosphingolipids are internalized by phagocytosis as described for the glycosaminoglycans (see p. 163). All of the enzymes required for the degradative process are present in lysosomes, which fuse with the phagosomes. The lysosomal enzymes hydrolytically and irreversibly cleave specific bonds in the glycosphingolipid. As seen with the glycosaminoglycans and glycoproteins (see p. 170), degradation is a sequential process following the rule "last on, first off," in which the last group added during synthesis is the first group removed in degradation. Therefore, defects in the degradation of the polysaccharide chains in these three glycoconjugates result in lysosomal storage diseases.

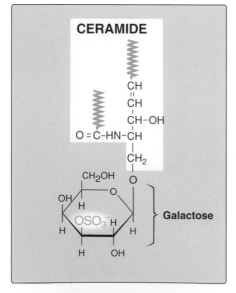

Figure 17.17
Structure of galactocerebroside 3-sulfate. (⋀⋀⋀⋀ is a hydrophobic hydrocarbon chain.)

D. Sphingolipidoses

In a normal individual, synthesis and degradation of glycosphingolipids are balanced, so that the amount of these compounds present in membranes is constant. If a specific lysosomal *acid hydrolase* required for degradation is partially or totally missing, a sphingolipid accumulates. Lysosomal lipid storage diseases caused by these deficiencies are called sphingolipidoses. The result of a specific *acid hydrolase* deficiency may be seen dramatically in nerve tissue, where neurologic deterioration can lead to early death. Figure 17.20 provides an outline of the pathway of sphingolipid degradation and descriptions of some sphingolipidoses. [Note: Some sphingolipidoses can also result from defects in lysosomal activator proteins (for example, the saposins)

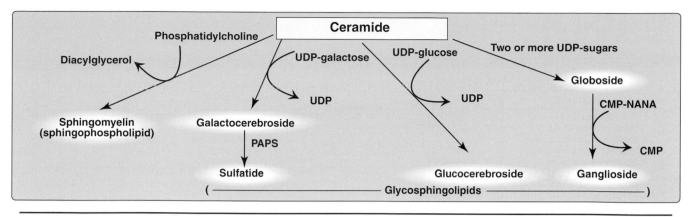

Figure 17.18
Overview of sphingolipid synthesis. UDP = uridine diphosphate; CMP = cytidine monophosphate; NANA = N-acetylneuraminic acid; PAPS = 3′-phosphoadenosine-5′-phosphosulfate.

that facilitate access of the *hydrolases* to short carbohydrate chains as degradation proceeds.]

1. **Common properties:** A specific lysosomal hydrolytic enzyme is deficient in the classic form of each disorder. Therefore, usually, only a single sphingolipid (the substrate for the deficient enzyme) accumulates in the involved organs in each disease. [Note: The rate of biosynthesis of the accumulating lipid is normal.] The disorders are progressive and, although many are fatal in childhood, extensive phenotypic variability is seen leading to the designation of different clinical types, such as types A and B in Niemann-Pick disease. Genetic variability is also seen because a given disorder can be caused by any one of a variety of mutations within a single gene. The sphingolipidoses are autosomal-recessive disorders, except for Fabry disease, which is X linked. The incidence of the sphingolipidoses is low in most populations, except for Gaucher and Tay-Sachs diseases, which, like Niemann-Pick disease, show a high frequency in the Ashkenazi Jewish population. [Note: Tay-Sachs also has a high frequency in Irish American, French Canadian, and Louisiana Cajun populations.]

2. **Diagnosis and treatment:** A specific sphingolipidosis can be diagnosed by measuring enzyme activity in cultured fibroblasts or peripheral leukocytes or by analyzing DNA (see Chapter 34). Histologic examination of the affected tissue is also useful. [Note: Shell-like inclusion bodies are seen in Tay-Sachs, and a crumpled tissue paper appearance of the cytosol is seen in Gaucher disease (Fig. 17.19).] Prenatal diagnosis, using cultured amniocytes or chorionic villi, is available. Gaucher disease, in which macrophages become engorged with glucocerebroside, and Fabry disease, in which globosides accumulate in the vascular endothelial lysosomes of the brain, heart, kidneys, and skin, are treated by recombinant human enzyme replacement therapy, but the monetary cost is extremely high. Gaucher has also been treated by bone marrow transplantation (because macrophages are derived from hematopoietic stem cells) and by substrate reduction therapy through pharmacologic reduction of glucosylceramide, the substrate for the deficient enzyme.

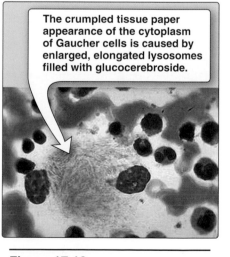

The crumpled tissue paper appearance of the cytoplasm of Gaucher cells is caused by enlarged, elongated lysosomes filled with glucocerebroside.

Figure 17.19
Aspirated bone marrow cells from a patient with Gaucher disease.

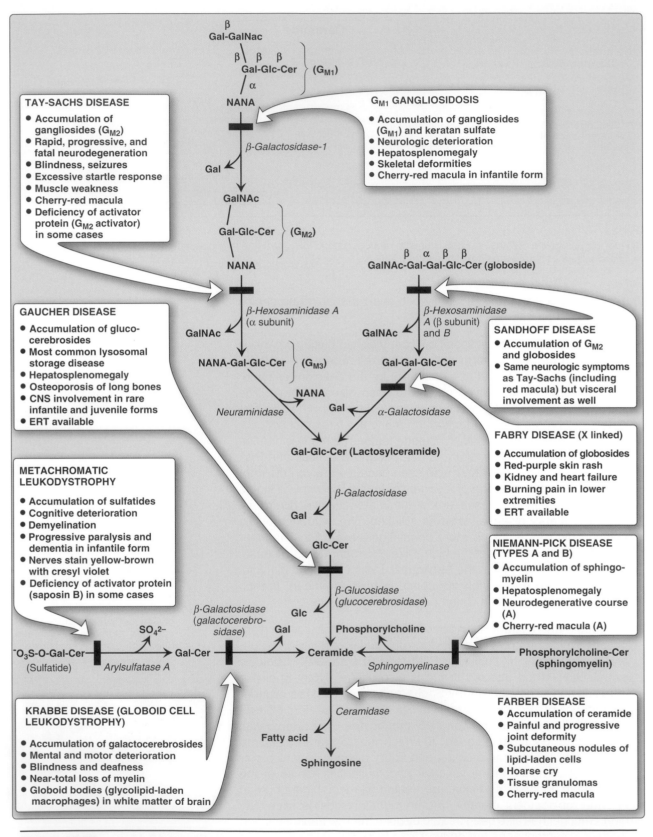

Figure 17.20

Degradation of sphingolipids showing the lysosomal enzymes affected in related genetic diseases, the sphingolipidoses. All are autosomal-recessive diseases except Fabry, which is X linked, and all can be fatal in early life. Cer = ceramide; Gal = galactose; Glc = glucose; GalNAc = N-acetylgalactosamine; NANA = N-acetylneuraminic acid; CNS = central nervous system. SO_4^{2-} = sulfate; ERT = enzyme replacement therapy.

VIII. EICOSANOIDS: PROSTAGLANDINS, THROMBOXANES, AND LEUKOTRIENES

Prostaglandins (PG), thromboxanes (TX), and leukotrienes (LT) are collectively known as eicosanoids to reflect their origin from ω-3 and ω-6 polyunsaturated FA with 20 carbons (eicosa = 20). They are extremely potent compounds that elicit a wide range of responses, both physiologic (inflammatory response) and pathologic (hypersensitivity). They insure gastric integrity and renal function, regulate smooth muscle contraction (the intestine and uterus are key sites) and blood vessel diameter, and maintain platelet homeostasis. Although they have been compared to hormones in terms of their actions, eicosanoids differ from endocrine hormones in that they are produced in very small amounts in almost all tissues rather than in specialized glands and act locally rather than after transport in the blood to distant sites. Eicosanoids are not stored, and they have an extremely short half-life, being rapidly metabolized to inactive products. Their biologic actions are mediated by plasma membrane GPCR (see p. 94), which are different in different organ systems and typically result in changes in cyclic adenosine monophosphate production. Examples of eicosanoid structures are shown in Figure 17.21.

A. Prostaglandin and thromboxane synthesis

Arachidonic acid, an ω-6 FA containing 20 carbons and four double bonds (an eicosatetraenoic FA), is the immediate precursor of the predominant type of human PG (series 2 or those with two double bonds, as shown in Fig. 17.22). It is derived by the elongation and desaturation of the essential FA linoleic acid, also an ω-6 FA. Arachidonic acid is incorporated into membrane phospholipids (typically PI) at carbon 2, from which it is released by *phospholipase A_2* (Fig. 17.23) in response to a variety of signals, such as a rise in calcium. [Note: Series 1 PG contain one double bond and are derived from an ω-6 eicosatrienoic FA, dihomo-γ-linolenic acid, whereas series 3 PG contain three double bonds and are derived from eicosapentaenoic acid (EPA), an ω-3 FA. See p. 363.]

1. **Prostaglandin H_2 synthase:** The first step in PG and TX synthesis is the oxidative cyclization of free arachidonic acid to yield PGH_2 by *PGH_2 synthase* (or, *prostaglandin endoperoxide synthase*). This enzyme is an ER membrane-bound protein that has two catalytic activities: *fatty acid cyclooxygenase (COX)*, which requires two molecules of O_2, and *peroxidase*, which requires reduced glutathione (see p. 148). PGH_2 is converted to a variety of PG and TX, as shown in Figure 17.23, by cell-specific *synthases*. [Note: PG contain a five-carbon ring, whereas TX contain a heterocyclic six-membered oxane ring (see Fig. 17.21).] Two isozymes of *PGH_2 synthase*, usually denoted as *COX-1* and *COX-2*, are known. *COX-1* is made constitutively in most tissues and is required for maintenance of healthy gastric tissue, renal homeostasis, and platelet aggregation. *COX-2* is inducible in a limited number of tissues in response to products of activated immune and inflammatory cells. [Note: The increase in PG synthesis subsequent to the induction of *COX-2* mediates the pain, heat, redness, and swelling of inflammation and the fever of infection.]

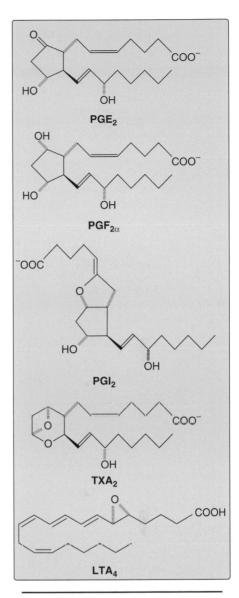

Figure 17.21
Examples of eicosanoid structures. [Note: Prostaglandins are named as follows: PG plus a third letter (for example, E), which designates the type and arrangement of functional groups in the molecule. The subscript number indicates the number of double bonds in the molecule. PGI_2 is also known as prostacyclin. Thromboxanes are designated by TX and leukotrienes by LT.]

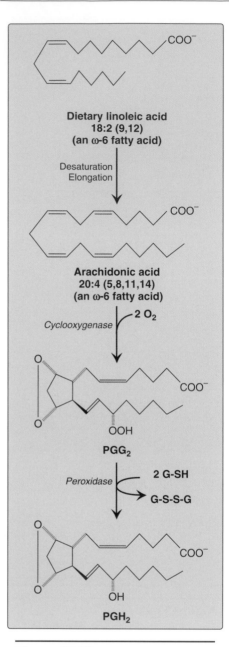

Figure 17.22

Oxidation and cyclization of arachidonic acid by the two catalytic activities (*cyclooxygenase* and *peroxidase*) of *PGH₂ synthase* (*prostaglandin endoperoxide synthase*). G-SH = reduced glutathione; G-S-S-G = oxidized glutathione; PG = prostaglandin.

2. Synthesis inhibition: The synthesis of PG and TX can be inhibited by unrelated compounds. For example, cortisol (a steroidal anti-inflammatory agent) inhibits *phospholipase A₂* activity (see Fig. 17.23) and, therefore, arachidonic acid, the substrate for PG and TX synthesis, is not released from membrane phospholipids. Aspirin, indomethacin, and phenylbutazone (all nonsteroidal anti-inflammatory drugs [NSAID]) inhibit both *COX-1* and *COX-2* and, thus, prevent the synthesis of the parent molecule, PGH₂. [Note: Systemic inhibition of *COX-1*, with subsequent damage to the stomach and the kidneys and impaired clotting of blood, is the basis of aspirin's toxicity.] Aspirin (but not other NSAID) also induces synthesis of lipoxins (anti-inflammatory mediators made from arachidonic acid) and resolvins and protectins (inflammation-resolving mediators made from EPA). Inhibitors specific for *COX-2* (the coxibs, for example, celecoxib) were designed to reduce pathologic inflammatory processes mediated by *COX-2* while maintaining the physiologic functions of *COX-1*. However, their use has been associated with increased risk of heart attacks, likely as a result of decreased PGI₂ synthesis (see B. below), and some have been withdrawn from the market.

B. Thromboxanes and prostaglandins in platelet homeostasis

Thromboxane A₂ (TXA₂) is produced by *COX-1* in activated platelets. It promotes platelet adhesion and aggregation and contraction of vascular smooth muscle, thereby promoting formation of blood clots (thrombi). (See online Chapter 35.) Prostacyclin (PGI₂), produced by *COX-2* in vascular endothelial cells, inhibits platelet aggregation and stimulates vasodilation and, so, impedes thrombogenesis. The opposing effects of TXA₂ and PGI₂ limit thrombi formation to sites of vascular injury. [Note: Aspirin has an antithrombogenic effect. It inhibits TXA₂ synthesis by *COX-1* in platelets and PGI₂ synthesis by *COX-2* in endothelial cells through irreversible acetylation of these isozymes (Fig. 17.24). *COX-1* inhibition cannot be overcome in platelets, which lack nuclei. However, *COX-2* inhibition can be overcome in endothelial cells because they have a nucleus and, therefore, can generate more of the enzyme. This difference is the basis of low-dose aspirin therapy used to lower the risk of stroke and heart attacks by decreasing formation of thrombi.]

C. Leukotriene synthesis

Arachidonic acid is converted to a variety of linear hydroperoxy (–OOH) acids by a separate pathway involving a family of *lipoxygenases* (*LOX*). For example, *5-LOX* converts arachidonic acid to 5-hydroperoxy-6,8,11,14 eicosatetraenoic acid ([5-HPETE]; see Fig. 17.23). 5-HPETE is converted to a series of LT containing four double bonds, the nature of the final products varying according to the tissue. LT are mediators of allergic response and inflammation. Inhibitors of *5-LOX* and LT-receptor antagonists are used in the treatment of asthma. [Note: LT synthesis is inhibited by cortisol and not by NSAID. Aspirin-exacerbated respiratory disease is a response to LT overproduction with NSAID use in ~10% of individuals with asthma.]

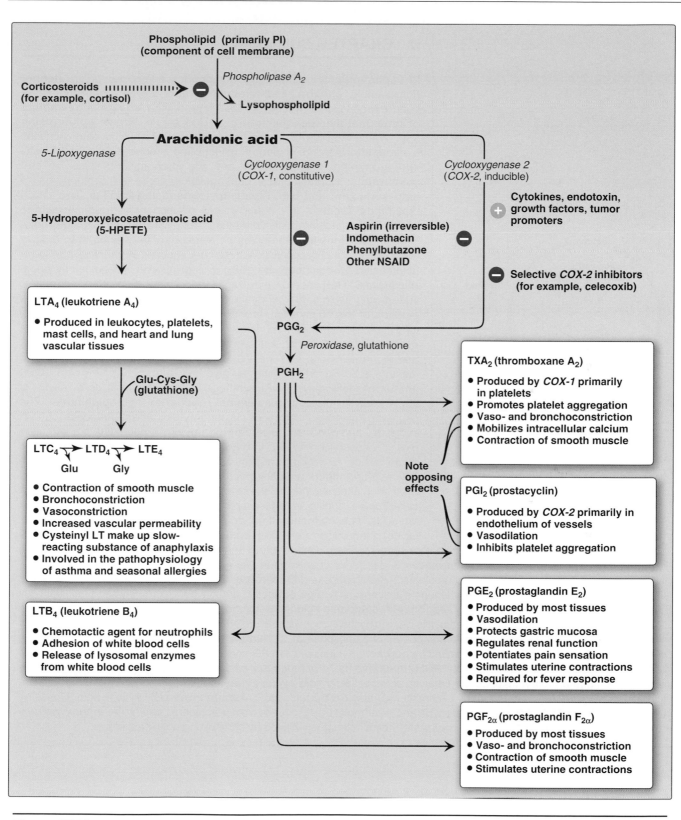

Figure 17.23
Overview of the biosynthesis and function of some important prostaglandins (PG), leukotrienes (LT), and a thromboxane (TX) from arachidonic acid. [Note: The arachidonic acid in the membrane phospholipid was derived from the ω-6 essential fatty acid (FA), linoleic, also an ω-6 FA.] PI = phosphatidylinositol; NSAID = nonsteroidal anti-inflammatory drugs; Glu = glutamate; Cys = cysteine; Gly = glycine.

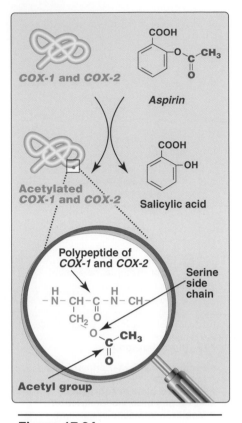

Figure 17.24
Irreversible acetylation of *cyclooxygenase (COX)-1* and *COX-2* by aspirin.

IX. CHAPTER SUMMARY

Phospholipids are polar, ionic compounds composed of an **alcohol** (for example, **choline** or **ethanolamine**) attached by a phosphodiester bond either to **diacylglycerol (DAG)**, producing **phosphatidylcholine** or **phosphatidylethanolamine**, or to the amino alcohol **sphingosine** (Fig. 17.25). Addition of a long-chain fatty acid to sphingosine produces a **ceramide**. Addition of **phosphorylcholine** produces the phospholipid **sphingomyelin**. Phospholipids are the predominant lipids of **cell membranes**. Nonmembrane phospholipids serve as components of **lung surfactant** and **bile**. **Dipalmitoylphosphatidylcholine**, also called **dipalmitoyl lecithin**, is the major lipid component of **lung surfactant**. Insufficient surfactant production causes **respiratory distress syndrome**. **Phosphatidylinositol (PI)** serves as a reservoir for **arachidonic acid** in membranes. The phosphorylation of membrane-bound PI produces **phosphatidylinositol 4,5-bisphosphate (PIP$_2$)**. This compound is degraded by *phospholipase C* in response to the binding of various neurotransmitters, hormones, and growth factors to membrane **G protein–coupled receptors**. The products of this degradation, **inositol 1,4,5-trisphosphate (IP$_3$)** and **DAG**, mediate the mobilization of intracellular **calcium** and the activation of *protein kinase C*, which act synergistically to evoke cellular responses. Specific proteins can be covalently attached via a carbohydrate bridge to membrane-bound PI, forming a **glycosyl phosphatidylinositol (GPI) anchor**. A deficiency in GPI synthesis in hematopoietic cells results in the hemolytic disease **paroxysmal nocturnal hemoglobinuria**. The degradation of phosphoglycerides is performed by *phospholipases* found in all tissues and pancreatic juice. **Sphingomyelin** is degraded to a ceramide plus phosphorylcholine by the lysosomal enzyme *sphingomyelinase*, a deficiency of which causes **Niemann-Pick (A and B) disease**. **Glycosphingolipids** are derivatives of **ceramides** to which carbohydrates have been attached. Adding one sugar molecule to the ceramide produces a **cerebroside**, adding an oligosaccharide produces a **globoside**, and adding an acidic **N-acetylneuraminic acid** molecule produces a **ganglioside**. Glycosphingolipids are found predominantly in cell membranes of the **brain** and **peripheral nervous tissue**, with high concentrations in the **myelin sheath**. They are **antigenic**. Glycolipids are degraded in the **lysosomes** by *acid hydrolases*. A deficiency of any one of these enzymes causes a **sphingolipidosis**, in which a characteristic sphingolipid accumulates. **Prostaglandins (PG)**, **thromboxanes (TX)**, and **leukotrienes (LT)**, the **eicosanoids**, are produced in very small amounts in almost all tissues, act locally, and have an extremely short half-life. They serve as mediators of the **inflammatory response**. **Arachidonic acid** is the immediate precursor of the predominant class of human PG (those with two double bonds). It is derived by the elongation and desaturation of the essential fatty acid **linoleic acid** and is stored in the membrane as a component of a phospholipid, generally PI. Arachidonic acid is released from the phospholipid by *phospholipase A$_2$* (inhibited by **cortisol**). Synthesis of the **PG** and **TX** begins with the oxidative cyclization of free arachidonic acid to yield PGH$_2$ by *PGH$_2$ synthase* (or, *prostaglandin endoperoxide synthase*), an endoplasmic reticular membrane protein that has two catalytic activities: *fatty acid cyclooxygenase (COX)* and *peroxidase*. There are two isozymes of *PGH$_2$ synthase*: **COX-1** (constitutive) and **COX-2** (inducible). **Aspirin** irreversibly inhibits both. Opposing effects of PGI$_2$ and TXA$_2$ limit clot formation. **LT** are linear molecules produced from arachidonic acid by the *5-lipoxygenase (5-LOX)* pathway. They mediate allergic response. Their synthesis is inhibited by cortisol and not by aspirin.

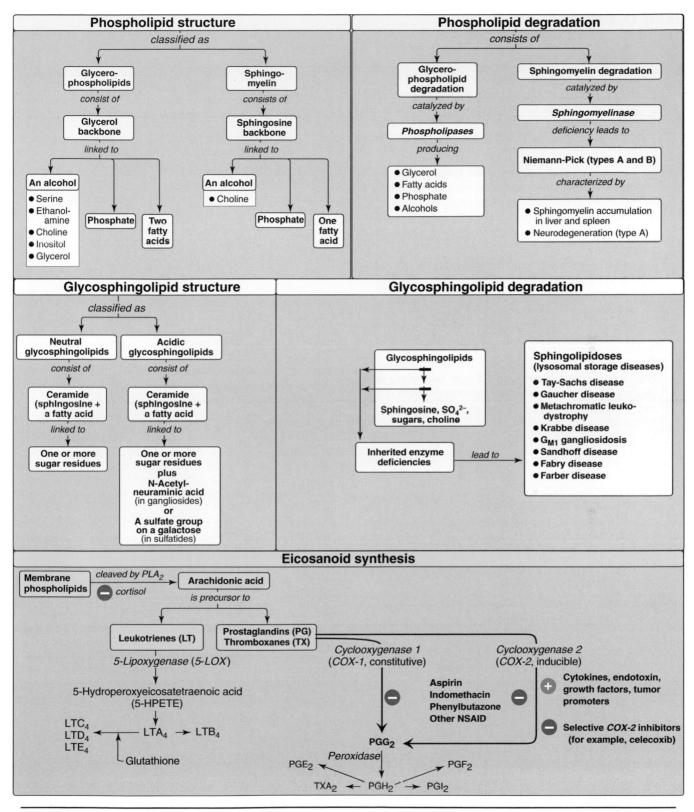

Figure 17.25

Key concept map for phospholipids, glycosphingolipids, and eicosanoids. *PLA₂ = phospholipase A₂*; SO_4^{2-} = sulfate ion; NSAID = nonsteroidal anti-inflammatory drugs.

Study Questions

Choose the ONE best answer.

17.1 Aspirin-exacerbated respiratory disease (AERD) is a severe reaction to nonsteroidal anti-inflammatory drugs (NSAID) characterized by bronchoconstriction 30 minutes to several hours after ingestion. Which of the following statements best explains the symptoms seen in patients with AERD? NSAID:

A. inhibit the activity of the cystic fibrosis transmembrane conductance regulator protein, resulting in thickened mucus that block airways.

B. inhibit cyclooxygenase but not lipoxygenase, resulting in the flow of arachidonic acid to leukotriene synthesis.

C. activate the cyclooxygenase activity of prostaglandin H_2 synthase, resulting in increased synthesis of prostaglandins that promote vasodilation.

D. activate phospholipases, resulting in decreased amounts of dipalmitoylphosphatidylcholine and alveolar collapse (atelectasis).

> Correct answer = B. NSAID inhibit cyclooxygenase but not lipoxygenase, so any arachidonic acid available is used for the synthesis of bronchoconstricting leukotrienes. NSAID have no effect on the cystic fibrosis (CF) transmembrane conductance regulator protein, defects in which are the cause of CF. Steroids, not NSAID, inhibit phospholipase A_2. Cyclooxygenase is inhibited by NSAID, not activated. NSAID have no effect on phospholipases.

17.2 An infant, born at 28 weeks' gestation, rapidly gave evidence of respiratory distress. Clinical laboratory and imaging results supported the diagnosis of infant respiratory distress syndrome. Which of the following statements about this syndrome is true?

A. It is unrelated to the baby's premature birth.

B. It is a consequence of too few type II pneumocytes.

C. The lecithin/sphingomyelin ratio in the amniotic fluid is likely to be high (>2).

D. The concentration of dipalmitoylphosphatidylcholine in the amniotic fluid would be expected to be lower than that of a full-term baby.

E. It is an easily treated disorder with low mortality.

F. It is treated by administering surfactant to the mother just before she gives birth.

> Correct answer = D. Dipalmitoylphosphatidylcholine (DPPC or, dipalmitoyl lecithin) is the lung surfactant found in mature, healthy lungs. Respiratory distress syndrome (RDS) can occur in lungs that make too little of this compound. If the lecithin/sphingomyelin (L/S) ratio in amniotic fluid is ≥2, a newborn's lungs are considered to be sufficiently mature (premature lungs would be expected to have a ratio <2). The RDS would not be due to too few type II pneumocytes, which would simply be secreting sphingomyelin rather than DPPC at 28 weeks' gestation. The mother is given a glucocorticoid, not surfactant, prior to giving birth (antenatally). Surfactant would be administered to the baby postnatally to reduce surface tension.

17.3 A 10-year-old boy was evaluated for burning sensations in his feet and clusters of small, red-purple spots on his skin. Laboratory studies revealed protein in his urine. Enzymatic analysis revealed a deficiency of α-galactosidase, and enzyme replacement therapy was recommended. The most likely diagnosis is:

A. Fabry disease.

B. Farber disease.

C. Gaucher disease.

D. Krabbe disease.

E. Niemann-Pick disease.

> Correct answer = A. Fabry disease, a deficiency of α-galactosidase, is the only X-linked sphingolipidosis. It is characterized by pain in the extremities, a red-purple skin rash (generalized angiokeratomas), and kidney and cardiac complications. Protein in his urine indicates kidney damage. Enzyme replacement therapy is available.

17.4 Current medical advice for individuals experiencing chest pain is to call emergency medical services and chew a regular strength, noncoated aspirin. What is the basis for recommending aspirin?

> Aspirin has an antithrombogenic effect: It prevents formation of blood clots that could occlude heart vessels. Aspirin inhibits thromboxane A_2 synthesis by cyclooxygenase-1 in platelets through irreversible acetylation, thereby inhibiting platelet activation and vasoconstriction. Chewing a noncoated aspirin increases the rate of its absorption.

Cholesterol, Lipoprotein, and Steroid Metabolism

18

I. OVERVIEW

Cholesterol, the characteristic steroid alcohol of animal tissues, performs a number of essential functions in the body. For example, cholesterol is a structural component of all cell membranes, modulating their fluidity, and, in specialized tissues, cholesterol is a precursor of bile acids, steroid hormones, and vitamin D. Therefore, it is critically important that the cells of the body be assured an appropriate supply of cholesterol. To meet this need, a complex series of transport, biosynthetic, and regulatory mechanisms has evolved. The liver plays a central role in the regulation of the body's cholesterol homeostasis. For example, cholesterol enters the hepatic cholesterol pool from a number of sources including dietary cholesterol as well as that synthesized de novo by extrahepatic tissues and by the liver itself. Cholesterol is eliminated from the liver as unmodified cholesterol in the bile, or it can be converted to bile salts that are secreted into the intestinal lumen. It can also serve as a component of plasma lipoproteins that carry lipids to the peripheral tissues. In humans, the balance between cholesterol influx and efflux is not precise, resulting in a gradual deposition of cholesterol in the tissues, particularly in the endothelial linings of blood vessels. This is a potentially life-threatening occurrence when the lipid deposition leads to plaque formation, causing the narrowing of blood vessels (atherosclerosis) and increased risk of cardio-, cerebro-, and peripheral vascular disease. Figure 18.1 summarizes the major sources of liver cholesterol and the routes by which cholesterol leaves the liver.

II. CHOLESTEROL STRUCTURE

Cholesterol is a very hydrophobic compound. It consists of four fused hydrocarbon rings (A–D) called the steroid nucleus, and it has an eight-carbon, branched hydrocarbon chain attached to carbon 17 of the D ring. Ring A has a hydroxyl group at carbon 3, and ring B has a double bond between carbon 5 and carbon 6 (Fig. 18.2).

A. Sterols

Steroids with 8 to 10 carbon atoms in the side chain at carbon 17 and a hydroxyl group at carbon 3 are classified as sterols. Cholesterol is

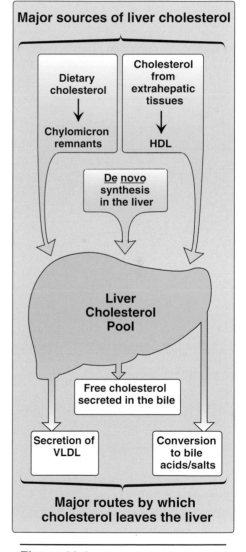

Figure 18.1
Sources of liver cholesterol (influx) and routes by which cholesterol leaves the liver (efflux). HDL and VLDL = high- and very-low-density lipoproteins.

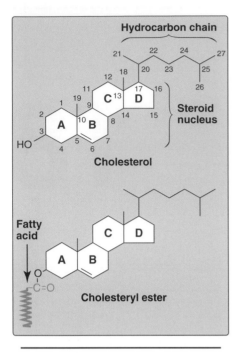

Figure 18.2
Structure of cholesterol and its ester.

the major sterol in animal tissues. It arises from <u>de novo</u> synthesis and absorption of dietary cholesterol. Intestinal uptake of cholesterol is mediated by the Niemann-Pick C1-like 1 protein, the target of the drug ezetimibe that reduces absorption of dietary cholesterol (see p. 176). [Note: Plant sterols (phytosterols), such as β-sitosterol, are poorly absorbed by humans (5% absorbed as compared to 40% for cholesterol). After entering the enterocytes, they are actively transported back into the intestinal lumen. Defects in the efflux transporter (ABCG5/8) result in the rare condition of sitosterolemia. Because some cholesterol is transported back as well, plant sterols reduce the absorption of dietary cholesterol. Daily ingestion of plant sterol esters supplied, for example, in spreads, is one of a number of dietary strategies to reduce plasma cholesterol levels (see p. 363).]

B. Cholesteryl esters

Most plasma cholesterol is in an esterified form (with a fatty acid [FA] attached at carbon 3, as shown in Fig. 18.2), which makes the structure even more hydrophobic than free (nonesterified) cholesterol. Cholesteryl esters are not found in membranes and are normally present only in low levels in most cells. Because of their hydrophobicity, cholesterol and its esters must be transported in association with protein as a component of a lipoprotein particle (see p. 227) or be solubilized by phospholipids and bile salts in the bile (see p. 226).

III. CHOLESTEROL SYNTHESIS

Cholesterol is synthesized by virtually all tissues in humans, although liver, intestine, adrenal cortex, and reproductive tissues, including ovaries, testes, and placenta, make the largest contributions to the cholesterol pool. As with FA, all the carbon atoms in cholesterol are provided by acetyl coenzyme A (CoA), and nicotinamide adenine dinucleotide phosphate (NADPH) provides the reducing equivalents. The pathway is endergonic, being driven by hydrolysis of the high-energy thioester bond of acetyl CoA and the terminal phosphate bond of ATP. Synthesis requires enzymes in the cytosol, the membrane of the smooth endoplasmic reticulum (SER), and the peroxisome. The pathway is responsive to changes in cholesterol concentration, and regulatory mechanisms exist to balance the rate of cholesterol synthesis against the rate of cholesterol excretion. An imbalance in this regulation can lead to an elevation in circulating levels of plasma cholesterol, with the potential for vascular disease.

A. 3-Hydroxy-3-methylglutaryl coenzyme A synthesis

The first two reactions in the cholesterol biosynthetic pathway are similar to those in the pathway that produces ketone bodies (see Fig. 16.22, p. 196). They result in the production of 3-hydroxy-3-methylglutaryl CoA ([HMG CoA], Fig. 18.3). First, two acetyl CoA molecules condense to form acetoacetyl CoA. Next, a third molecule of acetyl CoA is added by *HMG CoA synthase*, producing HMG CoA, a six-carbon compound. [Note: Liver parenchymal cells contain two isoenzymes of the *synthase*. The cytosolic enzyme participates in cholesterol synthesis, whereas the mitochondrial enzyme functions in the pathway for ketone body synthesis.]

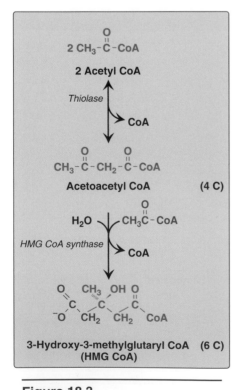

Figure 18.3
Synthesis of HMG CoA. CoA = coenzyme A.

B. Mevalonate synthesis

HMG CoA is reduced to mevalonate by *HMG CoA reductase*. This is the rate-limiting and key regulated step in cholesterol synthesis. It occurs in the cytosol, uses two molecules of NADPH as the reducing agent, and releases CoA, making the reaction irreversible (Fig. 18.4). [Note: *HMG CoA reductase* is an integral membrane protein of the SER, with its catalytic domain projecting into the cytosol. Regulation of *reductase* activity is discussed in D. below.]

C. Cholesterol synthesis from mevalonate

The reactions and enzymes involved in the synthesis of cholesterol from mevalonate are illustrated in Figure 18.5. [Note: The numbers shown in brackets below correspond to numbered reactions shown in this figure.]

[1] Mevalonate is converted to 5-pyrophosphomevalonate in two steps, each of which transfers a phosphate group from ATP.

[2] A five-carbon isoprene unit, isopentenyl pyrophosphate (IPP), is formed by the decarboxylation of 5-pyrophosphomevalonate. The reaction requires ATP. [Note: IPP is the precursor of a family of molecules with diverse functions, the isoprenoids. Cholesterol is a sterol isoprenoid. Nonsterol isoprenoids include dolichol (see p. 167) and ubiquinone (or, coenzyme Q; see p. 75).]

[3] IPP is isomerized to 3,3-dimethylallyl pyrophosphate (DPP).

[4] IPP and DPP condense to form 10-carbon geranyl pyrophosphate (GPP).

[5] A second molecule of IPP then condenses with GPP to form 15-carbon farnesyl pyrophosphate (FPP). [Note: Covalent attachment of farnesyl to proteins, a process known as prenylation, is one mechanism for anchoring proteins (for example, ras) to the inner face of plasma membranes.]

[6] Two molecules of FPP combine, releasing pyrophosphate, and are reduced, forming the 30-carbon compound squalene. [Note: Squalene is formed from six isoprenoid units. Because 3 ATP are hydrolyzed per mevalonate residue converted to IPP, a total of 18 ATP are required to make the polyisoprenoid squalene.]

[7] Squalene is converted to the sterol lanosterol by a sequence of two reactions catalyzed by SER-associated enzymes that use molecular oxygen (O_2) and NADPH. The hydroxylation of linear squalene triggers the cyclization of the structure to lanosterol.

[8] The conversion of lanosterol to cholesterol is a multistep process involving shortening of the side chain, oxidative removal of methyl groups, reduction of double bonds, and migration of a double bond. Smith-Lemli-Opitz syndrome (SLOS), an autosomal-recessive disorder of cholesterol biosynthesis, is caused by a partial deficiency in *7-dehydrocholesterol-7-reductase*, the enzyme that reduces the double bond in 7-dehydrocholesterol (7-DHC), thereby converting it to cholesterol. SLOS is one of several multisystem, embryonic malformation syndromes associated with impaired cholesterol synthesis. [Note: 7-DHC is converted to vitamin D_3 in the skin (see p. 390).]

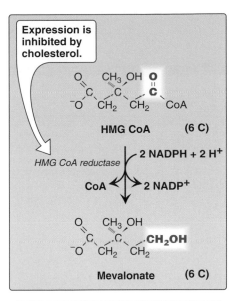

Figure 18.4
Synthesis of mevalonate. HMG CoA = hydroxymethylglutaryl coenzyme A; NADP(H) = nicotinamide adenine dinucleotide phosphate.

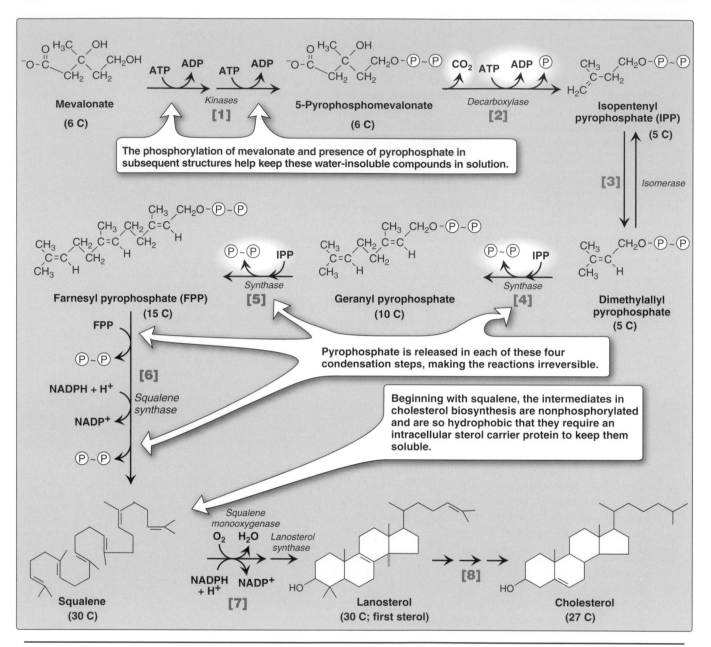

Figure 18.5
Synthesis of cholesterol from mevalonate. ADP = adenosine diphosphate; ℗ = phosphate; ℗ ~ ℗ = pyrophosphate; NADP(H) = nicotinamide adenine dinucleotide phosphate.

D. Cholesterol synthesis regulation

HMG CoA reductase is the major control point for cholesterol biosynthesis and is subject to different kinds of metabolic control.

1. **Sterol-dependent regulation of gene expression:** Expression of the gene for *HMG CoA reductase* is controlled by the trans-acting factor, sterol regulatory element–binding protein-2 (SREBP-2), which binds DNA at the cis-acting sterol regulatory element (SRE) upstream of the *reductase* gene. Inactive SREBP-2 is an integral protein of the SER membrane and associates with a second SER membrane protein, SREBP cleavage–activating protein (SCAP). When sterol levels

in the SER are low, the SREBP-2–SCAP complex moves from the ER to the Golgi. In the Golgi membrane, SREBP-2 is sequentially acted upon by two *proteases*, which generate a soluble fragment that enters the nucleus, binds the SRE, and functions as a transcription factor. This results in increased synthesis of *HMG CoA reductase* and, therefore, increased cholesterol synthesis (Fig. 18.6). However, if sterols are abundant, they bind SCAP at its sterol-sensing domain and induce the binding of SCAP to yet other ER membrane proteins, the insulin-induced gene proteins (INSIG). This results in the retention of the SCAP–SREBP complex in the SER, thereby preventing the activation of SREBP-2 and leading to downregulation of cholesterol synthesis. [Note: SREBP-1c upregulates expression of enzymes involved in FA synthesis in response to insulin (see p. 184).]

2. **Sterol-accelerated enzyme degradation:** The *reductase* itself is a sterol-sensing integral protein of the SER membrane. When sterol levels in the SER are high, the enzyme binds to INSIG proteins. Binding leads to cytosolic transfer, ubiquitination, and proteasomal degradation of the *reductase* (see p. 247).

3. **Sterol-independent phosphorylation/dephosphorylation:** *HMG CoA reductase* activity is controlled covalently through the actions of *adenosine monophosphate (AMP)–activated protein kinase* ([AMPK] see p. 183) and a *phosphoprotein phosphatase* (see Fig. 18.6). The phosphorylated form of the enzyme is inactive, whereas the dephosphorylated form is active. [Note: Because *AMPK* is activated by AMP, cholesterol synthesis, like FA synthesis, is decreased when ATP availability is decreased.]

4. **Hormonal regulation:** The activity of *HMG CoA reductase* is controlled hormonally. An increase in insulin favors dephosphorylation (activation) of the *reductase*, whereas an increase in glucagon and epinephrine has the opposite effect.

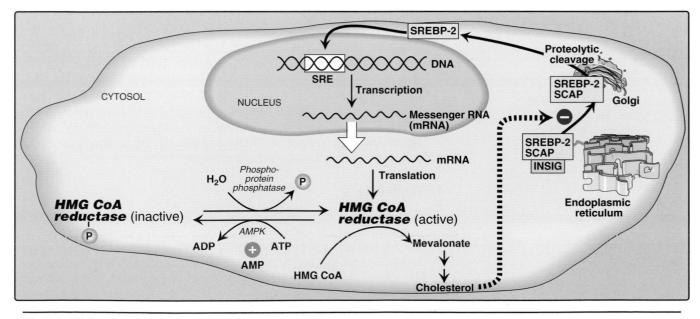

Figure 18.6
Regulation of *hydroxymethylglutaryl coenzyme A (HMG CoA) reductase*. SRE = sterol regulatory element; SREBP = SRE-binding protein; SCAP = SREBP cleavage–activating protein; *AMPK = adenosine monophosphate–activated protein kinase*; ADP = adenosine diphosphate; Ⓟ = phosphate; INSIG = insulin-induced gene protein.

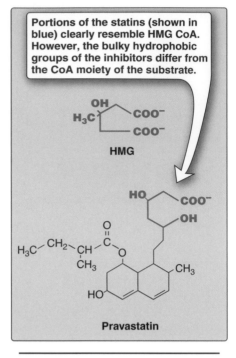

Figure 18.7
Structural similarity of hydroxymethyl-glutaric acid (HMG) and pravastatin, a clinically useful cholesterol-lowering drug of the statin family. CoA = coenzyme A.

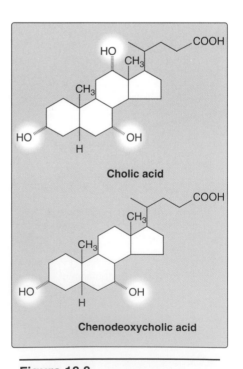

Figure 18.8
Bile acids. [Note: The ionized forms are bile salts.]

5. Drug inhibition: The statin drugs (atorvastatin, fluvastatin, lovastatin, pravastatin, rosuvastatin, and simvastatin) are structural analogs of HMG CoA and are (or are metabolized to) reversible, competitive inhibitors of *HMG CoA reductase* (Fig. 18.7). They are used to decrease plasma cholesterol levels in patients with hypercholesterolemia.

IV. CHOLESTEROL DEGRADATION

Humans cannot metabolize the cholesterol ring structure to carbon dioxide and water. Rather, the intact steroid nucleus is eliminated from the body by conversion to bile acids and bile salts, a small percentage of which is excreted in the feces, and by secretion of cholesterol into the bile, which transports it to the intestine for elimination. [Note: Some of the cholesterol in the intestine is modified by bacteria before excretion. The primary compounds made are the isomers coprostanol and cholestanol, which are reduced derivatives of cholesterol. Together with cholesterol, these compounds make up the bulk of neutral fecal sterols.]

V. BILE ACIDS AND BILE SALTS

Bile consists of a watery mixture of organic and inorganic compounds. Phosphatidylcholine (PC), or lecithin (see p. 202), and conjugated bile salts are quantitatively the most important organic components of bile. Bile can either pass directly from the liver, where it is synthesized, into the duodenum through the common bile duct, or be stored in the gallbladder when not immediately needed for digestion.

A. Structure

The bile acids contain 24 carbons, with two or three hydroxyl groups and a side chain that terminates in a carboxyl group. The carboxyl group has a pK_a (see p. 6) of ~6. In the duodenum (pH ~6), this group will be protonated in half of the molecules (the bile acids) and deprotonated in the rest (the bile salts). The terms bile acid and bile salt are frequently used interchangeably, however. Both forms have hydroxyl groups that are α in orientation (they lie below the plane of the rings) and methyl groups that are β (they lie above the plane of the rings). Therefore, the molecules have both a polar and a nonpolar surface and can act as emulsifying agents in the intestine, helping prepare dietary fat (triacylglycerol [TAG]) and other complex lipids for degradation by pancreatic digestive enzymes.

B. Synthesis

Bile acids are synthesized in the liver by a multistep, multiorganelle pathway in which hydroxyl groups are inserted at specific positions on the steroid structure; the double bond of the cholesterol B ring is reduced; and the hydrocarbon chain is shortened by three carbons, introducing a carboxyl group at the end of the chain. The most common resulting compounds, cholic acid (a triol) and chenodeoxycholic acid (a diol), as shown in Figure 18.8, are called primary bile acids. [Note: The rate-limiting step in bile acid synthesis is the introduction of a hydroxyl group at carbon 7 of the steroid nucleus by *7-α-hydroxylase*, a SER-associated *cytochrome P450 monooxygenase* found only in liver. Expression of the enzyme is downregulated by bile acids (Fig. 18.9)].

C. Conjugation

Before the bile acids leave the liver, they are conjugated to a molecule of either glycine or taurine (an end product of cysteine metabolism) by an amide bond between the carboxyl group of the bile acid and the amino group of the added compound. These new structures include glycocholic and glycochenodeoxycholic acids and taurocholic and taurochenodeoxycholic acids (Fig. 18.10). The ratio of glycine to taurine forms in the bile is ~3/1. Addition of glycine or taurine results in the presence of a carboxyl group with a lower pK_a (from glycine) or a sulfonate group (from taurine), both of which are fully ionized (negatively charged) at the alkaline pH of bile. The conjugated, ionized bile salts are more effective detergents than the unconjugated ones because of their enhanced amphipathic nature. Therefore, only the conjugated forms are found in the bile. Individuals with genetic deficiencies in the conversion of cholesterol to bile acids are treated with exogenously supplied chenodeoxycholic acid.

> ‖ Bile salts provide the only significant mechanism for cholesterol excretion, both as a metabolic product of cholesterol and as a solubilizer of cholesterol in bile.

D. Bacterial action on bile salts

Bacteria of the intestinal microbiota (see p. 372) can deconjugate (remove glycine and taurine) bile salts. They can also dehydroxylate carbon 7, producing secondary bile salts such as deoxycholic acid from cholic acid and lithocholic acid from chenodeoxycholic acid.

E. Enterohepatic circulation

Bile salts secreted into the intestine are efficiently reabsorbed (>95%) and reused. The liver actively secretes bile salts via the bile salt export pump. In the intestine, they are reabsorbed in the terminal ileum via the apical sodium (Na^+)–bile salt cotransporter and returned to the blood via a separate transport system. [Note: Lithocholic acid is only poorly absorbed.] They are efficiently taken up from blood by the hepatocytes via an isoform of the cotransporter and reused. [Note: Albumin binds bile salts and transports them through the blood as was seen with FA (see p. 181).] The continuous process of secretion of bile salts into the bile, their passage through the duodenum where some are deconjugated then dehydroxylated to secondary bile salts, their uptake in the ileum, and their subsequent return to the liver as a mixture of primary and secondary forms is termed the enterohepatic circulation (Fig. 18.11). Between 15 and 30 g of bile salts are secreted from the liver into the duodenum each day, yet only ~0.5 g (<3%) is lost daily in the feces. Approximately 0.5 g/day is synthesized from cholesterol in the liver to replace the amount lost. Bile acid sequestrants, such as cholestyramine, bind bile salts in the gut and prevent their reabsorption,

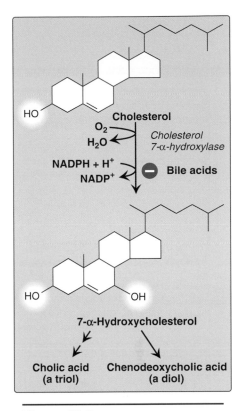

Figure 18.9
Synthesis of the bile acids cholic acid and chenodeoxycholic acid from cholesterol.

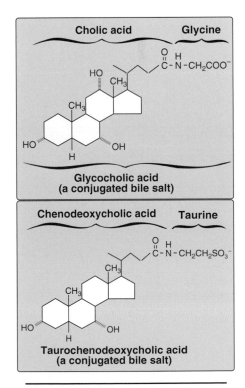

Figure 18.10
Conjugated bile salts. Note "cholic" in the names.

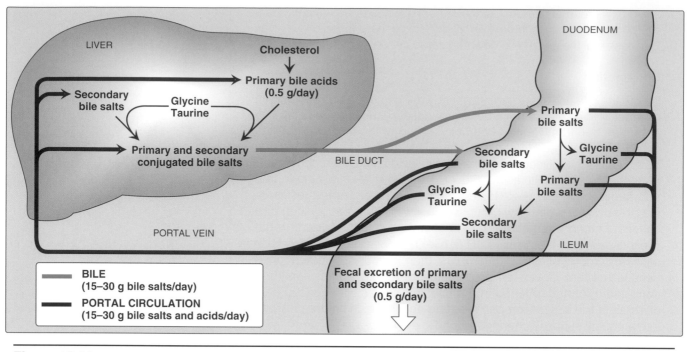

Figure 18.11
Enterohepatic circulation of bile salts. [Note: Ionized bile acids are called bile salts.]

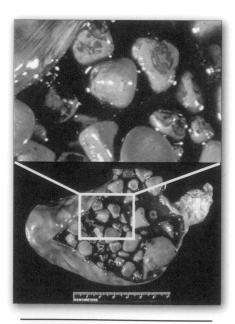

Figure 18.12
Gallbladder with gallstones.

thereby promoting their excretion. They are used in the treatment of hypercholesterolemia because the removal of bile salts relieves the inhibition on bile acid synthesis in the liver, thereby diverting additional cholesterol into that pathway. [Note: Dietary fiber also binds bile salts and increases their excretion (see p. 365).]

F. Bile salt deficiency: Cholelithiasis

The movement of cholesterol from the liver into the bile must be accompanied by the simultaneous secretion of phospholipid and bile salts. If this dual process is disrupted and more cholesterol is present than can be solubilized by the bile salts and PC present, the cholesterol may precipitate in the gallbladder, leading to cholesterol gallstone disease or cholelithiasis (Fig. 18.12). This disorder is typically caused by a decrease of bile acids in the bile. Cholelithiasis also may result from increased secretion of cholesterol into bile, as seen with the use of fibrates (for example, gemfibrozil) to reduce cholesterol (and TAG) in the blood. Laparoscopic cholecystectomy (surgical removal of the gallbladder through a small incision) is currently the treatment of choice. However, for patients who are unable to undergo surgery, oral administration of chenodeoxycholic acid to supplement the body's supply of bile acids results in a gradual (months to years) dissolution of the gallstones. [Note: Cholesterol stones account for >85% of cases of cholelithiasis, with bilirubin and mixed stones accounting for the rest].

VI. PLASMA LIPOPROTEINS

The plasma lipoproteins are spherical macromolecular complexes of lipids and proteins (apolipoproteins). The lipoprotein particles include chylomicrons, very-low-density lipoproteins (VLDL), low-density lipoproteins

(LDL), and high-density lipoproteins (HDL). They differ in lipid and protein composition, size, density (Fig. 18.13), and site of origin. [Note: Because lipoprotein particles constantly interchange lipids and apolipoproteins, the actual apolipoprotein and lipid content of each class of particles is somewhat variable.] Lipoproteins function both to keep their component lipids soluble as they transport them in the plasma and to provide an efficient mechanism for transporting their lipid contents to (and from) the tissues. In humans, the transport system is less perfect than in other animals and, as a result, humans experience a gradual deposition of lipid (especially cholesterol) in tissues.

A. Composition

Lipoproteins are composed of a neutral lipid core (containing TAG and cholesteryl esters) surrounded by a shell of amphipathic apolipoproteins, phospholipid, and nonesterified (free) cholesterol (Fig. 18.14). These amphipathic compounds are oriented such that their polar portions are exposed on the surface of the lipoprotein, thereby rendering the particle soluble in aqueous solution. The TAG and cholesterol carried by the lipoproteins are obtained either from the diet (exogenous source) or from de novo synthesis (endogenous source). [Note: The cholesterol (C) content of plasma lipoproteins is now routinely measured in fasting blood. Total C = LDL-C + HDL-C + VLDL-C, where VLDL-C is calculated by dividing TAG by 5 because the TAG/cholesterol ratio is 5/1 in VLDL. The goal value for total cholesterol is <200 mg/dl.]

1. **Size and density:** Chylomicrons are the lipoprotein particles lowest in density and largest in size and that contain the highest percentage of lipid (as TAG) and the lowest percentage of protein. VLDL and LDL are successively denser, having higher ratios of protein to lipid. HDL particles are the smallest and densest. Plasma lipoproteins can be separated on the basis of their electrophoretic mobility, as shown in Figure 18.15, or on the basis of their density by ultracentrifugation.

2. **Apolipoproteins:** The apolipoproteins associated with lipoprotein particles have a number of diverse functions, such as providing recognition sites for cell-surface receptors and serving as activators or coenzymes for enzymes involved in lipoprotein metabolism. Some of the apolipoproteins are required as essential structural components of the particles and cannot be removed (in fact, the particles cannot be produced without them), whereas others are transferred freely between lipoproteins. Apolipoproteins are divided by structure and function into several major classes, denoted by letters, with each class having subclasses (for example, apolipoprotein [apo] C-I, apo C-II, and apo C-III). [Note: The functions of all the apolipoproteins are not yet known.]

B. Chylomicron metabolism

Chylomicrons are assembled in intestinal mucosal cells and carry dietary (exogenous) TAG, cholesterol, fat-soluble vitamins, and cholesteryl esters to the peripheral tissues (Fig. 18.16). [Note: TAG account for close to 90% of the lipids in a chylomicron.]

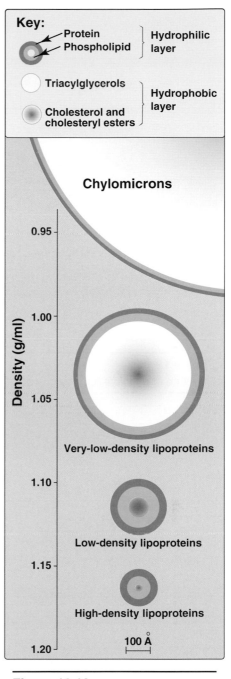

Figure 18.13
Plasma lipoprotein particles exhibit a range of sizes and densities, and typical values are shown. Ring widths approximate the amount of each component. [Note: Although cholesterol and its esters are shown as one component in the center of each particle, physically, cholesterol is on the surface, whereas cholesteryl esters are in the interior.]

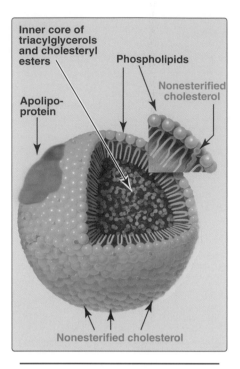

Figure 18.14
Structure of a typical lipoprotein particle.

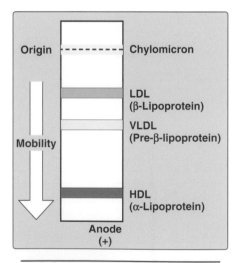

Figure 18.15
Electrophoretic mobility of plasma lipoprotein particles. [Note: The order of low-density lipoprotein (LDL) and very-low-density lipoprotein (VLDL) is reversed if ultracentrifugation is used as the separation technique.] HDL = high-density lipoprotein.

1. **Apolipoprotein synthesis:** Apo B-48 is unique to chylomicrons. Its synthesis begins on the rough ER (RER), and it is glycosylated as it moves through the RER and Golgi. [Note: Apo B-48 is so named because it constitutes the N-terminal 48% of the protein encoded by the gene for apo B. Apo B-100, which is synthesized by the liver and found in VLDL and LDL, represents the entire protein encoded by this gene. Posttranscriptional editing (see p. 474) of a cytosine to a uracil in intestinal apo B-100 messenger RNA (mRNA) creates a nonsense (stop) codon (see p. 449), allowing translation of only 48% of the mRNA.]

2. **Chylomicron assembly:** Many enzymes involved in TAG, cholesterol, and phospholipid synthesis are located in the SER. Assembly of the apolipoprotein and lipid into chylomicrons requires microsomal triglyceride transfer protein ([MTP] see p. 177), which loads apo B-48 with lipid. This occurs before transition from the ER to the Golgi, where the particles are packaged in secretory vesicles. These fuse with the plasma membrane releasing the lipoproteins, which then enter the lymphatic system and, ultimately, the blood. [Note: Chylomicrons leave the lymphatic system via the thoracic duct that empties into the left subclavian vein.]

3. **Nascent chylomicron modification:** The particle released by the intestinal mucosal cell is called a nascent chylomicron because it is functionally incomplete. When it reaches the plasma, the particle is rapidly modified, receiving apo E (which is recognized by hepatic receptors) and apo C. The latter includes apo C-II, which is necessary for the activation of *lipoprotein lipase* (*LPL*), the enzyme that degrades the TAG contained in the chylomicron. The source of these apolipoproteins is circulating HDL (see Fig. 18.16). [Note: Apo C-III on TAG-rich lipoproteins inhibits *LPL.*]

4. **Triacylglycerol degradation by lipoprotein lipase:** *LPL* is an extracellular enzyme that is anchored to the capillary walls of most tissues but predominantly those of adipose tissue and cardiac and skeletal muscle. The adult liver does not express this enzyme. [Note: A *hepatic lipase* is found on the surface of endothelial cells of the liver. It plays a role in TAG degradation in chylomicrons and VLDL and is important in HDL metabolism (see p. 234).] *LPL*, activated by apo C-II on circulating chylomicrons, hydrolyzes the TAG in these particles to FA and glycerol. The FA are stored (in adipose) or used for energy (in muscle). The glycerol is taken up by the liver, converted to dihydroxyacetone phosphate (an intermediate of glycolysis), and used in lipid synthesis or gluconeogenesis. [Note: Patients with a deficiency of *LPL* or apo C-II (type I hyperlipoproteinemia or familial chylomicronemia) show a dramatic accumulation (≥1,000 mg/dl) of chylomicron-TAG in the plasma (hypertriacylglycerolemia) even in the fasted state. They are at increased risk for acute pancreatitis. Treatment is the reduction of dietary fat.]

5. **Lipoprotein lipase expression:** *LPL* is synthesized by adipose tissue and by cardiac and skeletal muscle. Expression of the tissue-specific isozymes is regulated by nutritional state and hormonal level. For example, in the fed state (elevated insulin levels),

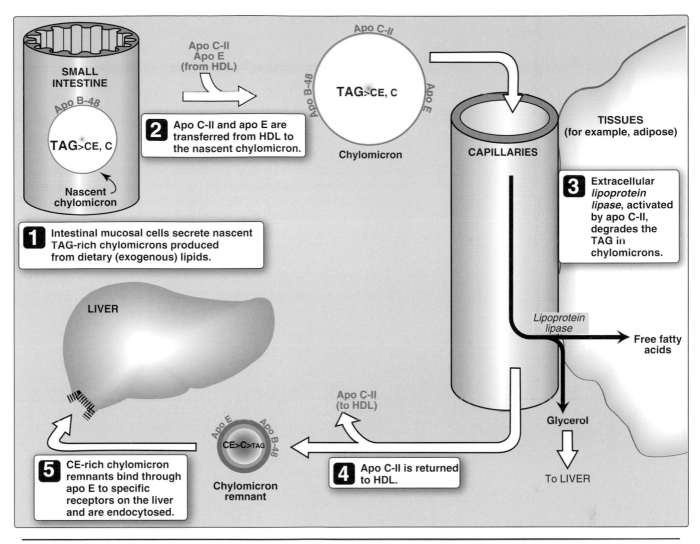

Figure 18.16
Metabolism of chylomicrons. Apo B-48, apo C-II, and apo E are apolipoproteins found as components of plasma lipoprotein particles. The particles are not drawn to scale (see Fig. 18.13 for details of their size and density). TAG = triacylglycerol; C = cholesterol; CE = cholesteryl ester; HDL = high-density lipoprotein.

LPL synthesis is increased in adipose but decreased in muscle tissue. Fasting (decreased insulin) favors LPL synthesis in muscle. [Note: The highest concentration of LPL is in cardiac muscle, reflecting the use of FA to provide much of the energy needed for cardiac function.]

6. **Chylomicron remnant formation:** As the chylomicron circulates, and >90% of the TAG in its core is degraded by LPL, the particle decreases in size and increases in density. In addition, the C apolipoproteins (but not apo B or E) are returned to HDL. The remaining particle, called a remnant, is rapidly removed from the circulation by the liver, whose cell membranes contain lipoprotein receptors that recognize apo E (see Fig. 18.16). Chylomicron remnants bind to these receptors and are taken into the hepatocytes by endocytosis. The endocytosed vesicle then fuses with a lysosome, and the

apolipoproteins, cholesteryl esters, and other components of the remnant are hydrolytically degraded, releasing amino acids, free cholesterol, and FA. The receptor is recycled. [Note: The mechanism of receptor-mediated endocytosis is illustrated for LDL in Fig. 18.20.]

C. Very-low-density lipoprotein metabolism

VLDL are produced in the liver (Fig. 18.17). They are composed predominantly of endogenous TAG (~60%), and their function is to carry this lipid from the liver (site of synthesis) to the peripheral tissues. There, the TAG is degraded by *LPL*, as discussed for chylomicrons (see p. 228). [Note: Nonalcoholic fatty liver (hepatic steatosis) occurs in conditions in which there is an imbalance between hepatic TAG synthesis and the secretion of VLDL. Such conditions include obesity and type 2 diabetes mellitus (see p. 343).]

1. **Release from the liver:** VLDL are secreted directly into the blood by the liver as nascent particles containing apo B-100. They must obtain apo C-II and apo E from circulating HDL (see Fig. 18.17).

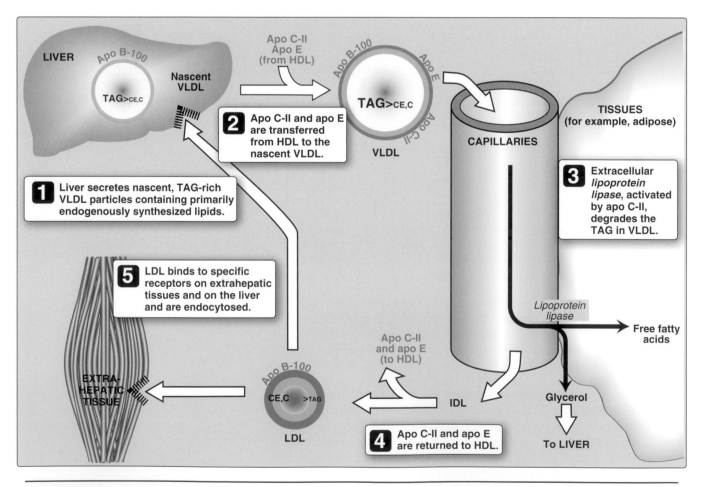

Figure 18.17

Metabolism of very-low-density lipoprotein (VLDL) and low-density lipoprotein (LDL) particles. Apo B-100, C-II, and E are apolipoproteins found as components of plasma lipoprotein particles. The particles are not drawn to scale (see Fig. 18.13 for details of their size and density). [Note: IDL can also be taken up by liver.] TAG = triacylglycerol; HDL and IDL = high- and intermediate-density lipoproteins; C = cholesterol; CE = cholesteryl ester.

As with chylomicrons, apo C-II is required for activation of *LPL*. [Note: Abetalipoproteinemia is a rare hypolipoproteinemia caused by a defect in MTP, leading to an inability to load apo B with lipid. Consequently, few VLDL or chylomicrons are formed, and TAG accumulates in the liver and intestine. Absorption of fat-soluble vitamins is decreased. LDL are low.]

2. **Modification in the circulation:** As VLDL pass through the circulation, TAG is degraded by *LPL*, causing the VLDL to decrease in size and become denser. Surface components, including the C and E apolipoproteins, are returned to HDL, but the particles retain apo B-100. Additionally, some TAG are transferred from VLDL to HDL in an exchange reaction that concomitantly transfers cholesteryl esters from HDL to VLDL. This exchange is accomplished by *cholesteryl ester transfer protein (CETP)*, as shown in Figure 18.18.

3. **Conversion to low-density lipoproteins:** With these modifications, the VLDL is converted in the plasma to LDL. Intermediate-density lipoproteins (IDL) of varying sizes are formed during this transition. IDL can also be taken up by liver cells through receptor-mediated endocytosis that uses apo E as the ligand. Apo E is normally present in three isoforms, E-2 (the least common), E-3 (the most common), and E-4. Apo E-2 binds poorly to receptors, and patients who are homozygotic for apo E-2 are deficient in the clearance of IDL and chylomicron remnants. These individuals have familial type III hyperlipoproteinemia (familial dysbetalipoproteinemia or broad beta disease), with hypercholesterolemia and premature atherosclerosis. [Note: The apo E-4 isoform confers increased susceptibility to an earlier age of onset of the late-onset form of Alzheimer disease. The effect is dose dependent, with homozygotes being at greatest risk. Estimates of the risk vary.]

D. Low-density lipoprotein metabolism

LDL particles contain much less TAG than their VLDL predecessors and have a high concentration of cholesterol and cholesteryl esters (Fig. 18.19). About 70% of plasma cholesterol is in LDL.

1. **Receptor-mediated endocytosis:** The primary function of LDL particles is to provide cholesterol to the peripheral tissues (or return it to the liver). They do so by binding to plasma membrane LDL receptors that recognize apo B-100 (but not apo B-48). Because these LDL receptors can also bind apo E, they are known as apo B-100/apo E receptors. A summary of the uptake and degradation of LDL particles is presented in Figure 18.20. [Note: The numbers in brackets below refer to corresponding numbers on that figure.] A similar mechanism of receptor-mediated endocytosis is used for the uptake and degradation of chylomicron remnants and IDL by the liver.

[1] LDL receptors are negatively charged glycoproteins that are clustered in pits on cell membranes. The cytosolic side of the pit is coated with the protein clathrin, which stabilizes the pit.

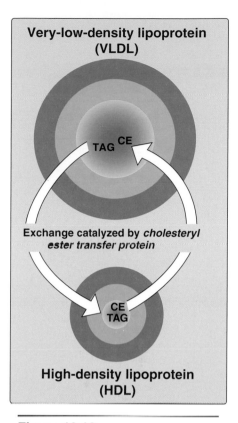

Very-low-density lipoprotein (VLDL)

TAG CE

Exchange catalyzed by *cholesteryl ester transfer protein*

CE TAG

High-density lipoprotein (HDL)

Figure 18.18
Transfer of cholesteryl ester (CE) from HDL to VLDL in exchange for triacylglycerol (TAG).

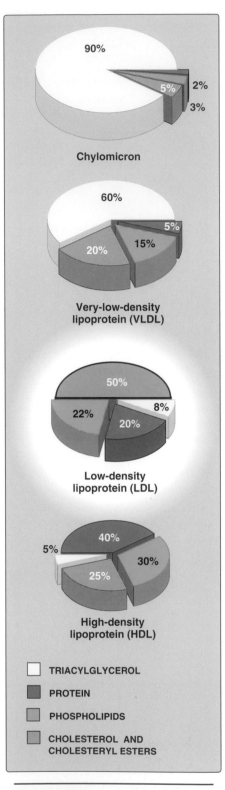

Figure 18.19

Composition of the plasma lipoprotein particles. Note the high concentration of cholesterol and cholesteryl esters in LDL.

[2]   After binding, the LDL–receptor complex is endocytosed. [Note: Defects in the synthesis of functional LDL receptors causes a significant elevation in plasma LDL-C. Patients with such deficiencies have type IIa hyperlipidemia (familial hypercholesterolemia [FH]) and premature atherosclerosis. Autosomal dominant hypercholesterolemia can also be caused by defects in apo B-100 that reduce its binding to the receptor and by increased activity of a *protease*, *proprotein convertase subtilisin/kexin type 9* (*PCSK9*), which promotes internalization and lysosomal degradation of the receptor. *PCSK9* inhibitors are now available for the treatment of hypercholesterolemia.]

[3]   The vesicle containing LDL loses its clathrin coat and fuses with other similar vesicles, forming larger vesicles called endosomes.

[4]   The pH of the endosome falls (due to the proton-pumping activity of endosomal *ATPase*), which allows separation of the LDL from its receptor. The receptors then migrate to one side of the endosome, whereas the LDL stay free within the lumen of the vesicle.

[5]   The receptors can be recycled, whereas the lipoprotein remnants in the vesicle are transferred to lysosomes and degraded by lysosomal *acid hydrolases*, releasing free cholesterol, amino acids, FA, and phospholipids. These compounds can be reutilized by the cell. [Note: Lysosomal storage diseases result from rare autosomal-recessive deficiencies in the ability to hydrolyze lysosomal cholesteryl esters (Wolman disease) or to transport free cholesterol out of the lysosome (Niemann-Pick disease, type C).]

2. **Endocytosed cholesterol and cholesterol homeostasis:** The chylomicron remnant–, IDL-, and LDL-derived cholesterol affects cellular cholesterol content in several ways (see Fig. 18.20). First, expression of the gene for *HMG CoA reductase* is inhibited by high cholesterol, and <u>de</u> <u>novo</u> cholesterol synthesis decreases as a result. Additionally, degradation of the *reductase* is accelerated. Second, synthesis of new LDL receptor protein is reduced by decreasing the expression of the LDL receptor gene, thus limiting further entry of LDL-C into cells. [Note: As was seen with the *reductase* gene (see p. 222), transcriptional regulation of the LDL receptor gene involves an SRE and SREBP-2. This allows coordinate regulation of the expression of these proteins.] Third, if the cholesterol is not required immediately for some structural or synthetic purpose, it is esterified by *acyl CoA:cholesterol acyltransferase* (*ACAT*). *ACAT* transfers a FA from a fatty acyl CoA to cholesterol, producing a cholesteryl ester that can be stored in the cell (Fig. 18.21). The activity of *ACAT* is enhanced in the presence of increased intracellular cholesterol.

3. **Uptake by macrophage scavenger receptors:** In addition to the highly specific and regulated receptor-mediated pathway for LDL uptake described above, macrophages possess high levels of scavenger receptor activity. These receptors, known as scavenger receptor class A (SR-A), can bind a broad range of ligands and mediate the endocytosis of chemically modified LDL in which the lipid or apo B component has been oxidized. Unlike the LDL receptor, the scavenger receptor is not downregulated in response

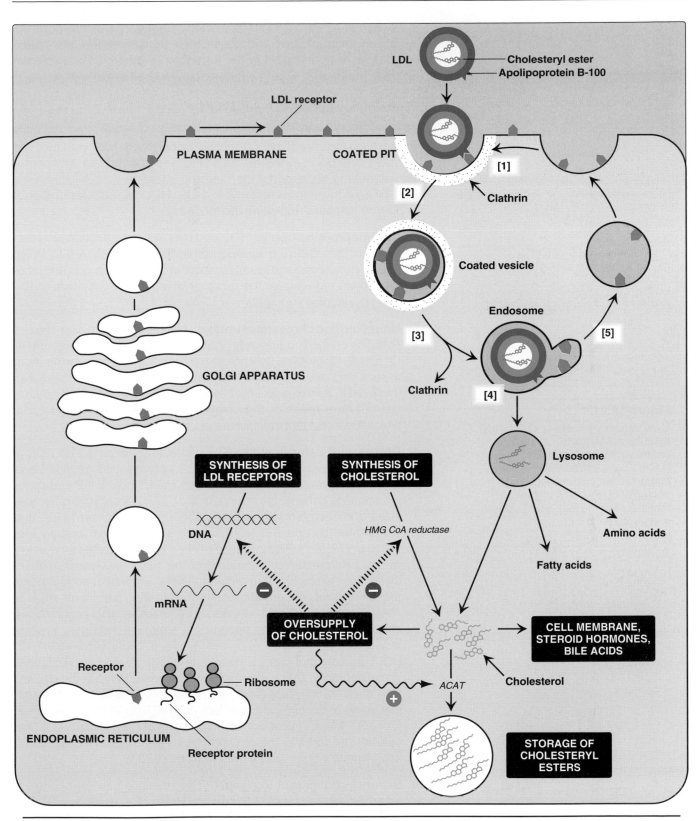

Figure 18.20
Cellular uptake and degradation of low-density lipoprotein (LDL) particles. [Note: Oversupply of cholesterol accelerates the degradation of *HMG CoA reductase*. It also decreases transcription of its gene as seen with the LDL receptor.] *ACAT = acyl CoA:cholesterol acyltransferase*; HMG CoA = hydroxymethylglutaryl coenzyme A; mRNA = messenger RNA.

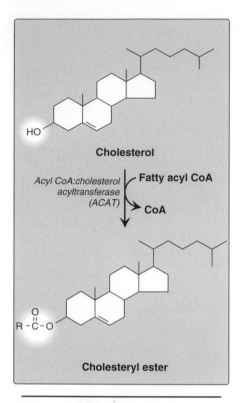

Figure 18.21
Synthesis of intracellular cholesteryl ester by *ACAT*. [Note: *Lecithin: cholesterol acyl transferase* (*LCAT*) is the extracellular enzyme that esterifies cholesterol using phosphatidylcholine (lecithin) as the source of the fatty acid.] CoA = coenzyme A.

to increased intracellular cholesterol. Cholesteryl esters accumulate in macrophages and cause their transformation into "foam" cells, which participate in the formation of atherosclerotic plaque (Fig. 18.22). LDL-C is the primary cause of atherosclerosis.

E. High-density lipoprotein metabolism

HDL comprise a heterogeneous family of lipoproteins with a complex metabolism that is not yet completely understood. HDL particles are formed in the blood by the addition of lipid to apo A-1, an apolipoprotein made and secreted by the liver and intestine. Apo A-1 accounts for ~70% of the apolipoproteins in HDL. HDL perform a number of important functions, including the following.

1. **Apolipoprotein supply:** HDL particles serve as a circulating reservoir of apo C-II (the apolipoprotein that is transferred to VLDL and chylomicrons and is an activator of *LPL*) and apo E (the apolipoprotein required for the receptor-mediated endocytosis of IDL and chylomicron remnants).

2. **Nonesterified cholesterol uptake:** Nascent HDL are disc-shaped particles containing primarily phospholipid (largely PC) and apo A, C, and E. They take up cholesterol from nonhepatic (peripheral) tissues and return it to the liver as cholesteryl esters (Fig. 18.23). [Note: HDL particles are excellent acceptors of nonesterified cholesterol as a result of their high concentration of phospholipids, which are important solubilizers of cholesterol.]

3. **Cholesterol esterification:** The cholesterol taken up by HDL is immediately esterified by the plasma enzyme *lecithin:cholesterol acyltransferase* (*LCAT*, also known as *PCAT*, in which P stands for phosphatidylcholine, the source of the FA). This enzyme is synthesized and secreted by the liver. *LCAT* binds to nascent HDL and is activated by apo A-I. *LCAT* transfers the FA from carbon 2 of PC to cholesterol. This produces a hydrophobic cholesteryl ester, which is sequestered in the core of the HDL, and lysophosphatidylcholine, which binds to albumin. [Note: Esterification maintains the cholesterol concentration gradient, allowing continued efflux of cholesterol to HDL.] As the discoidal nascent HDL accumulates cholesteryl esters, it first becomes a spherical, relatively cholesteryl ester–poor HDL3 and, eventually, a cholesteryl ester–rich HDL2 particle that carries these esters to the liver. *Hepatic lipase*, which degrades TAG and phospholipids, participates in the conversion of HDL2 to HDL3 (see Fig. 18.23). *CETP* (see p. 231) transfers some of the cholesteryl esters from HDL to VLDL in exchange for TAG, relieving product inhibition of *LCAT*. Because VLDL are catabolized to LDL, the cholesteryl esters transferred by *CETP* are ultimately taken up by the liver (see p. 231).

4. **Reverse cholesterol transport:** The selective transfer of cholesterol from peripheral cells to HDL and from HDL to the liver for bile acid synthesis or disposal via the bile is a key component of cholesterol homeostasis. This process of reverse cholesterol transport (RCT) is, in part, the basis for the inverse relationship seen between plasma HDL concentration and atherosclerosis and for

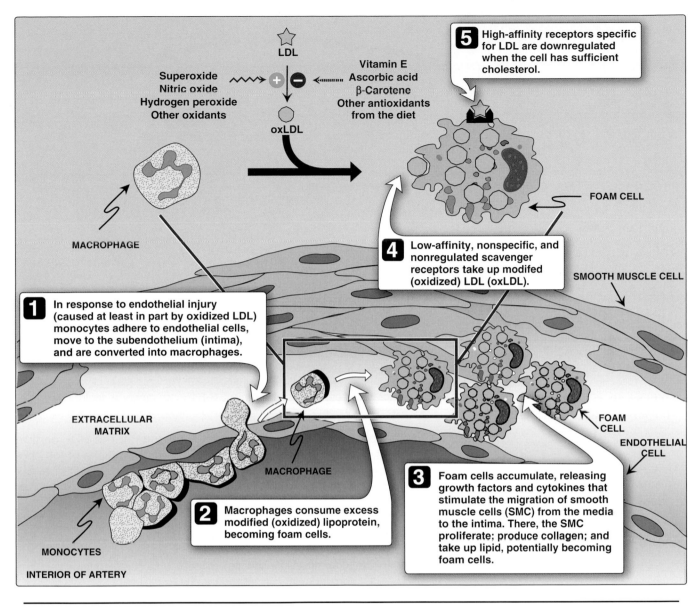

Figure 18.22
Role of oxidized low-density lipoprotein (LDL) particles in plaque formation in an arterial wall.

the designation of HDL as the "good" cholesterol carrier. [Note: Exercise and estrogen raise HDL levels.] RCT involves efflux of cholesterol from peripheral cells to HDL, esterification of the cholesterol by *LCAT*, binding of the cholesteryl ester–rich HDL (HDL2) to liver (and, perhaps, steroidogenic cells), selective transfer of the cholesteryl esters into these cells, and release of lipid-depleted HDL (HDL3). The efflux of cholesterol from peripheral cells is mediated primarily by the transport protein ABCA1. [Note: Tangier disease is a very rare deficiency of ABCA1 and is characterized by the virtual absence of HDL particles due to degradation of lipid-poor apo A-1.] Cholesteryl ester uptake by the liver is mediated by the cell-surface receptor SR-B1 (scavenger receptor class B type 1)

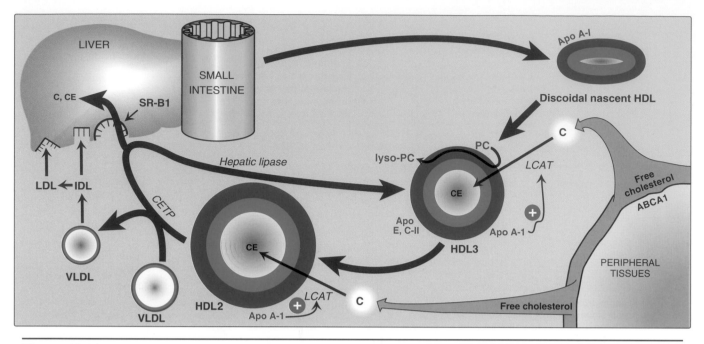

Figure 18.23
Metabolism of high-density lipoprotein (HDL) particles. Apo = apolipoprotein; ABCA1 = ATP-binding cassette transport protein; C = cholesterol; CE = cholesteryl ester; *LCAT = lecithin:cholesterol acyltransferase*; VLDL, IDL, and LDL = very-low-, intermediate-, and low-density lipoproteins; *CETP = cholesteryl ester transfer protein*; SR-B1 = scavenger receptor B1.

that binds HDL (see p. 232 for SR-A receptors). The HDL particle itself is not taken up. Instead, there is selective uptake of the cholesteryl ester from the HDL particle. [Note: Low HDL-C is a risk factor for atherosclerosis.]

> ABCA1 is an ATP-binding cassette (ABC) protein. ABC proteins use energy from ATP hydrolysis to transport materials, including lipids, in and out of cells and across intracellular compartments. In addition to Tangier disease, defects in specific ABC proteins result in sitosterolemia, cystic fibrosis, X-linked adrenoleukodystrophy, respiratory distress syndrome due to decreased surfactant secretion, and liver disease due to decreased bile salt secretion.

F. Lipoprotein (a) and heart disease

Lipoprotein (a), or Lp(a), is nearly identical in structure to an LDL particle. Its distinguishing feature is the presence of an additional apolipoprotein molecule, apo(a), which is covalently linked at a single site to apo B-100. Circulating levels of Lp(a) are determined primarily by genetics. However, factors such as diet may play some role, as trans FA have been reported to increase it. The physiologic function of Lp(a) is unknown. When present in large quantities in the plasma, Lp(a) is associated with an increased risk of coronary heart disease. [Note: Apo(a) is structurally homologous to plasminogen, the precursor of a blood *protease* whose target is fibrin, the main protein component of blood clots (see Chapter 35 online). It is hypothesized that elevated Lp(a) slows the breakdown of blood clots that trigger heart attacks because it competes with plasminogen for binding to fibrin.] Niacin reduces Lp(a), as well as LDL-C and TAG, and raises HDL-C.

VII. STEROID HORMONES

Cholesterol is the precursor of all classes of steroid hormones: glucocorticoids (for example, cortisol), mineralocorticoids (for example, aldosterone), and the sex hormones (that is, androgens, estrogens, and progestins), as shown in Figure 18.24. [Note: Glucocorticoids and mineralocorticoids are collectively called corticosteroids.] Synthesis and secretion occur in the adrenal cortex (cortisol, aldosterone, and androgens), ovaries and placenta (estrogens and progestins), and testes (testosterone). Steroid hormones are transported by the blood from their sites of synthesis to their target organs. Because of their hydrophobicity, they must be complexed with a plasma protein. Albumin can act as a nonspecific carrier and does carry aldosterone. However, specific steroid-carrier plasma proteins bind the steroid hormones more tightly than does albumin (for example, corticosteroid-binding globulin, or transcortin, is responsible for transporting cortisol). A number of genetic diseases are caused by deficiencies in specific steps in the biosynthesis of steroid hormones. Some representative diseases are described in Figure 18.25.

A. Synthesis

Synthesis involves shortening the hydrocarbon chain of cholesterol and hydroxylating the steroid nucleus. The initial and rate-limiting reaction converts cholesterol to the 21-carbon pregnenolone. It is catalyzed by the *cholesterol side-chain cleavage enzyme*, a *cytochrome P450 (CYP) mixed function oxidase* of the inner mitochondrial membrane (see p. 149) that is also known as *P450$_{scc}$* and *desmolase*. NADPH and O_2 are required for the reaction. The cholesterol substrate can be newly synthesized, taken up from lipoproteins, or released by an *esterase* from cholesteryl esters stored in the cytosol of steroidogenic tissues. The cholesterol moves to the outer mitochondrial membrane. An important control point is the subsequent movement from the outer to the inner mitochondrial membrane. This process is mediated by StAR (steroidogenic acute regulatory) protein. Pregnenolone is the parent compound for all steroid hormones (see Fig. 18.25). It is oxidized and then isomerized to progesterone, which is further modified to the other steroid hormones by CYP protein–catalyzed hydroxylation reactions in the SER and mitochondria. A defect in the activity or amount of an enzyme in this pathway can lead to a deficiency in the synthesis of hormones beyond the affected

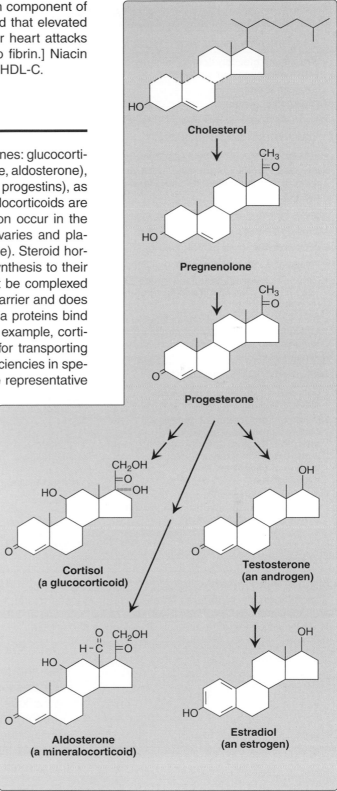

Figure 18.24
Key steroid hormones.

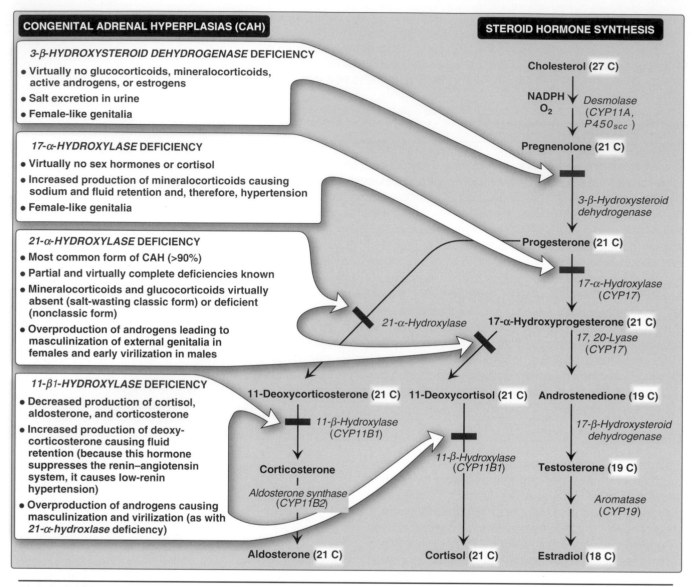

Figure 18.25
Steroid hormone synthesis and associated diseases. [Note: *3-β-Hydroxysteroid dehydrogenase*, *CYP17*, and *CYP11B2* are multifunctional enzymes. Synthesis of testosterone and the estrogens occurs primarily outside of the adrenal gland.] NADPH = nicotinamide adenine dinucleotide phosphate; CYP = cytochrome P450.

step and to an excess in the hormones or metabolites before that step. Because all members of the pathway have potent biologic activity, serious metabolic imbalances occur with enzyme deficiencies (see Fig. 18.25). Collectively, these disorders are known as the congenital adrenal hyperplasias (CAH), because they result in enlarged adrenals. [Note: Addison disease, due to autoimmune destruction of the adrenal cortex, is characterized by adrenocortical insufficiency.]

B. Adrenal cortical steroid hormones

Steroid hormones are synthesized and secreted in response to hormonal signals. The corticosteroids and androgens are made in different regions of the adrenal cortex and are secreted into blood in response to different signals. [Note: The adrenal medulla makes catecholamines (see p. 285).]

1. **Cortisol:** Its production in the middle layer (zona fasciculata) of the adrenal cortex is controlled by the hypothalamus, to which the pituitary gland is attached (Fig. 18.26). In response to severe stress (for example, infection), corticotropin-releasing hormone (CRH), produced by the hypothalamus, travels through capillaries to the anterior lobe of the pituitary, where it induces the production and secretion of adrenocorticotropic hormone (ACTH), a peptide. ACTH stimulates the adrenal cortex to synthesize and secrete the glucocorticoid cortisol, the stress hormone. [Note: ACTH binds to a membrane G protein–coupled receptor, resulting in cyclic AMP (cAMP) production and activation of *protein kinase A* ([*PKA*] see p. 94). *PKA* phosphorylates and activates both the *esterase* that converts cholesteryl ester to free cholesterol and StAR protein.] Cortisol allows the body to respond to stress through its effects on intermediary metabolism (for example, increased gluconeogenesis) and the inflammatory and immune responses (which are decreased). As cortisol levels rise, the release of CRH and ACTH is inhibited. [Note: The reduction of cortisol in CAH results in a rise in ACTH that causes adrenal hyperplasia.]

2. **Aldosterone:** Its production in the outer layer (zona glomerulosa) of the adrenal cortex is induced by a decrease in the plasma Na+/potassium (K+) ratio and by the hormone angiotensin II (Ang-II). Ang-II (an octapeptide) is produced from angiotensin I ([Ang-I] a decapeptide) by *angiotensin-converting enzyme* (*ACE*), an enzyme found predominantly in the lungs but also distributed widely in the body. [Note: Ang-I is produced in the blood by cleavage of an inactive precursor, angiotensinogen, secreted by the liver. Cleavage is catalyzed by *renin*, made and secreted by the kidneys.] Ang-II binds to cell surface receptors. However, in contrast to ACTH, its effects are mediated through the phosphatidylinositol 4,5-bisphosphate pathway (see p. 205) and not by cAMP. Aldosterone's primary effect is on the kidney tubules, where it stimulates Na+ and water uptake and K+ excretion (Fig. 18.27). [Note: An effect of aldosterone is an increase in blood pressure. Competitive inhibitors of *ACE* are used to treat *renin*-dependent hypertension.]

3. **Androgens:** Both the inner (zona reticularis) and middle layers of the adrenal cortex produce androgens, primarily dehydroepiandrosterone and androstenedione. Although adrenal androgens themselves are weak, they are converted by *aromatase* (*CYP19*) to testosterone, a stronger androgen, in the testes and to estrogens in the ovaries (primarily) of premenopausal women. [Note: Postmenopausal women produce estrogen at extragonadal sites such as the breast. *Aromatase* inhibitors are used in the treatment of estrogen-responsive breast cancer in these women.]

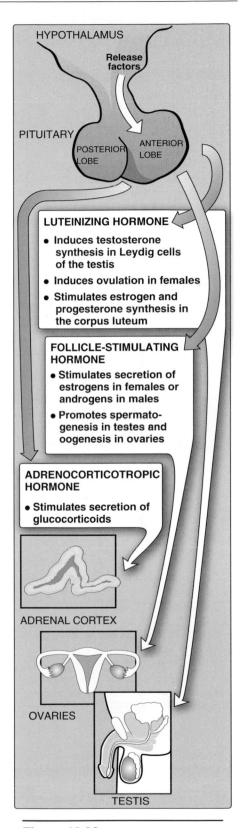

Figure 18.26
Pituitary hormone stimulation of steroid hormone synthesis and secretion.

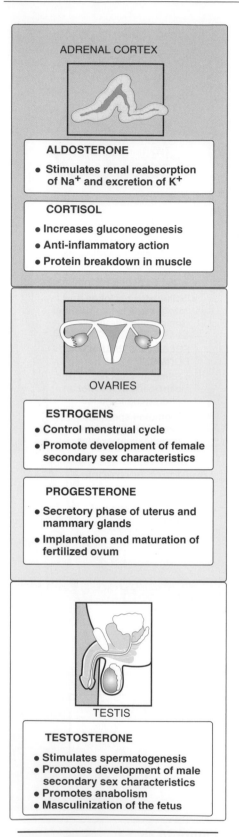

Figure 18.27
Actions of steroid hormones. Na⁺ = sodium; K⁺ = potassium.

C. Gonadal steroid hormones

The testes and ovaries (gonads) synthesize hormones necessary for sexual differentiation and reproduction. A single hypothalamic-releasing factor, gonadotropin-releasing hormone, stimulates the anterior pituitary to release the glycoproteins luteinizing hormone (LH) and follicle-stimulating hormone (FSH). Like ACTH, LH and FSH bind to surface receptors and cause an increase in cAMP. LH stimulates the testes to produce testosterone and the ovaries to produce estrogens and progesterone (see Fig. 18.27). FSH regulates the growth of ovarian follicles and stimulates testicular spermatogenesis.

D. Mechanism

Each steroid hormone diffuses across the plasma membrane of its target cell and binds to a specific cytosolic or nuclear receptor. These receptor–ligand complexes accumulate in the nucleus, dimerize, and bind to specific regulatory DNA sequences (hormone response elements [HRE]) in association with coactivator proteins, thereby causing increased transcription of targeted genes (Fig. 18.28). An HRE is found in the promoter or an enhancer element (see p. 440) for genes that respond to a specific steroid hormone, thus insuring coordinated regulation of these genes. Hormone–receptor complexes can also inhibit transcription in association with corepressors. [Note: The binding of a hormone to its receptor causes a conformational change in the receptor that uncovers its DNA-binding domain, allowing the complex to interact through a zinc finger motif with the appropriate DNA sequence. Receptors for the steroid hormones, plus those for thyroid hormone, retinoic acid (see p. 386), and 1,25-dihydroxycholecalciferol (vitamin D; see p. 390), are members of a superfamily of structurally related gene regulators that function in a similar way.]

E. Further metabolism

Steroid hormones are generally converted into inactive metabolic excretion products in the liver. Reactions include reduction of unsaturated bonds and the introduction of additional hydroxyl groups. The resulting structures are made more soluble by conjugation with glucuronic acid or sulfate (from 3′-phosphoadenosyl-5′-phosphosulfate; see p. 162). These conjugated metabolites are fairly water soluble and do not need protein carriers. They are eliminated in feces and urine.

VIII. CHAPTER SUMMARY

Cholesterol is a hydrophobic compound, with a single hydroxyl group located at carbon 3 of the A ring, to which a fatty acid (FA) can be attached, producing an even more hydrophobic **cholesteryl ester**. Cholesterol is synthesized by virtually all human tissues, although primarily by the **liver**, **intestine**, **adrenal cortex**, and **reproductive tissues** (Fig. 18.29). All the carbon atoms are provided by **acetyl coenzyme A (CoA)**, and **nicotinamide adenine dinucleotide phosphate** provides the reducing equivalents. The pathway is driven by hydrolysis of the high-energy thioester bond of acetyl CoA and the terminal phosphate bond of ATP. Synthesis requires enzymes of the **cytosol, smooth endoplasmic reticulum (SER)**, and **peroxisomes**. The rate-limiting and regulated step in cholesterol synthesis is catalyzed by the SER-membrane protein **hydroxymethylglutaryl coenzyme A (HMG CoA) reductase**, which produces **mevalonate** from HMG CoA. The enzyme is regulated by a number of mechanisms: 1) increased **expression** of the *reductase* gene when cholesterol levels are low, via the transcription factor, **sterol regulatory element–binding protein-2 (SREBP-2)**, bound to a **sterol regulatory element (SRE)**, resulting in increased enzyme and, therefore, cholesterol, synthesis; 2) accelerated **degradation** of the *reductase* protein when cholesterol levels are high; 3) **phosphorylation** (causing **inactivation** of *reductase* activity) by **adenosine monophosphate–activated protein kinase [AMPK]** and **dephosphorylation (activation)** by a *phosphoprotein phosphatase*; and 4) hormonal regulation by **insulin** and **glucagon**. **Statins** are **competitive inhibitors** of *HMG CoA reductase*. These drugs are used to decrease plasma cholesterol in patients with **hypercholesterolemia**. The ring structure of cholesterol cannot be degraded in humans.

Cholesterol is eliminated from the body either by conversion to bile salts or by secretion into the **bile**. **Bile salts** and **phosphatidylcholine (PC)** are quantitatively the most important organic components of bile. The rate-limiting step in bile acid synthesis is catalyzed by **cholesterol-7-α-hydroxylase**, which is inhibited by **bile acids**. Before the bile acids leave the liver, they are conjugated to a molecule of either **glycine** or **taurine**, producing the **conjugated bile salts glycocholic** or **taurocholic acid** and **glycochenodeoxycholic** or **taurochenodeoxycholic acid**. Bile salts (deprotonated) are more amphipathic than bile acids (protonated) and, therefore, are more effective **emulsifiers** of dietary fat. Intestinal **bacteria** can remove the glycine and taurine as well as a hydroxyl group from the steroid nucleus, producing the **secondary bile salts**, **deoxycholic** and **lithocholic acids**. Bile salts are efficiently reabsorbed (>95%) in the intestinal ileum by a **sodium–bile salt cotransporter**, returned to the blood, and carried by **albumin** back to the liver where they are taken up by the hepatic isoform of the cotransporter and reused (**enterohepatic circulation**, which **bile acid sequestrants** reduce). If more cholesterol enters the bile than can be solubilized by the available bile salts and PC, **cholesterol gallstone disease (cholelithiasis)** can occur.

The plasma lipoproteins (see Fig. 18.29) include **chylomicrons, very-low-density lipoproteins (VLDL), intermediate-density lipoproteins (IDL), low-density lipoproteins (LDL)**, and **high-density lipoproteins (HDL)**. They function to keep lipids (primarily **triacylglycerol [TAG]** and **cholesteryl esters**) soluble as they transport them between tissues. Lipoproteins are composed of a **neutral lipid (TAG, cholesteryl esters**, or both) core surrounded by a shell of **amphipathic apolipoproteins, phospholipid**, and **nonesterified cholesterol**. **Chylomicrons** are assembled in **intestinal mucosal cells** from **dietary lipids** (primarily TAG). Each nascent chylomicron particle has one molecule of **apolipoprotein (apo) B-48**. They are released from the cells into the lymphatic system and travel to the blood, where they receive **apo C-II** and **apo E** from HDL. Apo C-II activates endothelial **lipoprotein lipase (LPL)**, which degrades the TAG in chylomicrons to FA and glycerol. The **FA** that are released are stored (in **adipose tissue**) or used for energy (in **muscle**). The **glycerol** is

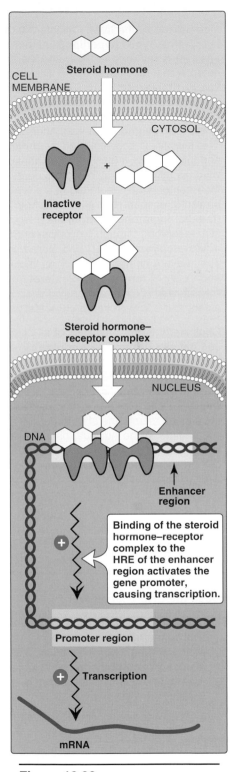

Figure 18.28
Activation of transcription by interaction of steroid hormone–receptor complex with hormone response element (HRE). The receptor contains domains that bind the hormone, DNA, and coactivating proteins. mRNA = messenger RNA.

metabolized by the **liver**. Patients with a **deficiency** of *LPL* or apo C-II show a dramatic accumulation of chylomicrons in the plasma (**type I hyperlipoproteinemia** or **familial chylomicronemia**) even if fasted. After most of the TAG is removed, apo C-II is returned to HDL, and the **chylomicron remnant**, carrying most of the **dietary cholesterol**, binds to a liver receptor that recognizes apo E. The particle is **endocytosed**, and its contents degraded by **lysosomal enzymes**. Defective uptake of these remnants (and IDL) causes **type III hyperlipoproteinemia** or **dysbetalipoproteinemia**. Nascent VLDL are produced in the liver and are composed predominantly of TAG. They contain a single molecule of **apo B-100**. Like chylomicrons, VLDL receive apo C-II and apo E from HDL in the plasma. VLDL carry hepatic TAG to the peripheral tissues where *LPL* degrades the lipid. Additionally, the VLDL particle receives **cholesteryl esters** from HDL in exchange for TAG. This process is accomplished by ***cholesteryl ester transfer protein*** (***CETP***). VLDL in the plasma is first converted to IDL and then to LDL, a much smaller, denser particle. Apo C-II and apo E are returned to HDL, but the LDL retains apo B-100, which is recognized by receptors on peripheral tissues and the liver. LDL undergo **receptor-mediated endocytosis**, and their contents are degraded in the **lysosomes**. The protease ***proprotein convertase subtilisin/kexin type 9*** (***PCSK9***) prevents receptor recycling. Defects in the synthesis of functional LDL receptors causes **type IIa hyperlipoproteinemia** (**familial hypercholesterolemia [FH]**). The endocytosed cholesterol decreases expression of *HMG CoA reductase* (and LDL receptors) through prevention of SREBP-2 binding to the SRE. Some of it can be esterified by ***acyl CoA:cholesterol acyltransferase*** (***ACAT***) and stored. HDL are created by **lipidation** of **apo A-1** synthesized in the liver and intestine. They have a number of functions, including 1) serving as a circulating **reservoir** of apo C-II and apo E for chylomicrons and VLDL; 2) removing **cholesterol** from peripheral tissues via ABCA1 and esterifying it using ***lecithin:cholesterol acyl transferase*** (***LCAT***), a liver-synthesized plasma enzyme that is activated by **apo A-1**; and 3) delivering these cholesteryl esters to the liver (**reverse cholesterol transport**) for uptake via **scavenger receptor-B1** (**SR-B1**).

Cholesterol is the precursor of all classes of **steroid hormones**, which include **glucocorticoids**, **mineralocorticoids**, and the **sex hormones** (**androgens**, **estrogens**, and **progestins**). Synthesis, using primarily ***cytochrome P450 mixed function oxidases***, occurs in the **adrenal cortex** (**cortisol** in the **zona fasciculata**, **aldosterone** in the **zona glomerulosa**, and **androgens** in the **zona reticularis**), **ovaries** and **placenta** (**estrogens** and **progestins**), and **testes** (**testosterone**). The initial and rate-limiting step is the conversion of cholesterol to **pregnenolone** by the side-chain cleavage enzyme $P450_{scc}$. Deficiencies in synthesis lead to **congenital adrenal hyperplasia** (**CAH**). Each steroid hormone diffuses across the plasma membrane of its target cell and binds to a specific intracellular receptor. These **receptor–hormone complexes** accumulate in the nucleus, dimerize, and bind to specific regulatory DNA sequences (**hormone response elements**) in association with coactivator proteins, thereby causing increased **transcription** of targeted genes. In association with corepressors, transcription is decreased.

Study Questions

Choose the ONE best answer.

18.1 Mice were genetically engineered to contain hydroxymethylglutaryl coenzyme A reductase in which serine 871, a phosphorylation site, was replaced by alanine. Which of the following statements concerning the modified form of the enzyme is most likely to be correct?

A. The enzyme is nonresponsive to ATP depletion.

B. The enzyme is nonresponsive to statin drugs.

C. The enzyme is nonresponsive to the sterol response element–sterol response element–binding protein system.

D. The enzyme is unable to be degraded by the ubiquitin–proteasome system.

Correct answer = A. The reductase is regulated by covalent phosphorylation and dephosphorylation. Depletion of ATP results in a rise in adenosine monophosphate (AMP), which activates AMP kinase (AMPK), thereby phosphorylating and inactivating the reductase. In the absence of the serine, a common phosphorylation site, the enzyme cannot be phosphorylated by AMPK. The enzyme is also regulated physiologically through changes in transcription and degradation and pharmacologically by statin drugs (competitive inhibitors), but none of these depends on serine phosphorylation.

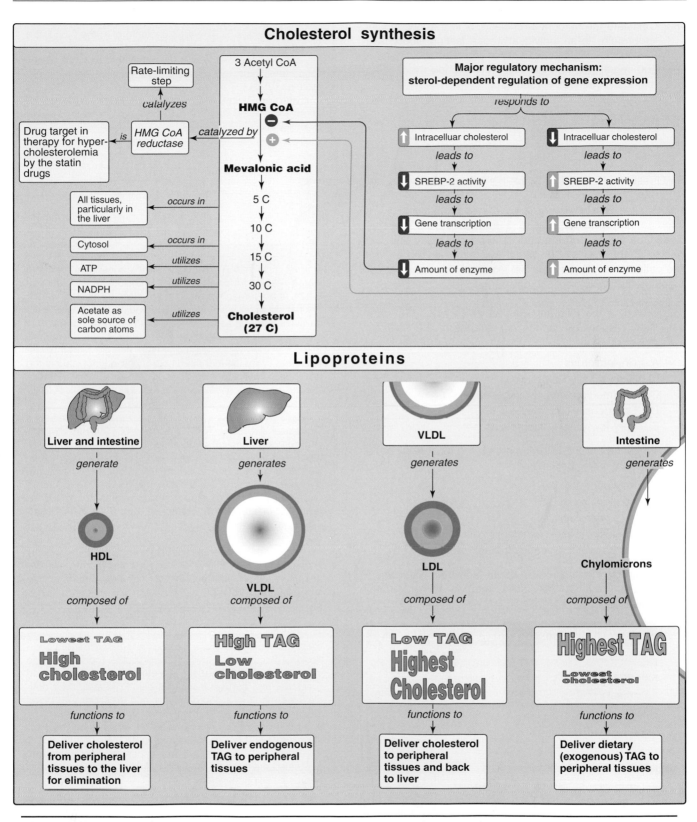

Figure 18.29
Concept map for cholesterol and the lipoproteins. HMG CoA = hydroxymethylglutaryl coenzyme A; SREBP = sterol regulatory element–binding protein; HDL, LDL, and VLDL = high-, low-, and very-low-density lipoproteins; TAG = triacylglycerol; NADPH = nicotinamide adenine dinucleotide phosphate; C = carbon.

18.2 Calculate the amount of cholesterol in the low-density lipoproteins in an individual whose fasting blood gave the following lipid-panel test results: total cholesterol = 300 mg/dl, high-density lipoprotein cholesterol = 25 mg/dl, triglycerides = 150 mg/dl.

A. 55 mg/dl
B. 95 mg/dl
C. 125 mg/dl
D. 245 mg/dl

Correct answer = D. The total cholesterol in the blood of a fasted individual is equal to the sum of the cholesterol in low-density lipoproteins plus the cholesterol in high-density lipoproteins plus the cholesterol in very-low-density lipoproteins (VLDL). This last term is calculated by dividing the triacylglycerol value by 5 because cholesterol accounts for about 1/5 of the volume of VLDL in fasted blood.

For Questions 18.3 and 18.4, use the following scenario.

A young girl with a history of severe abdominal pain was taken to her local hospital at 5 a.m. in severe distress. Blood was drawn, and the plasma appeared milky, with the triacylglycerol level >2,000 mg/dl (normal = 4–150 mg/dl). The patient was placed on a diet extremely limited in fat but supplemented with medium-chain triglycerides.

18.3 Which of the following lipoprotein particles are most likely responsible for the appearance of the patient's plasma?

A. Chylomicrons
B. High-density lipoproteins
C. Intermediate-density lipoproteins
D. Low-density lipoproteins
E. Very-low-density lipoproteins

Correct answer = A. The milky appearance of her plasma was a result of triacylglycerol-rich chylomicrons. Because 5 a.m. is presumably several hours after her evening meal, the patient must have difficulty degrading these lipoprotein particles. Intermediate-, low-, and high-density lipoproteins contain primarily cholesteryl esters, and, if one or more of these particles was elevated, it would cause hypercholesterolemia. Very-low-density lipoproteins do not cause the described milky appearance of plasma.

18.4 Which one of the following proteins is most likely to be deficient in this patient?

A. Apolipoprotein A-I
B. Apolipoprotein B-48
C. Apolipoprotein C-II
D. Cholesteryl ester transfer protein
E. Microsomal triglyceride transfer protein

Correct answer = C. The triacylglycerol (TAG) in chylomicrons is degraded by endothelial lipoprotein lipase (LPL), which requires apolipoprotein (apo) C-II as a coenzyme. Deficiency of LPL or apo C-II results in decreased ability to degrade chylomicrons to their remnants, which get cleared (via apo E) by liver receptors. Apo A-I is the coenzyme for lecithin:cholesterol acyltransferase; apo B-48 is the characteristic structural protein of chylomicrons; cholesteryl ester transfer protein catalyzes the cholesteryl ester–TAG exchange between high-density and very-low-density lipoproteins (VLDL); and microsomal triglyceride transfer protein is involved in the formation, not degradation, of chylomicrons (and VLDL).

18.5 Complete the table below for an individual with classic 21-α-hydroxylase deficiency relative to a normal individual.

Variable	Increased	Decreased
Aldosterone		
Androstenedione		
Cortisol		
Blood glucose		
Adrenocorticotropic hormone		
Blood pressure		

How might the results be changed if this individual were deficient in 17-α-hydroxylase, rather than 21-α-hydroxylase?

Classic 21-α-hydroxylase deficiency causes mineralocorticoids (aldosterone) and glucocorticoids (cortisol) to be virtually absent. Because aldosterone increases blood pressure, and cortisol increases blood glucose, their deficiencies result in a decrease in blood pressure and blood glucose, respectively. Cortisol normally feeds back to inhibit adrenocorticotropic hormone (ACTH) release by the pituitary, and, so, its absence results in an elevation in ACTH. The loss of 21-α-hydroxylase pushes progesterone and pregnenolone to androgen synthesis and, therefore, causes androstenedione levels to rise.

With 17-α-hydroxylase deficiency, sex hormone synthesis would be decreased. Mineralocorticoid production would be increased, leading to hypertension.

Amino Acids: Nitrogen Disposal

19

I. OVERVIEW

Unlike fats and carbohydrates, amino acids are not stored by the body. That is, no protein exists whose sole function is to maintain a supply of amino acids for future use. Therefore, amino acids must be obtained from the diet, synthesized de novo, or produced from the degradation of body protein. Any amino acids in excess of the biosynthetic needs of the cell are rapidly degraded. The first phase of catabolism involves the removal of the α-amino groups (usually by transamination and subsequent oxidative deamination), forming ammonia and the corresponding α-keto acids, the carbon skeletons of amino acids. A portion of the free ammonia is excreted in the urine, but most is used in the synthesis of urea (Fig. 19.1), which is quantitatively the most important route for disposing of nitrogen from the body. In the second phase of amino acid catabolism, described in Chapter 20, the carbon skeletons of the α-keto acids are converted to common intermediates of energy-producing metabolic pathways. These compounds can be metabolized to carbon dioxide (CO_2) and water (H_2O), glucose, fatty acids, or ketone bodies by the central pathways of metabolism described in Chapters 8–13 and 16.

II. OVERALL NITROGEN METABOLISM

Amino acid catabolism is part of the larger process of the metabolism of nitrogen-containing molecules. Nitrogen enters the body in a variety of compounds present in food, the most important being amino acids contained in dietary protein. Nitrogen leaves the body as urea, ammonia, and other products derived from amino acid metabolism (such as creatinine, see p. 287). The role of body proteins in these transformations involves two important concepts: the amino acid pool and protein turnover.

A. Amino acid pool

Free amino acids are present throughout the body, such as in cells, blood, and the extracellular fluids. For the purpose of this discussion,

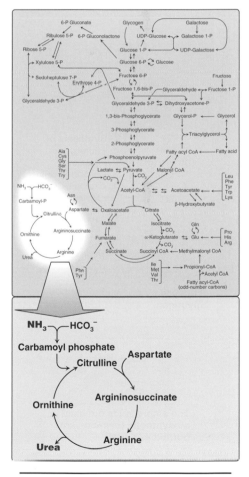

Figure 19.1
Urea cycle shown as part of the essential pathways of energy metabolism. [Note: See Fig. 8.2, p. 92, for a more detailed map of metabolism.] NH_3 = ammonia; CO_2 = carbon dioxide.

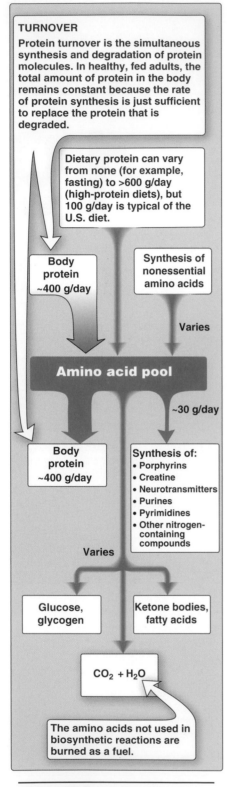

Figure 19.2
Sources and fates of amino acids. [Note: Nitrogen from amino acid degradation is released as ammonia, which is converted to urea and excreted.] CO_2 = carbon dioxide.

envision all of these amino acids as if they belonged to a single entity, called the amino acid pool. This pool is supplied by three sources: 1) amino acids provided by the degradation of endogenous (body) proteins, most of which are reutilized; 2) amino acids derived from exogenous (dietary) protein; and 3) nonessential amino acids synthesized from simple intermediates of metabolism (Fig. 19.2). Conversely, the amino acid pool is depleted by three routes: 1) synthesis of body protein, 2) consumption of amino acids as precursors of essential nitrogen-containing small molecules, and 3) conversion of amino acids to glucose, glycogen, fatty acids, and ketone bodies or oxidation to CO_2 + H_2O (see Fig. 19.2). Although the amino acid pool is small (comprising ~90–100 g of amino acids) in comparison with the amount of protein in the body (~12 kg in a 70-kg man), it is conceptually at the center of whole-body nitrogen metabolism.

> In healthy, well-fed individuals, the input to the amino acid pool is balanced by the output. That is, the amount of amino acids contained in the pool is constant. The amino acid pool is said to be in a steady state, and the individual is said to be in nitrogen balance (see p. 367).

B. Protein turnover

Most proteins in the body are constantly being synthesized and then degraded (turned over), permitting the removal of abnormal or unneeded proteins. For many proteins, regulation of synthesis determines the concentration of protein in the cell, with protein degradation assuming a minor role. For other proteins, the rate of synthesis is constitutive (that is, essentially constant), and cellular levels of the protein are controlled by selective degradation.

1. **Rate:** In healthy adults, the total amount of protein in the body remains constant because the rate of protein synthesis is just sufficient to replace the protein that is degraded. This process, called protein turnover, leads to the hydrolysis and resynthesis of 300–400 g of body protein each day. The rate of protein turnover varies widely for individual proteins. Short-lived proteins (for example, many regulatory proteins and misfolded proteins) are rapidly degraded, having half-lives measured in minutes or hours. Long-lived proteins, with half-lives of days to weeks, constitute the majority of proteins in the cell. Structural proteins, such as collagen, are metabolically stable and have half-lives measured in months or years.

2. **Protein degradation:** There are two major enzyme systems responsible for degrading proteins: the ATP-dependent ubiquitin (Ub)–proteasome system of the cytosol and the ATP-independent degradative enzyme system of the lysosomes. Proteasomes selectively degrade damaged or short-lived proteins. Lysosomes use *acid hydrolases* (see p. 162) to nonselectively degrade intracellular proteins (autophagy) and extracellular proteins (heterophagy), such as plasma proteins, that are taken into the cell by endocytosis.

a. **Ubiquitin–proteasome system:** Proteins selected for degradation by the cytosolic ubiquitin–proteasome system are first modified by the covalent attachment of Ub, a small, globular, nonenzymic protein that is highly conserved across eukaryotic species. Ubiquitination of the target substrate occurs through isopeptide linkage of the α-carboxyl group of the C-terminal glycine of Ub to the ε-amino group of a lysine in the protein substrate by a three-step, enzyme-catalyzed, ATP-dependent process. [Note: *Enzyme 1* (*E1*, an activating enzyme) activates Ub, which is then transferred to *E2* (a conjugating enzyme). *E3* (a *ligase*) identifies the protein to be degraded and interacts with *E2*-Ub. There are many more *E3* proteins than there are *E1* or *E2*.] The consecutive addition of four or more Ub molecules to the target protein generates a polyubiquitin chain. Proteins tagged with Ub chains are recognized by a large, barrel-shaped, macromolecular, proteolytic complex called a proteasome (Fig. 19.3). The proteasome unfolds, deubiquitinates, and cuts the target protein into fragments that are then further degraded by cytosolic *proteases* to amino acids, which enter the amino acid pool. The Ub is recycled. It is noteworthy that the selective degradation of proteins by the ubiquitin–proteosome complex (unlike simple hydrolysis by proteolytic enzymes) requires ATP hydrolysis.

b. **Degradation signals:** Because proteins have different half-lives, it is clear that protein degradation cannot be random but, rather, is influenced by some structural aspect of the protein that serves as a degradation signal, which is recognized and bound by an *E3*. The half-life of a protein is also influenced by the amino (N)-terminal residue, the so-called N-end rule, and ranges from minutes to hours. Destabilizing N-terminal amino acids include arginine and posttranslationally modified amino acids such as acetylated alanine. In contrast, serine is a stabilizing amino acid. Additionally, proteins rich in sequences containing proline, glutamate, serine, and threonine (called PEST sequences after the one-letter designations for these amino acids) are rapidly ubiquitinated and degraded and, therefore, have short half-lives.

III. DIETARY PROTEIN DIGESTION

Most of the nitrogen in the diet is consumed in the form of protein, typically amounting to 70–100 g/day in the American diet (see Fig. 19.2). Proteins are generally too large to be absorbed by the intestine. [Note: An example of an exception to this rule is that newborns can take up maternal antibodies in breast milk.] Therefore, proteins must be hydrolyzed to yield di- and tripeptides as well as individual amino acids, which can be absorbed. Proteolytic enzymes responsible for degrading proteins are produced by three different organs: the stomach, the pancreas, and the small intestine (Fig. 19.4).

A. Digestion by gastric secretion

The digestion of proteins begins in the stomach, which secretes gastric juice, a unique solution containing hydrochloric acid (HCl) and the proenzyme pepsinogen.

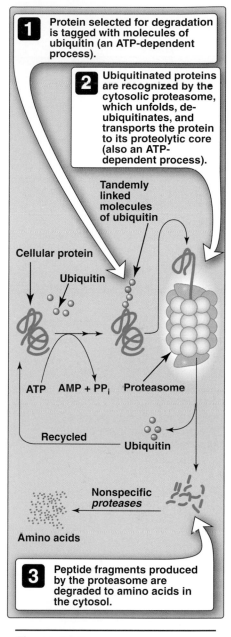

1 Protein selected for degradation is tagged with molecules of ubiquitin (an ATP-dependent process).

2 Ubiquitinated proteins are recognized by the cytosolic proteasome, which unfolds, de-ubiquitinates, and transports the protein to its proteolytic core (also an ATP-dependent process).

Tandemly linked molecules of ubiquitin

Cellular protein

Ubiquitin

ATP   AMP + PP_i   Proteasome

Recycled

Ubiquitin

Nonspecific *proteases*

Amino acids

3 Peptide fragments produced by the proteasome are degraded to amino acids in the cytosol.

Figure 19.3
The ubiquitin–proteasome degradation pathway of proteins. AMP = adenosine monophosphate; PP$_i$ = pyrophosphate.

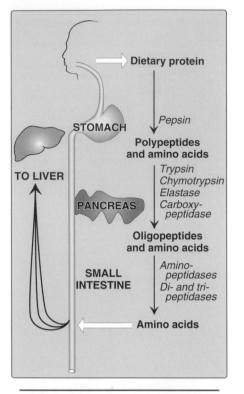

Figure 19.4
Digestion of dietary proteins by the proteolytic enzymes of the gastrointestinal tract.

1. **Hydrochloric acid:** Stomach HCl is too dilute (pH 2–3) to hydrolyze proteins. The acid, secreted by the parietal cells of the stomach, functions instead to kill some bacteria and to denature proteins, thereby making them more susceptible to subsequent hydrolysis by *proteases.*

2. **Pepsin:** This acid-stable *endopeptidase* is secreted by the chief cells of the stomach as an inactive zymogen (or proenzyme), pepsinogen. [Note: In general, zymogens contain extra amino acids in their sequences that prevent them from being catalytically active. Removal of these amino acids permits the proper folding required for an active enzyme.] In the presence of HCl, pepsinogen undergoes a conformational change that allows it to cleave itself (autocatalysis) to the active form, *pepsin,* which releases polypeptides and a few free amino acids from dietary proteins.

B. Digestion by pancreatic enzymes

On entering the small intestine, the polypeptides produced in the stomach by the action of *pepsin* are further cleaved to oligopeptides and amino acids by a group of pancreatic *proteases* that include both *endopeptidases* (that cleave within) and *exopeptidases* (that cut at an end). [Note: Bicarbonate (HCO_3^-), secreted by the pancreas in response to the intestinal hormone secretin, raises the intestinal pH.]

1. **Specificity:** Each of these enzymes has a different specificity for the amino acid R-groups adjacent to the susceptible peptide bond (Fig. 19.5). For example, *trypsin* cleaves only when the carbonyl group of the peptide bond is contributed by arginine or lysine. These enzymes, like *pepsin* described above, are synthesized and secreted as inactive zymogens.

2. **Zymogen release:** The release and activation of the pancreatic zymogens are mediated by the secretion of cholecystokinin, a polypeptide hormone of the small intestine (see p. 176).

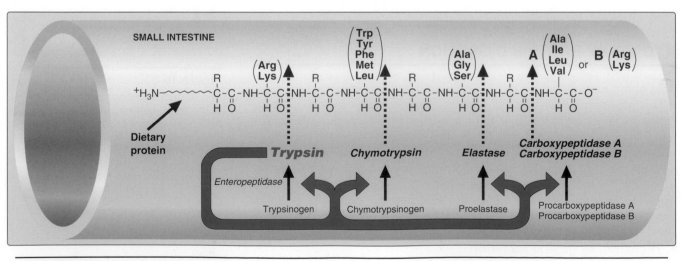

Figure 19.5
Cleavage of dietary protein in the small intestine by pancreatic *proteases.* The peptide bonds susceptible to hydrolysis are shown for each of the five major pancreatic *proteases.* [Note: The first three are serine *endopeptidases,* whereas the last two are *exopeptidases.* Each is produced from an inactive zymogen.]

3. **Zymogen activation:** *Enteropeptidase* (also called *enterokinase*), a *serine protease* synthesized by and present on the luminal (apical) surface of intestinal mucosal cells (enterocytes) of the brush border, converts the pancreatic zymogen trypsinogen to *trypsin* by removal of a hexapeptide from the N-terminus of trypsinogen. *Trypsin* subsequently converts other trypsinogen molecules to *trypsin* by cleaving a limited number of specific peptide bonds in the zymogen. Thus, *enteropeptidase* unleashes a cascade of proteolytic activity because *trypsin* is the common activator of all the pancreatic zymogens (see Fig. 19.5).

4. **Digestion abnormalities:** In individuals with a deficiency in pancreatic secretion (for example, because of chronic pancreatitis, cystic fibrosis, or surgical removal of the pancreas), the digestion and absorption of fat and protein are incomplete. This results in the abnormal appearance of lipids in the feces (a condition called steatorrhea; see p. 177) as well as undigested protein.

> Celiac disease (celiac sprue) is a disease of malabsorption resulting from immune-mediated damage to the small intestine in response to ingestion of gluten (or gliadin produced from gluten), a protein found in wheat, barley, and rye.

C. Digestion of oligopeptides by small intestine enzymes

The luminal surface of the enterocytes contains *aminopeptidase*, an *exopeptidase* that repeatedly cleaves the N-terminal residue from oligopeptides to produce even smaller peptides and free amino acids.

D. Amino acid and small peptide intestinal absorption

Most free amino acids are taken into enterocytes via sodium-dependent secondary active transport by solute carrier (SLC) proteins of the apical membrane. At least seven different transport systems with overlapping amino acid specificities are known. Di- and tripeptides, however, are taken up by a proton-linked peptide transporter (PepT1). The peptides are then hydrolyzed to free amino acids. Regardless of their source, free amino acids are released from enterocytes into the portal system by sodium-independent transporters of the basolateral membrane. Therefore, only free amino acids are found in the portal vein after a meal containing protein. These amino acids are either metabolized by the liver or released into the general circulation. [Note: Branched-chain amino acids (BCAA) are not metabolized by the liver but, instead, are sent from the liver to muscle via the blood.]

E. Absorption abnormalities

The small intestine and the proximal tubules of the kidneys have common transport systems for amino acid uptake. Consequently, a defect in any one of these systems results in an inability to absorb particular amino acids into the intestine and into the kidney tubules. For example, one system is responsible for the uptake of cystine and the dibasic amino acids ornithine, arginine, and lysine (represented as COAL). In the inherited disorder cystinuria, this carrier system is defective, and all four amino acids appear in the urine (Fig. 19.6).

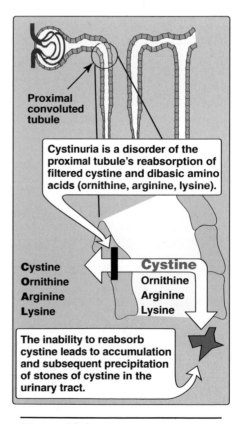

Proximal convoluted tubule

Cystinuria is a disorder of the proximal tubule's reabsorption of filtered cystine and dibasic amino acids (ornithine, arginine, lysine).

Cystine	Cystine
Ornithine	Ornithine
Arginine	Arginine
Lysine	Lysine

The inability to reabsorb cystine leads to accumulation and subsequent precipitation of stones of cystine in the urinary tract.

Figure 19.6
Genetic defect seen in cystinuria. [Note: Cystinuria is distinct from cystinosis, a rare defect in the transport of cystine out of lysosomes that results in the formation of cystine crystals within the lysosome and widespread tissue damage.]

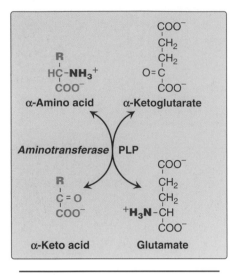

Figure 19.7
Aminotransferase reaction using
α-ketoglutarate as the amino group
acceptor. PLP = pyridoxal phosphate.

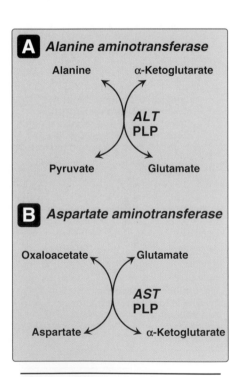

Figure 19.8
Reactions catalyzed during
amino acid catabolism. A. *Alanine
aminotransferase (ALT)*. B. *Aspartate
aminotransferase (AST)*. PLP =
pyridoxal phosphate.

Cystinuria occurs at a frequency of 1 in 7,000 individuals, making it one of the most common inherited diseases and the most common genetic error of amino acid transport. The disease expresses itself clinically by the precipitation of cystine to form kidney stones (calculi), which can block the urinary tract. Oral hydration is an important part of treatment for this disorder. [Note: Defects in the uptake of tryptophan by a neutral amino acid transporter can result in Hartnup disorder and pellagra-like (see p. 384) dermatologic and neurologic symptoms.]

IV. NITROGEN REMOVAL FROM AMINO ACIDS

The presence of the α-amino group keeps amino acids safely locked away from oxidative breakdown. Removing the α-amino group is essential for producing energy from any amino acid and is an obligatory step in the catabolism of all amino acids. Once removed, this nitrogen can be incorporated into other compounds or excreted as urea, with the carbon skeletons being metabolized. This section describes transamination and oxidative deamination, reactions that ultimately provide ammonia and aspartate, the two sources of urea nitrogen (see p. 253).

A. Transamination: Funneling amino groups to glutamate

The first step in the catabolism of most amino acids is the transfer of their α-amino group to α-ketoglutarate (Fig. 19.7), producing an α-keto acid (derived from the original amino acid) and glutamate. α-Ketoglutarate plays a pivotal role in amino acid metabolism by accepting the amino groups from most amino acids, thereby becoming glutamate. Glutamate produced by transamination can be oxidatively deaminated (see B. below) or used as an amino group donor in the synthesis of nonessential amino acids. This transfer of amino groups from one carbon skeleton to another is catalyzed by a family of enzymes called *aminotransferases* (also called *transaminases*). These enzymes are found in the cytosol and mitochondria of cells throughout the body. All amino acids, with the exception of lysine and threonine, participate in transamination at some point in their catabolism. [Note: These two amino acids lose their α-amino groups by deamination (see pp. 265–266).]

1. **Substrate specificity:** Each *aminotransferase* is specific for one or, at most, a few amino group donors. *Aminotransferases* are named after the specific amino group donor, because the acceptor of the amino group is almost always α-ketoglutarate. Two important *aminotransferase* reactions are catalyzed by *alanine aminotransferase (ALT)* and *aspartate aminotransferase (AST)*, as shown in Figure 19.8.

   a. **Alanine aminotransferase:** *ALT* is present in many tissues. The enzyme catalyzes the transfer of the amino group of alanine to α-ketoglutarate, resulting in the formation of pyruvate and glutamate. The reaction is readily reversible. However, during amino acid catabolism, this enzyme (like most *aminotransferases*) functions in the direction of glutamate synthesis. [Note: In effect, glutamate acts as a collector of nitrogen from most amino acids.]

b. Aspartate aminotransferase: *AST* is an exception to the rule that *aminotransferases* funnel amino groups to form glutamate. During amino acid catabolism, *AST* primarily transfers amino groups from glutamate to oxaloacetate, forming aspartate, which is used as a source of nitrogen in the urea cycle (see p. 255). Like other transaminations, the *AST* reaction is reversible.

2. **Mechanism:** All *aminotransferases* require the coenzyme pyridoxal phosphate (a derivative of vitamin B₆; see p. 382), which is covalently linked to the ε-amino group of a specific lysine residue at the active site of the enzyme. *Aminotransferases* act by transferring the amino group of an amino acid to the pyridoxal part of the coenzyme to generate pyridoxamine phosphate. The pyridoxamine form of the coenzyme then reacts with an α-keto acid to form an amino acid, at the same time regenerating the original aldehyde form of the coenzyme. Figure 19.9 shows these two component reactions for the transamination catalyzed by *AST*.

3. **Equilibrium:** For most transamination reactions, the equilibrium constant is near 1. This allows the reaction to function in both amino acid degradation through removal of α-amino groups (for example, after consumption of a protein-rich meal) and biosynthesis of nonessential amino acids through addition of amino groups to the carbon skeletons of α-keto acids (for example, when the supply of amino acids from the diet is not adequate to meet the synthetic needs of cells).

4. **Diagnostic value:** *Aminotransferases* are normally intracellular enzymes, with the low levels found in the plasma representing the release of cellular contents during normal cell turnover. Elevated plasma levels of *aminotransferases* indicate damage to cells rich in these enzymes. For example, physical trauma or a disease process can cause cell lysis, resulting in release of intracellular enzymes into the blood. Two *aminotransferases*, *AST* and *ALT*, are of particular diagnostic value when they are found in the plasma.

a. Hepatic disease: Plasma *AST* and *ALT* are elevated in nearly all hepatic diseases but are particularly high in conditions that cause extensive cell necrosis, such as severe viral hepatitis, toxic injury, and prolonged circulatory collapse. *ALT* is more specific than *AST* for liver disease, but the latter is more sensitive because the liver contains larger amounts of *AST*. Serial measurements of *AST* and *ALT* (liver function tests) are often useful in determining the course of liver damage. Figure 19.10 shows the early release of *ALT* into the blood, following ingestion of a liver toxin. [Note: The elevation in bilirubin results from hepatocellular damage that decreases the hepatic conjugation and excretion of bilirubin (see p. 282).]

b. Nonhepatic disease: *Aminotransferases* may be elevated in nonhepatic diseases such as those that cause damage to cardiac or skeletal muscle. However, these disorders can usually be distinguished clinically from liver disease.

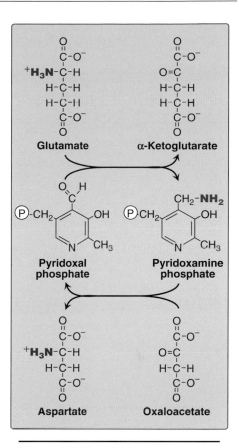

Figure 19.9
Cyclic interconversion of pyridoxal phosphate and pyridoxamine phosphate during the *aspartate aminotransferase* reaction.
Ⓟ = phosphate group.

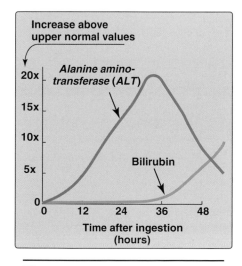

Figure 19.10
Pattern of *ALT* and bilirubin in the plasma, following poisoning by ingestion of the toxic mushroom <u>Amanita phalloides</u>.

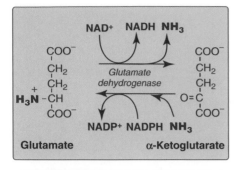

Figure 19.11
Oxidative deamination by *glutamate dehydrogenase*. [Note: The enzyme is unusual in that it uses both NAD$^+$ (nicotinamide adenine dinucleotide) and NADPH (nicotinamide adenine dinucleotide phosphate).] NH$_3$ = ammonia.

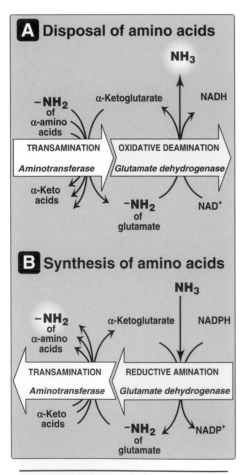

Figure 19.12
A, B. Combined actions of *aminotransferase* and *glutamate dehydrogenase* reactions. [Note: Reductive amination occurs only when ammonia (NH$_3$) level is high.] NAD(H) = nicotinamide adenine dinucleotide; NADP(H) = nicotinamide adenine dinucleotide phosphate.

B. Oxidative deamination: Amino group removal

In contrast to transamination reactions that transfer amino groups, oxidative deamination reactions result in the liberation of the amino group as free ammonia (Fig. 19.11). These reactions occur primarily in the liver and kidney. They provide α-keto acids that can enter the central pathways of energy metabolism and ammonia, which is a source of nitrogen in hepatic urea synthesis. [Note: Ammonia exists primarily as ammonium (NH$_4^+$) in aqueous solution, but it is the unionized form (NH$_3$) that crosses membranes.]

1. **Glutamate dehydrogenase:** As described above, the amino groups of most amino acids are ultimately funneled to glutamate by means of transamination with α-ketoglutarate. Glutamate is unique in that it is the only amino acid that undergoes rapid oxidative deamination, a reaction catalyzed by *glutamate dehydrogenase* ([*GDH*], see Fig. 19.11). Therefore, the sequential action of transamination (resulting in the transfer of amino groups from most amino acids to α-ketoglutarate to produce glutamate) and the oxidative deamination of that glutamate (regenerating α-ketoglutarate) provide a pathway whereby the amino groups of most amino acids can be released as ammonia.

   a. **Coenzymes:** *GDH*, a mitochondrial enzyme, is unusual in that it can use either nicotinamide adenine dinucleotide (NAD$^+$) or its phosphorylated reduced form (NADPH) as a coenzyme (see Fig. 19.11). NAD$^+$ is used primarily in oxidative deamination (the simultaneous loss of ammonia coupled with the oxidation of the carbon skeleton, as shown in Fig. 19.12A), whereas NADPH is used in reductive amination (the simultaneous gain of ammonia coupled with the reduction of the carbon skeleton, as shown in Fig. 19.12B).

   b. **Reaction direction:** The direction of the reaction depends on the relative concentrations of glutamate, α-ketoglutarate, and ammonia and the ratio of oxidized to reduced coenzymes. For example, after ingestion of a meal containing protein, glutamate levels in the liver are elevated, and the reaction proceeds in the direction of amino acid degradation and the formation of ammonia (see Fig. 19.12A). High ammonia levels are required to drive the reaction to glutamate synthesis.

   c. **Allosteric regulators:** Guanosine triphosphate is an allosteric inhibitor of *GDH*, whereas adenosine diphosphate is an activator. Therefore, when energy levels are low in the cell, amino acid degradation by *GDH* is high, facilitating energy production from the carbon skeletons derived from amino acids.

2. **D-Amino acid oxidase:** D-Amino acids (see p. 5) are supplied by the diet but are not used in the synthesis of mammalian proteins. They are, however, efficiently metabolized to α-keto acids, ammonia, and hydrogen peroxide in the peroxisomes of liver and kidney cells by flavin adenine dinucleotide–dependent *D-amino acid oxidase* (*DAO*). The α-keto acids can enter the general pathways of amino acid metabolism and be reaminated to L-isomers or catabolized for energy. [Note: *DAO* degrades D-serine, the isomeric form of serine that modulates N-methyl-D-aspartate (NMDA)-type

glutamate receptors. Increased *DAO* activity has been linked to increased susceptibility to schizophrenia. *DAO* also converts glycine to glyoxylate (see p. 263).] *L-Amino acid oxidases* are found in snake venom.

C. Ammonia transport to the liver

Two mechanisms are available in humans for the transport of ammonia from peripheral tissues to the liver for conversion to urea. Both are important in, but not exclusive to, skeletal muscle. The first uses *glutamine synthetase* to combine ammonia with glutamate to form glutamine, a nontoxic transport form of ammonia (Fig. 19.13). The glutamine is transported in the blood to the liver where it is cleaved by *glutaminase* to glutamate and ammonia (see p. 256). The glutamate is oxidatively deaminated to ammonia and α-ketoglutarate by *GDH*. The ammonia is converted to urea. The second transport mechanism involves the formation of alanine by the transamination of pyruvate produced from both aerobic glycolysis and metabolism of the succinyl coenzyme A (CoA) generated by the catabolism of the BCAA isoleucine and valine. Alanine is transported in the blood to the liver, where it is transaminated by *ALT* to pyruvate. The pyruvate is used to synthesize glucose, which can enter the blood and be used by muscle, a pathway called the glucose–alanine cycle. The glutamate product of *ALT* can be deaminated by *GDH*, generating ammonia. Thus, both alanine and glutamine carry ammonia to the liver.

V. UREA CYCLE

Urea ($H_2N\overset{O}{\overset{\|}{C}}NH_2$) is the major disposal form of amino groups derived from amino acids and accounts for ~90% of the nitrogen-containing components of urine. One nitrogen of the urea molecule is supplied by free ammonia and the other nitrogen by aspartate. [Note: Glutamate is the immediate precursor of both ammonia (through oxidative deamination by *GDH*) and aspartate nitrogen (through transamination of oxaloacetate by *AST*).] The carbon and oxygen of urea are derived from CO_2 (as HCO_3^-). Urea is produced by the liver and then is transported in the blood to the kidneys for excretion in the urine.

A. Reactions

The first two reactions leading to the synthesis of urea occur in the mitochondrial matrix, whereas the remaining cycle enzymes are located in the cytosol (Fig. 19.14). [Note: Gluconeogenesis (see p. 117) and heme synthesis (see p. 278) also involve both the mitochondrial matrix and the cytosol.]

1. **Carbamoyl phosphate formation:** Formation of carbamoyl phosphate by *carbamoyl phosphate synthetase I (CPS I)* is driven by cleavage of two molecules of ATP. Ammonia incorporated into carbamoyl phosphate is provided primarily by the oxidative deamination of glutamate by mitochondrial *GDH* (see Fig. 19.11). Ultimately, the nitrogen atom derived from this ammonia becomes one of the nitrogens of urea. *CPS I* requires N-acetylglutamate (NAG) as a positive allosteric activator (see Fig. 19.14). [Note: *Carbamoyl phosphate synthetase II* participates in the biosynthesis

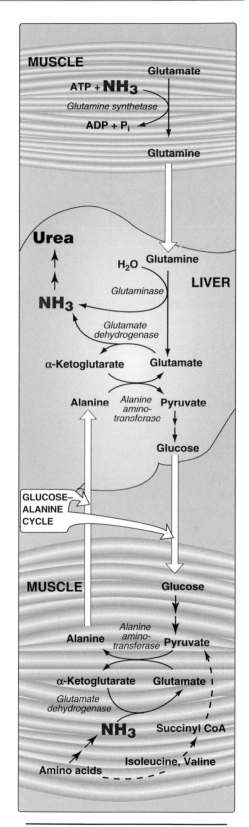

Figure 19.13
Transport of ammonia (NH_3) from muscle to the liver. ADP = adenosine diphosphate; P_i = inorganic phosphate; CoA = coenzyme A.

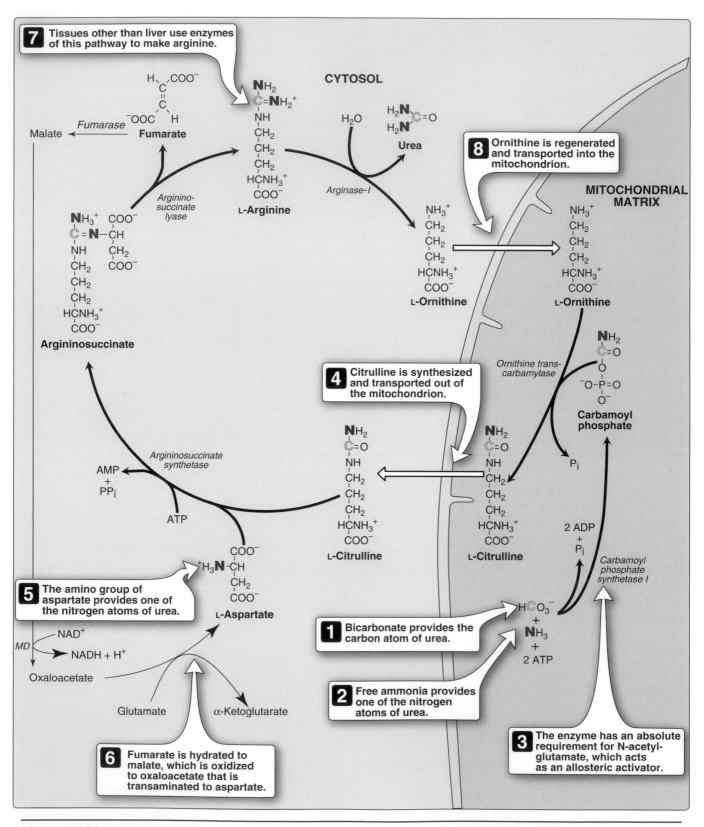

Figure 19.14

Reactions of the urea cycle. [Note: An antiporter transports citrulline and ornithine across the inner mitochondrial membrane.] ADP = adenosine diphosphate; AMP = adenosine monophosphate; PP$_i$ = pyrophosphate; P$_i$ = inorganic phosphate; NAD(H) = nicotinamide adenine dinucleotide; *MD = malate dehydrogenase*.

of pyrimidines (see p. 302). It does not require NAG, uses glutamine as the nitrogen source, and occurs in the cytosol.]

2. **Citrulline formation:** The carbamoyl portion of carbamoyl phosphate is transferred to ornithine by *ornithine transcarbamylase* (*OTC*) as the phosphate is released as inorganic phosphate. The reaction product, citrulline, is transported to the cytosol. [Note: Ornithine and citrulline move across the inner mitochondrial membrane via an antiporter. These basic amino acids are not incorporated into cellular proteins because there are no codons for them (see p. 447).] Ornithine is regenerated with each turn of the urea cycle, much in the same way that oxaloacetate is regenerated by the reactions of the tricarboxylic acid (TCA) cycle (see p. 109).

3. **Argininosuccinate formation:** *Argininosuccinate synthetase* combines citrulline with aspartate to form argininosuccinate. The α-amino group of aspartate provides the second nitrogen that is ultimately incorporated into urea. The formation of argininosuccinate is driven by the cleavage of ATP to adenosine monophosphate and pyrophosphate. This is the third and final molecule of ATP consumed in the formation of urea.

4. **Argininosuccinate cleavage:** Argininosuccinate is cleaved by *argininosuccinate lyase* to yield arginine and fumarate. The arginine serves as the immediate precursor of urea. The fumarate is hydrated to malate, providing a link with several metabolic pathways. Malate can be oxidized by *malate dehydrogenase* to oxaloacetate, which can be transaminated to aspartate (see Fig. 19.8) and enter the urea cycle (see Fig. 19.14). Alternatively, malate can be transported into mitochondria via the malate–aspartate shuttle (see p. 80), reenter the TCA cycle, and get oxidized to oxaloacetate, which can be used for gluconeogenesis (see p. 120). [Note: Malate oxidation generates NADH for oxidative phosphorylation (see p. 77), thereby reducing the energy cost of the urea cycle.]

5. **Arginine cleavage to ornithine and urea:** *Arginase-I* hydrolyzes arginine to ornithine and urea and is virtually exclusive to the liver. Therefore, only the liver can cleave arginine, thereby synthesizing urea, whereas other tissues, such as the kidney, can synthesize arginine from citrulline. [Note: *Arginase-II* in kidneys controls arginine availability for nitric oxide synthesis (see p. 150).]

6. **Fate of urea:** Urea diffuses from the liver and is transported in the blood to the kidneys, where it is filtered and excreted in the urine (see Fig. 19.19). A portion of the urea diffuses from the blood into the intestine and is cleaved to CO_2 and ammonia by bacterial *urease*. The ammonia is partly lost in the feces and is partly reabsorbed into the blood. In patients with kidney failure, plasma urea levels are elevated, promoting a greater transfer of urea from blood into the gut. The intestinal action of *urease* on this urea becomes a clinically important source of ammonia, contributing to the hyperammonemia often seen in these patients. Oral administration of antibiotics reduces the number of intestinal bacteria responsible for this ammonia production.

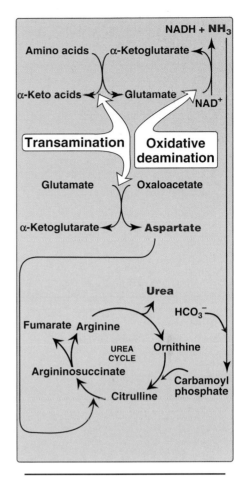

Figure 19.15
Flow of nitrogen from amino acids to urea. Amino groups for urea synthesis are collected in the form of ammonia (NH_3) and aspartate. NAD(H) = nicotinamide adenine dinucleotide; HCO_3^- = bicarbonate.

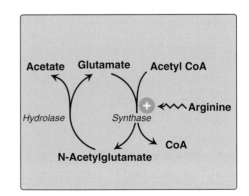

Figure 19.16
Formation and degradation of N-acetylglutamate, an allosteric activator of *carbamoyl phosphate synthetase I*. CoA = coenzyme A.

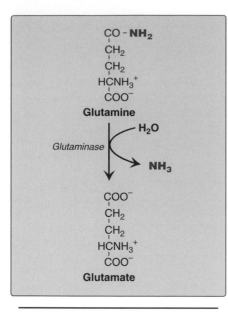

Figure 19.17
Hydrolysis of glutamine to form
ammonia (NH_3).

B. Overall stoichiometry

$$\text{Aspartate} + NH_3 + HCO_3^- + 3\ ATP + H_2O \rightarrow$$
$$\text{urea} + \text{fumarate} + 2\ ADP + AMP + 2\ P_i + PP_i$$

Because four high-energy phosphate bonds are consumed in the synthesis of each molecule of urea, the synthesis of urea is irreversible, with a large, negative ΔG (see p. 70). One nitrogen of the urea molecule is supplied by free ammonia and the other nitrogen by aspartate. Glutamate is the immediate precursor of both ammonia (through oxidative deamination by *GDH*) and aspartate nitrogen (through transamination of oxaloacetate by *AST*). In effect, both nitrogen atoms of urea arise from glutamate, which, in turn, gathers nitrogen from other amino acids (Fig. 19.15).

C. Regulation

NAG is an essential activator for *CPS I*, the rate-limiting step in the urea cycle. It increases the affinity of *CPS I* for ATP. NAG is synthesized from acetyl CoA and glutamate by *N-acetylglutamate synthase* (*NAGS*), as shown in Figure 19.16, in a reaction for which arginine is an activator. The cycle is also regulated by substrate availability (short-term regulation) and enzyme induction (long term).

VI. AMMONIA METABOLISM

Ammonia is produced by all tissues during the metabolism of a variety of compounds, and it is disposed of primarily by formation of urea in the liver. However, the blood ammonia level must be kept very low, because even slightly elevated concentrations (hyperammonemia) are toxic to the central nervous system (CNS). Therefore, a mechanism is required for the transport of nitrogen from the peripheral tissues to the liver for ultimate disposal as urea while keeping circulating levels of free ammonia low.

A. Sources

Amino acids are quantitatively the most important source of ammonia because most Western diets are high in protein and provide excess amino acids, which travel to the liver and undergo transdeamination (that is, the linking of the *aminotransferase* and *GDH* reactions), producing ammonia. [Note: The liver catabolizes straight-chain amino acids, primarily.] However, substantial amounts of ammonia can be obtained from other sources.

1. **Glutamine:** An important source of plasma glutamine is from the catabolism of BCAA in skeletal muscle. This glutamine is taken up by cells of the intestine, the liver, and the kidneys. The liver and kidneys generate ammonia from glutamine by the actions of *glutaminase* (Fig. 19.17) and *GDH*. In the kidneys, most of this ammonia is excreted into the urine as NH_4^+, which provides an important mechanism for maintaining the body's acid–base balance through the excretion of protons. In the liver, the ammonia is detoxified to urea and excreted. [Note: α-Ketoglutarate, the second product of *GDH*, is a glucogenic precursor in the liver and kidneys.]

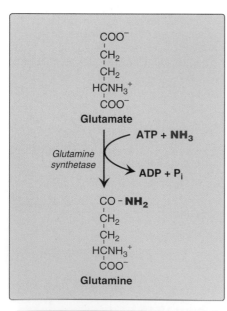

Figure 19.18
Synthesis of glutamine. ADP =
adenosine diphosphate; P_i =
inorganic phosphate; NH_3 =
ammonia.

Ammonia is also generated by intestinal *glutaminase*. Enterocytes obtain glutamine either from the blood or from digestion of dietary protein. [Note: Intestinal glutamine metabolism also produces alanine, which is used by the liver for gluconeogenesis, and citrulline, which is used by the kidneys to synthesize arginine.]

2. **Intestinal bacteria:** Ammonia is formed from urea by the action of bacterial *urease* in the lumen of the intestine. This ammonia is absorbed from the intestine by way of the portal vein, and virtually all is removed by the liver via conversion to urea.

3. **Amines:** Amines obtained from the diet and monoamines that serve as hormones or neurotransmitters give rise to ammonia by the action of *monoamine oxidase* (see p. 286).

4. **Purines and pyrimidines:** In the catabolism of purines and pyrimidines, amino groups attached to the ring atoms are released as ammonia (see Fig. 22.15 on p. 300).

B. Transport in the circulation

Although ammonia is constantly produced in the tissues, it is present at very low levels in blood. This is due both to the rapid removal of blood ammonia by the liver and to the fact that several tissues, particularly muscle, release amino acid nitrogen in the form of glutamine and alanine, rather than as free ammonia (see Fig. 19.13).

1. **Urea:** Formation of urea in the liver is quantitatively the most important disposal route for ammonia. Urea travels in the blood from the liver to the kidneys, where it passes into the glomerular filtrate.

2. **Glutamine:** This amide of glutamate provides a nontoxic storage and transport form of ammonia (Fig. 19.18). The ATP-requiring formation of glutamine from glutamate and ammonia by *glutamine synthetase* occurs primarily in skeletal muscle and the liver but is also important in the CNS, where it is the major mechanism for the removal of ammonia in the brain. Glutamine is found in plasma at concentrations higher than other amino acids, a finding consistent with its transport function. [Note: The liver keeps blood ammonia levels low through *glutaminase*, *GDH*, and the urea cycle in periportal (close to inflow of blood) hepatocytes and through *glutamine synthetase* as an ammonia scavenger in the perivenous hepatocytes.] Ammonia metabolism is summarized in Figure 19.19.

C. Hyperammonemia

The capacity of the hepatic urea cycle exceeds the normal rates of ammonia generation, and the levels of blood ammonia are normally low (5–35 μmol/l). However, when liver function is compromised, due either to genetic defects of the urea cycle or liver disease, blood levels can be >1,000 μmol/l. Such hyperammonemia is a medical emergency, because ammonia has a direct neurotoxic effect on the CNS. For example, elevated concentrations of ammonia in the blood cause the symptoms of ammonia intoxication, which include tremors, slurring of speech, somnolence (drowsiness), vomiting, cerebral edema, and blurring of vision. At high concentrations,

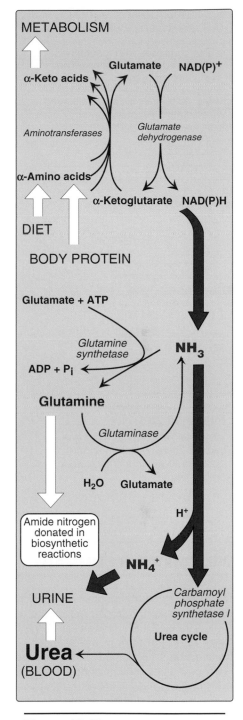

Figure 19.19
Ammonia (NH₃) metabolism. Urea content in the urine is reported as urinary urea nitrogen, or UUN. Urea in blood is reported as BUN (blood urea nitrogen). [Note: The enzymes *glutamate dehydrogenase*, *glutamine synthetase*, and *carbamoyl phosphate synthetase I* fix NH₃ into organic molecules.]

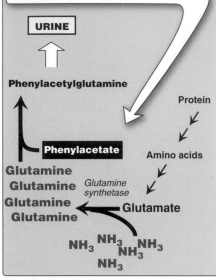

Phenylbutyrate is a prodrug that is rapidly converted to phenylacetate, which combines with glutamine to form phenylacetylglutamine. The phenylacetylglutamine, containing two atoms of nitrogen, is excreted in the urine, thereby assisting in clearance of nitrogenous waste.

Figure 19.20
Treatment of patients with urea cycle defects by administration of phenylbutyrate to aid in excretion of ammonia (NH_3).

ammonia can cause coma and death. There are two major types of hyperammonemia.

1. **Acquired:** Liver disease is a common cause of acquired hyperammonemia in adults and may be due, for example, to viral hepatitis or to hepatotoxins such as alcohol. Cirrhosis of the liver may result in formation of collateral circulation around the liver. As a result, portal blood is shunted directly into the systemic circulation and does not have access to the liver. Therefore, the conversion of ammonia to urea is severely impaired, leading to elevated levels of ammonia.

2. **Congenital:** Genetic deficiencies of each of the five enzymes of the urea cycle (and of *NAGS*) have been described, with an overall incidence of ~1:25,000 live births. X-linked *OTC* deficiency is the most common of these disorders, predominantly affecting males, although female carriers may become symptomatic. All of the other urea cycle disorders follow an autosomal-recessive inheritance pattern. In each case, the failure to synthesize urea leads to hyperammonemia during the first weeks following birth. [Note: The hyperammonemia seen with *arginase* deficiency is less severe because arginine contains two waste nitrogens and can be excreted in the urine.] Historically, urea cycle defects had high morbidity (neurologic manifestations) and mortality. Treatment included restriction of dietary protein in the presence of sufficient calories to prevent protein catabolism. Administration of compounds that bind covalently to nonessential amino acids, producing nitrogen-containing molecules that are excreted in the urine, has improved survival. For example, phenylbutyrate given orally is converted to phenylacetate. This condenses with glutamine to form phenylacetylglutamine, which is excreted (Fig. 19.20).

VII. CHAPTER SUMMARY

Nitrogen enters the body in a variety of compounds present in food, the most important being **amino acids** contained in **dietary protein**. Nitrogen leaves the body as **urea**, **ammonia**, and other products derived from amino acid metabolism (Fig. 19.21). Free amino acids in the body are produced by hydrolysis of dietary protein by *proteases* activated from their **zymogen** form in the stomach and intestine, degradation of tissue proteins, and de novo synthesis. This **amino acid pool** is consumed in the synthesis of body protein, metabolized for energy, or its members used as precursors for other nitrogen-containing compounds. Free amino acids from digestion are taken up by intestinal **enterocytes** via **sodium-dependent secondary active transport**. Small peptides are taken up via **proton-linked transport**. Note that body protein is simultaneously degraded and resynthesized, a process known as **protein turnover**. The concentration of a cellular protein may be determined by regulation of its synthesis or degradation. The ATP-dependent, cytosolic, selective **ubiquitin–proteasome** and ATP-independent, relatively nonselective **lysosomal** *acid hydrolases* are the two major enzyme systems that are responsible for degrading proteins. Nitrogen cannot be stored, and amino acids in excess of the biosynthetic needs of the cell are quickly degraded. The first phase of **catabolism** involves the transfer of the α-amino groups through **transamination** by **pyridoxal phosphate**–dependent *aminotransferases* (*transaminases*), followed by **oxidative deamination** of **glutamate** by *glutamate dehydrogenase*, forming **ammonia** and the corresponding α-keto **acids**. A portion of the free ammonia is excreted in the **urine**. Some ammonia is used in converting glutamate to **glutamine** for safe transport, but most is used in the hepatic synthesis of **urea**, which is quantitatively the most important route for disposing of nitrogen from the body. **Alanine** also carries nitrogen to the liver for disposal as urea. The two major causes of **hyperammonemia** (with its neurologic effects) are acquired liver disease and congenital deficiencies of urea cycle enzymes such as X-linked *ornithine transcarbamylase*.

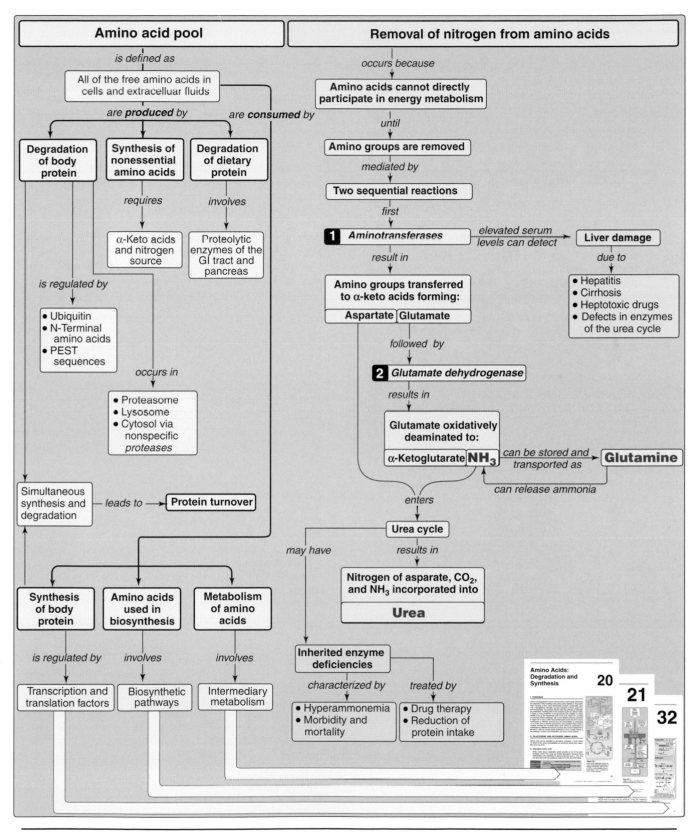

Figure 19.21

Key concept map for nitrogen metabolism. GI = gastrointestinal; PEST = proline, glutamate, serine, threonine; NH_3 = ammonia; CO_2 = carbon dioxide.

Study Questions

Choose the ONE best answer.

19.1 In this transamination reaction (right), which of the following are the products X and Y?

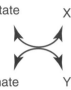

Oxaloacetate   X

Glutamate   Y

    A. Alanine, α-ketoglutarate
    B. Aspartate, α-ketoglutarate
    C. Glutamate, alanine
    D. Pyruvate, aspartate

19.2 Which one of the following statements about amino acids and their metabolism is correct?

    A. Free amino acids are taken into the enterocytes by a single proton-linked transport system.
    B. In healthy, well-fed individuals, the input to the amino acid pool exceeds the output.
    C. The liver uses ammonia to buffer protons.
    D. Muscle-derived glutamine is metabolized in liver and kidney tissue to ammonia + a gluconeogenic precursor.
    E. The first step in the catabolism of most amino acids is their oxidative deamination.
    F. The toxic ammonia generated from the amide nitrogen of amino acids is transported through blood as arginine.

For Questions 19.3–19.5, use the following scenario.

A female neonate appeared healthy until age ~24 hours, when she became lethargic. A sepsis workup proved negative. At 56 hours, she started showing focal seizure activity. The plasma ammonia level was found to be 887 μmol/l (normal 5–35 μmol/l). Quantitative plasma amino acid levels revealed a marked elevation of citrulline but not argininosuccinate.

19.3 Which one of the following enzymic activities is most likely to be deficient in this patient?

    A. Arginase
    B. Argininosuccinate lyase
    C. Argininosuccinate synthetase
    D. Carbamoyl phosphate synthetase I
    E. Ornithine transcarbamylase

19.4 Which one of the following would also be elevated in the blood of this patient?

    A. Asparagine
    B. Glutamine
    C. Lysine
    D. Urea

19.5 Why might supplementation with arginine be of benefit to this patient?

Correct answer = B. Transamination reactions always have an amino acid and an α-keto acid as substrates. The products of the reaction are also an amino acid (corresponding to the α-keto substrate) and an α-keto acid (corresponding to the amino acid substrate). Three amino acid α-keto acid pairs commonly encountered in metabolism are alanine/pyruvate, aspartate/oxaloacetate, and glutamate/α-ketoglutarate. In this question, glutamate is deaminated to form α-ketoglutarate, and oxaloacetate is aminated to form aspartate.

Correct answer = D. Glutamine, produced by the catabolism of branched-chain amino acids in muscle, is deaminated by glutaminase to ammonia + glutamate. The glutamate is deaminated by glutamate dehydrogenase to ammonia + α-ketoglutarate, which can be used for gluconeogenesis. Free amino acids are taken into enterocytes by several different sodium-linked transport systems. Healthy, well-fed individuals are in nitrogen balance, in which nitrogen input equals output. The liver converts ammonia to urea, and the kidneys use ammonia to buffer protons. Amino acid catabolism begins with transamination that generates glutamate. The glutamate undergoes oxidative deamination. Toxic ammonia is transported as glutamine and alanine. Arginine is synthesized and hydrolyzed in the hepatic urea cycle.

Correct answer = C. Genetic deficiencies of each of the five enzymes of the urea cycle, as well as deficiencies in N-acetylglutamate synthase, have been described. The accumulation of citrulline (but not argininosuccinate) in the plasma of this patient means that the enzyme required for the conversion of citrulline to argininosuccinate (argininosuccinate synthetase) is defective, whereas the enzyme that cleaves argininosuccinate (argininosuccinate lyase) is functional.

Correct answer = B. Deficiencies of the enzymes of the urea cycle result in the failure to synthesize urea and lead to hyperammonemia in the first few weeks after birth. Glutamine will also be elevated because it acts as a nontoxic storage and transport form of ammonia. Therefore, elevated glutamine accompanies hyperammonemia. Asparagine and lysine do not serve this sequestering role. Urea would be decreased because of impaired activity of the urea cycle. [Note: Alanine would also be elevated in this patient.]

The arginine will be cleaved by arginase to urea and ornithine. Ornithine will be combined with carbamoyl phosphate by ornithine transcarbamylase to form citrulline. Citrulline, containing one waste nitrogen, will be excreted.

Amino Acids: Degradation and Synthesis

20

I. OVERVIEW

Amino acid degradation involves removal of the α-amino group, followed by the catabolism of the resulting α-keto acids (carbon skeletons). These pathways converge to form seven intermediate products: oxaloacetate, pyruvate, α-ketoglutarate, fumarate, succinyl coenzyme A (CoA), acetyl CoA, and acetoacetate. The products directly enter the pathways of intermediary metabolism, resulting either in the synthesis of glucose, ketone bodies, or lipids or in the production of energy through their oxidation to carbon dioxide (CO_2) by the tricarboxylic acid (TCA) cycle. Figure 20.1 provides an overview of these pathways, with a more detailed summary presented in Figure 20.15 (see p. 269). Nonessential amino acids (Fig. 20.2) can be synthesized in sufficient amounts from the intermediates of metabolism or, as in the case of cysteine and tyrosine, from essential amino acids. In contrast, because the essential amino acids cannot be synthesized (or synthesized in sufficient amounts) by humans, they must be obtained from the diet in order for normal protein synthesis to occur. Genetic defects in the pathways of amino acid metabolism can cause serious disease.

II. GLUCOGENIC AND KETOGENIC AMINO ACIDS

Amino acids can be classified as glucogenic, ketogenic, or both, based on which of the seven intermediates are produced during their catabolism (see Fig. 20.2).

A. Glucogenic amino acids

Amino acids whose catabolism yields pyruvate or one of the intermediates of the TCA cycle are termed glucogenic. Because these intermediates are substrates for gluconeogenesis (see p. 118), they can give rise to the net synthesis of glucose in the liver and kidney.

Color-coding used in this chapter:	• **BLUE CAPS TEXT** = names of seven products of amino acid metabolism • **Red text** = names of glucogenic amino acids • **Brown text** = names of glucogenic and ketogenic amino acids • **Green text** = names of ketogenic amino acids • **Cyan text** = one-carbon compounds

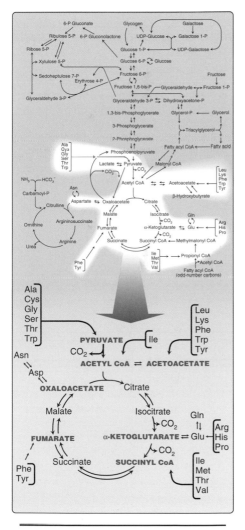

Figure 20.1

Amino acid metabolism shown as a part of the essential pathways of energy metabolism. (See Fig. 8.2, p. 92, for a more detailed map of metabolism.) CoA = coenzyme A; CO_2 = carbon dioxide.

Glucogenic	Glucogenic and Ketogenic	Ketogenic
Nonessential Alanine Arginine Asparagine Aspartate Cysteine Glutamate Glutamine Glycine Proline Serine	Tyrosine	
Essential Histidine Methionine Threonine Valine	Isoleucine Phenyl- alanine Tryptophan	Leucine Lysine

Figure 20.2
Classification of amino acids. [Note: Some amino acids can become conditionally essential. For example, supplementation with glutamine and arginine has been shown to improve outcomes in patients with trauma, postoperative infections, and immunosuppression.]

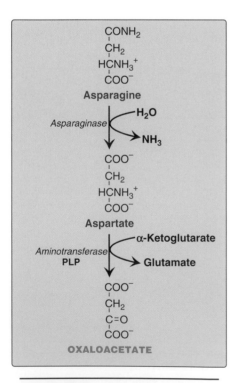

Figure 20.3
Metabolism of asparagine and aspartate. PLP = pyridoxal phosphate; NH_3 = ammonia.

B. Ketogenic amino acids

Amino acids whose catabolism yields either acetoacetate or one of its precursors (acetyl CoA or acetoacetyl CoA) are termed ketogenic (see Fig. 20.2). Acetoacetate is one of the ketone bodies, which also include 3-hydroxybutyrate and acetone (see p. 195). Leucine and lysine are the only exclusively ketogenic amino acids found in proteins. Their carbon skeletons are not substrates for gluconeogenesis and, therefore, cannot give rise to the net synthesis of glucose.

III. AMINO ACID CARBON SKELETON CATABOLISM

The pathways by which amino acids are catabolized are conveniently organized according to which one (or more) of the seven intermediates listed above is produced from a particular amino acid.

A. Amino acids that form oxaloacetate

Asparagine is hydrolyzed by *asparaginase*, liberating ammonia and aspartate (Fig. 20.3). Aspartate loses its amino group by transamination to form oxaloacetate (see Fig. 20.3). [Note: Some rapidly dividing leukemic cells are unable to synthesize sufficient asparagine to support their growth. This makes asparagine an essential amino acid for these cells, which, therefore, require asparagine from the blood. *Asparaginase*, which hydrolyzes asparagine to aspartate, can be administered systemically to treat leukemia. *Asparaginase* lowers the level of asparagine in the plasma, thereby depriving cancer cells of a required nutrient.]

B. Amino acids that form α-ketoglutarate via glutamate

1. **Glutamine:** This amino acid is hydrolyzed to glutamate and ammonia by the enzyme *glutaminase* (see p. 256). Glutamate is converted to α-ketoglutarate by transamination or through oxidative deamination by *glutamate dehydrogenase* (see p. 252).

2. **Proline:** This amino acid is oxidized to glutamate. Glutamate is transaminated or oxidatively deaminated to form α-ketoglutarate.

3. **Arginine:** This amino acid is hydrolyzed by *arginase* to produce ornithine (and urea). [Note: The reaction occurs primarily in the liver as part of the urea cycle (see p. 255).] Ornithine is subsequently converted to α-ketoglutarate, with glutamate semialdehyde as an intermediate.

4. **Histidine:** This amino acid is oxidatively deaminated by *histidase* to urocanic acid, which subsequently forms N-formiminoglutamate ([FIGlu], Fig. 20.4). FIGlu donates its formimino group to tetrahydrofolate (THF), leaving glutamate, which is degraded as described above. [Note: Individuals deficient in folic acid excrete increased amounts of FIGlu in the urine, particularly after ingestion of a large dose of histidine. The FIGlu excretion test has been used in diagnosing a deficiency of folic acid. See p. 267 for a discussion of folic acid, THF, and one-carbon metabolism.]

C. Amino acids that form pyruvate

1. **Alanine:** This amino acid loses its amino group by transamination to form pyruvate (Fig. 20.5). [Note: Tryptophan catabolism produces alanine and, therefore, pyruvate (see Fig. 20.10 on p. 265).]

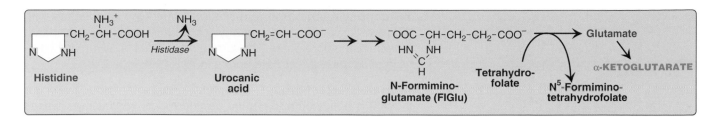

Figure 20.4
Degradation of histidine. NH$_3$ = ammonia.

2. **Serine:** This amino acid can be converted to glycine as THF becomes N^5,N^{10}-methylenetetrahydrofolate (N^5,N^{10}-MTHF), as shown in Figure 20.6A. Serine can also be converted to pyruvate (see Fig. 20.6B).

3. **Glycine:** This amino acid can be converted to serine by the reversible addition of a methylene group from N^5,N^{10}-MTHF (see Fig. 20.6A) or oxidized to CO$_2$ and ammonia by the glycine cleavage system. [Note: Glycine can be deaminated to glyoxylate (by a *D-amino acid oxidase*; see p. 253), which can be oxidized to oxalate or transaminated to glycine. Deficiency of the *transaminase* in liver peroxisomes causes overproduction of oxalate, the formation of oxalate stones, and kidney damage (primary oxaluria type 1).]

4. **Cysteine:** This sulfur-containing amino acid undergoes desulfurization to yield pyruvate. [Note: The sulfate released can be used to synthesize 3′-phosphoadenosine-5′-phosphosulfate (PAPS), an activated sulfate donor to a variety of acceptors.] Cysteine can also be oxidized to its disulfide derivative, cystine.

5. **Threonine:** This amino acid is converted to pyruvate in most organisms but is a minor pathway (at best) in humans.

D. Amino acids that form fumarate

1. **Phenylalanine and tyrosine:** Hydroxylation of phenylalanine produces tyrosine (Fig. 20.7). This irreversible reaction, catalyzed by tetrahydrobiopterin-requiring *phenylalanine hydroxylase* (*PAH*), initiates the catabolism of phenylalanine. Thus, phenylalanine metabolism and tyrosine metabolism merge, leading ultimately to fumarate and acetoacetate formation. Therefore, phenylalanine and tyrosine are both glucogenic and ketogenic.

2. **Inherited deficiencies:** Inherited deficiencies in the enzymes of phenylalanine and tyrosine metabolism lead to the diseases phenylketonuria (PKU) (see p. 270), tyrosinemia (see p. 274), and alkaptonuria (see p. 274) as well as the condition of albinism (see p. 273).

E. Amino acids that form succinyl CoA: Methionine

Methionine is one of four amino acids that form succinyl CoA. This sulfur-containing amino acid deserves special attention because it is converted to S-adenosylmethionine (SAM), the major methyl group donor in one-carbon metabolism (Fig. 20.8). Methionine is also the source of homocysteine (Hcy), a metabolite associated with atherosclerotic vascular disease and thrombosis (see p. 265).

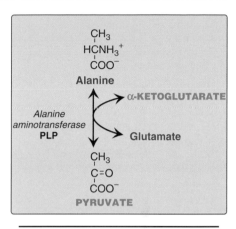

Figure 20.5
Transamination of alanine to pyruvate. PLP = pyridoxal phosphate.

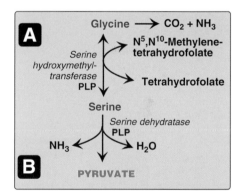

Figure 20.6
A. Interconversion of serine and glycine and oxidation of glycine. B. Dehydration of serine to pyruvate. PLP = pyridoxal phosphate; NH$_3$ = ammonia.

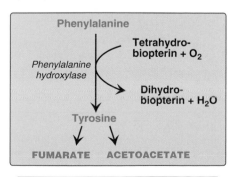

Figure 20.7
Degradation of phenylalanine.

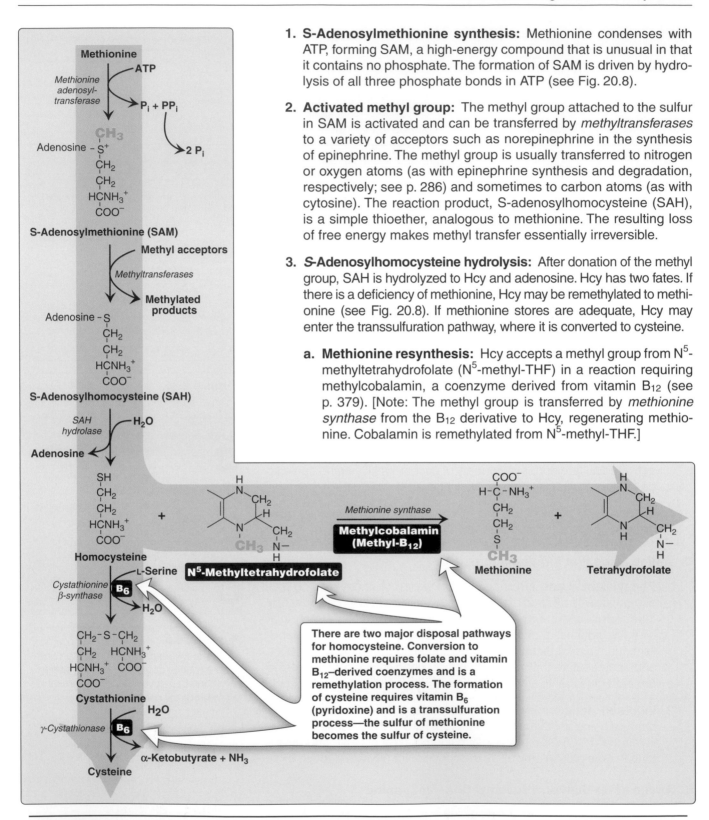

1. **S-Adenosylmethionine synthesis:** Methionine condenses with ATP, forming SAM, a high-energy compound that is unusual in that it contains no phosphate. The formation of SAM is driven by hydrolysis of all three phosphate bonds in ATP (see Fig. 20.8).

2. **Activated methyl group:** The methyl group attached to the sulfur in SAM is activated and can be transferred by *methyltransferases* to a variety of acceptors such as norepinephrine in the synthesis of epinephrine. The methyl group is usually transferred to nitrogen or oxygen atoms (as with epinephrine synthesis and degradation, respectively; see p. 286) and sometimes to carbon atoms (as with cytosine). The reaction product, S-adenosylhomocysteine (SAH), is a simple thioether, analogous to methionine. The resulting loss of free energy makes methyl transfer essentially irreversible.

3. *S*-**Adenosylhomocysteine hydrolysis:** After donation of the methyl group, SAH is hydrolyzed to Hcy and adenosine. Hcy has two fates. If there is a deficiency of methionine, Hcy may be remethylated to methionine (see Fig. 20.8). If methionine stores are adequate, Hcy may enter the transsulfuration pathway, where it is converted to cysteine.

   a. **Methionine resynthesis:** Hcy accepts a methyl group from N^5-methyltetrahydrofolate (N^5-methyl-THF) in a reaction requiring methylcobalamin, a coenzyme derived from vitamin B_{12} (see p. 379). [Note: The methyl group is transferred by *methionine synthase* from the B_{12} derivative to Hcy, regenerating methionine. Cobalamin is remethylated from N^5-methyl-THF.]

Figure 20.8

Degradation and resynthesis of methionine. [Note: The resynthesis of methionine from homocysteine is the only reaction in which tetrahydrofolate both carries and donates a methyl ($-CH_3$) group. In all other reactions, SAM is the methyl group carrier and donor.] PP_i = pyrophosphate; P_i = inorganic phosphate; NH_3 = ammonia.

b. Cysteine synthesis: Hcy condenses with serine, forming cystathionine, which is hydrolyzed to α-ketobutyrate and cysteine (see Fig. 20.8). This vitamin B6–requiring sequence has the net effect of converting serine to cysteine and Hcy to α-ketobutyrate, which is oxidatively decarboxylated to form propionyl CoA. Propionyl CoA is converted to succinyl CoA (see Fig. 16.20 on p. 195). Because Hcy is synthesized from the essential amino acid methionine, cysteine is not an essential amino acid as long as sufficient methionine is available.

4. **Relationship of homocysteine to vascular disease:** Elevations in plasma Hcy levels promote oxidative damage, inflammation, and endothelial dysfunction and are an independent risk factor for occlusive vascular diseases such as cardiovascular disease (CVD) and stroke (Fig. 20.9). Mild elevations (hyperhomocysteinemia) are seen in ~7% of the population. Epidemiologic studies have shown that plasma Hcy levels are inversely related to plasma levels of folate, B12, and B6, the three vitamins involved in the conversion of Hcy to methionine and cysteine. Supplementation with these vitamins has been shown to reduce circulating levels of Hcy. However, in patients with established CVD, vitamin therapy does not decrease cardiovascular events or death. This raises the question as to whether Hcy is a cause of the vascular damage or merely a marker of such damage. [Note: Large elevations in plasma Hcy as a result of rare deficiencies in *cystathionine β-synthase* of the transsulfuration pathway are seen in patients with classic homocystinuria (resulting from severe hyperhomocysteinemia [>100 μmol/l], see p. 273).] Deficiencies in the remethylation reaction also result in a rise in Hcy.

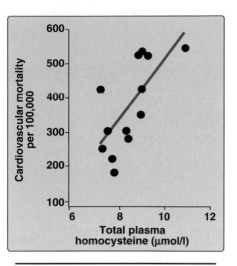

Figure 20.9
Association between cardiovascular disease mortality and total plasma homocysteine.

||| Elevated homocysteine and decreased folic acid levels in pregnant women are associated with increased incidence of neural tube defects (improper closure, as in spina bifida) in the fetus. Periconceptual supplementation with folate reduces the risk of such defects.

F. Other amino acids that form succinyl CoA

Degradation of valine, isoleucine, and threonine also results in the production of succinyl CoA, a TCA cycle intermediate and gluconeogenic compound. [Note: It is metabolized to pyruvate.]

1. **Valine and isoleucine:** These amino acids are branched-chain amino acids (BCAA) that generate propionyl CoA, which is converted to methylmalonyl CoA and then succinyl CoA by biotin- and vitamin B12–requiring reactions.

2. **Threonine:** This amino acid is dehydrated to α-ketobutyrate, which is converted to propionyl CoA and then to succinyl CoA. Propionyl CoA, then, is generated by the catabolism of the amino acids methionine, valine, isoleucine, and threonine. [Note: Propionyl CoA also is generated by the oxidation of odd-numbered fatty acids (see p. 193).]

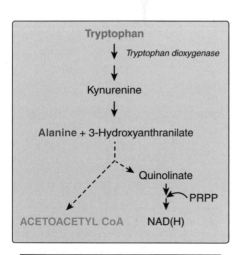

Figure 20.10
Metabolism of tryptophan by the kynurenine pathway (abbreviated). CoA = coenzyme A; PRPP = phosphoribosyl pyrophosphate; NAD(H) = nicotinamide adenine dinucleotide.

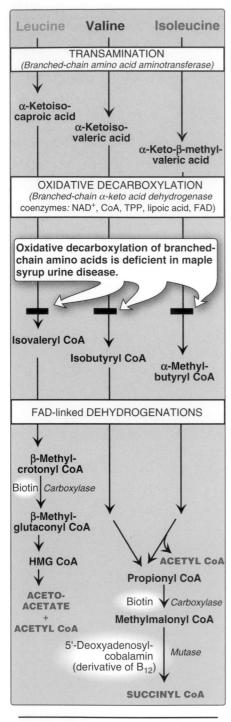

Figure 20.11
Degradation of leucine, valine, and isoleucine. [Note: *β-Methylcrotonyl CoA carboxylase* is one of four biotin-requiring *carboxylases* discussed in this book. The other three are *pyruvate carboxylase*, *acetyl CoA carboxylase*, and *propionyl CoA carboxylase*.] TPP = thiamine pyrophosphate; FAD = flavin adenine dinucleotide; CoA = coenzyme A; NAD = nicotinamide adenine dinucleotide; HMG = hydroxymethylglutarate.

G. Amino acids that form acetyl CoA or acetoacetyl CoA

Tryptophan, leucine, isoleucine, and lysine form acetyl CoA or acetoacetyl CoA directly, without pyruvate serving as an intermediate. As noted earlier, phenylalanine and tyrosine also give rise to acetoacetate during their catabolism (see Fig. 20.7). Therefore, there are a total of six partly or wholly ketogenic amino acids.

1. **Tryptophan:** This amino acid is both glucogenic and ketogenic, because its catabolism yields alanine and acetoacetyl CoA (Fig. 20.10). [Note: Quinolinate from tryptophan catabolism is used in the synthesis of nicotinamide adenine dinucleotide ([NAD], see p. 383).]

2. **Leucine:** This amino acid is exclusively ketogenic, because its catabolism yields acetyl CoA and acetoacetate (Fig. 20.11). The first two reactions in the catabolism of leucine and the other BCAA, isoleucine and valine, are catalyzed by enzymes that use all three BCAA (or their derivatives) as substrates (see H. below).

3. **Isoleucine:** This amino acid is both ketogenic and glucogenic, because its metabolism yields acetyl CoA and propionyl CoA.

4. **Lysine:** This amino acid is exclusively ketogenic and is unusual in that neither of its amino groups undergoes transamination as the first step in catabolism. Lysine is ultimately converted to acetoacetyl CoA.

H. Branched-chain amino acid degradation

The BCAA isoleucine, leucine, and valine are essential amino acids. In contrast to other amino acids, they are catabolized primarily by the peripheral tissues (particularly muscle), rather than by the liver. Because these three amino acids have a similar route of degradation, it is convenient to describe them as a group (see Fig. 20.11).

1. **Transamination:** Transfer of the amino groups of all three BCAA to α-ketoglutarate is catalyzed by a single, vitamin B₆–requiring enzyme, *branched-chain amino acid aminotransferase*, that is expressed primarily in skeletal muscle.

2. **Oxidative decarboxylation:** Removal of the carboxyl group of the α-keto acids derived from leucine, valine, and isoleucine is catalyzed by a single multienzyme complex, *branched-chain α-keto acid dehydrogenase (BCKD) complex.* This complex uses thiamine pyrophosphate, lipoic acid, oxidized flavin adenine dinucleotide (FAD), NAD⁺, and CoA as its coenzymes and produces NADH. [Note: This reaction is similar to the conversion of pyruvate to acetyl CoA by the *pyruvate dehydrogenase* (*PDH*) *complex* (see p. 109) and α-ketoglutarate to succinyl CoA by the *α-ketoglutarate dehydrogenase complex* (see p. 112). The *dihydrolipoyl dehydrogenase* (*Enzyme 3*, or *E3*) component is identical in all three complexes.]

3. **Dehydrogenations:** Oxidation of the products formed in the *BCKD* reaction produces α-β-unsaturated acyl CoA derivatives and FADH₂. These reactions are analogous to the FAD-linked dehydrogenation in the β-oxidation of fatty acids (see p. 192). [Note: Deficiency in the *dehydrogenase* specific for isovaleryl CoA causes neurologic problems and is associated with a "sweaty feet" odor in body fluids.]

4. **End products:** The catabolism of isoleucine ultimately yields acetyl CoA and succinyl CoA, rendering it both ketogenic and glucogenic. Valine yields succinyl CoA and is glucogenic. Leucine is ketogenic, being metabolized to acetoacetate and acetyl CoA. In addition, NADH and $FADH_2$ are produced in the decarboxylation and dehydrogenation reactions, respectively. [Note: BCAA catabolism also results in glutamine and alanine being synthesized and sent out into the blood from muscle (see p. 253).]

IV. FOLIC ACID AND AMINO ACID METABOLISM

Some synthetic pathways require the addition of single-carbon groups that exist in a variety of oxidation states, including formyl, methenyl, methylene, and methyl. These single-carbon groups can be transferred from carrier compounds such as THF and SAM to specific structures that are being synthesized or modified. The "one-carbon pool" refers to the single-carbon units attached to this group of carriers. [Note: CO_2, coming from bicarbonate (HCO_3^-), is carried by the vitamin biotin (see p. 385), which is a prosthetic group for most carboxylation reactions but is not considered a member of the one-carbon pool. Defects in the ability to add or remove biotin from *carboxylases* result in multiple *carboxylase* deficiency. Treatment is supplementation with biotin.]

A. Folic acid and one-carbon metabolism

The active form of folic acid, THF, is produced from folate by *dihydrofolate reductase* in a two-step reaction requiring two nicotinamide adenine dinucleotide phosphate (NADPH). The one-carbon unit carried by THF is bound to N^5 or N^{10} or to both N^5 and N^{10}. Figure 20.12 shows the structures of the various members of the THF family and their interconversions and indicates the sources of the one-carbon units and the synthetic reactions in which the specific members participate. [Note: Folate deficiency presents as a megaloblastic anemia because of decreased availability of the purines and of the thymidine monophosphate needed for DNA synthesis (see p. 303).]

V. BIOSYNTHESIS OF NONESSENTIAL AMINO ACIDS

Nonessential amino acids are synthesized from intermediates of metabolism or, as in the case of tyrosine and cysteine, from the essential amino acids phenylalanine and methionine, respectively. The synthetic reactions for the nonessential amino acids are described below and are summarized in Figure 20.15. [Note: Some amino acids found in proteins, such as hydroxyproline and hydroxylysine (see p. 45), are produced by posttranslational modification (after incorporation into a protein) of their precursor (parent) amino acids.]

A. Synthesis from α-keto acids

Alanine, aspartate, and glutamate are synthesized by transfer of an amino group to the α-keto acids pyruvate, oxaloacetate, and α-ketoglutarate, respectively. These transamination reactions (Fig. 20.13; also see p. 250) are the most direct of the biosynthetic pathways. Glutamate is unusual in that it can also be synthesized by reversal of oxidative deamination, catalyzed by *glutamate dehydrogenase*, when ammonia levels are high (see p. 252).

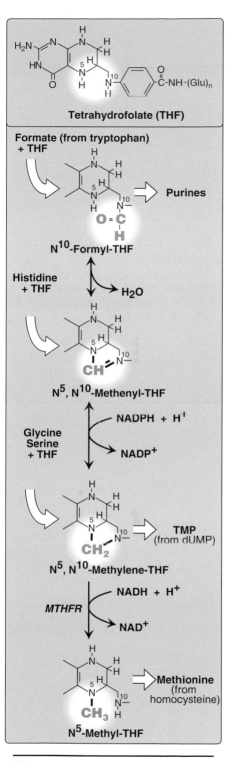

Figure 20.12
Summary of the interconversions and uses of THF. [Note: N^5,N^{10}-Methenyl-THF also arises from N^5-formimino-THF (see Fig. 20.4).] NADP(H) = nicotinamide adenine dinucleotide phosphate; NAD(H) = nicotinamide adenine dinucleotide; TMP = thymidine monophosphate; dUMP = deoxyuridine monophosphate; *MTHFR* = N^5,N^{10}-methylene-THF reductase.

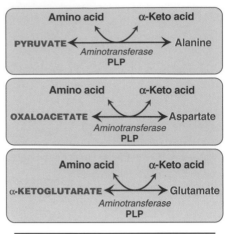

Figure 20.13
Formation of alanine, aspartate, and glutamate from the corresponding α-keto acids by transamination. PLP = pyridoxal phosphate.

B. Synthesis by amidation

1. **Glutamine:** This amino acid, which contains an amide linkage with ammonia at the γ-carboxyl, is formed from glutamate by *glutamine synthetase* (see Fig. 19.18, p. 256). The reaction is driven by the hydrolysis of ATP. In addition to producing glutamine for protein synthesis, the reaction also serves as a major mechanism for the transport of ammonia in a nontoxic form. (See p. 256 for a discussion of ammonia metabolism.)

2. **Asparagine:** This amino acid, which contains an amide linkage with ammonia at the β-carboxyl, is formed from aspartate by *asparagine synthetase,* using glutamine as the amide donor. Like the synthesis of glutamine, the reaction requires ATP and has an equilibrium far in the direction of amide synthesis.

C. Proline

Glutamate via glutamate semialdehyde is converted to proline by cyclization and reduction reactions. [Note: The semialdehyde can also be transaminated to ornithine.]

D. Serine, glycine, and cysteine

The pathways of synthesis for these amino acids are interconnected.

1. **Serine:** This amino acid arises from 3-phosphoglycerate, a glycolytic intermediate (see Fig. 8.18, p. 101), which is first oxidized to 3-phosphopyruvate and then transaminated to 3-phosphoserine. Serine is formed by hydrolysis of the phosphate ester. Serine can also be formed from glycine through transfer of a hydroxymethyl group by *serine hydroxymethyltransferase* using N^5,N^{10}-MTHF as the one-carbon donor (see Fig. 20.6A). [Note: Selenocysteine (Sec), the 21st genetically encoded amino acid, is synthesized from serine and selenium (see p. 407), while serine is attached to transfer RNA. Sec is found in ~25 human proteins including *glutathione peroxidase* (see p. 148) and *thioredoxin reductase* (see p. 297).]

2. **Glycine:** This amino acid is synthesized from serine by removal of a hydroxymethyl group, also by *serine hydroxymethyltransferase* (see Fig. 20.6A). THF is the one-carbon acceptor.

3. **Cysteine:** This amino acid is synthesized by two consecutive reactions in which Hcy combines with serine, forming cystathionine, which, in turn, is hydrolyzed to α-ketobutyrate and cysteine (see Fig. 20.8). [Note: Hcy is derived from methionine, as described on p. 264. Because methionine is an essential amino acid, cysteine synthesis requires adequate dietary intake of methionine.]

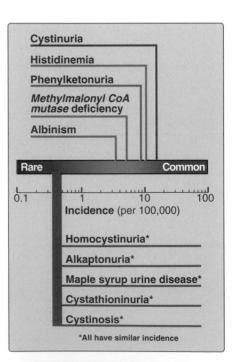

Figure 20.14
Incidence of inherited diseases of amino acid metabolism. [Note: Cystinuria is the most common inborn error of amino acid transport.]

E. Tyrosine

Tyrosine is formed from phenylalanine by *PAH* (see p. 263). The reaction requires molecular oxygen and the coenzyme tetrahydrobiopterin (BH₄), which is synthesized from guanosine triphosphate. One atom of molecular oxygen becomes the hydroxyl group of tyrosine, and the other atom is reduced to water. During the reaction, BH₄ is oxidized to dihydrobiopterin (BH₂). BH₄ is regenerated from BH₂ by NADH-requiring *dihydropteridine reductase.* Tyrosine, like cysteine, is formed from an essential amino acid and is, therefore, nonessential only in the presence of adequate dietary phenylalanine.

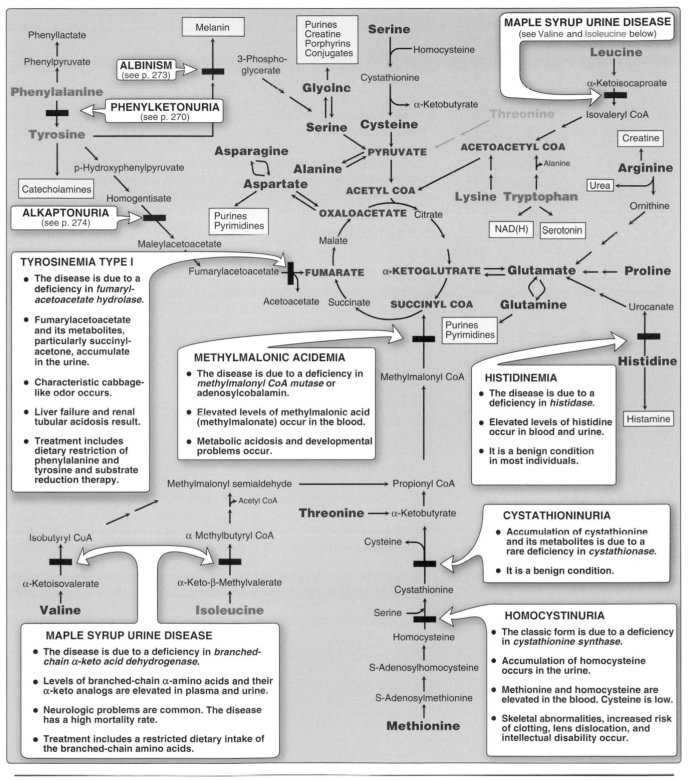

Figure 20.15

Summary of the metabolism of amino acids in humans. Genetically determined enzyme deficiencies are summarized in white boxes. Nitrogen-containing compounds derived from amino acids are shown in small, yellow boxes. Classification of amino acids is color coded: **Red** = glucogenic; **brown** = glucogenic and ketogenic; **green** = ketogenic. Compounds in **BLUE ALL CAPS** are the seven metabolites to which all amino acid metabolism converges. CoA = coenzyme A; NAD(H) = nicotinamide adenine dinucleotide.

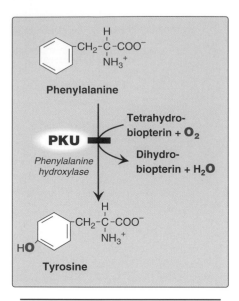

Figure 20.16
A deficiency in *phenylalanine hydroxylase* results in the disease phenylketonuria (PKU).

VI. AMINO ACID METABOLISM DISORDERS

These single gene disorders, a subset of the inborn errors of metabolism, are caused by mutations that generally result in abnormal proteins, most often enzymes. The inherited defects may be expressed as a total loss of enzyme activity or, more frequently, as a partial deficiency in catalytic activity. Without treatment, the amino acid disorders almost invariably result in intellectual disability or other developmental abnormalities as a consequence of harmful accumulation of metabolites. Although >50 of these disorders have been described, many are rare, occurring in <1 per 250,000 in most populations (Fig. 20.14). Collectively, however, they constitute a very significant portion of pediatric genetic diseases (Fig. 20.15).

A. Phenylketonuria

PKU is the most common clinically encountered inborn error of amino acid metabolism (incidence 1:15,000). It is caused by a deficiency of *PAH* (Fig. 20.16). Biochemically, PKU is characterized by hyperphenylalaninemia. Phenylalanine is present in high concentrations (ten times normal) not only in plasma but also in urine and body tissues. Tyrosine, which normally is formed from phenylalanine by *PAH*, is deficient. Treatment includes dietary restriction of phenylalanine and supplementation with tyrosine. [Note: Hyperphenylalaninemia may also be caused by rare deficiencies in any of the several enzymes required to synthesize BH_4 or in *dihydropteridine reductase*, which regenerates BH_4 from BH_2 (Fig. 20.17). Such deficiencies indirectly raise phenylalanine concentrations, because *PAH* requires BH_4 as a coenzyme. BH_4 is also required for *tyrosine hydroxylase* and *tryptophan hydroxylase*, which catalyze reactions leading to the synthesis of neurotransmitters, such as serotonin and the catecholamines. Simply restricting dietary phenylalanine does not reverse the central nervous system effects due to deficiencies in neurotransmitters. Supplementation with BH_4 and replacement therapy with L-3,4-dihydroxyphenylalanine and 5-hydroxytryptophan (products of the affected

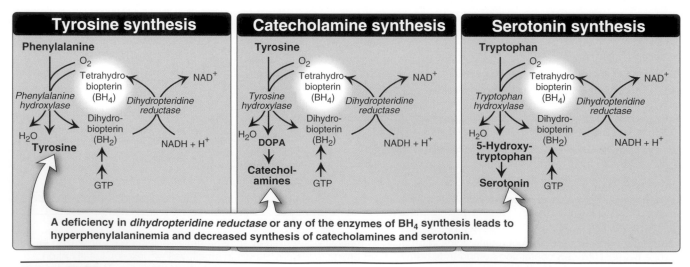

Figure 20.17
Biosynthetic reactions involving amino acids and tetrahydrobiopterin. [Note: Aromatic amino acid *hydroxylases* use BH_4 and not PLP (pyridoxal phosphate).] NAD(H) = nicotinamide adenine dinucleotide; GTP = guanosine triphosphate; DOPA = L-3,4-dihydroxyphenylalanine; O_2 = oxygen.

tyrosine hydroxylase– and *tryptophan hydroxylase*–catalyzed reactions) improves the clinical outcome in these variant forms of hyperphenylalaninemia, although the response is unpredictable.]

| Screening of newborns for a number of treatable disorders, including inborn errors of amino acid metabolism, is done by tandem mass spectrometry of blood obtained from a heel prick. By law, all states must screen for >20 disorders, with some screening for >50. All states screen for PKU. |

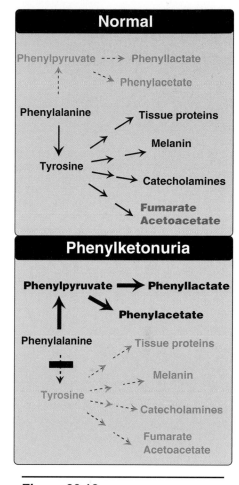

Figure 20.18
Pathways of phenylalanine metabolism in normal individuals and in patients with phenylketonuria.

1. **Additional characteristics:** As the name suggests, PKU is also characterized by elevated levels of a phenylketone in the urine.

   a. **Elevated phenylalanine metabolites:** Phenylpyruvate (a phenylketone), phenylacetate, and phenyllactate, which are not normally produced in significant amounts in the presence of functional *PAH*, are elevated in PKU (Fig. 20.18). These metabolites give urine a characteristic musty ("mousy") odor.

   b. **Central nervous system effects:** Severe intellectual disability, developmental delay, microcephaly, and seizures are characteristic findings in untreated PKU. The affected individual typically shows symptoms of intellectual disability by age 1 year and rarely achieves an intelligence quotient (IQ) >50 (Fig. 20.19). [Note: These clinical manifestations are now rarely seen as a result of newborn screening programs, which allow early diagnosis and treatment.]

   c. **Hypopigmentation:** Patients with untreated PKU may show a deficiency of pigmentation (fair hair, light skin color, and blue eyes). The hydroxylation of tyrosine by copper-requiring *tyrosinase*, which is the first step in the formation of the pigment melanin, is decreased in PKU because tyrosine is decreased.

2. **Newborn screening and diagnosis:** Early diagnosis of PKU is important because the disease is treatable by dietary means. Because of the lack of neonatal symptoms, laboratory testing for elevated blood levels of phenylalanine is mandatory for detection. However, the infant with PKU frequently has normal blood levels of phenylalanine at birth because the mother clears increased blood phenylalanine in her affected fetus through the placenta. Normal levels of phenylalanine may persist until the newborn is exposed to 24–48 hours of protein feeding. Thus, screening tests are typically done after this time to avoid false negatives. For newborns with a positive screening test, diagnosis is confirmed through quantitative determination of phenylalanine levels.

3. **Prenatal diagnosis:** Classic PKU is caused by any of 100 or more different mutations in the gene that encodes *PAH*. The frequency of any given mutation varies among populations, and the disease is often doubly heterozygous (that is, the *PAH* gene has a different mutation in each allele). Despite this complexity, prenatal diagnosis is possible (see p. 493).

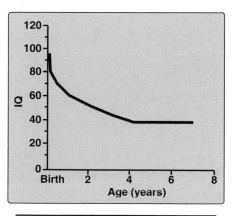

Figure 20.19
Typical intellectual ability in untreated patients of different ages with phenylketonuria. IQ = intelligence quotient.

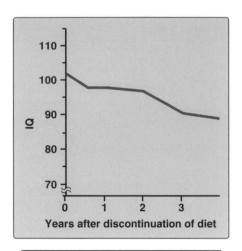

Figure 20.20
Changes in intelligence quotient (IQ) scores after discontinuation of low-phenylalanine diet in patients with phenylketonuria.

4. **Treatment:** Because most natural protein contains phenylalanine, an essential amino acid, it is impossible to satisfy the body's protein requirement without exceeding the phenylalanine limit when ingesting a normal diet. Therefore, in PKU, blood phenylalanine level is maintained close to the normal range by feeding synthetic amino acid preparations free of phenylalanine, supplemented with some natural foods (such as fruits, vegetables, and certain cereals) selected for their low phenylalanine content. The amount is adjusted according to the tolerance of the individual as measured by blood phenylalanine levels. The earlier treatment is started, the more completely neurologic damage can be prevented. Individuals who are appropriately treated can have normal intelligence. [Note: Treatment must begin during the first 7–10 days of life to prevent cognitive impairment.] Because phenylalanine is an essential amino acid, overzealous treatment that results in blood phenylalanine levels below normal is avoided. In patients with PKU, tyrosine cannot be synthesized from phenylalanine, and, therefore, it becomes an essential amino acid and must be supplied in the diet. Discontinuance of the phenylalanine-restricted diet in early childhood is associated with poor performance on IQ tests. Adult PKU patients show deterioration of IQ scores after discontinuation of the diet (Fig. 20.20). Therefore, lifelong restriction of dietary phenylalanine is recommended. [Note: Individuals with PKU are advised to avoid aspartame, an artificial sweetener that contains phenylalanine.]

5. **Maternal phenylketonuria:** If women with PKU who are not on a low-phenylalanine diet become pregnant, the offspring can be affected with maternal PKU syndrome. High blood phenylalanine in the mother has a teratogenic effect, causing microcephaly and congenital heart abnormalities in the fetus. Because these developmental responses to high phenylalanine occur during the first months of pregnancy, dietary control of blood phenylalanine must begin prior to conception and be maintained throughout the pregnancy.

B. **Maple syrup urine disease**

Maple syrup urine disease (MSUD) is a rare (1:185,000), autosomal-recessive disorder in which there is a partial or complete deficiency in *BCKD*, the mitochondrial enzyme complex that oxidatively decarboxylates leucine, isoleucine, and valine (see Fig. 20.11). These BCAA and their corresponding α-keto acids accumulate in the blood, causing a toxic effect that interferes with brain functions. The disease is characterized by feeding problems, vomiting, ketoacidosis, changes in muscle tone, neurologic problems that can result in coma (primarily because of the rise in leucine), and a characteristic maple syrup–like odor of the urine because of the rise in isoleucine. If untreated, the disease is fatal. If treatment is delayed, intellectual disability results.

1. **Classification:** MSUD includes a classic type and several variant forms. The classic, neonatal-onset form is the most common type of MSUD. Leukocytes or cultured skin fibroblasts from these patients show little or no *BCKD* activity. Infants with classic MSUD show symptoms within the first several days of life. If not diagnosed and treated, classic MSUD is lethal in the first weeks of life. Patients

with intermediate forms have a higher level of enzyme activity (up to 30% of normal). The symptoms are milder and show an onset from infancy to adolescence. Patients with the rare thiamine-dependent variant of MSUD respond to large doses of this vitamin.

2. **Screening and diagnosis:** As with PKU, prenatal diagnosis and newborn screening are available, and most affected individuals are compound heterozygotes.

3. **Treatment:** MSUD is treated with a synthetic formula that is free of BCAA, supplemented with limited amounts of leucine, isoleucine, and valine to allow for normal growth and development without producing toxic levels. [Note: Elevated leucine is the cause of the neurologic damage in MSUD, and its level is carefully monitored.] Early diagnosis and lifelong dietary treatment are essential if the child with MSUD is to develop normally. [Note: BCAA are an important energy source in times of metabolic need, and individuals with MSUD are at risk of decompensation during periods of increased protein catabolism.]

C. Albinism

Albinism refers to a group of conditions in which a defect in tyrosine metabolism results in a deficiency in the production of melanin. These defects result in the partial or full absence of pigment from the skin, hair, and eyes. Albinism appears in different forms, and it may be inherited by one of several modes: autosomal recessive (primary mode), autosomal dominant, or X linked. Total absence of pigment from the hair, eyes, and skin (Fig. 20.21), *tyrosinase*-negative oculocutaneous albinism (type 1 albinism), results from an absent or defective copper-requiring *tyrosinase*. It is the most severe form of the condition. In addition to hypopigmentation, affected individuals have vision defects and photophobia (sunlight hurts their eyes). They are at increased risk for skin cancer.

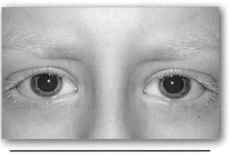

Figure 20.21
Patient with oculocutaneous albinism, showing white eyebrows and lashes and eyes that appear red in color.

D. Homocystinuria

The homocystinurias are a group of disorders involving defects in the metabolism of Hcy. These autosomal-recessive diseases are characterized by high urinary levels of Hcy, high plasma levels of Hcy and methionine, and low plasma levels of cysteine. The most common cause of homocystinuria is a defect in the enzyme *cystathionine β-synthase*, which converts Hcy to cystathionine (Fig. 20.22). Individuals homozygous for *cystathionine β-synthase* deficiency exhibit dislocation of the lens (ectopia lentis), skeletal anomalies (long limbs and fingers), intellectual disability, and an increased risk for developing thrombi (blood clots). Thrombosis is the major cause of early death in these individuals. Treatment includes restriction of methionine and supplementation with vitamin B_{12} and folate. Additionally, some patients are responsive to oral administration of pyridoxine (vitamin B_6), which is converted to pyridoxal phosphate, the coenzyme of *cystathionine β-synthase*. These patients usually have a milder and later onset of clinical symptoms compared with B_6-nonresponsive patients. [Note: Deficiencies in methylcobalamin (see Fig. 20.8) or N^5,N^{10}-*MTHF reductase* ([*MTHFR*]; see Fig. 20.12) also result in elevated Hcy.]

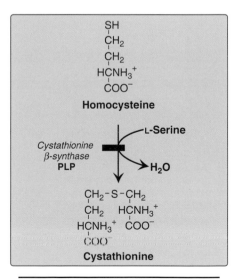

Figure 20.22
Enzyme deficiency in homocystinuria. PLP = pyridoxal phosphate.

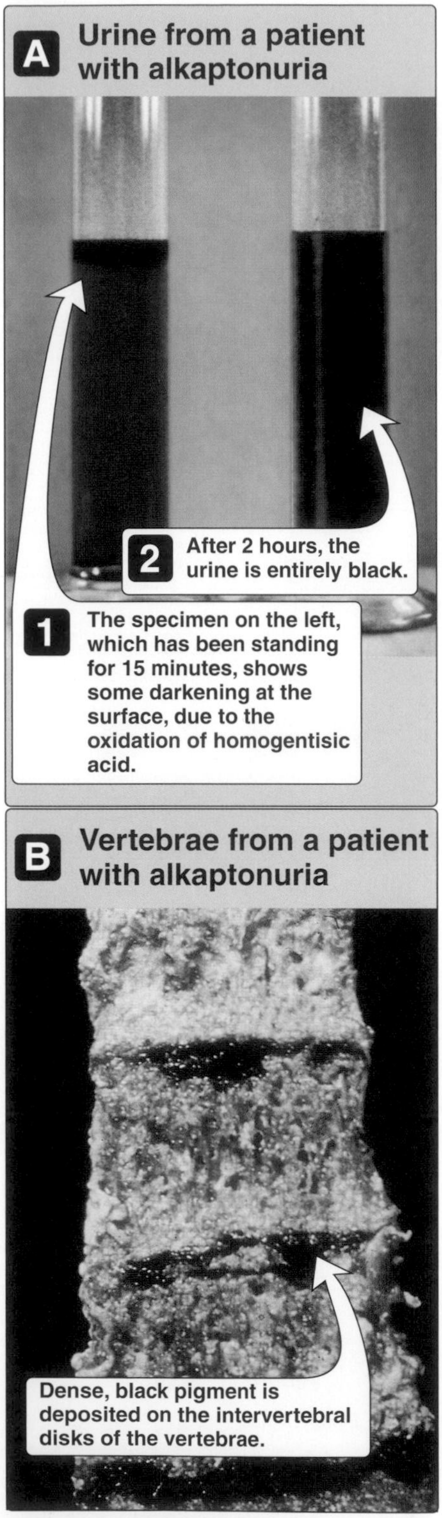

A Urine from a patient with alkaptonuria

2 After 2 hours, the urine is entirely black.

1 The specimen on the left, which has been standing for 15 minutes, shows some darkening at the surface, due to the oxidation of homogentisic acid.

B Vertebrae from a patient with alkaptonuria

Dense, black pigment is deposited on the intervertebral disks of the vertebrae.

Figure 20.23
Specimens from a patient with alkaptonuria. A. Urine. B. Vertebrae.

E. Alkaptonuria

Alkaptonuria is a rare organic aciduria involving a deficiency in *homogentisic acid oxidase*, resulting in the accumulation of homogentisic acid (HA), an intermediate in the degradative pathway of tyrosine (see Fig. 20.15 on p. 269). The condition has three characteristic symptoms: homogentisic aciduria (the urine contains elevated levels of HA, which is oxidized to a dark pigment on standing, as shown in Fig. 20.23A), early onset of arthritis in the large joints, and deposition of black pigment (ochronosis) in cartilage and collagenous tissue (see Fig. 20.23B). Dark staining of diapers can indicate the disease in infants, but usually no symptoms are present until about age 40 years. Treatment includes dietary restriction of phenylalanine and tyrosine to reduce HA levels. Although alkaptonuria is not life threatening, the associated arthritis may be severely crippling. [Note: Deficiencies in *fumarylacetoacetate hydrolase*, the terminal enzyme of tyrosine metabolism, result in tyrosinemia type I (see Fig. 20.15) and a characteristic cabbage-like odor to urine.]

VII. CHAPTER SUMMARY

Amino acids whose catabolism yields **pyruvate** or an **intermediate** of the **tricarboxylic acid cycle** are termed **glucogenic** (Fig. 20.24). They can give rise to the net formation of **glucose** in the **liver** and **kidneys**. The solely glucogenic amino acids are glutamine, glutamate, proline, arginine, histidine, alanine, serine, glycine, cysteine, methionine, valine, threonine, aspartate, and asparagine. Amino acids whose catabolism yields either **acetoacetate** or one of its precursors, **acetyl coenzyme A (CoA)** or **acetoacetyl CoA**, are termed **ketogenic**. Leucine and lysine are solely ketogenic. Tyrosine, phenylalanine, tryptophan, and isoleucine are both ketogenic and glucogenic. **Nonessential amino acids** can be synthesized from metabolic intermediates or from the carbon skeletons of essential amino acids. **Essential amino acids** need to be obtained from the **diet**. They include histidine, methionine, threonine, valine, isoleucine, phenylalanine, tryptophan, leucine, and lysine. **Phenylketonuria** (**PKU**) is caused by a deficiency of *phenylalanine hydroxylase* (*PAH*), which converts phenylalanine to tyrosine. **Hyperphenylalaninemia** may also be caused by deficiencies in the enzymes that synthesize or regenerate the coenzyme for *PAH*, **tetrahydrobiopterin**. Untreated individuals with PKU suffer from severe intellectual disability, developmental delay, microcephaly, seizures, and a characteristic musty (mousy) smell of the urine. Treatment involves controlling dietary phenylalanine. **Tyrosine** becomes an essential dietary component for people with PKU. **Maple syrup urine disease** (**MSUD**) is caused by a partial or complete deficiency in *branched-chain α-keto acid dehydrogenase*, the enzyme that decarboxylates the branched-chain amino acids (BCAA) **leucine**, **isoleucine**, and **valine**. Symptoms include feeding problems, vomiting, ketoacidosis, changes in muscle tone, and a characteristic sweet smell of the urine. If untreated, the disease leads to neurologic problems that result in death. Treatment involves controlling BCAA intake. Other important genetic diseases associated with amino acid metabolism include **albinism**, **homocystinuria**, **methylmalonic acidemia**, **alkaptonuria**, **histidinemia**, **tyrosinemia**, and **cystathioninuria**.

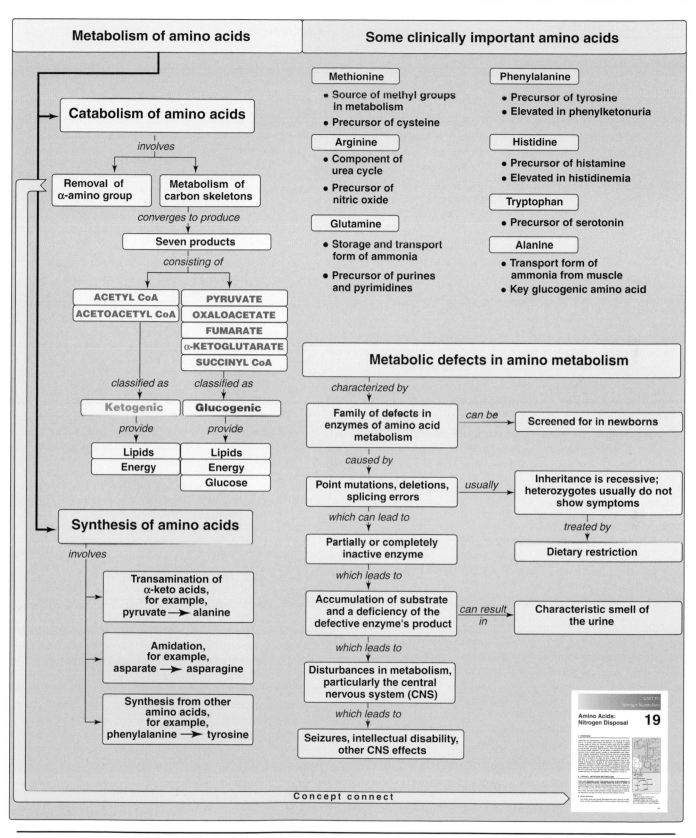

Figure 20.24
Key concept map for amino acid metabolism. CoA = coenzyme A.

Study Questions

Choose the ONE best answer.

For Questions 20.1–20.3, match the deficient enzyme with the associated clinical sign or laboratory finding in urine.

A. Black pigmentation of cartilage	E. Increased branched-chain amino acids
B. Sweaty feet–like odor of fluids	F. Increased homocysteine
C. Cystine crystals in urine	G. Increased methionine
D. White hair, red eye color	H. Increased phenylalanine

20.1 Cystathionine β-synthase

20.2 Homogentisic acid oxidase

20.3 Tyrosinase

20.4 A 1-week-old infant, who was born at home in a rural, medically-underserved area, has undetected classic phenylketonuria. Which statement about this baby and/or her treatment is correct?

A. A diet devoid of phenylalanine should be initiated immediately.
B. Dietary treatment will be discontinued in adulthood.
C. Supplementation with vitamin B$_6$ is required.
D. Tyrosine is an essential amino acid.

20.5 Which one of the following statements concerning amino acids is correct?

A. Alanine is ketogenic.
B. Amino acids that are catabolized to acetyl coenzyme A are glucogenic.
C. Branched-chain amino acids are catabolized primarily in the liver.
D. Cysteine is essential for individuals consuming a diet severely limited in methionine.

20.6 In an individual with the dihydrolipoyl dehydrogenase (E3)-deficient form of maple syrup urine disease, why would lactic acidosis be an expected finding?

20.7 In contrast to the vitamin B$_6$–derived pyridoxal phosphate required in most enzymic reactions involving amino acids, what coenzyme is required by the aromatic amino acid hydroxylases?

Correct answers = F, A, D. A deficiency in cystathionine β-synthase of methionine degradation results in a rise in homocysteine. A deficiency in homogentisic acid oxidase of tyrosine degradation results in a rise in homogentisic acid, which forms a black pigment that is deposited in connective tissue (ochronosis). A deficiency in tyrosinase results in decreased formation of melanin from tyrosine in the skin, hair, and eyes. A sweaty feet–like odor is characteristic of isovaleryl coenzyme A dehydrogenase deficiency. Cystine crystals in urine are seen with cystinuria, a defect in intestinal and renal cystine absorption. Increased branched-chain amino acids are seen in maple syrup urine disease, increased methionine is seen in defects in homocysteine metabolism, and increased phenylalanine is seen in phenylketonuria.

Correct answer = D. In patients with phenylketonuria, tyrosine cannot be synthesized from phenylalanine and, hence, becomes essential and must be supplied in the diet. Phenylalanine in the diet must be controlled but cannot be eliminated entirely because it is an essential amino acid. Dietary treatment must begin during the first 7–10 days of life to prevent intellectual disability, and lifelong restriction of phenylalanine is recommended to prevent cognitive decline. Additionally, elevated levels of phenylalanine are teratogenic to a developing fetus.

Correct answer = D. Methionine is the precursor of cysteine, which becomes essential if methionine is severely restricted. Alanine is a key glucogenic amino acid. Acetyl coenzyme A (CoA) cannot be used for the net synthesis of glucose. Amino acids catabolized to acetyl CoA are ketogenic. Branched-chain amino acids are catabolized primarily in skeletal muscle.

The three α-keto acid dehydrogenase complexes (pyruvate dehydrogenase [PDH], α-ketoglutarate dehydrogenase, and branched-chain α-keto acid dehydrogenase [BCKD]) have dihydrolipoyl dehydrogenase (Enzyme 3, or E3) in common. In E3-deficient maple syrup urine disease, in addition to the branched-chain amino acids and their α-keto acid derivatives accumulating as a result of decreased activity of BCKD, lactate will also be increased because of decreased activity of PDH.

Tetrahydrobiopterin, made from guanosine triphosphate, is the required coenzyme.

Amino Acids: Conversion to Specialized Products

21

I. OVERVIEW

In addition to serving as building blocks for proteins, amino acids are precursors of many nitrogen-containing compounds that have important physiologic functions (Fig. 21.1). These molecules include porphyrins, neurotransmitters, hormones, purines, and pyrimidines. [Note: See p. 151 for the synthesis of nitric oxide from arginine.]

II. PORPHYRIN METABOLISM

Porphyrins are cyclic compounds that readily bind metal ions, usually ferrous (Fe^{2+}) or ferric (Fe^{3+}) iron. The most prevalent metalloporphyrin in humans is heme, which consists of one Fe^{2+} coordinated in the center of the tetrapyrrole ring of protoporphyrin IX (see p. 279). Heme is the prosthetic group for hemoglobin (Hb), myoglobin, the cytochromes, the *cytochrome P450* (*CYP*) *monooxygenase* system, *catalase*, *nitric oxide synthase*, and *peroxidase*. These hemeproteins are rapidly synthesized and degraded. For example, 6–7 g of Hb is synthesized each day to replace heme lost through the normal turnover of erythrocytes. The synthesis and degradation of the associated porphyrins and recycling of the iron are coordinated with the turnover of hemeproteins.

A. Structure

Porphyrins are cyclic planar molecules formed by the linkage of four pyrrole rings through methenyl bridges (Fig. 21.2). Three structural features of these molecules are relevant to understanding their medical significance.

1. **Side chains:** Different porphyrins vary in the nature of the side chains attached to each of the four pyrrole rings. Uroporphyrin contains acetate (–CH_2–COO–) and propionate (–CH_2–CH_2–COO–) side chains; coproporphyrin contains methyl (–CH_3) and propionate groups; and protoporphyrin IX (and heme b, the most common heme)

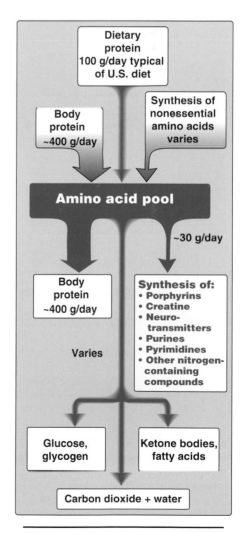

Figure 21.1
Amino acids as precursors of nitrogen-containing compounds.

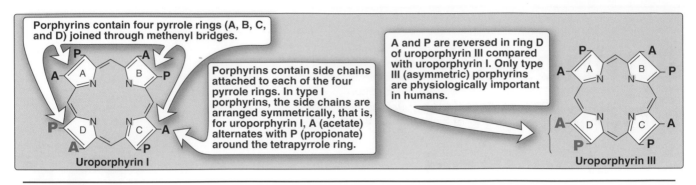

Figure 21.2
Structures of uroporphyrin I and uroporphyrin III.

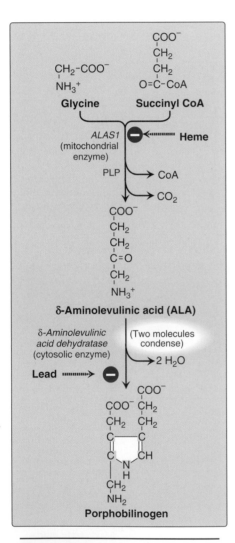

Figure 21.3
Pathway of porphyrin synthesis: Formation of porphobilinogen. [Note: *ALAS2* is regulated by iron.] *ALAS* = δ-*aminolevulinic acid synthase*; CoA = coenzyme A; CO_2 = carbon dioxide; PLP = pyridoxal phosphate. (Continued in Figs. 21.4 and 21.5.)

contains vinyl ($–CH=CH_2$), methyl, and propionate groups. [Note: The methyl and vinyl groups are produced by decarboxylation of acetate and propionate side chains, respectively.]

2. **Side chain distribution:** The side chains of porphyrins can be ordered around the tetrapyrrole nucleus in four different ways, designated by Roman numerals I to IV. Only type III porphyrins, which contain an asymmetric substitution on ring D (see Fig. 21.2), are physiologically important in humans. [Note: Protoporphyrin IX is a member of the type III series.]

3. **Porphyrinogens:** These porphyrin precursors (for example, uroporphyrinogen) exist in a chemically reduced, colorless form and serve as intermediates between porphobilinogen (PBG) and the oxidized, colored protoporphyrins in heme biosynthesis.

B. Heme biosynthesis

The major sites of heme biosynthesis are the liver, which synthesizes a number of heme proteins (particularly the *CYP* proteins), and the erythrocyte-producing cells of the bone marrow, which are active in Hb synthesis. In the liver, the rate of heme synthesis is highly variable, responding to alterations in the cellular heme pool caused by fluctuating demands for hemeproteins. In contrast, heme synthesis in erythroid cells is relatively constant and is matched to the rate of globin synthesis. [Note: Over 85% of all heme synthesis occurs in erythroid tissue. Mature red blood cells (RBC) lack mitochondria and are unable to synthesize heme.] The initial reaction and the last three steps in the formation of porphyrins occur in mitochondria, whereas the intermediate steps of the biosynthetic pathway occur in the cytosol. [Note: Fig. 21.8 summarizes heme synthesis.]

1. **δ-Aminolevulinic acid formation:** All the carbon and nitrogen atoms of the porphyrin molecule are provided by glycine (a nonessential amino acid) and succinyl coenzyme A (a tricarboxylic acid cycle intermediate) that condense to form δ-aminolevulinic acid (ALA) in a reaction catalyzed by *ALA synthase* ([*ALAS*], Fig. 21.3). This reaction requires pyridoxal phosphate ([PLP] see p. 382) as a coenzyme and is the committed and rate-limiting step in porphyrin biosynthesis. [Note: There are two *ALAS* isoforms, each produced by different genes and controlled by different mechanisms. *ALAS1* is found in all tissues, whereas *ALAS2* is erythroid specific.

Loss-of-function mutations in *ALAS2* result in X-linked sideroblastic anemia and iron overload.]

a. **Heme (hemin) effects:** When porphyrin production exceeds the availability of the apoproteins that require it, heme accumulates and is converted to hemin by the oxidation of Fe^{2+} to Fe^{3+}. Hemin decreases the amount (and, thus, the activity) of *ALAS1* by repressing transcription of its gene, increasing degradation of its messenger RNA, and decreasing import of the enzyme into mitochondria. [Note: In erythroid cells, *ALAS2* is controlled by the availability of intracellular iron (see p. 475).]

b. **Drug effects:** Administration of any of a large number of drugs results in a significant increase in hepatic *ALAS1* activity. These drugs are metabolized by the *microsomal CYP monooxygenase* system, a hemeprotein *oxidase* system found in the liver (see p. 149). In response to these drugs, the synthesis of *CYP* proteins increases, leading to an enhanced consumption of heme, a component of these proteins. This, in turn, causes a decrease in the concentration of heme in liver cells. The lower intracellular heme concentration leads to an increase in the synthesis of *ALAS1* and prompts a corresponding increase in the synthesis of ALA.

2. **Porphobilinogen formation:** The cytosolic condensation of two ALA to form PBG by zinc-containing *ALA dehydratase (PBG synthase)* is extremely sensitive to inhibition by heavy metal ions (for example, lead) that replace the zinc (see Fig. 21.3). This inhibition is, in part, responsible for the elevation in ALA and the anemia seen in lead poisoning.

3. **Uroporphyrinogen formation:** The condensation of four PBG produces the linear tetrapyrrole hydroxymethylbilane, which is cyclized and isomerized by *uroporphyrinogen III synthase* to produce the asymmetric uroporphyrinogen III. This cyclic tetrapyrrole undergoes decarboxylation of its acetate groups by *uroporphyrinogen III decarboxylase (UROD)*, generating coproporphyrinogen III (Fig. 21.4). The reactions occur in the cytosol.

4. **Heme formation:** Coproporphyrinogen III enters the mitochondrion, and two propionate side chains are decarboxylated by *coproporphyrinogen III oxidase* to vinyl groups generating protoporphyrinogen IX, which is oxidized to protoporphyrin IX. The introduction of iron (as Fe^{2+}) into protoporphyrin IX produces heme. This step can occur spontaneously, but the rate is enhanced by *ferrochelatase*, an enzyme that, like *ALA dehydratase*, is inhibited by lead (Fig. 21.5).

C. Porphyrias

Porphyrias are rare, inherited (or sometimes acquired) defects in heme synthesis, resulting in the accumulation and increased excretion of porphyrins or porphyrin precursors (see Fig. 21.8). [Note: Inherited porphyrias are autosominal-dominant (AD) or autosomal-recessive (AR) disorders.] Each porphyria results in the accumulation of a unique pattern of intermediates caused by the deficiency of an enzyme in the heme synthetic pathway. [Note: Porphyria, derived from the Greek for purple, refers to the red-blue color caused by pigment-like porphyrins in the urine of some patients with defects in heme synthesis.]

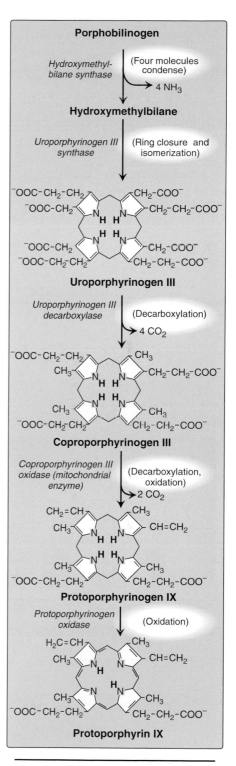

Figure 21.4

Pathway of porphyrin synthesis: formation of protoporphyrin IX. (Continued from Fig. 21.3.) The prefixes -uro (urine) and -copro (feces) reflect initial sites of discovery. [Note: Deficiency in *uroporphyrinogen III synthase* prevents isomerization, resulting in production of type I porphyrins.]

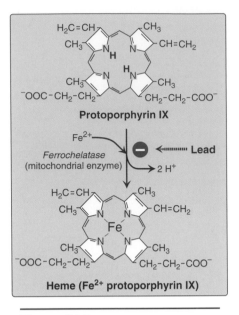

Protoporphyrin IX

Fe^{2+}

Ferrochelatase
(mitochondrial enzyme)

$\ominus$ $\longleftarrow$ **Lead**

$\rightarrow 2\ H^+$

Heme (Fe^{2+} protoporphyrin IX)

Figure 21.5
Pathway of porphyrin synthesis:
formation of heme b. (Continued
from Figs. 21.3 and 21.4.)
Fe^{2+} = ferrous iron.

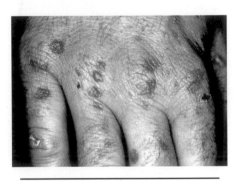

Figure 21.6
Skin eruptions in a patient with
porphyria cutanea tarda.

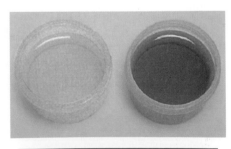

Figure 21.7
Urine from a patient with porphyria
cutanea tarda (right) and from a patient
with normal porphyrin excretion (left).

1. **Clinical manifestations:** The porphyrias are classified as erythropoietic or hepatic, depending on whether the enzyme deficiency occurs in the erythropoietic cells of the bone marrow or in the liver. Hepatic porphyrias can be further classified as chronic or acute. In general, individuals with an enzyme defect prior to the synthesis of the tetrapyrroles manifest abdominal and neuropsychiatric signs, whereas those with enzyme defects leading to the accumulation of tetrapyrrole intermediates show photosensitivity (that is, their skin itches and burns [pruritus] when exposed to sunlight). [Note: Photosensitivity is a result of the oxidation of colorless porphyrinogens to colored porphyrins, which are photosensitizing molecules thought to participate in the formation of superoxide radicals from oxygen. These radicals can oxidatively damage membranes and cause the release of destructive enzymes from lysosomes.]

   a. **Chronic hepatic porphyria:** Porphyria cutanea tarda, the most common porphyria, is a chronic disease of the liver. The disease is associated with severe deficiency of *UROD*, but clinical expression of the deficiency is influenced by various factors, such as hepatic iron overload, exposure to sunlight, alcohol ingestion, estrogen therapy, and the presence of hepatitis B or C or HIV infections. [Note: Mutations to *UROD* are found in only 20% of affected individuals. Inheritance is AD.] Clinical onset is typically during the fourth or fifth decade of life. Porphyrin accumulation leads to cutaneous symptoms (Fig. 21.6) as well as urine that is red to brown in natural light (Fig. 21.7) and pink to red in fluorescent light.

   b. **Acute hepatic porphyrias:** Acute hepatic porphyrias (*ALA dehydratase*–deficiency porphyria, acute intermittent porphyria, hereditary coproporphyria, and variegate porphyria) are characterized by acute attacks of gastrointestinal (GI), neuropsychiatric, and motor symptoms that may be accompanied by photosensitivity (Fig. 21.8). Porphyrias leading to accumulation of ALA and PBG, such as acute intermittent porphyria, cause abdominal pain and neuropsychiatric disturbances, ranging from anxiety to delirium. Symptoms of the acute hepatic porphyrias are often precipitated by use of drugs, such as barbiturates and ethanol, which induce the synthesis of the heme-containing *CYP* microsomal drug-oxidation system. This further decreases the amount of available heme, which, in turn, promotes increased synthesis of *ALAS1*.

   c. **Erythropoietic porphyrias:** The chronic erythropoietic porphyrias (congenital erythropoietic porphyria and erythropoietic protoporphyria) cause photosensitivity characterized by skin rashes and blisters that appear in early childhood (see Fig. 21.8).

2. **Increased δ-aminolevulinic acid synthase activity:** One common feature of the hepatic porphyrias is decreased synthesis of heme. In the liver, heme normally functions as a repressor of the *ALAS1* gene. Therefore, the absence of this end product results in an increase in the synthesis of *ALAS1* (derepression). This causes an increased synthesis of intermediates that occur prior to the genetic block. The accumulation of these toxic intermediates is the major pathophysiology of the porphyrias.

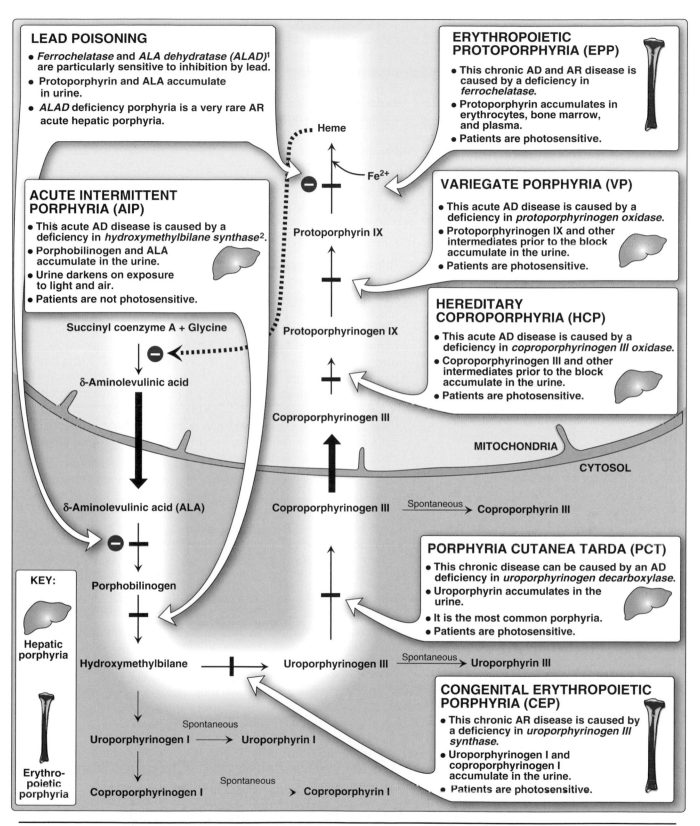

LEAD POISONING

- *Ferrochelatase* and *ALA dehydratase (ALAD)*[1] are particularly sensitive to inhibition by lead.
- Protoporphyrin and ALA accumulate in urine.
- *ALAD* deficiency porphyria is a very rare AR acute hepatic porphyria.

ERYTHROPOIETIC PROTOPORPHYRIA (EPP)

- This chronic AD and AR disease is caused by a deficiency in *ferrochelatase*.
- Protoporphyrin accumulates in erythrocytes, bone marrow, and plasma.
- Patients are photosensitive.

ACUTE INTERMITTENT PORPHYRIA (AIP)

- This acute AD disease is caused by a deficiency in *hydroxymethylbilane synthase*[2].
- Porphobilinogen and ALA accumulate in the urine.
- Urine darkens on exposure to light and air.
- Patients are not photosensitive.

VARIEGATE PORPHYRIA (VP)

- This acute AD disease is caused by a deficiency in *protoporphyrinogen oxidase*.
- Protoporphyrinogen IX and other intermediates prior to the block accumulate in the urine.
- Patients are photosensitive.

HEREDITARY COPROPORPHYRIA (HCP)

- This acute AD disease is caused by a deficiency in *coproporphyrinogen III oxidase*.
- Coproporphyrinogen III and other intermediates prior to the block accumulate in the urine.
- Patients are photosensitive.

Heme

Fe^{2+}

Protoporphyrin IX

Protoporphyrinogen IX

Succinyl coenzyme A + Glycine

δ-Aminolevulinic acid

δ-Aminolevulinic acid (ALA)

Coproporphyrinogen III

Coproporphyrinogen III   Spontaneous → Coproporphyrin III

MITOCHONDRIA

CYTOSOL

PORPHYRIA CUTANEA TARDA (PCT)

- This chronic disease can be caused by an AD deficiency in *uroporphyrinogen decarboxylase*.
- Uroporphyrin accumulates in the urine.
- It is the most common porphyria.
- Patients are photosensitive.

KEY:

Hepatic porphyria

Erythro-poietic porphyria

Porphobilinogen

Hydroxymethylbilane

Uroporphyrinogen III   Spontaneous → Uroporphyrin III

Uroporphyrinogen I → Uroporphyrin I   Spontaneous

Coproporphyrinogen I   Spontaneous → Coproporphyrin I

CONGENITAL ERYTHROPOIETIC PORPHYRIA (CEP)

- This chronic AR disease is caused by a deficiency in *uroporphyrinogen III synthase*.
- Uroporphyrinogen I and coproporphyrinogen I accumulate in the urine.
- Patients are photosensitive.

Figure 21.8

Summary of heme synthesis. [1]Also referred to as *porphobilinogen synthase*. [2]Also referred to as *porphobilinogen deaminase*. [Note: Symptomatic deficiencies in *ALA synthase-1* (*ALAS1*) are unknown. Deficiencies in X-linked *ALAS2* result in an anemia.] ALA = δ-aminolevulinic acid; AD = autosomal dominant; AR = autosomal recessive; Fe = iron.

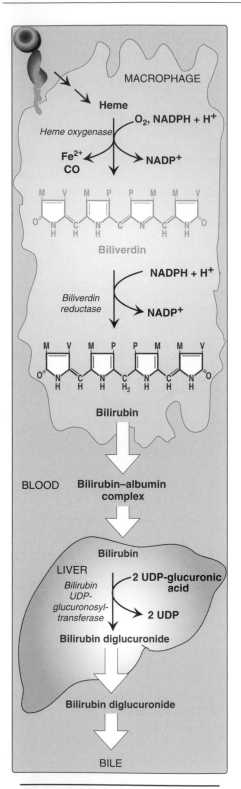

Figure 21.9
Formation of bilirubin from heme and its conversion to bilirubin diglucuronide. UDP = uridine diphosphate; Fe = iron; CO = carbon monoxide; NADP(H) = nicotinamide adenine dinucleotide phosphate.

3. **Treatment:** During acute porphyria attacks, patients require medical support, particularly treatment for pain and vomiting. The severity of acute symptoms of the porphyrias can be diminished by intravenous injection of hemin and glucose, which decreases the synthesis of *ALAS1*. Protection from sunlight, ingestion of β-carotene (provitamin A; see p. 386) that scavenges free radicals, and phlebotomy (removes porphyrins) are helpful in porphyrias with photosensitivity.

D. Heme degradation

After ~120 days in the circulation, RBC are taken up and degraded by the mononuclear phagocyte system (MPS), particularly in the liver and spleen (Fig. 21.9). Approximately 85% of heme destined for degradation comes from senescent RBC. The remainder is from the degradation of hemeproteins other than Hb.

1. **Bilirubin formation:** The first step in the degradation of heme is catalyzed by microsomal *heme oxygenase* in macrophages of the MPS. In the presence of nicotinamide adenine dinucleotide phosphate and oxygen, the enzyme catalyzes three successive oxygenations that result in opening of the porphyrin ring (converting cyclic heme to linear biliverdin), production of carbon monoxide (CO), and release of Fe^{2+} (see Fig. 21.9). [Note: The CO has biologic function, acting as a signaling molecule and anti-inflammatory. Iron is discussed in Chapter 29.] Biliverdin, a green pigment, is reduced, forming the red-orange bilirubin. Bilirubin and its derivatives are collectively termed bile pigments. [Note: The changing colors of a bruise reflect the varying pattern of intermediates that occurs during heme degradation.]

> Bilirubin, unique to mammals, appears to function at low levels as an antioxidant. In this role, it is oxidized to biliverdin, which is then reduced by *biliverdin reductase*, regenerating bilirubin.

2. **Bilirubin uptake by the liver:** Because bilirubin is only slightly soluble in plasma, it is transported through blood to the liver by binding noncovalently to albumin. [Note: Certain anionic drugs, such as salicylates and sulfonamides, can displace bilirubin from albumin, permitting bilirubin to enter the central nervous system (CNS). This causes the potential for neural damage in infants (see p. 285).] Bilirubin dissociates from the carrier albumin molecule, enters a hepatocyte via facilitated diffusion, and binds to intracellular proteins, particularly the protein ligandin.

3. **Bilirubin diglucuronide formation:** In the hepatocyte, bilirubin solubility is increased by the sequential addition of two molecules of glucuronic acid in a process called conjugation. The reactions are catalyzed by microsomal *bilirubin UDP-glucuronosyltransferase* (*bilirubin UGT*) using uridine diphosphate (UDP)-glucuronic acid as the glucuronate donor. The bilirubin diglucuronide product is referred to as conjugated bilirubin (CB). [Note: Varying degrees of deficiency of *bilirubin UGT* result in Crigler-Najjar I and II and Gilbert syndrome, with Crigler-Najjar I being the most severe.]

4. **Bilirubin secretion into bile:** CB is actively transported against a concentration gradient into the bile canaliculi and then into the bile. This energy-dependent, rate-limiting step is susceptible to impairment in liver disease. [Note: A rare deficiency in the protein required for transport of CB out of the liver results in Dubin-Johnson syndrome.] Unconjugated bilirubin (UCB) is normally not secreted into bile.

5. **Urobilin formation in the intestine:** CB is hydrolyzed and reduced by gut bacteria to yield urobilinogen, a colorless compound. Most of the urobilinogen is further oxidized by bacteria to stercobilin, which gives feces the characteristic brown color. However, some is reabsorbed from the gut and enters the portal blood. A portion of this urobilinogen participates in the enterohepatic urobilinogen cycle in which it is taken up by the liver and then resecreted into the bile. The remainder of the urobilinogen is transported by the blood to the kidney, where it is converted to yellow urobilin and excreted, giving urine its characteristic color. The metabolism of bilirubin is summarized in Figure 21.10.

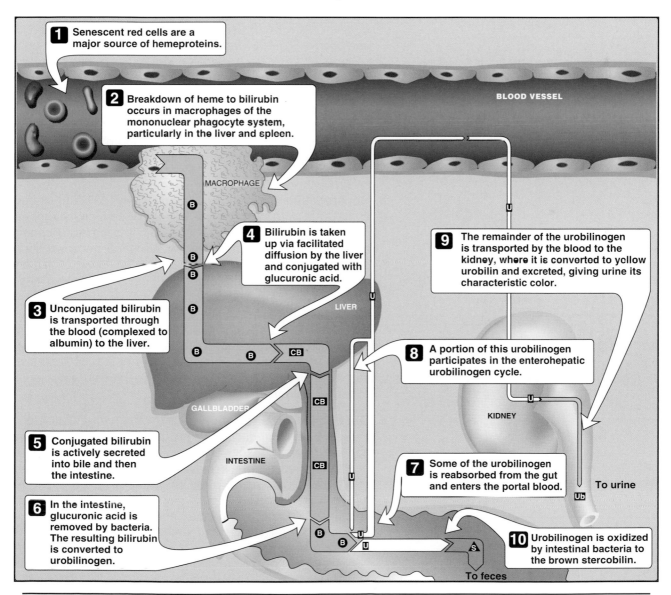

Figure 21.10

Catabolism of heme. Ⓑ = bilirubin; 🅲🅱 = conjugated bilirubin; 🆄 = urobilinogen; 🆄🅱 = urobilin; 🅰 = stercobilin.

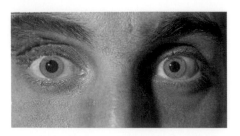

Figure 21.11
Jaundiced patient with the sclerae of his eyes appearing yellow.

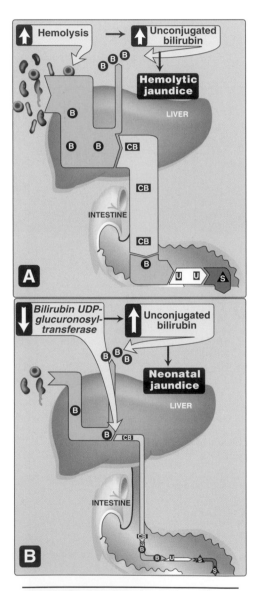

Figure 21.12
Alterations in the metabolism of heme. A. Hemolytic jaundice. B. Neonatal jaundice. CB = conjugated bilirubin; B = bilirubin; U = urobilinogen; S = stercobilin; UDP = uridine diphosphate.

E. Jaundice

Jaundice (or, icterus) refers to the yellow color of skin, nail beds, and sclerae (whites of the eyes) caused by bilirubin deposition, secondary to increased bilirubin levels in the blood (hyperbilirubinemia) as shown in Figure 21.11. Although not a disease, jaundice is usually a symptom of an underlying disorder. [Note: Blood bilirubin levels are normally ≤1 mg/dl. Jaundice is seen at 2–3 mg/dl.]

1. **Types:** Jaundice can be classified into three major types described below. However, in clinical practice, jaundice is often more complex than indicated in this simple classification. For example, the accumulation of bilirubin may be a result of defects at more than one step in its metabolism.

   a. **Hemolytic (prehepatic):** The liver has the capacity to conjugate and excrete >3,000 mg of bilirubin/day, whereas the normal production of bilirubin is only 300 mg/day. This excess capacity allows the liver to respond to increased heme degradation with a corresponding increase in conjugation and secretion of CB. However, extensive hemolysis (for example, in patients with sickle cell anemia or deficiency of *pyruvate kinase* or *glucose 6-phosphate dehydrogenase*) may produce bilirubin faster than it can be conjugated. UCB levels in the blood become elevated (unconjugated hyperbilirubinemia), causing jaundice (Fig. 21.12A). [Note: With hemolysis, more CB is made and excreted into the bile, the amount of urobilinogen entering the enterohepatic circulation is increased, and urinary urobilinogen is increased.]

   b. **Hepatocellular (hepatic):** Damage to liver cells (for example, in patients with cirrhosis or hepatitis) can cause unconjugated hyperbilirubinemia as a result of decreased conjugation. Urobilinogen is increased in the urine because hepatic damage decreases the enterohepatic circulation of this compound, allowing more to enter the blood, from which it is filtered into the urine. The urine consequently darkens, whereas stools may be a pale, clay color. Plasma levels of *alanine* and *aspartate transaminases* (*ALT* and *AST*, respectively; see p. 251) are elevated. If CB is made but is not efficiently secreted from the liver into bile (intrahepatic cholestasis), it can leak into the blood (regurgitation), causing a conjugated hyperbilirubinemia.

   c. **Obstructive (posthepatic):** In this instance, jaundice is not caused by overproduction of bilirubin or decreased conjugation but, instead, results from obstruction of the common bile duct (extrahepatic cholestasis). For example, the presence of a tumor or bile stones may block the duct, preventing passage of CB into the intestine. Patients with obstructive jaundice experience GI pain and nausea and produce stools that are a pale, clay color. The CB regurgitates into the blood (conjugated hyperbilirubinemia). The CB is eventually excreted in the urine (which darkens over time) and is referred to as urinary bilirubin. Urinary urobilinogen is absent.

2. **Jaundice in newborns:** Most newborn infants (60% of full term and 80% of preterm) show a rise in UCB in the first postnatal week (and a transient, physiologic jaundice) because the activity of hepatic *bilirubin UGT* is low at birth (it reaches adult levels in about 4 weeks), as shown in Figures 21.12B and 21.13. Elevated UCB, in excess of the binding capacity of albumin (20–25 mg/dl), can diffuse into the basal ganglia, causing toxic encephalopathy (kernicterus) and a pathologic jaundice. Therefore, newborns with significantly elevated bilirubin levels are treated with blue fluorescent light (phototherapy), as shown in Figure 21.14, which converts bilirubin to more polar and, therefore, water-soluble isomers. These photoisomers can be excreted into the bile without conjugation to glucuronic acid. [Note: Because of solubility differences, only UCB crosses the blood–brain barrier, and only CB appears in urine.]

3. **Bilirubin measurement:** Bilirubin is commonly measured by the van den Bergh reaction, in which diazotized sulfanilic acid reacts with bilirubin to form red azodipyrroles that are measured colorimetrically. In aqueous solution, the water-soluble CB reacts rapidly with the reagent (within 1 minute) and is said to be direct reacting. The UCB, which is much less soluble in aqueous solution, reacts more slowly. However, when the reaction is carried out in methanol, both CB and UCB are soluble and react with the reagent, providing the total bilirubin value. The indirect-reacting bilirubin, which corresponds to the UCB, is obtained by subtracting the direct-reacting bilirubin from the total bilirubin. [Note: In normal plasma, only ~4% of the total bilirubin is conjugated, or direct reacting, because most is secreted into bile.]

III. OTHER NITROGEN-CONTAINING COMPOUNDS

A. Catecholamines

Dopamine, norepinephrine (NE), and epinephrine (or, adrenaline) are biologically active (biogenic) amines that are collectively termed catecholamines. Dopamine and NE are synthesized in the brain and function as neurotransmitters. Epinephrine is synthesized from NE in the adrenal medulla.

1. **Function:** Outside the CNS, NE and its methylated derivative, epinephrine, are hormone regulators of carbohydrate and lipid metabolism. NE and epinephrine are released from storage vesicles in the adrenal medulla in response to fright, exercise, cold, and low levels of blood glucose. They increase the degradation of glycogen and triacylglycerol as well as increase blood pressure and the output of the heart. These effects are part of a coordinated response to prepare the individual for stress and are often called the "fight-or-flight" reactions.

2. **Synthesis:** The catecholamines are synthesized from tyrosine, as shown in Figure 21.15. Tyrosine is first hydroxylated by *tyrosine hydroxylase* to form L-3,4-dihydroxyphenylalanine (DOPA) in a reaction analogous to that described for the hydroxylation of phenylalanine (see p. 263). The tetrahydrobiopterin (BH$_4$)-requiring

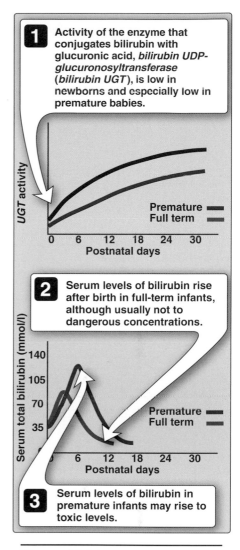

Figure 21.13
Neonatal jaundice. UDP = uridine diphosphate.

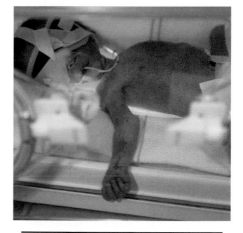

Figure 21.14
Phototherapy in neonatal jaundice.

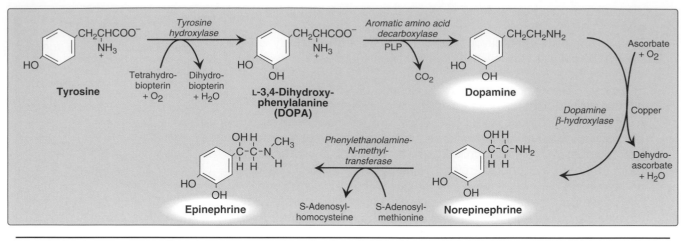

Figure 21.15
Synthesis of catecholamines. [Note: Catechols have two adjacent hydroxyl groups.] PLP = pyridoxal phosphate.

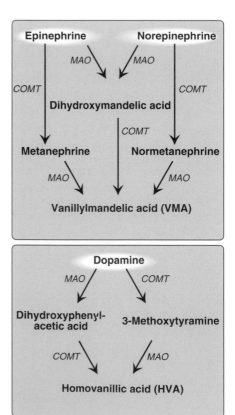

Figure 21.16
Metabolism of the catecholamines by *catechol-O-methyltranferase (COMT)* and *monoamine oxidase (MAO)*. [Note: *COMT* requires S-adenosylmethylamine.]

enzyme is abundant in the CNS, the sympathetic ganglia, and the adrenal medulla, and it catalyzes the rate-limiting step of the pathway. DOPA is decarboxylated in a reaction requiring PLP to form dopamine, which is hydroxylated by *dopamine β-hydroxylase* to yield NE in a reaction that requires ascorbic acid (vitamin C) and copper. Epinephrine is formed from NE by an N-methylation reaction using S-adenosylmethionine (SAM) as the methyl donor (see p. 264).

> Parkinson disease, a neurodegenerative movement disorder, is due to insufficient dopamine production as a result of the idiopathic loss of dopamine-producing cells in the brain. Administration of L-DOPA (levodopa) is the most common treatment, because dopamine cannot cross the blood–brain barrier.

3. **Degradation:** The catecholamines are inactivated by oxidative deamination catalyzed by *monoamine oxidase (MAO)* and by O-methylation catalyzed by *catechol-O-methyltransferase (COMT)* using SAM as the methyl donor (Fig. 21.16). The reactions can occur in either order. The aldehyde products of the *MAO* reaction are oxidized to the corresponding acids. The products of these reactions are excreted in the urine as vanillylmandelic acid (VMA) from epinephrine and NE and homovanillic acid (HVA) from dopamine. [Note: VMA and the metanephrines are increased with pheochromocytomas, rare tumors of the adrenal gland characterized by excessive production of catecholamines.]

4. **Monoamine oxidase inhibitors:** *MAO* is found in neural and other tissues, such as the intestine and liver. In the neuron, this enzyme oxidatively deaminates and inactivates any excess neurotransmitter molecules (NE, dopamine, or serotonin) that may leak out of synaptic vesicles when the neuron is at rest. *MAO* inhibitors (MAOI) may irreversibly or reversibly inactivate the enzyme, permitting

neurotransmitter molecules to escape degradation and, therefore, both to accumulate within the presynaptic neuron and to leak into the synaptic space. This causes activation of NE and serotonin receptors and may be responsible for the antidepressant action of MAOI. [Note: The interaction of MAOI with tyramine-containing foods is discussed on p. 373.]

B. Histamine

Histamine is a chemical messenger that mediates a wide range of cellular responses, including allergic and inflammatory reactions and gastric acid secretion. A powerful vasodilator, histamine is formed by decarboxylation of histidine in a reaction requiring PLP (Fig. 21.17). It is secreted by mast cells as a result of allergic reactions or trauma. Histamine has no clinical applications, but agents that interfere with the action of histamine have important therapeutic applications.

C. Serotonin

Serotonin, also called 5-hydroxytryptamine (5-HT), is synthesized and/or stored at several sites in the body (Fig. 21.18). The largest amount by far is found in the intestinal mucosa. Smaller amounts occur in the CNS, where it functions as a neurotransmitter, and in platelets (see online Chapter 35). Serotonin is synthesized from tryptophan, which is hydroxylated in a BH_4-requiring reaction analogous to that catalyzed by *phenylalanine hydroxylase*. The product, 5-hydroxytryptophan, is decarboxylated to 5-HT. Serotonin has multiple physiologic roles including pain perception and regulation of sleep, appetite, temperature, blood pressure, cognitive functions, and mood (causes a feeling of well-being). [Note: Selective serotonin reuptake inhibitors (SSRI) maintain serotonin levels, thereby functioning as antidepressants.] Serotonin is degraded by *MAO* to 5-hydroxy-3-indoleacetic acid (5-HIAA).

D. Creatine

Creatine phosphate (also called phosphocreatine), the phosphorylated derivative of creatine found in muscle, is a high-energy compound that provides a small but rapidly mobilized reserve of high-energy phosphates that can be reversibly transferred to adenosine diphosphate (Fig. 21.19) to maintain the intracellular level of ATP during the first few minutes of intense muscular contraction. [Note: The amount of creatine phosphate in the body is proportional to the muscle mass.]

1. **Synthesis:** Creatine is synthesized in the liver and kidneys from glycine and the guanidino group of arginine, plus a methyl group from SAM (see Fig. 21.19). Animal products are dietary sources. Creatine is reversibly phosphorylated to creatine phosphate by *creatine kinase*, using ATP as the phosphate donor. [Note: The presence of *creatine kinase* (*MB* isozyme) in the plasma is indicative of heart damage and is used in the diagnosis of myocardial infarction (see p. 65).]

2. **Degradation:** Creatine and creatine phosphate spontaneously cyclize at a slow but constant rate to form creatinine, which is excreted in the urine. The amount excreted is proportional to the

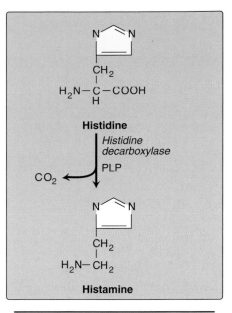

Figure 21.17
Biosynthesis of histamine.
PLP = pyridoxal phosphate.

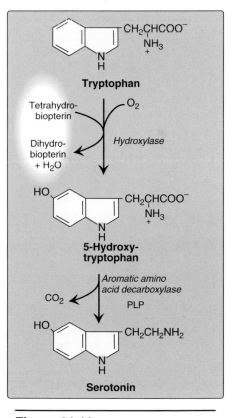

Figure 21.18
Synthesis of serotonin. [Note: Serotonin is converted to melatonin, a regulator of circadian rhythm, in the pineal gland.] PLP = pyridoxal phosphate; CO_2 = carbon dioxide.

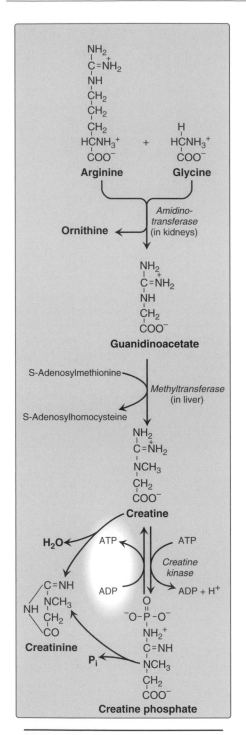

Figure 21.19
Synthesis of creatine.
ADP = adenosine diphosphate;
P_i = inorganic phosphate.

total creatine phosphate content of the body and, therefore, can be used to estimate muscle mass. When muscle mass decreases for any reason (for example, from paralysis or muscular dystrophy), the creatinine content of the urine falls. In addition, a rise in blood creatinine is a sensitive indicator of kidney malfunction, because creatinine normally is rapidly cleared from the blood and excreted. A typical adult male excretes ~1–2 g of creatinine/day.

E. Melanin

Melanin is a pigment that occurs in several tissues, particularly the eye, hair, and skin. It is synthesized from tyrosine in melanocytes (pigment-forming cells) of the epidermis. It functions to protect underlying cells from the harmful effects of sunlight. [Note: A defect in melanin production results in oculocutaneous albinism, the most common type being due to defects in copper-containing *tyrosinase* (see p. 273).]

IV. CHAPTER SUMMARY

Amino acids are **precursors** of many nitrogen (N)-containing compounds including **porphyrins**, which, in combination with **ferrous (Fe^{2+}) iron**, form **heme** (Fig. 21.20). The major sites of **heme biosynthesis** are the **liver**, which synthesizes a number of hemeproteins (particularly *cytochrome P450* **enzymes**), and the **erythrocyte-producing cells** of the bone marrow, which are active in **hemoglobin** synthesis. In the liver, the rate of heme synthesis is highly variable, responding to alterations in the cellular heme pool caused by fluctuating demands for hemeproteins. In contrast, heme synthesis in erythroid cells is relatively constant and is matched to the rate of globin synthesis. Heme synthesis starts with **glycine** and **succinyl coenzyme A**. The **committed step** is the formation of **δ-aminolevulinic acid (ALA)**. This mitochondrial reaction is catalyzed by *ALA synthase-1* (*ALAS1*) in the liver (inhibited by **hemin**, the oxidized form of heme that accumulates when heme is being underutilized) and *ALAS2* in erythroid tissues (regulated by iron). **Porphyrias** are caused by inherited or acquired (**lead poisoning**) defects in heme synthesis, resulting in the accumulation and increased excretion of porphyrins or porphyrin precursors. Enzymic defects early in the pathway cause **abdominal pain** and **neuropsychiatric symptoms**, whereas later defects cause **photosensitivity**. **Degradation** of heme occurs in the **mononuclear phagocyte system**, particularly in the **liver** and **spleen**. The first step is the production by *heme oxygenase* of **biliverdin**, which is subsequently reduced to **bilirubin**. Bilirubin is transported by **albumin** to the liver, where its solubility is increased by the addition of two molecules of **glucuronic acid** by *bilirubin uridine diphosphate-glucuronosyltransferase* (*bilirubin UGT*). Bilirubin diglucuronide (**conjugated bilirubin**) is transported into the **bile canaliculi**, where it is first hydrolyzed and reduced by gut bacteria to yield **urobilinogen**, which is further oxidized by bacteria to **stercobilin**. **Jaundice (icterus)** refers to the yellow color of the skin and sclerae that is caused by deposition of bilirubin, secondary to increased bilirubin levels in the blood. Three commonly encountered types of jaundice are **hemolytic (prehepatic)**, **obstructive (posthepatic)**, and **hepatocellular (hepatic)** (see Fig. 21.20). Other important N-containing compounds derived from amino acids include the **catecholamines** (**dopamine**, **norepinephrine**, and **epinephrine**), **creatine**, **histamine**, **serotonin**, **melanin**, and **nitric oxide**.

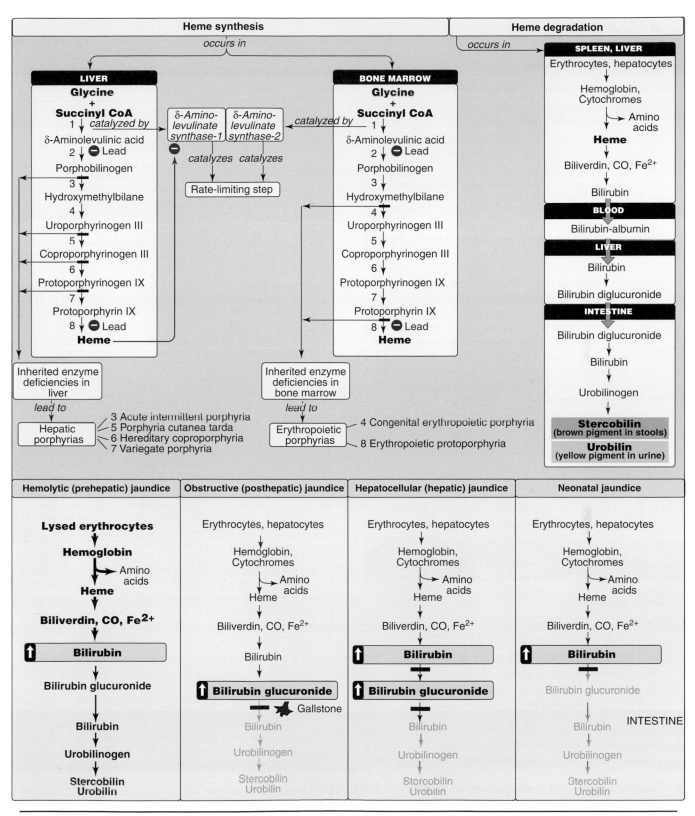

Figure 21.20

Key concept map for heme metabolism. ■■■■ = Block in the pathway. [Note: Hepatocellular jaundice can be caused by decreased conjugation of bilirubin or decreased secretion of conjugated bilirubin from the liver into bile.] CoA = coenzyme A; CO = carbon monoxide; Fe = iron.

Study Questions

Choose the ONE best answer.

21.1 δ-Aminolevulinic acid synthase activity:

    A. catalyzes the committed step in porphyrin biosynthesis.

    B. is decreased by iron in erythrocytes.

    C. is decreased in the liver in individuals treated with certain drugs such as the barbiturate phenobarbital.

    D. occurs in the cytosol.

    E. requires tetrahydrobiopterin as a coenzyme.

> Correct answer = A. δ-Aminolevulinic acid synthase is mitochondrial and catalyzes the rate-limiting and regulated step of porphyrin synthesis. It requires pyridoxal phosphate as a coenzyme. Iron increases production of the erythroid isozyme. The hepatic isozyme is increased in patients treated with certain drugs.

21.2 A 50-year-old man presented with painful blisters on the backs of his hands. He was a golf instructor and indicated that the blisters had erupted shortly after the golfing season began. He did not have recent exposure to common skin irritants. He had partial complex seizure disorder that had begun ~3 years earlier after a head injury. The patient had been taking phenytoin (his only medication) since the onset of the seizure disorder. He admitted to an average weekly ethanol intake of ~18 12-oz cans of beer. The patient's urine was reddish orange. Cultures obtained from skin lesions failed to grow organisms. A 24-hour urine collection showed elevated uroporphyrin (1,000 mg; normal, <27 mg). The most likely diagnosis is:

    A. acute intermittent porphyria.

    B. congenital erythropoietic porphyria.

    C. erythropoietic protoporphyria.

    D. hereditary coproporphyria.

    E. porphyria cutanea tarda.

> Correct answer = E. The disease is associated with a deficiency in uroporphyrinogen III decarboxylase (UROD), but clinical expression of the enzyme deficiency is influenced by hepatic injury caused by environmental (for example, ethanol) and infectious (for example, hepatitis B virus) agents. Exposure to sunlight can also be a precipitating factor. Clinical onset is typically during the fourth or fifth decade of life. Porphyrin accumulation leads to cutaneous symptoms and urine that is red to brown. Treatment of the patient's seizure disorder with phenytoin caused increased synthesis of δ-aminolevulinic acid synthase and, therefore, of uroporphyrinogen, the substrate of the deficient UROD. The laboratory and clinical findings are inconsistent with other porphyrias.

21.3 A patient presents with jaundice, abdominal pain, and nausea. Clinical laboratory results are shown below.

Plasma bilirubin	Urine urobilinogen	Urinary bilirubin
Increase in conjugated bilirubin	Not present	Present

What is the most likely cause of the jaundice?

    A. Decreased hepatic conjugation of bilirubin

    B. Decreased hepatic uptake of bilirubin

    C. Decreased secretion of bile into the intestine

    D. Increased hemolysis

> Correct answer = C. The data are consistent with an obstructive jaundice in which a block in the common bile duct decreases the secretion of bile containing conjugated bilirubin (CB) into the intestine (stool will be pale in color). The CB regurgitates into the blood (conjugated hyperbilirubinemia). The CB is excreted in the urine (which darkens) and is referred to as urinary bilirubin. Urinary urobilinogen is not present because its source is intestinal urobilinogen, which is low. The other choices do not match the data.

21.4 A 2-year-old child was brought to his pediatrician for evaluation of gastrointestinal problems. The parents report that the boy has been listless for the last few weeks. Lab tests reveal a microcytic, hypochromic anemia. Blood lead levels are elevated. Which of the enzymes listed below is most likely to have higher-than-normal activity in the liver of this child?

    A. δ-Aminolevulinic acid synthase

    B. Bilirubin UDP glucuronosyltransferase

    C. Ferrochelatase

    D. Heme oxygenase

    E. Porphobilinogen synthase

> Correct answer = A. This child has the acquired porphyria of lead poisoning. Lead inhibits both δ-aminolevulinic acid dehydratase and ferrochelatase and, consequently, heme synthesis. The decrease in heme derepresses δ-aminolevulinic acid synthase-1 (the hepatic isozyme), resulting in an increase in its activity. The decrease in heme also results in decreased hemoglobin synthesis, and anemia is seen. Ferrochelatase is directly inhibited by lead. The other choices are enzymes of heme degradation.

Nucleotide Metabolism

22

I. OVERVIEW

Ribonucleoside and deoxyribonucleoside phosphates (nucleotides) are essential for all cells. Without them, neither ribonucleic acid (RNA) nor deoxyribonucleic acid (DNA) can be produced, and, therefore, proteins cannot be synthesized or cells proliferate. Nucleotides also serve as carriers of activated intermediates in the synthesis of some carbohydrates, lipids, and conjugated proteins (for example, uridine diphosphate [UDP]-glucose and cytidine diphosphate [CDP]-choline) and are structural components of several essential coenzymes, such as coenzyme A, flavin adenine dinucleotide (FAD[H$_2$]), nicotinamide adenine dinucleotide (NAD[H]), and nicotinamide adenine dinucleotide phosphate (NADP[H]). Nucleotides, such as cyclic adenosine monophosphate (cAMP) and cyclic guanosine monophosphate (cGMP), serve as second messengers in signal transduction pathways. In addition, nucleotides play an important role as energy sources in the cell. Finally, nucleotides are important regulatory compounds for many of the pathways of intermediary metabolism, inhibiting or activating key enzymes. The purine and pyrimidine bases found in nucleotides can be synthesized de novo or can be obtained through salvage pathways that allow the reuse of the preformed bases resulting from normal cell turnover. [Note: Little of the purines and pyrimidines supplied by diet is utilized and is degraded instead.]

II. STRUCTURE

Nucleotides are composed of a nitrogenous base; a pentose monosaccharide; and one, two, or three phosphate groups. The nitrogen-containing bases belong to two families of compounds: the purines and the pyrimidines.

A. Purine and pyrimidine bases

Both DNA and RNA contain the same purine bases: adenine (A) and guanine (G). Both DNA and RNA contain the pyrimidine cytosine (C), but they differ in their second pyrimidine base: DNA contains thymine (T), whereas RNA contains uracil (U). T and U differ in that only T has a methyl group (Fig. 22.1). Unusual (modified) bases are occasionally found in some species of DNA (for example, in some viral DNA) and RNA (for example, in transfer RNA [tRNA]). Base modifications include methylation, glycosylation, acetylation, and reduction. Some examples

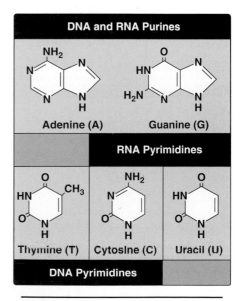

Figure 22.1
Purines and pyrimidines commonly found in DNA and RNA.

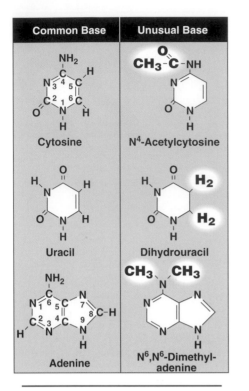

Figure 22.2
Examples of unusual bases.

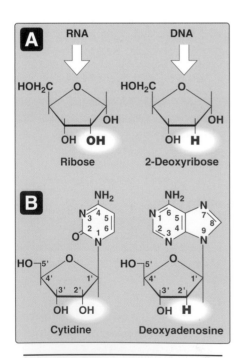

Figure 22.3
A. Pentoses found in nucleic acids.
B. Examples of the numbering systems for purine- and pyrimidine-containing nucleosides.

of unusual bases are shown in Figure 22.2. [Note: The presence of an unusual base in a nucleotide sequence may aid in its recognition by specific enzymes or protect it from being degraded by *nucleases*.]

B. Nucleosides

The addition of a pentose sugar to a base through an N-glycosidic bond (see p. 86) produces a nucleoside. If the sugar is ribose, a ribonucleoside is produced, and if the sugar is 2-deoxyribose, a deoxyribonucleoside is produced (Fig. 22.3A). The ribonucleosides of A, G, C, and U are named adenosine, guanosine, cytidine, and uridine, respectively. The deoxyribonucleosides of A, G, C, and T have the added prefix deoxy- (for example, deoxyadenosine). [Note: The compound deoxythymidine is often simply called thymidine, with the deoxy- prefix being understood, because it is incorporated into DNA only.] The carbon and nitrogen atoms in the rings of the base and the sugar are numbered separately (see Fig. 22.3B). [Note: Carbons in the pentose are numbered 1' to 5'. Thus, when the 5'-carbon of a nucleoside (or nucleotide) is referred to, a carbon atom in the pentose, rather than an atom in the base, is being specified.]

C. Nucleotides

The addition of one or more phosphate groups to a nucleoside produces a nucleotide. The first phosphate group is attached by an ester linkage to the 5'-OH of the pentose, forming a nucleoside 5'-phosphate or a 5'-nucleotide. The type of pentose is denoted by the prefix in the names 5'-ribonucleotide and 5'-deoxyribonucleotide. If one phosphate group is attached to the 5'-carbon of the pentose, the structure is a nucleoside monophosphate, like adenosine monophosphate (AMP, or adenylate). If a second or third phosphate is added to the nucleoside, a nucleoside diphosphate (for example, adenosine diphosphate [ADP] or triphosphate, for example, ATP) results (Fig. 22.4). The second and third phosphates are each connected to the nucleotide by a "high-energy bond" (a bond with a large, negative change in free energy [$-\Delta G$, see p. 70] of hydrolysis). [Note: The phosphate groups are responsible for the negative charges associated with nucleotides and cause DNA and RNA to be referred to as nucleic acids.]

III. PURINE NUCLEOTIDE SYNTHESIS

The atoms of the purine ring are contributed by a number of compounds, including amino acids (aspartate, glycine, and glutamine), carbon dioxide (CO_2), and N^{10}-formyltetrahydrofolate (N^{10}-formyl-THF), as shown in Figure 22.5. The purine ring is constructed primarily in the liver by a series of reactions that add the donated carbons and nitrogens to a preformed ribose 5-phosphate. [Note: Synthesis of ribose 5-phosphate from glucose 6-phosphate by the pentose phosphate pathway is discussed on p. 147.]

A. 5-Phosphoribosyl-1-pyrophosphate synthesis

5-Phosphoribosyl-1-pyrophosphate (PRPP) is an activated pentose that participates in the synthesis and salvage of purines and pyrimidines. Synthesis of PRPP from ATP and ribose 5-phosphate is catalyzed by *PRPP synthetase* (Fig. 22.6). This X-linked enzyme is activated by inorganic phosphate and inhibited by purine nucleotides (end-product inhibition). [Note: Because the sugar moiety of PRPP is ribose, ribonucleotides are the end products of <u>de novo</u> purine synthesis. When deoxyribonucleotides are required for DNA synthesis, the ribose sugar moiety is reduced (see p. 297).]

B. 5-Phosphoribosylamine synthesis

Synthesis of 5-phosphoribosylamine from PRPP and glutamine is shown in Figure 22.7. The amide group of glutamine replaces the pyrophosphate group attached to carbon 1 of PRPP. This is the committed step in purine nucleotide biosynthesis. The enzyme that catalyzes the reaction, *glutamine:phosphoribosylpyrophosphate amidotransferase* (*GPAT*), is inhibited by the purine 5′-nucleotides AMP and guanosine monophosphate (GMP, or guanylate), the end products of the pathway. The rate of the reaction is also controlled by the intracellular concentration of PRPP. [Note: The concentration of PRPP is normally far below the Michaelis constant (K_m) for the *GPAT*. Therefore, any small change in the PRPP concentration causes a proportional change in rate of the reaction (see p. 59).]

C. Inosine monophosphate synthesis

The next nine steps in purine nucleotide biosynthesis leading to the synthesis of inosine monophosphate ([IMP] whose base is hypoxanthine) are illustrated in Figure 22.7. IMP is the parent purine nucleotide for AMP and GMP. Four steps in this pathway require ATP as an energy source, and two steps in the pathway require N^{10}-formyl-THF as a one-carbon donor (see p. 267). [Note: Hypoxanthine is found in tRNA (see Fig. 32.9 on p. 453).]

D. Synthetic inhibitors

Some synthetic inhibitors of purine synthesis (for example, the sulfonamides) are designed to inhibit the growth of rapidly dividing microorganisms without interfering with human cell functions (see Fig. 22.7). Other purine synthesis inhibitors, such as structural analogs

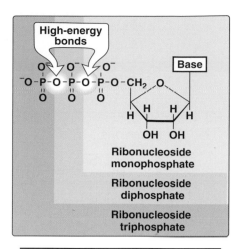

Figure 22.4
Ribonucleoside monophosphate, diphosphate, and triphosphate.

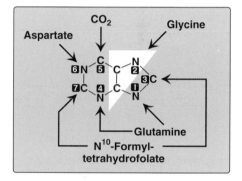

Figure 22.5
Sources of the individual atoms in the purine ring. The order in which the atoms are added is shown by the numbers in the black boxes (see Fig. 22.7). CO_2 = carbon dioxide.

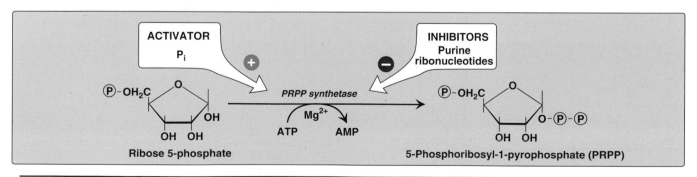

Figure 22.6
Synthesis of PRPP, showing the activator and inhibitors of the reaction. [Note: This is not the committed step of purine synthesis because PRPP is used in other pathways such as salvage (see p. 296).] Ⓟ = phosphate; P_i = inorganic phosphate; AMP = adenosine monophosphate; Mg = magnesium.

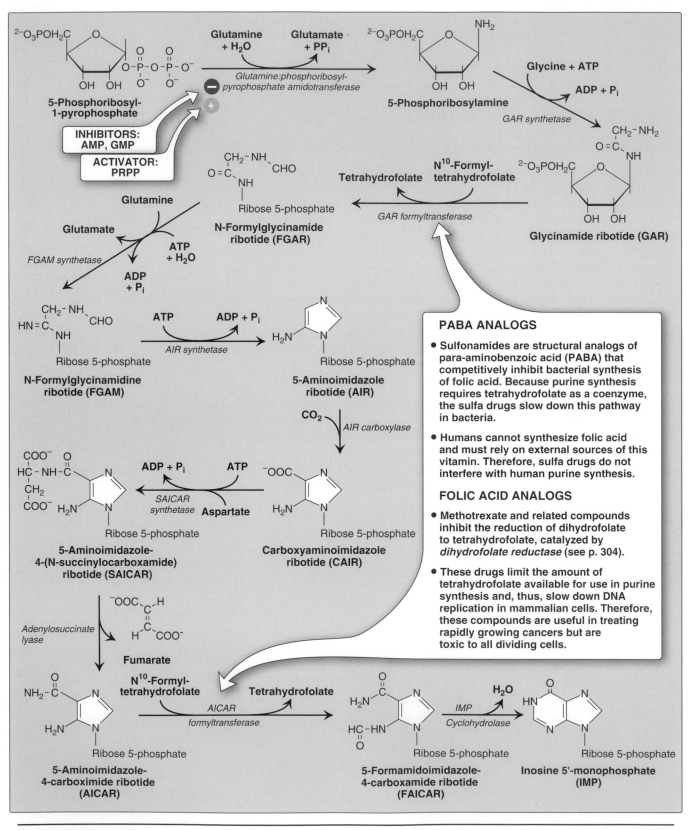

Figure 22.7

<u>De novo</u> synthesis of purine nucleotides, showing the inhibitory effect of some structural analogs. AMP and ADP = adenosine mono- and diphosphates; GMP = guanosine monophosphate; PRPP = 5-phosphoribosyl-1-pyrophosphate; P_i = inorganic phosphate; PP_i = pyrophosphate; CO_2 = carbon dioxide.

of folic acid (for example, methotrexate), are used pharmacologically to control the spread of cancer by interfering with the synthesis of nucleotides and, therefore, of DNA and RNA (see Fig. 22.7).

> Inhibitors of human purine synthesis are extremely toxic to tissues, especially to developing structures such as in a fetus, or to cell types that normally replicate rapidly, including those of bone marrow, skin, gastrointestinal (GI) tract, immune system, or hair follicles. As a result, individuals taking such anticancer drugs can experience adverse effects, including anemia, scaly skin, GI tract disturbance, immunodeficiency, and hair loss.

E. Adenosine and guanosine monophosphate synthesis

The conversion of IMP to either AMP or GMP uses a two-step, energy- and nitrogen-requiring pathway (Fig. 22.8). [Note: AMP synthesis requires guanosine triphosphate (GTP) as an energy source and aspartate as a nitrogen source, whereas GMP synthesis requires ATP and glutamine.] Also, the first reaction in each pathway is inhibited by the end product of that pathway. This provides a mechanism for diverting IMP to the synthesis of the purine present in lesser amounts.

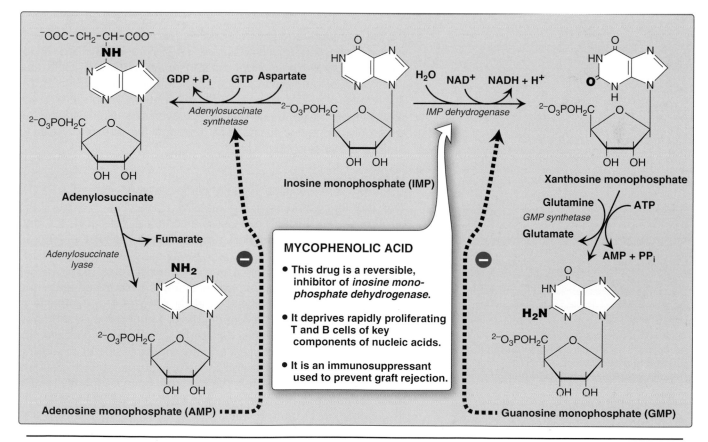

Figure 22.8
Conversion of IMP to AMP (or, adenylate) and GMP (or, guanylate) showing feedback inhibition. NAD(H) = nicotinamide adenine dinucleotide; GDP and GTP = guanosine di- and triphosphates; P_i = inorganic phosphate; PP_i = pyrophosphate.

Base-specific nucleoside monophosphate kinases		
AMP + ATP	$\xrightarrow{\text{Adenylate kinase}}$	2 ADP
GMP + ATP	$\xrightarrow{\text{Guanylate kinase}}$	GDP + ADP
Nucleoside diphosphate kinase		
GDP + ATP	$\rightleftharpoons$	GTP + ADP
CDP + ATP	$\rightleftharpoons$	CTP + ADP

Figure 22.9
Conversion of nucleoside monophosphates to di- and triphosphates. AMP and ADP = adenosine mono- and diphosphates; GMP, GDP, and GTP = guanosine mono-, di-, and triphosphates; CDP and CTP = cytidine di- and triphosphates.

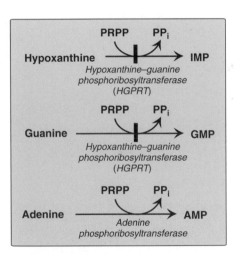

Figure 22.10
Salvage pathways of purine nucleotide synthesis. [Note: Virtually complete deficiency of *HGPRT* results in Lesch-Nyhan syndrome. Partial deficiencies of *HGPRT* are known. As the amount of functional enzyme increases, the severity of the symptoms decreases.] IMP, GMP, and AMP = inosine, guanosine, and adenosine monophosphates; PRPP = 5-phosphoribosyl-1-pyrophosphate; PP$_i$ = pyrophosphate.

If both AMP and GMP are present in adequate amounts, the de novo pathway of purine nucleotide synthesis is inhibited at the *GPAT* step.

F. Nucleoside di- and triphosphate synthesis

Nucleoside diphosphates are synthesized from the corresponding nucleoside monophosphates by base-specific *nucleoside monophosphate kinases* (Fig. 22.9). [Note: These *kinases* do not discriminate between ribose or deoxyribose in the substrate.] ATP is generally the source of the transferred phosphate because it is present in higher concentrations than the other nucleoside triphosphates. *Adenylate kinase* is particularly active in the liver and in muscle, where the turnover of energy from ATP is high. Its function is to maintain equilibrium among the adenine nucleotides (AMP, ADP, and ATP). Nucleoside diphosphates and triphosphates are interconverted by *nucleoside diphosphate kinase*, an enzyme that, unlike the *monophosphate kinases*, has broad substrate specificity.

G. Purine salvage pathway

Purines that result from the normal turnover of cellular nucleic acids, or the small amount that is obtained from the diet and not degraded, can be converted to nucleoside triphosphates and used by the body. This is referred to as the salvage pathway for purines. [Note: Salvage is particularly important in the brain.]

1. **Purine base salvage to nucleotides:** Two enzymes are involved: *adenine phosphoribosyltransferase* (*APRT*) and X-linked *hypoxanthine–guanine phosphoribosyltransferase* (*HGPRT*). Both use PRPP as the source of the ribose 5-phosphate group (Fig. 22.10). The release of pyrophosphate and its subsequent hydrolysis by *pyrophosphatase* makes these reactions irreversible. [Note: Adenosine is the only purine nucleoside to be salvaged. It is phosphorylated to AMP by *adenosine kinase*.]

2. **Lesch-Nyhan syndrome:** This is a rare, X-linked recessive disorder associated with a virtually complete deficiency of *HGPRT*. The deficiency results in an inability to salvage hypoxanthine or guanine, from which excessive amounts of uric acid, the end product of purine degradation, are then produced (see p. 298). In addition, the lack of this salvage pathway causes increased PRPP levels and decreased IMP and GMP levels. As a result, *GPAT* (the regulated step in purine synthesis) has excess substrate and decreased inhibitors available, and de novo purine synthesis is increased. The combination of decreased purine reutilization and increased purine synthesis results in increased degradation of purines and the production of large amounts of uric acid, making *HGPRT* deficiency an inherited cause of hyperuricemia. In patients with Lesch-Nyhan syndrome, the hyperuricemia frequently results in the formation of uric acid stones in the kidneys (urolithiasis) and the deposition of urate crystals in the joints (gouty arthritis) and soft tissues. In addition, the syndrome is characterized by motor dysfunction, cognitive deficits, and behavioral disturbances that include self-mutilation (for example, biting of lips and fingers), as shown in Figure 22.11.

IV. DEOXYRIBONUCLEOTIDE SYNTHESIS

The nucleotides described thus far all contain ribose (ribonucleotides). DNA synthesis, however, requires 2′-deoxyribonucleotides, which are produced from ribonucleoside diphosphates by the enzyme *ribonucleotide reductase* during the S-phase of the cell cycle (see p. 423). [Note: The same enzyme acts on pyrimidine ribonucleotides.]

A. Ribonucleotide reductase

Ribonucleotide reductase (*ribonucleoside diphosphate reductase*) is a dimer composed of two nonidentical subunits, R1 (or, α) and the smaller R2 (or, β), and is specific for the reduction of purine nucleoside diphosphates (ADP and GDP) and pyrimidine nucleoside diphosphates (CDP and UDP) to their deoxy forms (dADP, dGDP, dCDP, and dUDP). The immediate donors of the hydrogen atoms needed for the reduction of the 2′-hydroxyl group are two sulfhydryl (–SH) groups on the enzyme itself (R1 subunit), which form a disulfide bond during the reaction (see p. 19). [Note: R2 contains the stable tyrosyl radical required for catalysis at R1.]

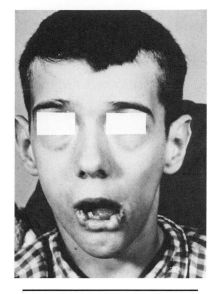

Figure 22.11
Lesions on the lips of a patient with Lesch-Nyhan syndrome.

1. **Reduced enzyme regeneration:** In order for *ribonucleotide reductase* to continue to produce deoxyribonucleotides at R1, the disulfide bond created during the production of the 2′-deoxy carbon must be reduced. The source of the reducing equivalents is thioredoxin, a protein coenzyme of *ribonucleotide reductase*. Thioredoxin contains two cysteine residues separated by two amino acids in the peptide chain. The two –SH groups of thioredoxin donate their hydrogen atoms to *ribonucleotide reductase*, forming a disulfide bond in the process (Fig. 22.12).

2. **Reduced thioredoxin regeneration:** Thioredoxin must be converted back to its reduced form in order to continue performing its function. The reducing equivalents are provided by NADPH + H$^+$, and the reaction is catalyzed by *thioredoxin reductase*, a selenoprotein (see p. 268).

B. Deoxyribonucleotide synthesis regulation

Ribonucleotide reductase is responsible for maintaining a balanced supply of the deoxyribonucleotides required for DNA synthesis. Consequently, the regulation of the enzyme is complex. In addition to the catalytic site, R1 contains two distinct allosteric sites involved in regulating enzymic activity (Fig. 22.13).

1. **Activity sites:** The binding of dATP to allosteric sites (known as activity sites) on R1 inhibits the overall catalytic activity of the enzyme and, therefore, prevents the reduction of any of the four nucleoside diphosphates. This effectively prevents DNA synthesis and explains the toxicity of increased levels of dATP seen in conditions such as *adenosine deaminase (ADA)* deficiency (see p. 301). In contrast, ATP bound to these sites activates the enzyme.

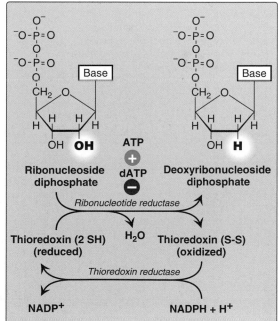

Figure 22.12
Conversion of ribonucleotides to deoxyribonucleotides. NADP(H) = nicotinamide adenine dinucleotide phosphate; dATP = deoxyadenosine triphosphate.

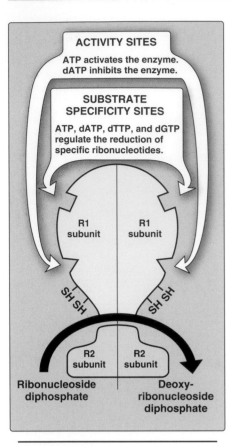

Figure 22.13
Regulation of *ribonucleotide reductase*. dATP, dTTP, and dGTP = deoxyadenosine, deoxythymidine, and deoxyguanosine triphosphates. [Note: The R1 subunit is also referred to as α and the R2 as β.]

2. **Substrate specificity sites:** The binding of nucleoside triphosphates to additional allosteric sites (known as substrate specificity sites) on R1 regulates substrate specificity, causing an increase in the conversion of different species of ribonucleotides to deoxyribonucleotides as they are required for DNA synthesis. For example, deoxythymidine triphosphate binding at the specificity site causes a conformational change that allows reduction of GDP to dGDP at the catalytic site when ATP is at the activity site.

The drug hydroxyurea (hydroxycarbamide) inhibits *ribonucleotide reductase*, thereby inhibiting the generation of substrates for DNA synthesis. The drug is an antineoplastic agent and is used in the treatment of cancers such as melanoma. Hydroxyurea is also used in the treatment of sickle cell anemia (see p. 36). However, the increase in fetal hemoglobin seen with hydroxyurea is because of changes in gene expression and not to *ribonucleotide reductase* inhibition.

V. PURINE NUCLEOTIDE DEGRADATION

Degradation of dietary nucleic acids occurs in the small intestine, where pancreatic *nucleases* hydrolyze them to nucleotides. The nucleotides are sequentially degraded by intestinal enzymes to nucleosides, phosphorylated sugars, and free bases. Uric acid is the end product of intestinal purine degradation. [Note: Purine nucleotides from <u>de novo</u> synthesis are degraded in the liver primarily. The free bases are sent out from the liver and salvaged by peripheral tissues.]

A. Degradation in the small intestine

Ribonucleases and *deoxyribonucleases*, secreted by the pancreas, hydrolyze dietary RNA and DNA to oligonucleotides that are further hydrolyzed by pancreatic *phosphodiesterases*, producing a mixture of 3′- and 5′-mononucleotides. At the intestinal mucosal surface, *nucleotidases* remove the phosphate groups hydrolytically, releasing nucleosides that are taken into enterocytes by sodium-dependent transporters and degraded by *nucleosidases* (*nucleoside phosphorylases*) to free bases plus (deoxy) ribose 1-phosphate. Dietary purine bases are not used to any appreciable extent for the synthesis of tissue nucleic acids. Instead, they are degraded to uric acid in the enterocytes. Most of the uric acid enters the blood and is eventually excreted in the urine. A summary of this pathway is shown in Figure 22.14. [Note: Mammals other than primates express *urate oxidase* (*uricase*), which cleaves the purine ring, generating allantoin. Modified recombinant *urate oxidase* is now used clinically to lower urate levels.]

B. Uric acid formation

A summary of the steps in the production of uric acid and the genetic diseases associated with deficiencies of specific degradative enzymes are shown in Figure 22.15. [Note: The bracketed numbers refer to specific reactions in the figure.]

[1] An amino group is removed from AMP to produce IMP by *AMP* (*adenylate*) *deaminase* or from adenosine to produce inosine (hypoxanthine-ribose) by *adenosine deaminase*.

[2] IMP and GMP are converted into their respective nucleoside forms, inosine and guanosine, by the action of *5'-nucleotidase*.

[3] *Purine nucleoside phosphorylase* converts inosine and guanosine into their respective purine bases, hypoxanthine and guanine. [Note: A *mutase* interconverts ribose 1- and ribose 5-phosphate.]

[4] Guanine is deaminated to form xanthine.

[5] Hypoxanthine is oxidized by molybdenum-containing *xanthine oxidase* (*XO*) to xanthine, which is further oxidized by *XO* to uric acid, the final product of human purine degradation. Uric acid is excreted primarily in the urine.

C. Diseases associated with purine degradation

1. Gout: Gout is a disorder initiated by high levels of uric acid (the end product of purine catabolism) in blood (hyperuricemia), as a result of either the overproduction or underexcretion of uric acid. The hyperuricemia can lead to the deposition of monosodium urate (MSU) crystals in the joints and an inflammatory response to the crystals, causing first acute and then progressing to chronic gouty arthritis. Nodular masses of MSU crystals (tophi) may be deposited in the soft tissues, resulting in chronic tophaceous gout (Fig. 22.16). Formation of uric acid stones in the kidney (urolithiasis) may also be seen. [Note: Hyperuricemia is not sufficient to cause gout, but gout is always preceded by hyperuricemia. Hyperuricemia is typically asymptomatic but may be indicative of comorbid conditions such as hypertension.] The definitive diagnosis of gout requires aspiration and examination of synovial fluid (Fig. 22.17) from an affected joint (or material from a tophus) using polarized light microscopy to confirm the presence of needle-shaped MSU crystals (Fig. 22.18).

a. Uric acid underexcretion: In >90% of individuals with hyperuricemia, the cause is underexcretion of uric acid. Underexcretion can be primary, because of as-yet-unidentified inherent excretory defects, or secondary to known disease processes that affect how the kidney handles urate (for example, in lactic acidosis, lactate increases renal urate reabsorption, thereby decreasing its excretion) and to environmental factors such as the use of drugs (for example, thiazide diuretics) or exposure to lead (saturnine gout).

b. Uric acid overproduction: A less common cause of hyperuricemia is from the overproduction of uric acid. Primary hyperuricemia is, for the most part, idiopathic (having no known cause). However, several identified mutations in the gene for X-linked *PRPP synthetase* result in the enzyme having an increased maximal velocity ($[V_{max}]$ see p. 57) for the production of PRPP, a lower K_m (see p. 59) for ribose 5-phosphate, or a decreased sensitivity to purine nucleotides, its allosteric inhibitors (see p. 62). In each case, increased availability of PRPP increases purine production,

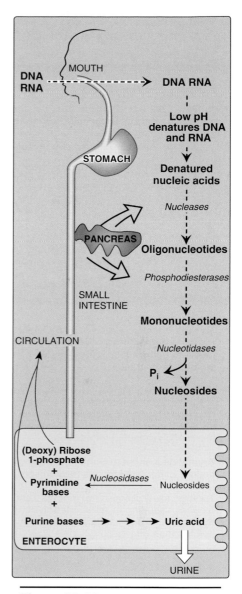

Figure 22.14
Digestion of dietary nucleic acids.
P_i = inorganic phosphate.

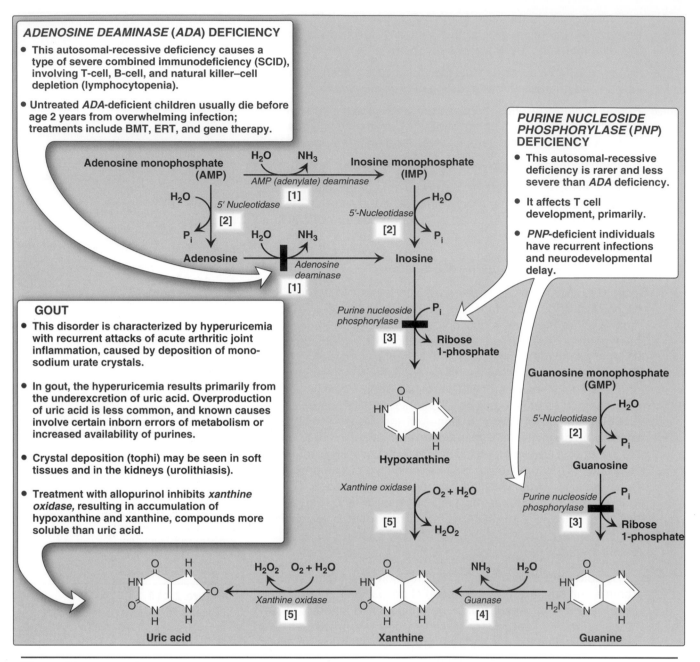

Figure 22.15
The degradation of purine nucleotides to uric acid, illustrating some of the genetic diseases associated with this pathway. [Note: The numbers in brackets refer to the corresponding numbered citations in the text.] BMT = bone marrow transplantation; ERT = enzyme replacement therapy; P_i = inorganic phosphate; H_2O_2 = hydrogen peroxide; NH_3 = ammonia.

resulting in elevated levels of plasma uric acid. Lesch-Nyhan syndrome (see p. 296) also causes hyperuricemia as a result of the decreased salvage of hypoxanthine and guanine and the subsequent increased availability of PRPP. Secondary hyperuricemia is typically the consequence of increased availability of purines (for example, in patients with myeloproliferative disorders or who are undergoing chemotherapy and so have a high rate of cell turnover). Hyperuricemia can also be the result of seemingly unrelated metabolic diseases, such as von Gierke disease (see Fig. 11.8 on p. 130) or hereditary fructose intolerance (see p. 138).

> | A diet rich in meat, seafood (particularly shellfish), and ethanol is associated with increased risk of gout, whereas a diet rich in low-fat dairy products is associated with a decreased risk.

c. **Treatment:** Acute attacks of gout are treated with anti-inflammatory agents. Colchicine, steroidal drugs such as prednisone, and nonsteroidal drugs such as indomethacin are used. [Note: Colchicine prevents formation of microtubules, thereby decreasing the movement of neutrophils into the affected area. Like the other anti-inflammatory drugs, it has no effect on uric acid levels.] Long-term therapeutic strategies for gout involve lowering the uric acid level below its saturation point (6.5 mg/dl), thereby preventing the deposition of MSU crystals. Uricosuric agents, such as probenecid or sulfinpyrazone, that increase renal excretion of uric acid, are used in patients who are under-excretors of uric acid. Allopurinol, a structural analog of hypoxanthine, inhibits uric acid synthesis and is used in patients who are overproducers of uric acid. Allopurinol is oxidized to oxypurinol, a long-lived inhibitor of *XO*. This results in an accumulation of hypoxanthine and xanthine (see Fig. 22.15), compounds more soluble than uric acid and, therefore, less likely to initiate an inflammatory response. In patients with normal levels of *HGPRT*, the hypoxanthine can be salvaged, reducing the levels of PRPP and, therefore, de novo purine synthesis. Febuxostat, a nonpurine inhibitor of *XO*, is also available. [Note: Uric acid levels in the blood normally are close to the saturation point. One reason for this may be the strong antioxidant effects of uric acid.]

2. **Adenosine deaminase deficiency:** *ADA* is expressed in a variety of tissues, but, in humans, lymphocytes have the highest activity of this cytoplasmic enzyme. A deficiency of *ADA* results in an accumulation of adenosine, which is converted to its ribonucleotide or deoxyribonucleotide forms by cellular *kinases*. As dATP levels rise, *ribonucleotide reductase* is inhibited, thereby preventing the production of all deoxyribose-containing nucleotides (see p. 297). Consequently, cells cannot make DNA and divide. [Note: The dATP and adenosine that accumulate in *ADA* deficiency lead to developmental arrest and apoptosis of lymphocytes.] In its most severe form, this autosomal-recessive disorder causes a type of severe combined immunodeficiency disease (SCID), involving a decrease in T cells, B cells, and natural killer cells. *ADA* deficiency accounts for ~14% of cases of SCID in the United States. Treatments include bone marrow transplantation, enzyme replacement therapy, and gene therapy (see p. 501). Without appropriate treatment, children with this disorder usually die from infection by age 2 years. [Note: *Purine nucleoside phosphorylase* deficiency results in a less severe immunodeficiency primarily involving T cells.]

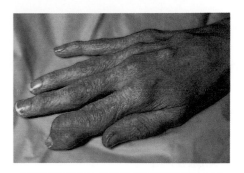

Figure 22.16
Tophaceous gout.

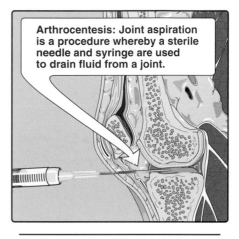

Figure 22.17
Analysis of joint fluid can help to define causes of joint swelling and arthritis, such as infection, gout, and rheumatoid disease.

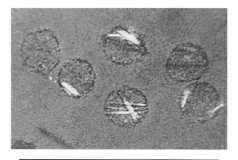

Figure 22.18
Gout can be diagnosed by the presence of negatively birefringent monosodium urate crystals in aspirated synovial fluid examined by polarized light microscopy. Here, crystals are seen within polymorphonuclear leukocytes.

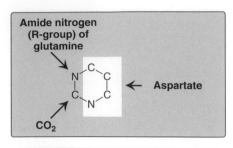

Figure 22.19
Sources of the individual atoms in the pyrimidine ring. CO_2 = carbon dioxide.

Variable	*CPS I*	*CPS II*
Cellular location	Mitochondria	Cytosol
Pathway involved	Urea cycle	Pyrimidine synthesis
Source of nitrogen	Ammonia	γ-Amide group of glutamine
Regulators	Activator: N-acetyl-glutamate	Activator: PRPP Inhibitor: UTP

Figure 22.20
Summary of the differences between *carbamoyl phosphate synthetase* (*CPS*) I and II. PRPP = 5-phosphoribosyl-1-pyrophosphate; UTP = uridine triphosphate.

VI. PYRIMIDINE SYNTHESIS AND DEGRADATION

Unlike the synthesis of the purine ring, which is constructed on a pre-existing ribose 5-phosphate, the pyrimidine ring is synthesized before being attached to ribose 5-phosphate, which is donated by PRPP. The sources of the atoms in the pyrimidine ring are glutamine, CO_2, and aspartate (Fig. 22.19).

A. Carbamoyl phosphate synthesis

The regulated step of this pathway in mammalian cells is the synthesis of carbamoyl phosphate from glutamine and CO_2, catalyzed by *carbamoyl phosphate synthetase* (*CPS*) *II*. *CPS II* is inhibited by uridine triphosphate (the end product of this pathway, which can be converted into the other pyrimidine nucleotides) and is activated by PRPP. [Note: Carbamoyl phosphate, synthesized by *CPS I*, is also a precursor of urea (see p. 253). Defects in *ornithine transcarbamylase* of the urea cycle promote pyrimidine synthesis because of increased availability of carbamoyl phosphate. A comparison of the two enzymes is presented in Figure 22.20.]

B. Orotic acid synthesis

The second step in pyrimidine synthesis is the formation of carbamoylaspartate, catalyzed by *aspartate transcarbamoylase*. The pyrimidine ring is then closed by *dihydroorotase*. The resulting dihydroorotate is oxidized to produce orotic acid (orotate), as shown in Figure 22.21. The human enzyme that produces orotate, *dihydroorotate dehydrogenase*, is a flavin mononucleotide-containing protein of the inner mitochondrial membrane. All other enzymes in pyrimidine biosynthesis are cytosolic. [Note: The first three enzymic activities in this pathway (*CPS II*, *aspartate transcarbamoylase*, and *dihydroorotase*) are actually three different catalytic domains of a single polypeptide known as *CAD* from the first letter in the name of each domain. (See p. 18 for a discussion of domains.) This is an example of a multifunctional or multicatalytic polypeptide that facilitates the ordered synthesis of an important compound. Synthesis of the purine nucleotide IMP also involves multifunctional proteins.]

C. Pyrimidine nucleotide synthesis

The completed pyrimidine ring is converted to the nucleotide orotidine monophosphate (OMP) in the second stage of pyrimidine nucleotide synthesis (see Fig. 22.21). As seen with the purines, PRPP is the ribose 5-phosphate donor. The enzyme *orotate phosphoribosyltransferase* produces OMP and releases pyrophosphate, thereby making the reaction biologically irreversible. [Note: Both purine and pyrimidine synthesis require glutamine, aspartic acid, and PRPP as essential precursors.] OMP (orotidylate) is decarboxylated to uridine monophosphate (UMP) by *orotidylate decarboxylase*. The *phosphoribosyltransferase* and *decarboxylase* activities are separate catalytic domains of a single polypeptide called *UMP synthase*. Hereditary orotic aciduria (a very rare disorder) may be caused by a deficiency of one or both activities of this bifunctional enzyme, resulting in orotic acid in the urine (see Fig. 22.21). UMP is sequentially phosphorylated

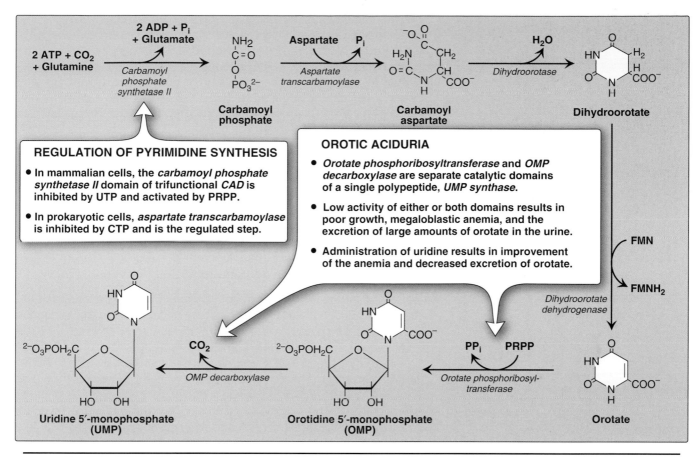

Figure 22.21

<u>De</u> <u>novo</u> pyrimidine synthesis. ADP = adenosine diphosphate; P_i = inorganic phosphate; FMN(H_2) = flavin mononucleotide; CTP = cytidine triphosphate; PRPP = 5-phosphoribosyl-1-pyrophosphate; PP_i = pyrophosphate.

to UDP and UTP. [Note: The UDP is a substrate for *ribonucleotide reductase*, which generates dUDP. The dUDP is phosphorylated to dUTP, which is rapidly hydrolyzed to dUMP by *UTP diphosphatase* (*dUTPase*). Thus, *dUTPase* plays an important role in reducing availability of dUTP as a substrate for DNA synthesis, thereby preventing erroneous incorporation of uracil into DNA.]

D. Cytidine triphosphate synthesis

Cytidine triphosphate (CTP) is produced by amination of UTP by *CTP synthetase* (Fig. 22.22), with glutamine providing the nitrogen. Some of this CTP is dephosphorylated to CDP, which is a substrate for *ribonucleotide reductase*. The dCDP product can be phosphorylated to dCTP for DNA synthesis or dephosphorylated to dCMP that is deaminated to dUMP.

E. Deoxythymidine monophosphate synthesis

dUMP is converted to deoxythymidine monophosphate (dTMP) by *thymidylate synthase*, which uses N^5,N^{10}-methylene-THF as the source of the methyl group (see p. 267). This is an unusual reaction in that THF contributes not only a one-carbon unit but also two hydrogen atoms from the pteridine ring, resulting in the oxidation of THF to dihydrofolate

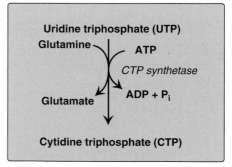

Figure 22.22

Synthesis of CTP from UTP. [Note: CTP, required for RNA synthesis, is converted to dCTP for DNA synthesis.] ADP = adenosine diphosphate; P_i = inorganic phosphate.

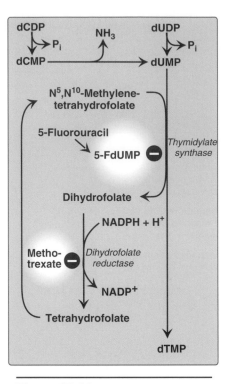

Figure 22.23
Synthesis of dTMP from dUMP,
illustrating sites of action of
antineoplastic drugs.

([DHF], Fig. 22.23). Inhibitors of *thymidylate synthase* include thymine analogs such as 5-fluorouracil, which serve as antitumor agents. 5-Fluorouracil is metabolically converted to 5-fluorodeoxyuridine monophosphate (5-FdUMP), which becomes permanently bound to the inactivated *thymidylate synthase*, making the drug a suicide inhibitor (see p. 60). DHF can be reduced to THF by *dihydrofolate reductase* (see Fig. 28.2, p. 378), an enzyme that is inhibited by folate analogs such as methotrexate. By decreasing the supply of THF, these drugs not only inhibit purine synthesis (see Fig. 22.7), but, by preventing methylation of dUMP to dTMP, they also decrease the availability of this essential component of DNA. DNA synthesis is inhibited and cell growth slowed. Thus, these drugs are used to treat cancer. [Note: Acyclovir (a purine analog) and AZT (3′-azido-3′-deoxythymidine, a pyrimidine analog) are used to treat infections of herpes simplex virus and human immunodeficiency virus, respectively. Each inhibits the viral *DNA polymerase*.]

F. Pyrimidine salvage and degradation

Unlike the purine ring, which is not cleaved in humans and is excreted as poorly soluble uric acid, the pyrimidine ring is opened and degraded to highly soluble products, β-alanine (from the degradation of CMP and UMP) and β-aminoisobutyrate (from TMP degradation), with the production of ammonia and CO_2. Pyrimidine bases can be salvaged to nucleosides, which are phosphorylated to nucleotides. However, their high solubility makes pyrimidine salvage less significant clinically than purine salvage. [Note: The salvage of pyrimidine nucleosides is the basis for using uridine in the treatment of hereditary orotic aciduria (see p. 302).]

VII. CHAPTER SUMMARY

Nucleotides are composed of a **nitrogenous base** (adenine = **A**, guanine = **G**, cytosine = **C**, uracil = **U**, and thymine = **T**); a **pentose sugar**; and one, two, or three **phosphate groups** (Fig. 22.24). A and G are **purines**, and C, U, and T are **pyrimidines**. If the sugar is **ribose**, the nucleotide is a **ribonucleoside phosphate** (for example, adenosine monophosphate [AMP]), and it can have several functions in the cell, including being a component of **RNA**. If the sugar is **deoxyribose**, the nucleotide is a **deoxyribonucleoside phosphate** (for example, deoxyAMP) and will be found almost exclusively as a component of **DNA**. The committed step in **purine synthesis** uses **5-phosphoribosyl-1-pyrophosphate** ([PRPP], an activated pentose that provides the **ribose 5-phosphate** for de novo purine and pyrimidine synthesis and salvage) and nitrogen from **glutamine** to produce phosphoribosylamine. The enzyme is **glutamine:phosphoribosylpyrophosphate amidotransferase** and is inhibited by AMP and guanosine monophosphate (the end products of the pathway) and activated by PRPP. Purine nucleotides can also be produced from preformed purine bases by using **salvage reactions** catalyzed by **adenine phosphoribosyltransferase** (**APRT**) and **hypoxanthine–guanine phosphoribosyltransferase** (**HGPRT**). A near-total deficiency of *HGPRT* causes **Lesch-Nyhan syndrome**, a severe, inherited form of hyperuricemia accompanied by compulsive self-mutilation. All deoxyribonucleotides are synthesized from ribonucleotides by the enzyme **ribonucleotide reductase**. This enzyme is highly regulated (for example, it is strongly inhibited by **deoxyadenosine triphosphate [dATP]**, a compound that is overproduced in bone marrow cells in individuals with **adenosine deaminase** [**ADA**] deficiency). *ADA* deficiency causes **severe combined immunodeficiency disease**. The end product of purine degradation is **uric acid**, a compound of low solubility whose overproduction or undersecretion causes **hyperuricemia** that, if accompanied by the deposition of **monosodium urate crystals** in joints and soft tissues and an inflammatory response to those crystals, results in **gout**. The first step in **pyrimidine synthesis**, the production of carbamoyl phosphate by **carbamoyl phosphate synthetase II**, is the regulated step in this pathway (it is inhibited by **uridine triphosphate** [**UTP**] and activated by PRPP). The UTP produced by this pathway can be converted to cytidine triphosphate. **Deoxyuridine monophosphate** can be converted to **deoxythymidine monophosphate** by **thymidylate synthase**, an enzyme targeted by anticancer drugs such as **5-fluorouracil**. The regeneration of **tetrahydrofolate** from dihydrofolate produced in the *thymidylate synthase* reaction requires **dihydrofolate reductase**, an enzyme targeted by the drug **methotrexate**. Pyrimidine degradation results in soluble products.

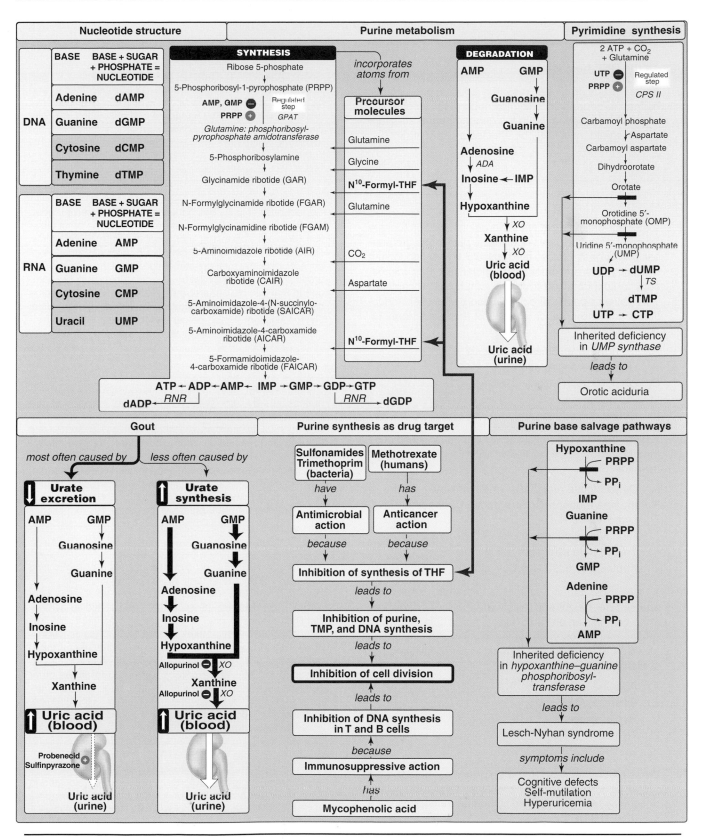

Figure 22.24

Key concept map for nucleotide metabolism. THF = tetrahydrofolate; *GPAT = glutamine:phosphoribosylpyrophosphate amidotransferase; ADA = adenosine deaminase*; XO = *xanthine oxidase*; TS = *thymidylate synthase*; RNR = *ribonucleotide reductase*; CPS II = *carbamoyl phosphate synthetase II*; AMP, GMP, CMP, TMP, and IMP = adenosine, guanosine, cytidine, thymidine, and inosine monophosphates; d = deoxy; PP$_i$ = pyrophosphate; PRPP = 5-phosphoribosyl-1-pyrophosphate.

Study Questions

Choose the ONE best answer.

22.1 Azaserine, a drug with research applications, inhibits glutamine-dependent enzymes. Incorporation of which of the ring nitrogens (N) in the generic purine structure shown would most likely be affected by azaserine?

  A. 1
  B. 3
  C. 7
  D. 9

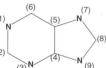

> Correct answer = D. The N at position 9 is supplied by glutamine in the first step of purine de novo synthesis, and its incorporation would be affected by azaserine. The N at position 1 is supplied by aspartate and at position 7 by glycine. The N at position 3 is also supplied by glutamine, but azaserine would have inhibited purine synthesis prior to this step.

22.2 A 42-year-old male patient undergoing radiation therapy for prostate cancer develops severe pain in the metatarsal phalangeal joint of his right big toe. Monosodium urate crystals are detected by polarized light microscopy in fluid obtained from this joint by arthrocentesis. This patient's pain is directly caused by the overproduction of the end product of which of the following metabolic pathways?

  A. De novo pyrimidine biosynthesis
  B. Pyrimidine degradation
  C. De novo purine biosynthesis
  D. Purine salvage
  E. Purine degradation

> Correct answer = E. The patient's pain is caused by gout, resulting from an inflammatory response to the crystallization of excess urate (as monosodium urate) in his joints. Radiation therapy caused cell death, with degradation of nucleic acids and their constituent purines. Uric acid, the end product of purine degradation, is a relatively insoluble compound that can cause gout (and kidney stones). Pyrimidine metabolism is not associated with uric acid production. Overproduction of purines can indirectly result in hyperuricemia. Purine salvage decreases uric acid production.

22.3 Which one of the following enzymes of nucleotide metabolism is correctly paired with its pharmacologic inhibitor?

  A. Dihydrofolate reductase—methotrexate
  B. Inosine monophosphate dehydrogenase—hydroxyurea
  C. Ribonucleotide reductase—5-fluorouracil
  D. Thymidylate synthase—allopurinol
  E. Xanthine oxidase—probenecid

> Correct answer = A. Methotrexate interferes with folate metabolism by acting as a competitive inhibitor of the enzyme dihydrofolate reductase. This starves cells for tetrahydrofolate and makes them unable to synthesize purines and thymidine monophosphate. Inosine monophosphate dehydrogenase is inhibited by mycophenolic acid. Ribonucleotide reductase is inhibited by hydroxyurea. Thymidylate synthase is inhibited by 5-fluorouracil. Xanthine oxidase is inhibited by allopurinol. Probenecid increases renal excretion of urate but does not inhibit its production.

22.4 A 1-year-old female patient is lethargic, weak, and anemic. Her height and weight are low for her age. Her urine contains an elevated level of orotic acid. Activity of uridine monophosphate synthase is low. Administration of which of the following is most likely to alleviate her symptoms?

  A. Adenine
  B. Guanine
  C. Hypoxanthine
  D. Thymidine
  E. Uridine

> Correct answer = E. The elevated excretion of orotic acid and low activity of uridine monophosphate (UMP) synthase indicate that the patient has orotic aciduria, a very rare genetic disorder affecting de novo pyrimidine synthesis. Deficiencies in one or both catalytic domains of UMP synthase leave the patient unable to synthesize pyrimidines. Uridine, a pyrimidine nucleoside, is a useful treatment because it bypasses the missing activities and can be salvaged to UMP, which can be converted to all the other pyrimidines. Although thymidine is a pyrimidine nucleoside, it cannot be converted to other pyrimidines. Hypoxanthine, guanine, and adenine are all purine bases and cannot be converted to pyrimidines.

22.5 What laboratory test would help in distinguishing an orotic aciduria caused by ornithine transcarbamylase deficiency from that caused by uridine monophosphate synthase deficiency?

> Blood ammonia level would be expected to be elevated in ornithine transcarbamylase deficiency that affects the urea cycle but not in uridine monophosphate synthase deficiency.

Metabolic Effects of Insulin and Glucagon

23

I. OVERVIEW

Four major tissues play a dominant role in fuel metabolism: liver, adipose, muscle, and brain. These tissues contain unique sets of enzymes, such that each tissue is specialized for the storage, use, or generation of specific fuels. These tissues do not function in isolation but rather form part of a network in which one tissue may provide substrates to another or process compounds produced by other tissues. Communication between tissues is mediated by the nervous system, by the availability of circulating substrates, and by variation in the levels of plasma hormones (Fig. 23.1). The integration of energy metabolism is controlled primarily by the actions of two peptide hormones, insulin and glucagon (secreted in response to changing substrate levels in the blood), with the catecholamines epinephrine and norepinephrine (secreted in response to neural signals) playing a supporting role. Changes in the circulating levels of these hormones allow the body to store energy when food is abundant or to make stored energy available such as during survival crises (for example, famine, severe injury, and "fight-or-flight" situations). This chapter describes the structure, secretion, and metabolic effects of the two hormones that most profoundly affect energy metabolism.

II. INSULIN

Insulin is a peptide hormone produced by the β cells of the islets of Langerhans, which are clusters of cells embedded in the endocrine portion of the pancreas (Fig. 23.2). [Note: "Insulin" is from the Latin for island.] The islets make up only about 1%–2% of the total cells of the pancreas. Insulin is the most important hormone coordinating the use of fuels by tissues. Its metabolic effects are anabolic, favoring, for example, synthesis of glycogen, triacylglycerol (TAG), and protein.

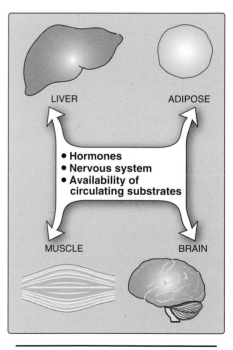

Figure 23.1
Mechanisms of communication between four major tissues.

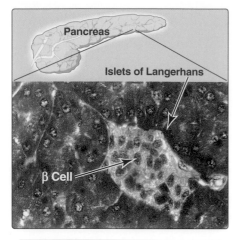

Figure 23.2
Islets of Langerhans.

A. Structure

Insulin is composed of 51 amino acids arranged in two polypeptide chains, designated A (21 amino acids) and B, which are linked together by two disulfide bonds (Fig. 23.3A). The insulin molecule also contains an intramolecular disulfide bond between amino acid residues of the A chain. [Note: Insulin was the first peptide for which the primary structure was determined and the first therapeutic molecule made by recombinant DNA technology (see p. 486).]

B. Synthesis

The processing and transport of intermediates that occur during the synthesis of insulin are shown in Figures 23.3B and 23.4. Biosynthesis involves production of two inactive precursors, preproinsulin and proinsulin, which are sequentially cleaved to form the active hormone plus the connecting or C-peptide in a 1:1 ratio (see Fig. 23.4). [Note: The C-peptide is essential for proper insulin folding. Also, because its half-life in plasma is longer than that of insulin, the C-peptide level is a good indicator of insulin production and secretion.] Insulin is stored in cytosolic granules that, given the proper stimulus (see C.1. below), are released by exocytosis. (See p. 459 for a discussion of the synthesis of secreted proteins.) Insulin is degraded by *insulin-degrading enzyme*, which is present in the liver and, to a lesser extent, in the kidneys. Insulin has a plasma half-life of ~6 minutes. This short duration of action permits rapid changes in circulating levels of the hormone.

C. Secretion regulation

Secretion of insulin is regulated by bloodborne fuels and hormones.

1. **Increased secretion:** Insulin secretion by the pancreatic β cells is closely coordinated with the secretion of glucagon by pancreatic

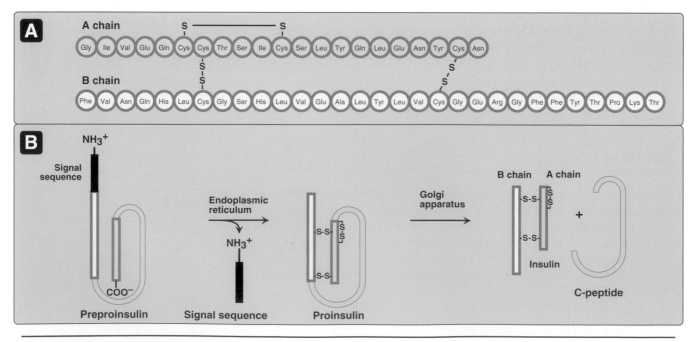

Figure 23.3
A. Structure of insulin. B. Formation of human insulin from preproinsulin. S-S = disulfide bond.

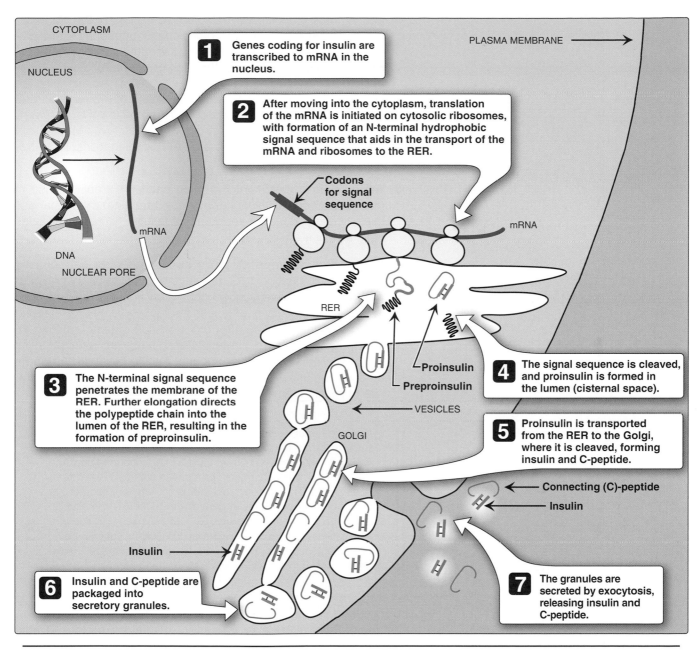

Figure 23.4

Intracellular movements of insulin and its precursors. mRNA = messenger RNA; RER = rough endoplasmic reticulum.

α cells (Fig. 23.5). The relative amounts of glucagon and insulin released are normally regulated such that the rate of hepatic glucose production is kept equal to the use of glucose by peripheral tissues. This maintains blood glucose between 70 and 140 mg/dl. In view of its coordinating role, it is not surprising that the β cell responds to a variety of stimuli. In particular, insulin secretion is increased by glucose, amino acids, and gastrointestinal peptide hormones.

a. Glucose: Ingestion of a carbohydrate-rich meal leads to a rise in blood glucose, the primary stimulus for insulin secretion (see Fig. 23.5). The β cells are the most important glucose-sensing cells in the body. Like the liver, β cells contain GLUT-2 transporters

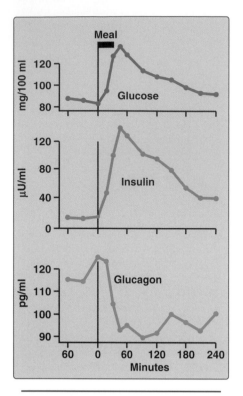

Figure 23.5
Changes in blood levels of glucose, insulin, and glucagon after ingestion of a carbohydrate-rich meal.

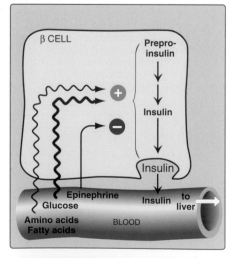

Figure 23.6
Regulation of insulin release from pancreatic β cells. [Note: Gastrointestinal peptide hormones also stimulate insulin release.]

and express *glucokinase* (*hexokinase IV*; see p. 98). At blood glucose levels >45 mg/dl, *glucokinase* phosphorylates glucose in amounts proportional to the glucose concentration. Proportionality results from the lack of direct inhibition of *glucokinase* by glucose 6-phosphate, its product. Additionally, the sigmoidal relationship between the velocity of the reaction and substrate concentration (see p. 98) maximizes the enzyme's responsiveness to changes in blood glucose level. Metabolism of glucose 6-phosphate generates ATP, leading to insulin secretion (see blue box below).

b. **Amino acids:** Ingestion of protein causes a transient rise in plasma amino acid levels (for example, arginine) that enhances the glucose-stimulated secretion of insulin. [Note: Fatty acids have a similar effect.]

c. **Gastrointestinal peptide hormones:** The intestinal peptides glucagon-like peptide-1 (GLP-1) and gastric inhibitory polypeptide ([GIP] also called glucose-dependent insulinotropic peptide) increase the sensitivity of β cells to glucose. They are released from the small intestine after the ingestion of food, causing an anticipatory rise in insulin levels and, thus, are referred to as incretins. Their action may account for the fact that the same amount of glucose given orally induces a much greater secretion of insulin than if given intravenously (IV).

> Glucose-dependent release of insulin into blood is mediated through a rise in calcium (Ca^{2+}) concentration in the β cell. Glucose taken into β cells by GLUT-2 is phosphorylated and metabolized, with subsequent production of ATP. ATP-sensitive potassium (K^+) channels close, causing depolarization of the plasma membrane, opening of voltage-gated Ca^{2+} channels, and influx of Ca^{2+} into the cell. Ca^{2+} causes vesicles containing insulin to be exocytosed from the β cell. Sulfonylureas, oral agents used to treat type 2 diabetes, increase insulin secretion by closing ATP-sensitive K^+ channels.

2. **Decreased secretion:** The synthesis and release of insulin are decreased when there is a scarcity of dietary fuels and also during periods of physiologic stress (for example, infection, hypoxia, and vigorous exercise), thereby preventing hypoglycemia. These effects are mediated primarily by the catecholamines norepinephrine and epinephrine, which are made from tyrosine in the sympathetic nervous system (SNS) and the adrenal medulla and then secreted. Secretion is largely controlled by neural signals. The catecholamines (primarily epinephrine) have a direct effect on energy metabolism, causing a rapid mobilization of energy-yielding fuels, including glucose from the liver (produced by glycogenolysis or gluconeogenesis; see p. 121) and fatty acids (FA) from adipose tissue (produced by lipolysis; see p. 189). In addition, these biogenic amines can override the normal glucose-stimulated release of insulin. Thus, in emergency situations, the SNS largely replaces the plasma glucose concentration as the controlling influence over β-cell secretion. The regulation of insulin secretion is summarized in Figure 23.6.

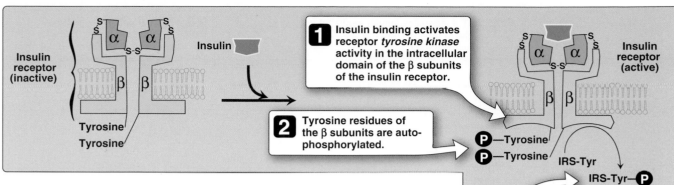

D. Metabolic effects

Insulin promotes the storage of nutrients as glycogen, TAG, and protein and inhibits their mobilization.

1. **Effects on carbohydrate metabolism:** The effects of insulin on glucose metabolism promote its storage and are most prominent in three tissues: liver, muscle, and adipose. In liver and muscle, insulin increases glycogen synthesis. In muscle and adipose, insulin increases glucose uptake by increasing the number of glucose transporters (GLUT-4; see p. 97) in the cell membrane. Thus, the IV administration of insulin causes an immediate decrease in blood glucose level. In the liver, insulin decreases the production of glucose through the inhibition of glycogenolysis and gluconeogenesis. [Note: The effects of insulin are due not just to changes in enzyme activity but also in enzyme amount insofar as insulin alters gene transcription.]

2. **Effects on lipid metabolism:** A rise in insulin rapidly causes a significant reduction in the release of FA from adipose tissue by inhibiting the activity of *hormone-sensitive lipase*, a key enzyme of TAG degradation in adipocytes. Insulin acts by promoting the dephosphorylation and, hence, inactivation of the enzyme (see p. 190). Insulin also increases the transport and metabolism of glucose into adipocytes, providing the glycerol 3-phosphate substrate for TAG synthesis (see p. 188). Expression of the gene for *lipoprotein lipase*, which degrades TAG in circulating chylomicrons and very-low-density lipoproteins ([VLDL] see p. 229), is increased by insulin in adipose, thereby providing FA for esterification to the glycerol. [Note: Insulin also promotes the conversion of glucose to TAG in the liver. The TAG are secreted in VLDL.]

3. **Effects on protein synthesis:** In most tissues, insulin stimulates both the entry of amino acids into cells and protein synthesis (translation). [Note: Insulin stimulates protein synthesis through covalent activation of factors required for translation initiation.]

E. Mechanism

Insulin binds to specific, high-affinity receptors in the cell membrane of most tissues, including liver, muscle, and adipose. This is the first step in a cascade of reactions ultimately leading to a diverse array of biologic actions (Fig. 23.7).

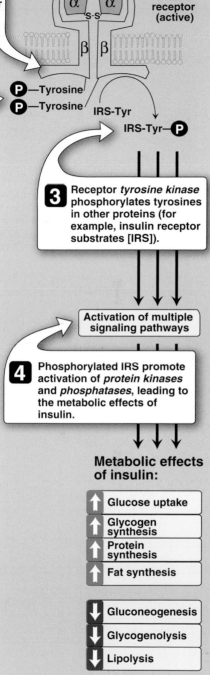

Figure 23.7
Mechanism of action of insulin. ⓟ = phosphate; Tyr – tyrosine; S-S = disulfide bond.

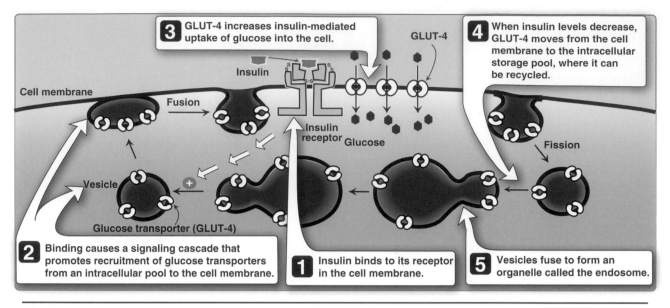

Figure 23.8
Insulin-mediated recruitment of GLUT-4 from intracellular stores to the cell membrane in skeletal and cardiac muscle and adipose tissue. S-S = disulfide bond.

1. **Insulin receptor:** The insulin receptor is synthesized as a single polypeptide that is glycosylated and cleaved into α and β subunits, which are then assembled into a tetramer linked by disulfide bonds (see Fig. 23.7). The extracellular α subunits contain the insulin-binding site. A hydrophobic domain in each β subunit spans the plasma membrane. The cytosolic domain of the β subunit is a *tyrosine kinase*, which is activated by insulin. As a result, the insulin receptor is classified as a *tyrosine kinase* receptor.

2. **Signal transduction:** The binding of insulin to the α subunits of the insulin receptor induces conformational changes that are transmitted to the β subunits. This promotes a rapid autophosphorylation of specific tyrosine residues on each β subunit (see Fig. 23.7). Autophosphorylation initiates a cascade of cell-signaling responses, including phosphorylation of a family of proteins called insulin receptor substrates (IRS). At least four IRS have been identified that show similar structures but different tissue distributions. Phosphorylated IRS proteins interact with other signaling molecules through specific domains (known as SH2), activating a number of pathways that affect gene expression, cell metabolism, and growth. The actions of insulin are terminated by dephosphorylation of the receptor.

3. **Membrane effects:** Glucose transport in some tissues, such as muscle and adipose, increases in the presence of insulin (Fig. 23.8). Insulin promotes movement of insulin-sensitive glucose transporters (GLUT-4) from a pool located in intracellular vesicles to the cell membrane. [Note: Movement is the result of a signaling cascade in which an IRS binds to and activates a *kinase* (*phosphoinositide 3-kinase*), leading to phosphorylation of the membrane phospholipid phosphatidylinositol 4,5-bisphosphate (PIP₂) to the 3,4,5-trisphosphate form (PIP₃) that binds to and activates *phosphoinositide-dependent kinase 1*. This *kinase*, in turn, activates *Akt* (or *protein kinase B*), resulting in GLUT-4 movement.] In contrast, other tissues have insulin-insensitive systems for glucose

	Active transport	Facilitated transport
Insulin sensitive		Skeletal and cardiac muscle and adipose tissue (together account for largest tissue mass)
Insulin insensitive	Epithelia of intestine Renal tubules Choroid plexus	Erythrocytes Leukocytes Lens of eye Cornea Liver Brain

Figure 23.9
Characteristics of glucose transport in various tissues.

transport (Fig. 23.9). For example, hepatocytes, erythrocytes, and cells of the nervous system, intestinal mucosa, renal tubules, and cornea do not require insulin for glucose uptake.

4. **Receptor regulation:** Binding of insulin is followed by internalization of the hormone–receptor complex. Once inside the cell, insulin is degraded in the lysosomes. The receptors may be degraded, but most are recycled to the cell surface. [Note: Elevated levels of insulin promote the degradation of receptors, thereby decreasing the number of surface receptors. This is one type of downregulation.]

5. **Time course:** The binding of insulin provokes a wide range of actions. The most immediate response is an increase in glucose transport into adipocytes and skeletal and cardiac muscle cells that occurs within seconds of insulin binding to its membrane receptor. Insulin-induced changes in enzymic activity in many cell types occur over minutes to hours and reflect changes in the phosphorylation states of existing proteins. Insulin-induced increase in the amount of many enzymes, such as *glucokinase*, liver *pyruvate kinase*, *acetyl coenzyme A* (*CoA*) *carboxylase* (*ACC*), and *fatty acid synthase*, requires hours to days. These changes reflect an increase in gene expression through increased transcription (mediated by sterol regulatory element–binding protein-1c; see p. 184) and translation.

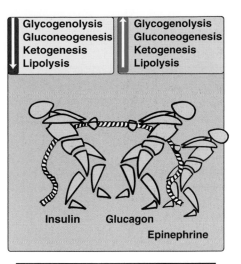

Figure 23.10
Opposing actions of insulin and glucagon plus epinephrine.

III. GLUCAGON

Glucagon is a peptide hormone secreted by the α cells of the pancreatic islets of Langerhans. Glucagon, along with epinephrine, norepinephrine, cortisol, and growth hormone (the counterregulatory hormones), opposes many of the actions of insulin (Fig. 23.10). Most importantly, glucagon acts to maintain blood glucose levels by activation of hepatic glycogenolysis and gluconeogenesis. Glucagon is composed of 29 amino acids arranged in a single polypeptide chain. [Note: Unlike insulin, the amino acid sequence of glucagon is the same in all mammalian species examined to date.] Glucagon is synthesized as a large precursor molecule (preproglucagon) that is converted to glucagon through a series of selective proteolytic cleavages, similar to those described for insulin biosynthesis (see Fig. 23.3). In contrast to insulin, preproglucagon is processed to different products in different tissues, for example, GLP-1 in intestinal L cells. Like insulin, glucagon has a short half-life.

A. Increased secretion

The α cell is responsive to a variety of stimuli that signal actual or potential hypoglycemia (Fig. 23.11). Specifically, glucagon secretion is increased by low blood glucose, amino acids, and catecholamines.

1. **Low blood glucose:** A decrease in plasma glucose concentration is the primary stimulus for glucagon release. During an overnight or prolonged fast, elevated glucagon levels prevent hypoglycemia (see Section IV below for a discussion of hypoglycemia).

2. **Amino acids:** Amino acids (for example, arginine) derived from a meal containing protein stimulate the release of glucagon. The glucagon effectively prevents the hypoglycemia that would otherwise occur as a result of the increased insulin secretion that also occurs after a protein meal.

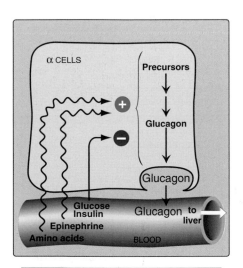

Figure 23.11
Regulation of glucagon release from pancreatic α cells. [Note: Amino acids increase release of insulin and glucagon, whereas glucose increases release of insulin and decreases release of glucagon.]

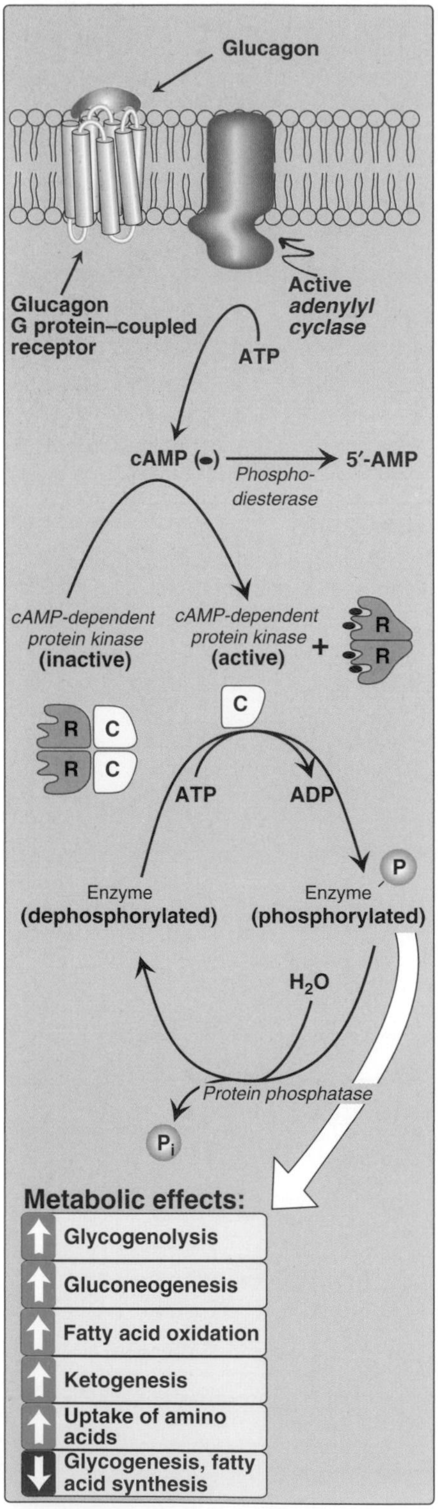

Figure 23.12
Mechanism of action of glucagon.
[Note: For clarity, G-protein activation
of *adenylyl cyclase* has been omitted.]
R = regulatory subunit; C = catalytic
subunit; cAMP = cyclic adenosine
monophosphate; ADP = adenosine
diphosphate; (P) = phosphate.

3. **Catecholamines:** Elevated levels of circulating epinephrine (from the adrenal medulla), norepinephrine (from sympathetic innervation of the pancreas), or both stimulate the release of glucagon. Thus, during periods of physiologic stress, the elevated catecholamine levels can override the effect on the α cell of circulating substrates. In these situations, regardless of the concentration of blood glucose, glucagon levels are elevated in anticipation of increased glucose use. In contrast, insulin levels are depressed.

B. Decreased secretion

Glucagon secretion is significantly decreased by elevated blood glucose and by insulin. Both substances are increased following ingestion of glucose or a carbohydrate-rich meal (see Fig. 23.5). The regulation of glucagon secretion is summarized in Figure 23.11.

C. Metabolic effects

Glucagon is a catabolic hormone that promotes the maintenance of blood glucose levels. Its primary target is the liver.

1. **Effects on carbohydrate metabolism:** The IV administration of glucagon leads to an immediate rise in blood glucose. This results from an increase in the degradation of liver glycogen and an increase in hepatic gluconeogenesis.

2. **Effects on lipid metabolism:** The primary effect of glucagon on lipid metabolism is inhibition of FA synthesis through phosphorylation and subsequent inactivation of *ACC* by *adenosine monophosphate* (*AMP*)–*activated protein kinase* (see p. 184). The resulting decrease in malonyl CoA production removes the inhibition on long-chain FA β-oxidation (see p. 191). Glucagon also plays a role in lipolysis in adipocytes, but the major activators of *hormone-sensitive lipase* (via phosphorylation by *protein kinase A*) are the catecholamines. The free FA released are taken up by liver and oxidized to acetyl CoA, which is used in ketone body synthesis.

3. **Effects on protein metabolism:** Glucagon increases uptake by the liver of amino acids supplied by muscle, resulting in increased availability of carbon skeletons for gluconeogenesis. As a consequence, plasma levels of amino acids are decreased.

D. Mechanism

Glucagon binds to high-affinity G protein–coupled receptors (GPCR) on the cell membrane of hepatocytes. The GPCR for glucagon is distinct from the GPCR that bind epinephrine. [Note: Glucagon receptors are not found on skeletal muscle.] Glucagon binding results in activation of *adenylyl cyclase* in the plasma membrane (Fig. 23.12; also see p. 94). This causes a rise in cyclic AMP (cAMP), which, in turn, activates *cAMP-dependent protein kinase A* and increases the phosphorylation of specific enzymes or other proteins. This cascade of increasing enzymic activities results in the phosphorylation-mediated activation or inhibition of key regulatory enzymes involved in carbohydrate and lipid metabolism. An example of such a cascade in glycogen degradation is shown in Figure 11.9 on p. 131. [Note: Glucagon, like insulin, affects gene transcription. For example, glucagon induces expression of *phosphoenolpyruvate carboxykinase* (see p. 122).]

IV. HYPOGLYCEMIA

Hypoglycemia is characterized by 1) central nervous system (CNS) symptoms, including confusion, aberrant behavior, or coma; 2) a simultaneous blood glucose level ≤50 mg/dl; and 3) symptoms being resolved within minutes following glucose administration (Fig. 23.13). Hypoglycemia is a medical emergency because the CNS has an absolute requirement for a continuous supply of bloodborne glucose to serve as a metabolic fuel. Transient hypoglycemia can cause cerebral dysfunction, whereas severe, prolonged hypoglycemia causes brain damage. Therefore, it is not surprising that the body has multiple overlapping mechanisms to prevent or correct hypoglycemia. The most important hormone changes in combating hypoglycemia are increased secretion of glucagon and the catecholamines, combined with decreased insulin secretion.

A. Symptoms

The symptoms of hypoglycemia can be divided into two categories. Adrenergic (neurogenic, autonomic) symptoms, such as anxiety, palpitation, tremor, and sweating, are mediated by catecholamine release

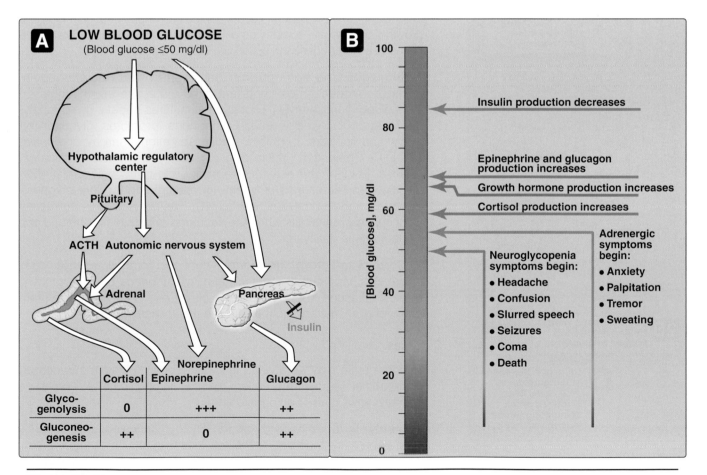

Figure 23.13
A. Actions of some of the glucoregulatory hormones in response to low blood glucose. B. Glycemic thresholds for the various responses to hypoglycemia. [Note: Normal fasted blood glucose is 70–99 mg/dl.] + = weak stimulation; ++ = moderate stimulation; +++ = strong stimulation; 0 = no effect; ACTH = adrenocorticotropic hormone.

(primarily epinephrine) regulated by the hypothalamus in response to hypoglycemia. Adrenergic symptoms typically occur when blood glucose levels fall abruptly. The second category of hypoglycemic symptoms is neuroglycopenic. The impaired delivery of glucose to the brain (neuroglycopenia) results in impairment of brain function, causing headache, confusion, slurred speech, seizures, coma, and death. Neuroglycopenic symptoms often result from a gradual decline in blood glucose, often to levels <50 mg/dl. The slow decline in glucose deprives the CNS of fuel but fails to trigger an adequate adrenergic response.

B. Glucoregulatory systems

Humans have two overlapping glucose-regulating systems that are activated by hypoglycemia: 1) the pancreatic α cells, which release glucagon, and 2) receptors in the hypothalamus, which respond to abnormally low concentrations of blood glucose. The hypothalamic glucoreceptors can trigger both the secretion of catecholamines (mediated by the sympathetic division of the autonomic nervous system) and release of adrenocorticotropic hormone (ACTH) and growth hormone by the anterior pituitary (see Fig. 23.13). [Note: ACTH increases cortisol synthesis and secretion in the adrenal cortex (see p. 239).] Glucagon, the catecholamines, cortisol, and growth hormone are sometimes called the counterregulatory hormones because each opposes the action of insulin on glucose use.

1. **Glucagon and epinephrine:** Secretion of these counterregulatory hormones is most important in the acute, short-term regulation of blood glucose levels. Glucagon stimulates hepatic glycogenolysis and gluconeogenesis. Epinephrine promotes glycogenolysis and lipolysis. It inhibits insulin secretion, thereby preventing GLUT-4–mediated uptake of glucose by muscle and adipose tissues. Epinephrine assumes a critical role in hypoglycemia when glucagon secretion is deficient, for example, in the late stages of type 1 diabetes mellitus (see p. 340). The prevention or correction of hypoglycemia fails when the secretion of both glucagon and epinephrine is deficient.

2. **Cortisol and growth hormone:** These counterregulatory hormones are less important in the short-term maintenance of blood glucose concentrations. They do, however, play a role in the long-term (transcriptional) management of glucose metabolism.

C. Types

Hypoglycemia may be divided into four types: 1) insulin induced, 2) postprandial (sometimes called reactive hypoglycemia), 3) fasting hypoglycemia, and 4) alcohol related.

1. **Insulin-induced hypoglycemia:** Hypoglycemia occurs frequently in patients with diabetes who are receiving insulin treatment, particularly those striving to achieve tight control of blood glucose levels. Mild hypoglycemia in fully conscious patients is treated by oral administration of carbohydrate. Unconscious patients are typically given glucagon subcutaneously or intramuscularly (Fig. 23.14).

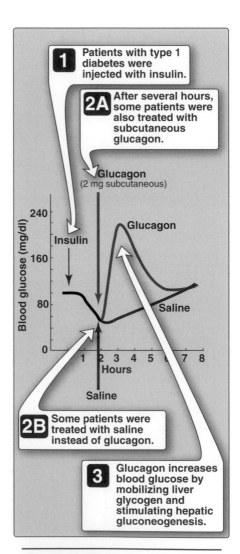

Figure 23.14
Reversal of insulin-induced hypoglycemia by administration of subcutaneous glucagon.

2. **Postprandial hypoglycemia:** This is the second most common form of hypoglycemia. It is caused by an exaggerated insulin release following a meal, prompting transient hypoglycemia with mild adrenergic symptoms. The plasma glucose level returns to normal even if the patient is not fed. The only treatment usually required is that the patient eats frequent small meals rather than the usual three large meals.

3. **Fasting hypoglycemia:** Low blood glucose during fasting is rare but is more likely to present as a serious medical problem. Fasting hypoglycemia, which tends to produce neuroglycopenic symptoms, may result from a reduction in the rate of glucose production by hepatic glycogenolysis or gluconeogenesis. Thus, low blood glucose levels are often seen in patients with hepatocellular damage or adrenal insufficiency or in fasting individuals who have consumed large quantities of ethanol (see 4. below). Alternately, fasting hypoglycemia may be the result of an increased rate of glucose use by the peripheral tissues because of overproduction of insulin by rare pancreatic tumors. If left untreated, a patient with fasting hypoglycemia may lose consciousness and experience convulsions and coma. [Note: Certain inborn errors of metabolism, for example, defects in FA oxidation, result in fasting hypoglycemia.]

4. **Alcohol-related hypoglycemia:** Alcohol (ethanol) is metabolized in the liver by two oxidation reactions (Fig. 23.15). Ethanol is first converted to acetaldehyde by zinc-containing *alcohol dehydrogenase*. Acetaldehyde is subsequently oxidized to acetate by *aldehyde dehydrogenase* (*ALDH*). [Note: *ALDH* is inhibited by disulfiram, a drug that is used in the treatment of chronic alcoholism. The resulting rise in acetaldehyde results in flushing, tachycardia, hyperventilation, and nausea.] In each reaction, electrons are transferred to oxidized nicotinamide adenine dinucleotide (NAD$^+$), resulting in an increase in the ratio of the reduced form (NADH) to NAD$^+$. The abundance of NADH favors the reduction of pyruvate to lactate and of oxaloacetate (OAA) to malate. Recall from p. 118 that pyruvate and OAA are substrates

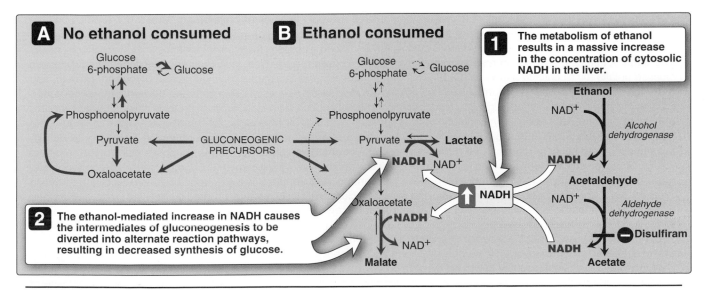

Figure 23.15
A. Normal gluconeogenesis in the absence of ethanol consumption. B. Inhibition of gluconeogenesis resulting from hepatic metabolism of ethanol. NAD(H) = nicotinamide adenine dinucleotide.

in the synthesis of glucose. Thus, the ethanol-mediated increase in NADH causes these gluconeogenic precursors to be diverted into alternate pathways, resulting in the decreased synthesis of glucose. This can precipitate hypoglycemia, particularly in individuals who have depleted their stores of liver glycogen. [Note: Decreased availability of OAA allows acetyl CoA to be diverted to ketone body synthesis in the liver (see p. 195) and can result in alcoholic ketosis that may result in ketoacidosis.] Hypoglycemia can produce many of the behaviors associated with alcohol intoxication, such as agitation, impaired judgment, and combativeness. Therefore, alcohol consumption in vulnerable individuals (such as those who are fasted or have engaged in prolonged, strenuous exercise) can produce hypoglycemia that may contribute to the behavioral effects of alcohol. Because alcohol consumption can also increase the risk for hypoglycemia in patients using insulin, those in an intensive insulin treatment protocol (see p. 340) are counseled about the increased risk of hypoglycemia that generally occurs many hours after alcohol ingestion.

> Chronic alcohol consumption can also result in alcoholic fatty liver because of increased hepatic synthesis of TAG coupled with impaired formation or release of VLDL. This occurs as a result of decreased FA oxidation because of a fall in the NAD^+/NADH ratio and increased lipogenesis because of the increased availability of FA (decreased catabolism) and of glyceraldehyde 3-phosphate (the *dehydrogenase* is inhibited by the low NAD^+/NADH ratio; see p. 101). With continued alcohol consumption, alcoholic fatty liver can progress first to alcoholic hepatitis and then to alcoholic cirrhosis.

V. CHAPTER SUMMARY

The integration of **energy metabolism** is controlled primarily by **insulin** and the opposing actions of **glucagon** and the catecholamines, particularly **epinephrine** (Fig. 23.16). Changes in the circulating levels of these hormones allow the body to store energy when food is abundant or to make stored energy available in times of **physiologic stress** (for example, during survival crises, such as famine). Insulin is a peptide hormone produced by the β **cells** of the **islets of Langerhans** of the **pancreas**. It consists of disulfide-linked A and B chains. A rise in blood glucose is the most important signal for insulin secretion. The **catecholamines**, secreted in response to stress, trauma, or extreme exercise, inhibit insulin secretion. Insulin increases glucose uptake (by glucose transporters (**GLUT-4**) in muscle and adipose tissue) and the synthesis of **glycogen**, **protein**, and **triacylglycerol**: It is an **anabolic** hormone. These actions are mediated by binding to its membrane *tyrosine kinase* receptor. Binding initiates a cascade of cell-signaling responses, including phosphorylation of a family of proteins called **insulin receptor substrate proteins**. **Glucagon** is a monomeric peptide hormone produced by the α **cells** of the pancreatic islets (both insulin and glucagon synthesis involve formation of inactive precursors that are cleaved to form the active hormones). Glucagon, along with epinephrine, norepinephrine, cortisol, and growth hormone (the **counterregulatory hormones**), opposes many of the actions of insulin. Glucagon acts to maintain blood glucose during periods of potential hypoglycemia. Glucagon increases **glycogenolysis**, **gluconeogenesis**, **fatty acid oxidation**, **ketogenesis**, and **amino acid uptake**: It is a **catabolic** hormone. Glucagon secretion is stimulated by low blood glucose, amino acids, and the catecholamines. Its secretion is inhibited by elevated blood glucose and by insulin. Glucagon binds to high-affinity **G protein–coupled receptors** on the cell membrane of hepatocytes. Binding results in the activation of *adenylyl cyclase*, which produces the second messenger **cyclic adenosine monophosphate** (cAMP). Subsequent activation of *cAMP-dependent protein kinase A* results in the **phosphorylation**-mediated activation or inhibition of key regulatory enzymes involved in carbohydrate and lipid metabolism. Both insulin and glucagon affect **gene transcription**. **Hypoglycemia** is characterized by low blood glucose accompanied by **adrenergic** and **neuroglycopenic symptoms** that are rapidly resolved by the administration of glucose. Insulin-induced, postprandial, and fasting hypoglycemia result in release of glucagon and epinephrine. The rise in **nicotinamide adenine dinucleotide** (**NADH**) that accompanies **ethanol** metabolism inhibits gluconeogenesis, leading to hypoglycemia in individuals with depleted stores. Alcohol consumption also increases the risk for hypoglycemia in patients using insulin. Chronic alcohol consumption can cause **fatty liver disease**.

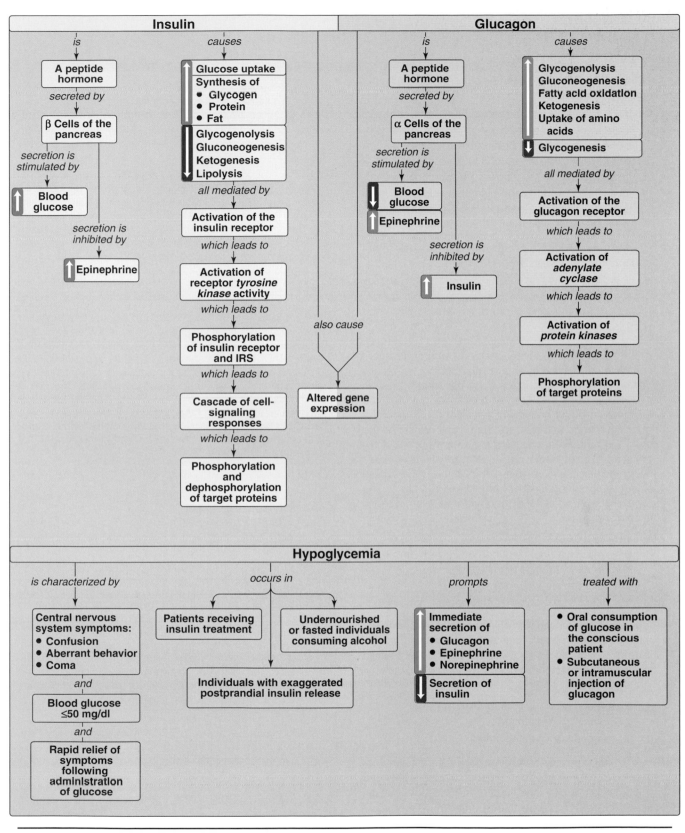

Figure 23.16
Key concept map for the metabolic effects of insulin and glucagon as well as hypoglycemia. IRS = insulin receptor substrates.

Study Questions

Choose the ONE best answer.

23.1 Which of the following statements is true for insulin but not for glucagon?

    A. It is a peptide hormone secreted by pancreatic cells.

    B. Its actions are mediated by binding to a receptor found on the cell membrane of liver cells.

    C. Its effects include alterations in gene expression.

    D. Its secretion is decreased by the catecholamines.

    E. Its secretion is increased by amino acids.

    F. Its synthesis involves a nonfunctional precursor that gets cleaved to yield a functional molecule.

23.2 In which one of the following tissues is glucose transport into the cell insulin dependent?

    A. Adipose

    B. Brain

    C. Liver

    D. Red blood cells

23.3 A 39-year-old woman is brought to the emergency room complaining of weakness and dizziness. She recalls getting up early that morning to do her weekly errands and had skipped breakfast. She drank a cup of coffee for lunch and had nothing to eat during the day. She met with friends at 8 p.m. and had a few drinks. As the evening progressed, she soon became weak and dizzy and was taken to the hospital. Laboratory tests revealed her blood glucose to be 45 mg/dl (normal = 70–99). She was given orange juice and immediately felt better. The biochemical basis of her alcohol-induced hypoglycemia is an increase in:

    A. fatty acid oxidation.

    B. the ratio of the reduced oxidized forms of nicotinamide adenine dinucleotide.

    C. oxaloacetate and pyruvate.

    D. use of acetyl coenzyme A in fatty acid synthesis.

23.4 A patient is diagnosed with an insulinoma, a rare neuroendocrine tumor, the cells of which are derived primarily from pancreatic β cells. Which of the following would logically be characteristic of an insulinoma?

    A. Decreased body weight

    B. Decreased connecting peptide in the blood

    C. Decreased glucose in the blood

    D. Decreased insulin in the blood

23.5 In a patient with an even rarer glucagon-secreting tumor derived from the α cells of the pancreas, how would the presentation be expected to differ relative to the patient in Question 23.4?

Correct answer = D. Secretion of insulin by pancreatic β cells is inhibited by the catecholamines, whereas glucagon secretion by the α cells is stimulated by them. All of the other statements are true for both insulin and glucagon.

Correct answer = A. The glucose transporter (GLUT-4) in adipose (and muscle) tissue is dependent on insulin. Insulin results in movement of GLUT-4 from intracellular vesicles to the cell membrane. The other tissues in the list contain GLUT that are independent of insulin because they are always located on the cell membrane.

Correct answer = B. The oxidation of ethanol to acetate by dehydrogenases is accompanied by the reduction of nicotinamide adenine dinucleotide (NAD^+) to NADH. The rise in the $NADH/NAD^+$ ratio shifts pyruvate to lactate and oxaloacetate (OAA) to malate, decreasing the availability of substrates for gluconeogenesis and resulting in hypoglycemia. The rise in NADH also reduces the NAD^+ needed for fatty acid (FA) oxidation. The decrease in OAA shunts any acetyl coenzyme A produced to ketogenesis. Note that the inhibition of FA degradation results in their reesterification into triacylglycerol that can result in fatty liver.

Correct answer = C. Insulinomas are characterized by constant production of insulin (and, therefore, of C-peptide) by the tumor cells. The increase in insulin drives glucose uptake by tissues such as muscle and adipose that have insulin-dependent glucose transporters, resulting in hypoglycemia. However, the hypoglycemia is insufficient to suppress insulin production and secretion. Insulinomas, then, are characterized by increased blood insulin and decreased blood glucose. Insulin, as an anabolic hormone, results in weight gain.

A glucagon-secreting tumor of the pancreas (glucagonoma) would result in hyperglycemia, not hypoglycemia. The constant production of glucagon would result in constant gluconeogenesis, using amino acids from proteolysis as substrates. This results in loss of body weight.

The Feed–Fast Cycle   24

I. OVERVIEW OF THE ABSORPTIVE STATE

The absorptive (well-fed) state is the 2- to 4-hour period after ingestion of a normal meal. During this interval, transient increases in plasma glucose, amino acids, and triacylglycerols (TAG) occur, the latter primarily as components of chylomicrons synthesized and secreted by the intestinal mucosal cells (see p. 228). Islet tissue of the pancreas responds to the elevated level of glucose with increased secretion of insulin and decreased secretion of glucagon. The elevated insulin/glucagon ratio and the ready availability of circulating substrates make the absorptive state an anabolic period characterized by increased synthesis of TAG and glycogen to replenish fuel stores as well as increased synthesis of protein. During this absorptive period, virtually all tissues use glucose as a fuel, and the metabolic response of the body is dominated by alterations in the metabolism of liver, adipose tissue, skeletal muscle, and brain. In this chapter, an "organ map" is introduced that traces the movement of metabolites between tissues. The goal is to create an expanded and clinically useful vision of whole-body metabolism.

II. REGULATORY MECHANISMS

The flow of intermediates through metabolic pathways is controlled by four mechanisms: 1) the availability of substrates, 2) allosteric regulation of enzymes, 3) covalent modification of enzymes, and 4) induction-repression of enzyme synthesis, primarily through regulation of transcription. Although this scheme may at first seem redundant, each mechanism operates on a different timescale (Fig. 24.1) and allows the body to adapt to a wide variety of physiologic situations. In the absorptive state, these regulatory mechanisms insure that available nutrients are captured as glycogen, TAG, and protein.

A. Allosteric effectors

Allosteric changes usually involve rate-determining reactions. For example, glycolysis in the liver is stimulated following a meal by an increase in fructose 2,6-bisphosphate, an allosteric activator of *phosphofructokinase-1* ([*PFK-1*] see p. 99). In contrast, gluconeogenesis is decreased by fructose 2,6-bisphosphate, an allosteric inhibitor of *fructose 1,6-bisphosphatase* (see p. 122).

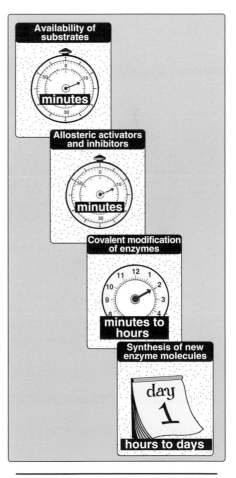

Figure 24.1
Control mechanisms of metabolism and some typical response times. [Note: Response times may vary according to the nature of the stimulus and from tissue to tissue.]

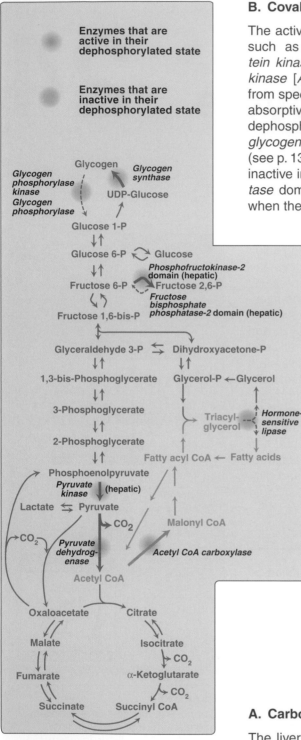

Figure 24.2
Important reactions of intermediary metabolism regulated by enzyme phosphorylation. **Blue text** = intermediates of carbohydrate metabolism; brown text = intermediates of lipid metabolism; P = phosphate; CoA = coenzyme A; CO_2 = carbon dioxide.

B. Covalent modification

The activity of many enzymes is regulated by the addition (via *kinases*, such as *cyclic adenosine monophosphate* [*cAMP*]–*dependent protein kinase A* [*PKA*] and *adenosine monophosphate–activated protein kinase* [*AMPK*]) or removal (via *phosphatases*) of phosphate groups from specific serine, threonine, or tyrosine residues of the protein. In the absorptive state, most of the covalently regulated enzymes are in the dephosphorylated form and are active (Fig. 24.2). Three exceptions are *glycogen phosphorylase kinase* (see p. 132), *glycogen phosphorylase* (see p. 132), and *hormone-sensitive lipase* (*HSL*) (see p. 189), which are inactive in their dephosphorylated form. [Note: In the liver, the *phosphatase* domain of bifunctional *phosphofructokinase-2* (*PFK-2*) is inactive when the protein is dephosphorylated (see p. 100).]

C. Induction and repression of enzyme synthesis

Increased (induction of) or decreased (repression of) enzyme synthesis leads to changes in the number of enzyme molecules, rather than changing the activity of existing enzyme molecules. Enzymes subject to synthesis regulation are often those that are needed under specific physiologic conditions. For example, in the well-fed state, elevated insulin levels result in an increase in the synthesis of key enzymes, such as *acetyl coenzyme A (CoA) carboxylase* (*ACC*) and *fatty acid synthase* (see p. 313), involved in anabolic metabolism. In the fasted state, glucagon induces expression of *phosphoenolpyruvate carboxykinase* (*PEPCK*) of gluconeogenesis (see p. 314). [Note: Both hormones affect gene transcription.]

III. LIVER: NUTRIENT DISTRIBUTION CENTER

The liver is uniquely situated to process and distribute dietary nutrients because the venous drainage of the gut and pancreas passes through the hepatic portal vein before entry into the general circulation. Thus, after a meal, the liver is bathed in blood containing absorbed nutrients and elevated levels of insulin secreted by the pancreas. During the absorptive period, the liver takes up carbohydrates, lipids, and most amino acids. These nutrients are then metabolized, stored, or routed to other tissues. In this way, the liver smooths out potentially broad fluctuations in the availability of nutrients for the peripheral tissues.

A. Carbohydrate metabolism

The liver is normally a glucose-producing rather than a glucose-using organ. However, after a meal containing carbohydrate, the liver becomes a net consumer, retaining roughly 60 g of every 100 g of glucose presented by the portal system. This increased use reflects increased glucose uptake by the hepatocytes. Their insulin-independent glucose transporter (GLUT-2) has a low affinity (high K_m [Michaelis constant]) for glucose and, therefore, takes up glucose only when blood glucose is high (see p. 98). Processes that are upregulated when hepatic glucose is increased include the following.

1. **Increased glucose phosphorylation:** The elevated levels of glucose within the hepatocyte (as a result of elevated extracellular levels) allow *glucokinase* to phosphorylate glucose to glucose 6-phosphate (Fig. 24.3, **❶**). [Note: *Glucokinase* has a high K_m for glucose, is not subject to direct product inhibition, and has a sigmoidal reaction curve (see p. 98).]

2. **Increased glycogenesis:** The conversion of glucose 6-phosphate to glycogen is favored by the activation of *glycogen synthase*, both by dephosphorylation and by increased availability of glucose 6-phosphate, its positive allosteric effector (see Fig. 24.3, **❷**).

3. **Increased pentose phosphate pathway activity:** The increased availability of glucose 6-phosphate, combined with the active use of nicotinamide adenine dinucleotide phosphate (NADPH) in hepatic lipogenesis, stimulates the pentose phosphate pathway (see p. 145). This pathway typically accounts for 5%–10% of the glucose metabolized by the liver (see Fig. 24.3, **❸**).

4. **Increased glycolysis:** In the liver, glycolysis is significant only during the absorptive period following a carbohydrate-rich meal. The conversion of glucose to pyruvate is stimulated by the elevated insulin/glucagon ratio that results in increased amounts of the regulated enzymes of glycolysis: *glucokinase, PFK-1,* and *pyruvate kinase* ([PK] see p. 105). Additionally, *PFK-1* is allosterically activated by fructose 2,6-bisphosphate generated by the active (dephosphorylated) *kinase* domain of bifunctional *PFK-2. PK* is dephosphorylated and active. *Pyruvate dehydrogenase* (*PDH*), which converts pyruvate to acetyl CoA, is active (dephosphorylated) because pyruvate inhibits *PDH kinase* (see Fig. 24.3, **❹**).

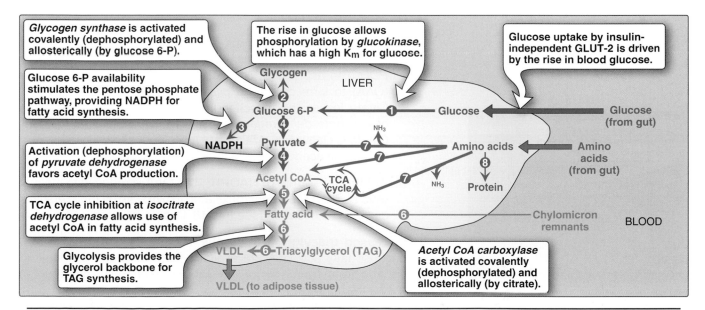

Figure 24.3
Major metabolic pathways in the liver in the absorptive state. [Note: The acetyl coenzyme A (CoA) is also used for cholesterol synthesis.] The numbers in circles, which appear both in the figure and in the text, indicate important pathways for carbohydrate, fat, or protein metabolism. **Blue text** = intermediates of carbohydrate metabolism; **brown text** = intermediates of lipid metabolism; **green text** = intermediates of protein metabolism; P = phosphate; TCA = tricarboxylic acid; VLDL = very-low-density lipoprotein; GLUT = glucose transporter; NADPH = nicotinamide adenine dinucleotide phosphate; NH_3 = ammonia.

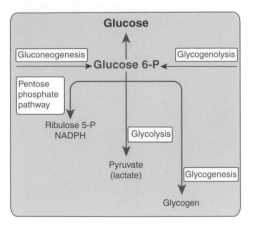

Figure 24.4
Central role of glucose 6-phosphate in metabolism. [Note: The presence of *glucose 6-phosphatase* in the liver allows the production of free glucose from the glucose 6-phosphate produced in glycogenolysis and gluconeogenesis.] NADPH = nicotinamide adenine dinucleotide phosphate; P = phosphate.

The acetyl CoA either is used as a substrate for fatty acid (FA) synthesis or is oxidized for energy in the tricarboxylic acid (TCA) cycle. (See Fig. 24.4 for the central role of glucose 6-phosphate.)

5. **Decreased glucose production:** While glycolysis and glycogenesis (pathways that promote glucose storage) are being stimulated in the liver in the absorptive state, gluconeogenesis and glycogenolysis (pathways that generate glucose) are being inhibited. *Pyruvate carboxylase* (*PC*), which catalyzes the first step in gluconeogenesis, is largely inactive because of low levels of acetyl CoA, its allosteric activator (see p. 119). [Note: The acetyl CoA is being used for FA synthesis.] The high insulin/glucagon ratio also favors inactivation of other gluconeogenic enzymes such as *fructose 1,6-bisphosphatase* (see Fig. 8.17, p. 100). Glycogenolysis is inhibited by dephosphorylation of *glycogen phosphorylase* and *phosphorylase kinase*. [Note: The increased uptake and decreased production of blood glucose in the absorptive period prevents hyperglycemia.]

B. **Fat metabolism**

1. **Increased fatty acid synthesis:** Liver is the primary site of de novo synthesis of FA (see Fig. 24.3, ❺). FA synthesis, a cytosolic process, is favored in the absorptive period by availability of the substrates acetyl CoA (from glucose and amino acid metabolism) and NADPH (from glucose metabolism in the pentose phosphate pathway) and by the activation of *ACC*, both by dephosphorylation and by the presence of its allosteric activator, citrate. [Note: Inactivity of *AMPK* favors dephosphorylation.] *ACC* catalyzes the formation of malonyl CoA from acetyl CoA, the rate-limiting reaction for FA synthesis (see p. 183). [Note: Malonyl CoA inhibits *carnitine palmitoyltransferase-I* (*CPT-I*) of FA oxidation (see p. 191). Thus, citrate directly activates FA synthesis and indirectly inhibits FA degradation.]

   a. **Source of cytosolic acetyl coenzyme A:** Pyruvate from aerobic glycolysis enters mitochondria and is decarboxylated by *PDH*. The acetyl CoA product is combined with oxaloacetate (OAA) to form citrate via *citrate synthase* of the TCA cycle. Citrate leaves the mitochondria (as a result of the inhibition of *isocitrate dehydrogenase* by ATP) and enters the cytosol. Citrate is cleaved by *ATP citrate lyase* (induced by insulin), producing the acetyl CoA substrate of *ACC* plus OAA.

   b. **Additional source of NADPH:** The OAA is reduced to malate, which is oxidatively decarboxylated to pyruvate by *malic enzyme* as NADPH is formed (see Fig. 16.11 on p. 187).

2. **Increased triacylglycerol synthesis:** TAG synthesis is favored because fatty acyl CoA are available both from de novo synthesis and from hydrolysis of the TAG component of chylomicron remnants removed from the blood by hepatocytes (see p. 178). Glycerol 3-phosphate, the backbone for TAG synthesis, is provided by glycolysis (see p. 189). The liver packages these endogenous TAG into very-low-density lipoprotein (VLDL) particles that are secreted into the blood for use by extrahepatic tissues, particularly adipose and muscle tissues (see Fig. 24.3, ❻).

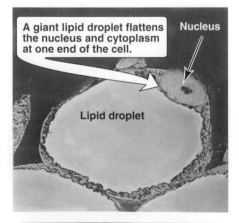

Figure 24.5
Colorized transmission electron micrograph of adipocytes.

C. Amino acid metabolism

1. **Increased amino acid degradation:** In the absorptive period, more amino acids are present than the liver can use in the synthesis of proteins and other nitrogen-containing molecules. The surplus amino acids are not stored but are either released into the blood for other tissues to use in protein synthesis or deaminated, with the resulting carbon skeletons being degraded by the liver to pyruvate, acetyl CoA, or TCA cycle intermediates. These metabolites can be oxidized for energy or used in FA synthesis (see Fig. 24.3, **7**). The liver has limited capacity to initiate degradation of the branched-chain amino acids (BCAA) leucine, isoleucine, and valine. They pass through the liver essentially unchanged and are metabolized in muscle (see p. 266).

2. **Increased protein synthesis:** The body does not store protein for energy in the same way that it maintains glycogen or TAG reserves. However, a transient increase in the synthesis of hepatic proteins does occur in the absorptive state, resulting in replacement of any proteins that may have been degraded during the previous period of fasting (see Fig. 24.3, **8**).

IV. ADIPOSE TISSUE: ENERGY STORAGE DEPOT

Adipose tissue is second only to the liver in its ability to distribute fuel molecules. In a 70-kg man, white adipose tissue (WAT) weighs ~14 kg, or about half as much as the total muscle mass. Nearly the entire volume of each adipocyte in WAT can be occupied by a droplet of anhydrous, calorically dense TAG (Fig. 24.5).

A. Carbohydrate metabolism

1. **Increased glucose transport:** Circulating insulin levels are elevated in the absorptive state, resulting in an influx of glucose into adipocytes via insulin-sensitive GLUT-4 recruited to the cell surface from intracellular vesicles (Fig. 24.6, **1**). The glucose is phosphorylated by *hexokinase*.

2. **Increased glycolysis:** The increased intracellular availability of glucose results in an enhanced rate of glycolysis (see Fig. 24.6, **2**). In adipose tissue, glycolysis serves a synthetic function by supplying glycerol 3-phosphate for TAG synthesis (see p. 188). [Note: Adipose tissue lacks *glycerol kinase*.]

3. **Increased pentose phosphate pathway activity:** Adipose tissue can metabolize glucose by means of the pentose phosphate pathway, thereby producing NADPH, which is essential for FA synthesis (see p. 186 and Fig. 24.6, **3**). However, in humans, de novo synthesis is not a major source of FA in adipose tissue, except when refeeding a previously fasted individual (see Fig. 24.6, **4**).

B. Fat metabolism

Most of the FA added to the TAG stores of adipocytes after consumption of a lipid-containing meal are provided by the degradation of exogenous (dietary) TAG in chylomicrons sent out by the intestine and

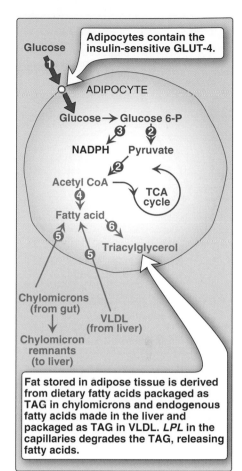

Figure 24.6
Major metabolic pathways in adipose tissue in the absorptive state. [Note: The numbers in the circles, which appear both in the figure and in the corresponding text, indicate important pathways for adipose tissue metabolism.] GLUT = glucose transporter; P = phosphate; NADPH = nicotinamide adenine dinucleotide; CoA = coenzyme A; TCA = tricarboxylic acid; TAG = triacylglycerol; VLDL = very-low-density lipoprotein; *LPL = lipoprotein lipase.*

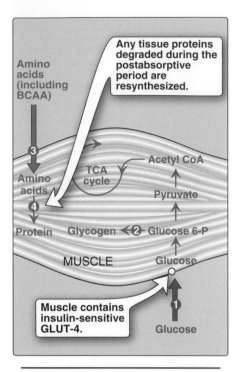

Figure 24.7
Major metabolic pathways in skeletal muscle in the absorptive state. [Note: The numbers in circles, which appear both in the figure and in the text, indicate important pathways for carbohydrate or protein metabolism.] CoA = coenzyme A; P = phosphate; GLUT = glucose transporter; BCAA = branched-chain amino acids; TCA = tricarboxylic acid.

endogenous TAG in VLDL sent out by the liver (see Fig. 24.6, ⑤). The FA are released from the lipoproteins by *lipoprotein lipase* (*LPL*), an extracellular enzyme attached to the endothelial cells of capillary walls in many tissues, particularly adipose and muscle (see p. 228). In adipose tissue, *LPL* is upregulated by insulin. Thus, in the fed state, elevated levels of glucose and insulin favor storage of TAG (see Fig. 24.6, ⑥), all the carbons of which are supplied by glucose. [Note: Elevated insulin favors the dephosphorylated (inactive) form of *HSL* (see p. 189), thereby inhibiting lipolysis in the well-fed state.]

V. RESTING SKELETAL MUSCLE

Skeletal muscle accounts for ~40% of the body mass in individuals of healthy weight, and it can use glucose, amino acids, FA, and ketone bodies as fuel. In the well-fed state, muscle takes up glucose via GLUT-4 (for energy and glycogen synthesis) and amino acids (for energy and protein synthesis). In contrast to liver, there is no covalent regulation of *PFK-2* in skeletal muscle. However, in the cardiac isozyme, the *kinase* domain is activated by epinephrine-mediated phosphorylation (see p. 100).

> Skeletal muscle is unique in being able to respond to substantial changes in the demand for ATP that accompanies contraction. At rest, muscle accounts for ~25% of the oxygen (O_2) consumption of the body, whereas during vigorous exercise, it is responsible for up to 90%. This underscores the fact that skeletal muscle, despite its potential for transient periods of anaerobic glycolysis, is an oxidative tissue.

A. Carbohydrate metabolism

1. **Increased glucose transport:** The transient increase in plasma glucose and insulin after a carbohydrate-rich meal leads to an increase in glucose transport into muscle cells (myocytes) by GLUT-4 (see p. 97 and Fig. 24.7, ①), thereby reducing blood glucose. Glucose is phosphorylated to glucose 6-phosphate by *hexokinase* and metabolized to meet the energy needs of myocytes.

2. **Increased glycogenesis:** The increased insulin/glucagon ratio and the availability of glucose 6-phosphate favor glycogen synthesis, particularly if glycogen stores have been depleted as a result of exercise (see p. 126 and Fig. 24.7, ②).

B. Fat metabolism

FA are released from chylomicrons and VLDL by the action of *LPL* (see pp. 228 and 231). However, FA are of secondary importance as a fuel for resting muscle during the well-fed state, in which glucose is the primary source of energy.

C. Amino acid metabolism

1. **Increased protein synthesis:** An increase in amino acid uptake and protein synthesis occurs in the absorptive period after ingestion

of a meal containing protein (see Fig. 24.7, **❸** and **❹**). This synthesis replaces protein degraded since the previous meal.

2. **Increased branched-chain amino acid uptake:** Muscle is the principal site for degradation of the BCAA because it contains the required *transaminase* (see p. 266). The dietary BCAA escape metabolism by the liver and are taken up by muscle, where they are used for protein synthesis (see Fig. 24.7, **❸**) and as energy sources.

VI. BRAIN

Although contributing only 2% of the adult weight, the brain accounts for a consistent 20% of the basal O_2 consumption of the body at rest. Because the brain is vital to the proper functioning of all organs of the body, special priority is given to its fuel needs. To provide energy, substrates must be able to cross the endothelial cells that line the blood vessels in the brain (the blood–brain barrier [BBB]). In the fed state, the brain exclusively uses glucose as a fuel (GLUT-1 of the BBB is insulin independent), completely oxidizing ~140 g/day to carbon dioxide and water. Because the brain contains no significant stores of glycogen, it is completely dependent on the availability of blood glucose (Fig. 24.8, **❶**). [Note: If blood glucose levels fall to <50 mg/dl (normal fasted blood glucose is 70–99 mg/dl), cerebral function is impaired (see p. 315).] The brain also lacks significant stores of TAG, and the FA circulating in the blood make little contribution to energy production for reasons that are unclear. The intertissue exchanges characteristic of the absorptive period are summarized in Figure 24.9.

VII. OVERVIEW OF THE FASTED STATE

Fasting begins if no food is ingested after the absorptive period. It may result from an inability to obtain food, the desire to lose weight rapidly, or clinical situations in which an individual cannot eat (for example, because of trauma, surgery, cancer, or burns). In the absence of food, plasma levels of glucose, amino acids, and TAG fall, triggering a decline in insulin secretion and an increase in glucagon, epinephrine, and cortisol secretion. The decreased insulin/counterregulatory hormone ratio and the decreased availability of circulating substrates make the postabsorptive period of nutrient deprivation a catabolic period characterized by degradation of TAG, glycogen, and protein. This sets into motion an exchange of substrates among the liver, adipose tissue, skeletal muscle, and brain that is guided by two priorities: 1) the need to maintain adequate plasma levels of glucose to sustain energy metabolism in the brain, red blood cells, and other glucose-requiring tissues and 2) the need to mobilize FA from TAG in WAT for the synthesis and release of ketone bodies by the liver to supply energy to other tissues and spare body protein. As a result, blood glucose levels are maintained within a narrow range in fasting, while FA and ketone body levels increase. [Note: Maintaining glucose requires that the substrates for gluconeogenesis (such as pyruvate, alanine, and glycerol) be available.]

A. Fuel stores

The metabolic fuels available in a normal 70-kg man at the beginning of a fast are shown in Figure 24.10. Observe the enormous caloric stores available in the form of TAG compared with those contained

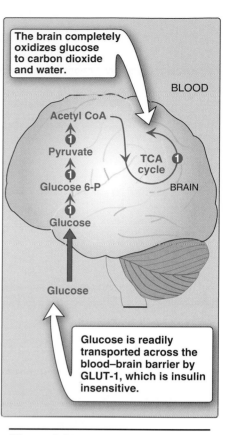

Figure 24.8
Major metabolic pathways in the brain in the absorptive state. [Note: The numbers in circles, which appear both in the figure and in the text, indicate important pathways for carbohydrate metabolism.] CoA = coenzyme A; TCA = tricarboxylic acid; P = phosphate; GLUT = glucose transporter.

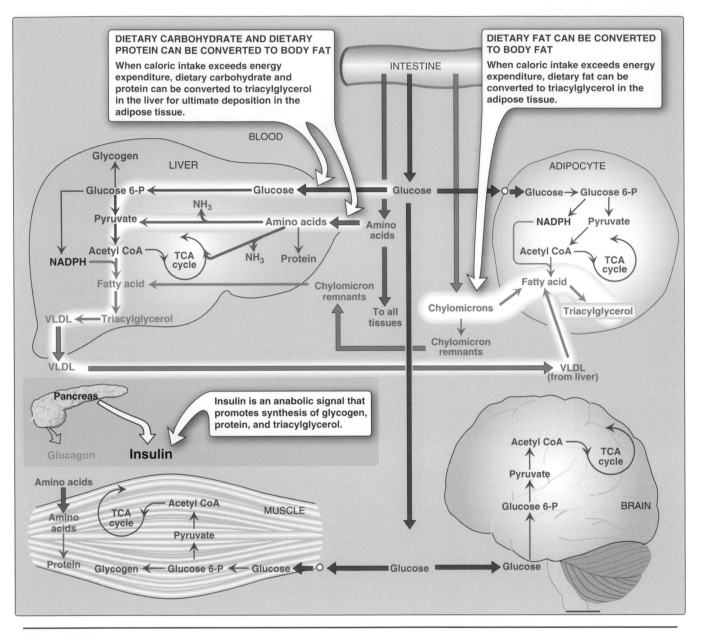

Figure 24.9
Intertissue relationships in the absorptive state and the hormonal signals that promote them. [Note: Small circles on the perimeter of muscle and the adipocyte indicate insulin-dependent glucose transporters.] P = phosphate; CoA = coenzyme A; NADPH = nicotinamide adenine dinucleotide phosphate; TCA = tricarboxylic acid; VLDL = very-low-density lipoprotein.

in glycogen. [Note: Although protein is listed as an energy source, each protein also has a function unrelated to energy metabolism (for example, as a structural component of the body or as an enzyme). Therefore, only about one third of the body's protein can be used for energy production without fatally compromising vital functions.]

B. Enzymic changes

In fasting (as in the well-fed state), the flow of intermediates through the pathways of energy metabolism is controlled by four mechanisms: 1) the availability of substrates, 2) allosteric regulation of enzymes, 3) covalent modification of enzymes, and 4) induction-repression of enzyme synthesis. The metabolic changes observed in fasting are generally opposite those described for the absorptive state (see Fig. 24.9). For example, although most of the enzymes regulated by covalent modification are dephosphorylated and active in the well-fed state, they are phosphorylated and inactive in the fasted state. Three exceptions are *glycogen phosphorylase* (see p. 132), *glycogen phosphorylase kinase* (see p. 132), and *HSL* (see p. 189), which are active in their phosphorylated states. In fasting, substrates are not provided by the diet but are available from the breakdown of stores and/or tissues, such as glycogenolysis with release of glucose from the liver, lipolysis with release of FA and glycerol from TAG in adipose tissue, and proteolysis with release of amino acids from muscle. Recognition that the changes in fasting are the reciprocal of those in the fed state is helpful in understanding the ebb and flow of metabolism.

VIII. LIVER IN FASTING

The primary role of the liver in fasting is maintenance of blood glucose through the production of glucose (from glycogenolysis and gluconeogenesis) for glucose-requiring tissues and the synthesis and distribution of ketone bodies for use by other tissues. Therefore, hepatic metabolism is distinguished from peripheral (or extrahepatic) metabolism.

A. Carbohydrate metabolism

The liver first uses glycogen degradation and then gluconeogenesis to maintain blood glucose levels to sustain energy metabolism of the brain and other glucose-requiring tissues in the fasted state. [Note: Recall that the presence of *glucose-6-phosphatase* in the liver allows the production of free glucose both from glycogenolysis and from gluconeogenesis (see Fig. 24.4).]

1. **Increased glycogenolysis:** Figure 24.11 shows the sources of blood glucose after ingestion of 100 g of glucose. During the brief absorptive period, ingested glucose is the major source of blood glucose. Several hours later, blood glucose levels have declined sufficiently to cause increased secretion of glucagon and decreased secretion of insulin. The increased glucagon/insulin ratio causes a rapid mobilization of liver glycogen stores (which contain ~80 g of glycogen in the fed state) because of *PKA*-mediated phosphorylation (and activation) of *glycogen phosphorylase kinase* that phosphorylates (and activates) *glycogen phosphorylase* (see p. 132). Figure 24.11 shows that because liver glycogen is exhausted by 24 hours of fasting, hepatic glycogenolysis is a transient response to early fasting. Figure 24.12, ❶, shows glycogen degradation as part of the overall metabolic response of the liver during fasting. [Note: Phosphorylation of *glycogen synthase* simultaneously inhibits glycogenesis.]

2. **Increased gluconeogenesis:** The synthesis of glucose and its release into the circulation are vital hepatic functions during short- and long-term fasting (see Fig. 24.12, ❷). The carbon skeletons for gluconeogenesis are derived primarily from glucogenic amino acids and lactate from muscle and glycerol from adipose tissue. Gluconeogenesis, favored by activation of *fructose*

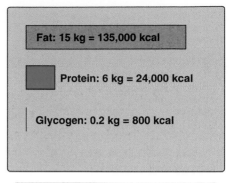

Figure 24.10
Metabolic fuels present in a 70-kg man at the beginning of a fast. The fat stores are sufficient to meet energy needs for ~80 days.

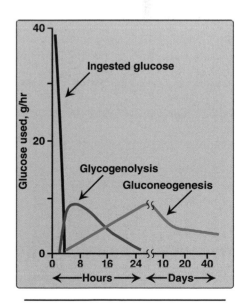

Figure 24.11
Sources of blood glucose after ingestion of 100 g of glucose. [Note: See Section B.2 for an explanation of the decline in gluconeogenesis.]

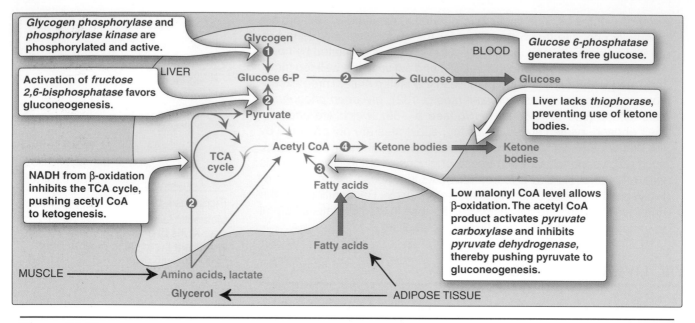

Figure 24.12

Major metabolic pathways in the liver during fasting. [Note: The numbers in circles, which appear both in the figure and in the corresponding citation in the text, indicate important metabolic pathways for carbohydrate or fat.] P = phosphate; CoA = coenzyme A; TCA = tricarboxylic acid; NADH = nicotinamide adenine dinucleotide.

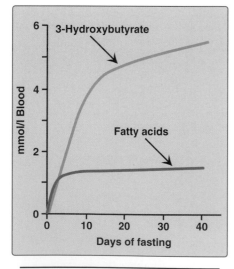

Figure 24.13

Concentrations of fatty acids and 3-hydroxybutyrate in the blood during fasting. [Note: 3-Hydroxybutyrate is made from the NADH-requiring reduction of acetoacetate.]

1,6-bisphosphatase (because of decreased availability of its inhibitor fructose 2,6-bisphosphate; see p. 121) and by induction of *PEPCK* by glucagon (see p. 122), begins 4–6 hours after the last meal and becomes fully active as stores of liver glycogen are depleted (see Fig. 24.11). [Note: The decrease in fructose 2,6-bisphosphate simultaneously inhibits glycolysis at *PFK-1* (see p. 99).]

B. Fat metabolism

1. **Increased fatty acid oxidation:** The oxidation of FA obtained from TAG hydrolysis in adipose tissue is the major source of energy in hepatic tissue in the fasted state (see Fig. 24.12, ❸). The fall in malonyl CoA because of phosphorylation (inactivation) of *ACC* by *AMPK* removes the brake on *CPT-I*, allowing β-oxidation to occur (see p. 191). FA oxidation generates NADH, flavin adenine dinucleotide (FADH$_2$), and acetyl CoA. The NADH inhibits the TCA cycle and shifts OAA to malate. This results in acetyl CoA being available for ketogenesis. The acetyl CoA is also an allosteric activator of *PC* and an allosteric inhibitor of *PDH*, thereby favoring use of pyruvate in gluconeogenesis (see Fig. 10.9, p. 122). [Note: Acetyl CoA cannot be used as a substrate for gluconeogenesis, in part because the *PDH* reaction is irreversible.] Oxidation of NADH and FADH$_2$ coupled with oxidative phosphorylation supplies the energy required by the *PC* and *PEPCK* reactions of gluconeogenesis.

2. **Increased ketogenesis:** The liver is unique in being able to synthesize and release ketone bodies, primarily 3-hydroxybutyrate but also acetoacetate, for use as fuel by peripheral tissues but not by the liver itself because liver lacks *thiophorase* (see p. 197). Ketogenesis, which starts during the first days of fasting (Fig. 24.13), is favored when the concentration of acetyl CoA from

FA oxidation exceeds the oxidative capacity of the TCA cycle. [Note: Ketogenesis releases CoA, insuring its availability for continued FA oxidation.] The availability of circulating water-soluble ketone bodies is important in fasting because they can be used for fuel by most tissues, including the brain, once their blood level is high enough. Ketone body concentration in blood increases from ~50 µM to ~6 mM in fasting. This reduces the need for gluconeogenesis from amino acid carbon skeletons, thus preserving essential protein (see Fig. 24.11). Ketogenesis as part of the overall hepatic response to fasting is shown in Figure 24.12, ❹. [Note: Ketone bodies are organic acids and, when present at high concentrations, can cause ketoacidosis.]

IX. ADIPOSE TISSUE IN FASTING

A. Carbohydrate metabolism

Glucose transport by insulin-sensitive GLUT-4 into the adipocyte and its subsequent metabolism are decreased because of low levels of circulating insulin. This results in decreased TAG synthesis.

B. Fat metabolism

1. **Increased fat degradation:** The *PKA*-mediated phosphorylation and activation of *HSL* (see p. 189) and subsequent hydrolysis of stored fat (TAG) are enhanced by the elevated catecholamines norepinephrine and epinephrine. These hormones, which are secreted from the sympathetic nerve endings in adipose tissue and/or from the adrenal medulla, are physiologically important activators of *HSL* (Fig. 24.14, ❶).

2. **Increased fatty acid release:** FA obtained from hydrolysis of TAG stored in adipocytes are primarily released into the blood (see Fig. 24.14, ❷). Bound to albumin, they are transported to a variety of tissues for use as fuel. The glycerol produced from TAG degradation is used as a gluconeogenic precursor by the liver, which contains *glycerol kinase*. [Note: FA can also be oxidized to acetyl CoA, which can enter the TCA cycle, thereby producing energy for the adipocyte. They also can be reesterified to glycerol 3-phosphate (from glyceroneogenesis, see p. 190), generating TAG and reducing plasma FA concentration.]

3. **Decreased fatty acid uptake:** In fasting, *LPL* activity of adipose tissue is low. Consequently, FA in circulating TAG of lipoproteins are less available to adipose tissue than to muscle.

X. RESTING SKELETAL MUSCLE IN FASTING

Resting muscle switches from glucose to FA as its major fuel source in fasting. [Note: By contrast, exercising muscle initially uses creatine phosphate and its glycogen stores. During intense exercise, glucose 6-phosphate from glycogenolysis is converted to lactate by anaerobic glycolysis (see p. 118). The lactate is used by the liver for gluconeogenesis (Cori

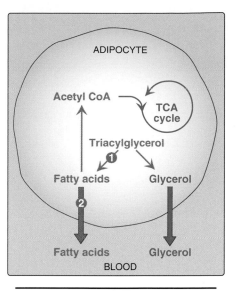

Figure 24.14
Major metabolic pathways in adipose tissue during fasting. [Note: The numbers in the circles, which appear both in the figure and in the corresponding citation in the text, indicate important pathways for fat metabolism.] CoA = coenzyme A; TCA = tricarboxylic acid.

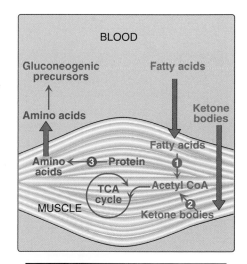

Figure 24.15
Major metabolic pathways in skeletal muscle during fasting. [Note: The numbers in the circles, which appear both in the figure and in the corresponding citation in the text, indicate important pathways for fat or protein metabolism.] CoA = coenzyme A; TCA = tricarboxylic acid.

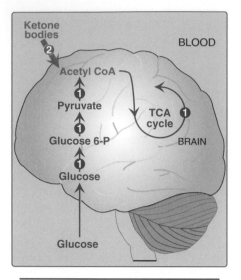

Figure 24.16
Major metabolic pathways in the brain during fasting. [Note: The numbers in the circles, which appear both in the figure and in the corresponding citation in the text, indicate important pathways for metabolism of fat or carbohydrates.] CoA = coenzyme A; TCA = tricarboxylic acid; P = phosphate.

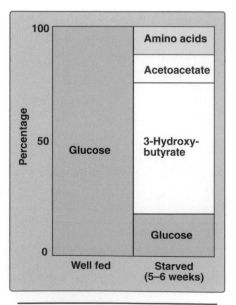

Figure 24.17
Fuel sources used by the brain to meet energy needs in the well-fed and starved states.

cycle; see p. 118). As these glycogen reserves are depleted, free FA provided by the degradation of TAG in adipose tissue become the dominant energy source. The contraction-based rise in AMP activates *AMPK* that phosphorylates and inactivates the muscle isozyme of *ACC*, decreasing malonyl CoA and allowing FA oxidation (see p. 183).]

A. Carbohydrate metabolism

Glucose transport into skeletal myocytes via insulin-sensitive GLUT-4 (see p. 97) and subsequent glucose metabolism are decreased because circulating insulin levels are low. Therefore, the glucose from hepatic gluconeogenesis is unavailable to muscle and adipose.

B. Lipid metabolism

Early in fasting, muscle uses FA from adipose tissue and ketone bodies from the liver as fuels (Fig. 24.15, ❶ and ❷). In prolonged fasting, muscle decreases its use of ketone bodies (thus sparing them for the brain) and oxidizes FA almost exclusively. [Note: The acetyl CoA from FA oxidation indirectly inhibits *PDH* (by activation of *PDH kinase*) and spares pyruvate, which is transaminated to alanine and used by the liver for gluconeogenesis (glucose–alanine cycle; see p. 253).]

C. Protein metabolism

During the first few days of fasting, there is a rapid breakdown of muscle protein (for example, glycolytic enzymes), providing amino acids that are used by the liver for gluconeogenesis (see Fig. 24.15, ❸). Because muscle does not have glucagon receptors, muscle proteolysis is initiated by a fall in insulin and sustained by a rise in glucocorticoids. [Note: Alanine and glutamine are quantitatively the most important glucogenic amino acids released from muscle. They are produced by the catabolism of BCAA (see p. 267). The glutamine is used as a fuel by enterocytes, for example, which send out alanine that is used in hepatic gluconeogenesis (glucose–alanine cycle)]. In the second week of fasting, the rate of muscle proteolysis decreases, paralleling a decline in the need for glucose as a fuel for the brain, which has begun using ketone bodies as a source of energy.

XI. BRAIN IN FASTING

During the early days of fasting, the brain continues to use only glucose as a fuel (Fig. 24.16, ❶). Blood glucose is maintained by hepatic gluconeogenesis from glucogenic precursors, such as amino acids from proteolysis and glycerol from lipolysis. In prolonged fasting (beyond 2–3 weeks), plasma ketone bodies (see Fig. 24.12) reach significantly elevated levels and replace glucose as the primary fuel for the brain (see Figs. 24.16, ❷ and 24.17). This reduces the need for protein catabolism for gluconeogenesis: Ketone bodies spare glucose and, thus, muscle protein. [Note: As the duration of a fast extends from overnight to days to weeks, blood glucose levels initially drop and then are maintained at the lower level (65–70 mg/dl).] The metabolic changes that occur during fasting insure that all tissues have an adequate supply of fuel molecules. The response of the major tissues involved in energy metabolism during fasting is summarized in Figure 24.18.

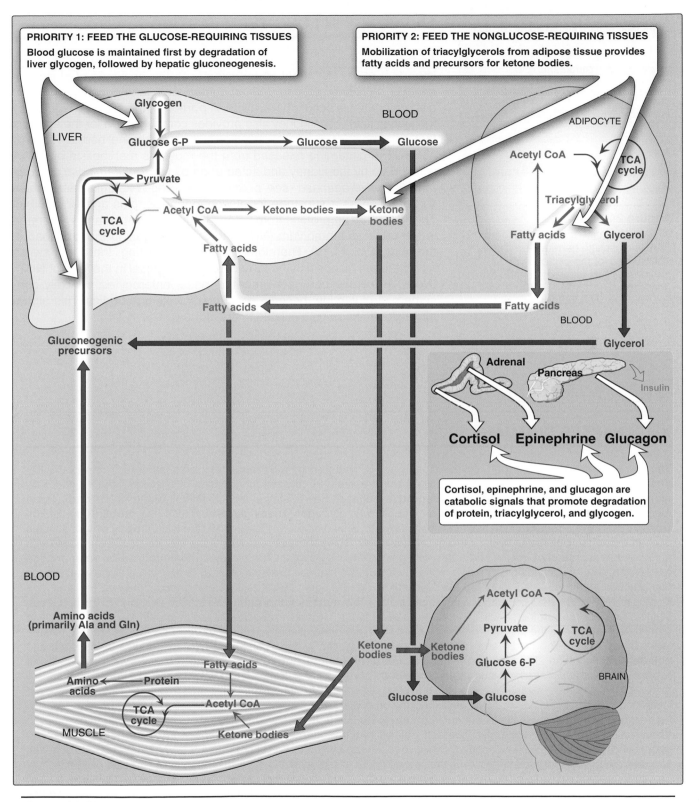

Figure 24.18
Intertissue relationships during fasting and the hormonal signals that promote them. P = phosphate; TCA = tricarboxylic acid; CoA = coenzyme A; Ala = alanine; Gln = glutamine.

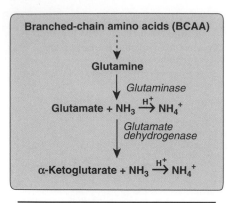

Figure 24.19
Use of glutamine from BCAA catabolism in muscle to generate ammonia (NH$_3$) used for the excretion of protons (H$^+$) as ammonium (NH$_4^+$) in the kidneys.

XII. KIDNEY IN LONG-TERM FASTING

As fasting continues into early starvation and beyond, the kidney plays important roles. The renal cortex expresses the enzymes of gluconeogenesis, including *glucose 6-phosphatase*, and, in late fasting, ~50% of gluconeogenesis occurs here. [Note: A portion of this glucose is used by the kidney itself.] The kidney also provides compensation for the acidosis that accompanies the increased production of ketone bodies (organic acids). The glutamine released from the muscle's metabolism of BCAA is taken up by the kidney and acted upon by renal *glutaminase* and *glutamate dehydrogenase* (see p. 256), producing α-ketoglutarate, which can be used as a substrate for gluconeogenesis, plus ammonia (NH$_3$). The NH$_3$ picks up protons from ketone body dissociation and is excreted in the urine as ammonium (NH$_4^+$), thereby decreasing the acid load in the body (Fig. 24.19). Therefore, in long-term fasting, there is a switch from nitrogen disposal in the form of urea to disposal in the form of NH$_4^+$. [Note: As ketone body concentration rises, enterocytes, typically consumers of glutamine, become consumers of ketone bodies. This allows more glutamine to be available to the kidney.]

XIII. CHAPTER SUMMARY

The flow of intermediates through metabolic pathways is controlled by **four regulatory mechanisms**: 1) the availability of substrates, 2) allosteric activation and inhibition of enzymes, 3) covalent modification of enzymes, and 4) induction-repression of enzyme synthesis. In the **absorptive state**, the 2- to 4-hour period after ingestion of a meal, these mechanisms insure that available nutrients are captured as **glycogen, triacylglycerol** (**TAG**), and **protein** (Fig. 24.20). During this interval, transient increases in plasma glucose, amino acids, and TAG occur, the last primarily as components of **chylomicrons** synthesized by the intestinal mucosal cells. The **pancreas** responds to the elevated levels of glucose with an increased secretion of insulin and a decreased secretion of glucagon. The elevated **insulin/glucagon ratio** and the ready availability of circulating substrates make the absorptive state an **anabolic period** during which virtually all tissues use **glucose** as a fuel. In addition, the **liver** replenishes its glycogen stores, replaces any needed hepatic proteins, and increases TAG synthesis. The latter are packaged in **very-low-density lipoproteins**, which are exported to the peripheral tissues. **Adipose tissue** increases TAG synthesis and storage, whereas **muscle** increases protein synthesis to replace protein degraded since the previous meal. In the fed state, the **brain** uses glucose exclusively as a fuel. In **fasting**, plasma levels of glucose, amino acids, and TAG fall, triggering a decline in insulin secretion and an increase in glucagon and **epinephrine** secretion. The decreased **insulin/counterregulatory hormone ratio** and the decreased availability of circulating substrates make the fasting state a **catabolic period**. This sets into motion an **exchange of substrates** among the liver, adipose tissue, skeletal muscle, and brain that is guided by two priorities: 1) the need to maintain adequate plasma levels of glucose to sustain energy metabolism of the brain and other glucose-requiring tissues and 2) the need to mobilize fatty acids (FA) from adipose tissue and release **ketone bodies** from liver to supply energy to other tissues. To accomplish these goals, the liver degrades glycogen and initiates **gluconeogenesis**, using increased **FA oxidation** to supply the energy and reducing equivalents needed for gluconeogenesis and the acetyl coenzyme A building blocks for **ketogenesis**. The adipose tissue degrades stored TAG, thus providing FA and **glycerol** to the liver. The muscle can also use FA as fuel as well as ketone bodies supplied by the liver. The liver uses the glycerol for gluconeogenesis. **Muscle protein** is degraded to supply amino acids for the liver to use in gluconeogenesis but decreases as ketone bodies increase. The brain can use both glucose and ketone bodies as fuels. From late fasting into starvation, the **kidneys** play important roles by synthesizing glucose and excreting the **protons** from ketone body dissociation as **ammonium** (NH$_4^+$).

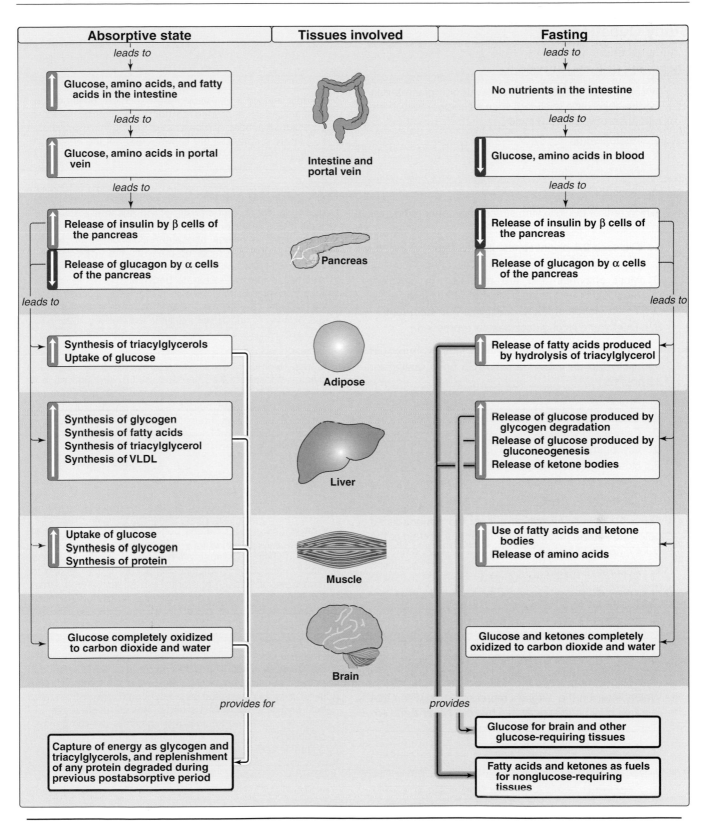

Figure 24.20
Key concept map for the feed–fast cycle. VLDL = very-low-density lipoprotein.

Study Questions

Choose the ONE best answer.

24.1 Which one of the following is elevated in plasma during the absorptive (well-fed) state as compared with the postabsorptive (fasted) state?

- A. Acetoacetate
- B. Chylomicrons
- C. Free fatty acids
- D. Glucagon

Correct answer = B. Triacylglycerol-rich chylomicrons are synthesized in (and released from) the intestine following ingestion of a meal. Acetoacetate, free fatty acids, and glucagon are elevated in the fasted state, not the absorptive state.

24.2 Which one of the following statements concerning liver in the absorptive state is correct?

- A. Fructose 2,6-bisphosphate is elevated.
- B. Insulin stimulates the uptake of glucose.
- C. Most enzymes that are regulated by covalent modification are in the phosphorylated state.
- D. The oxidation of acetyl coenzyme A is increased.
- E. The synthesis of glucokinase is repressed.

Correct answer = A. The increased insulin and decreased glucagon levels characteristic of the absorptive state promote the synthesis of fructose 2,6-bisphosphate, which allosterically activates phosphofructokinase-1 of glycolysis. Most covalently modified enzymes are in the dephosphorylated state and are active. Acetyl coenzyme A is not oxidized in the well-fed state because it is being used in fatty acid synthesis. Uptake of glucose (by glucose transporter-2) into the liver is insulin independent. Synthesis of glucokinase is induced by insulin in the well-fed state.

24.3 Which one of the following enzymes is phosphorylated and active in an individual who has been fasting for 12 hours?

- A. Arginase
- B. Carnitine palmitoyltransferase-I
- C. Fatty acid synthase
- D. Glycogen synthase
- E. Hormone-sensitive lipase
- F. Phosphofructokinase-1
- G. Pyruvate dehydrogenase

Correct answer = E. Hormone-sensitive lipase of adipocytes is phosphorylated and activated by protein kinase A in response to epinephrine. Choices A, B, C, and F are not regulated covalently. Choices D and G are regulated covalently but are inactive if phosphorylated.

24.4 For a 70-kg man, in which one of the periods listed below do ketone bodies supply the major portion of the caloric needs of brain?

- A. Absorptive period
- B. Overnight fast
- C. Three-day fast
- D. Four-week fast
- E. Five-month fast

Correct answer = D. Ketone bodies, made from the acetyl coenzyme A product of fatty acid oxidation, increase in the blood in fasting but must reach a critical level to cross the blood–brain barrier. Typically, this occurs in the second to third week of a fast. Fat stores in a 70-kg (~154-lb) man would not be able to supply his energy needs for 5 months.

24.5 The diagram below shows inputs to and outputs from pyruvate, a central molecule in energy metabolism.

Which letter on the diagram represents a reaction that requires biotin and is activated by acetyl coenzyme A?

Correct answer = C. Pyruvate carboxylase, a mitochondrial enzyme of gluconeogenesis, requires biotin (and ATP) and is allosterically activated by acetyl coenzyme A from fatty acid oxidation. None of the other choices meets these criteria. A = pyruvate kinase; B = pyruvate dehydrogenase complex; D = aspartate aminotransferase; E = alanine aminotransferase; F = lactate dehydrogenase.

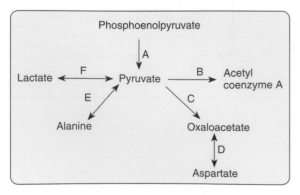

Diabetes Mellitus

25

I. OVERVIEW

Diabetes mellitus (diabetes) is not one disease but rather is a heterogeneous group of multifactorial, primarily polygenic syndromes characterized by an elevated fasting blood glucose (FBG) caused by a relative or absolute deficiency in insulin. Over 29 million people in the United States (~9% of the population) have diabetes. Of this number, ~8 million are as yet undiagnosed. Diabetes is the leading cause of adult blindness and amputation and a major cause of renal failure, nerve damage, heart attacks, and strokes. Most cases of diabetes mellitus can be separated into two groups (Fig. 25.1), type 1 ([T1D] formerly called insulin-dependent diabetes mellitus) and type 2 ([T2D] formerly called non–insulin-dependent diabetes

Characteristics	Type 1 Diabetes	Type 2 Diabetes
AGE OF ONSET	Usually during childhood or puberty; symptoms develop rapidly	Frequently after age 35 years; symptoms develop gradually
NUTRITIONAL STATUS AT TIME OF DISEASE ONSET	Frequently undernourished	Obesity usually present
PREVALENCE	<10% of diagnosed diabetics	>90% of diagnosed diabetics
GENETIC PREDISPOSITION	Moderate	Very strong
DEFECT OR DEFICIENCY	β-Cell destruction, eliminating production of insulin	Insulin resistance combined with inability of β cells to produce appropriate quantities of insulin
FREQUENCY OF KETOSIS	Common	Rare
PLASMA INSULIN	Low to absent	High early in disease; low to absent in disease of long duration
ACUTE COMPLICATIONS	Ketoacidosis	Hyperosmolar hyperglycemic state
RESPONSE TO ORAL HYPOGLYCEMIC DRUGS	Unresponsive	Responsive
TREATMENT	Insulin always necessary	Diet, exercise, oral hypoglycemic drugs, insulin (may or may not be necessary); reduction of risk factors (weight reduction, smoking cessation, blood pressure control, treatment of dyslipidemia) essential to therapy

Figure 25.1
Comparison of type 1 and type 2 diabetes mellitus. [Note: The name of the disease reflects the clinical presentation of copious amounts of glucose-containing urine and is derived from the Greek word for siphon (diabetes) and the Latin word for honey-sweet (mellitus).]

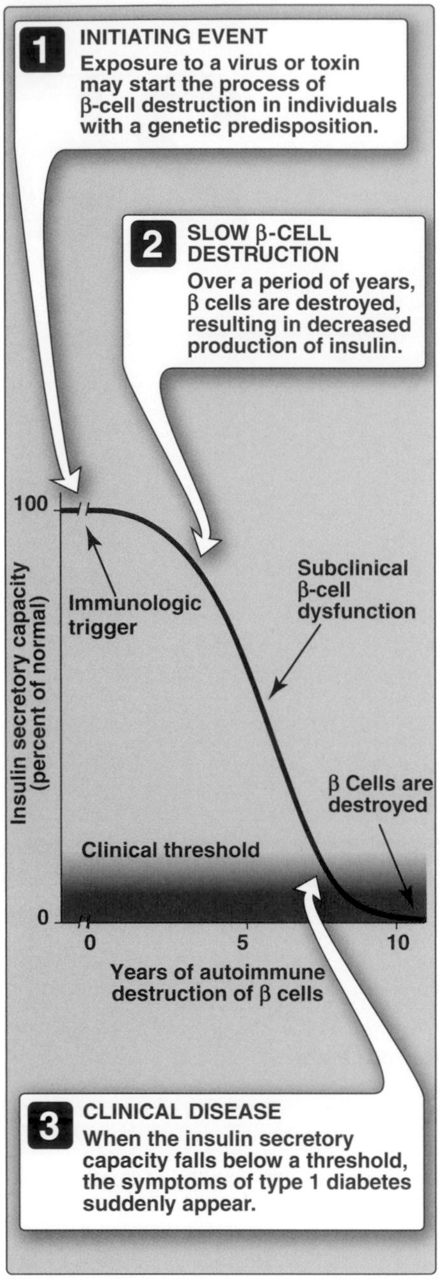
1
INITIATING EVENT
Exposure to a virus or toxin may start the process of β-cell destruction in individuals with a genetic predisposition.
2
SLOW β-CELL DESTRUCTION
Over a period of years, β cells are destroyed, resulting in decreased production of insulin.
100
Immunologic trigger
Subclinical β-cell dysfunction
Insulin secretory capacity (percent of normal)
β Cells are destroyed
Clinical threshold
0
0
5
10
Years of autoimmune destruction of β cells
3
CLINICAL DISEASE
When the insulin secretory capacity falls below a threshold, the symptoms of type 1 diabetes suddenly appear.

Figure 25.2
Insulin secretory capacity during onset of type 1 diabetes. [Note: Rate of autoimmune destruction of β cells may be faster or slower than shown.]

mellitus). The incidence and prevalence of T2D is increasing because of the aging of the U.S. population and the increasing prevalence of obesity and sedentary lifestyles (see p. 349). The increase in children with T2D is particularly disturbing.

II. TYPE 1

T1D constitutes <10% of the ~21 million known cases of diabetes in the United States. The disease is characterized by an absolute deficiency of insulin caused by an autoimmune attack on the islet β cells of the pancreas. In T1D, the islets of Langerhans become infiltrated with activated T lymphocytes, leading to a condition called insulitis. Over a period of years, this autoimmune attack on the β cells leads to gradual depletion of the β-cell population (Fig. 25.2). However, symptoms appear abruptly when 80%–90% of the β cells have been destroyed. At this point, the pancreas fails to respond adequately to ingestion of glucose, and insulin therapy is required to restore metabolic control and prevent life-threatening ketoacidosis. β-Cell destruction requires both a stimulus from the environment (such as a viral infection) and a genetic determinant that causes the β cells to be mistakenly identified as "nonself." [Note: Among monozygotic (identical) twins, if one sibling develops T1D, the other twin has only a 30%–50% chance of developing the disease. This contrasts with T2D (see p. 341), in which the genetic influence is stronger and, in virtually all monozygotic twinships, the disease eventually develops in both individuals.]

A. Diagnosis

The onset of T1D is typically during childhood or puberty, and symptoms develop suddenly. Individuals with T1D can usually be recognized by the abrupt appearance of polyuria (frequent urination), polydipsia (excessive thirst), and polyphagia (excessive hunger), often triggered by physiologic stress such as an infection. These symptoms are usually accompanied by fatigue and weight loss. The diagnosis is confirmed by a FBG ≥126 mg/dl (normal is 70–99). [Note: Fasting is defined as no caloric intake for at least 8 hours.] A FBG of 100–125 mg/dl is categorized as an impaired FBG. Individuals with impaired FBG are considered prediabetic and are at increased risk for developing T2D. Diagnosis can also be made on the basis of a nonfasting (random) blood glucose level >200 mg/dl or a glycated hemoglobin (see p. 340) concentration ≥6.5 mg/dl (normal is <5.7) in an individual with symptoms of hyperglycemia. [Note: The oral glucose tolerance test, in which blood glucose is measured 2 hours after ingestion of a solution containing 75 g of glucose, also is used but is less convenient. It is most typically used to screen pregnant women for gestational diabetes (see p. 342).]

> When blood glucose is >180 mg/dl, the ability of renal sodium-dependent glucose transporters (SGLT) to reclaim glucose is impaired, and glucose "spills" into urine. The loss of glucose is accompanied by the loss of water, resulting in the characteristic polyuria (with dehydration) and polydipsia of diabetes.

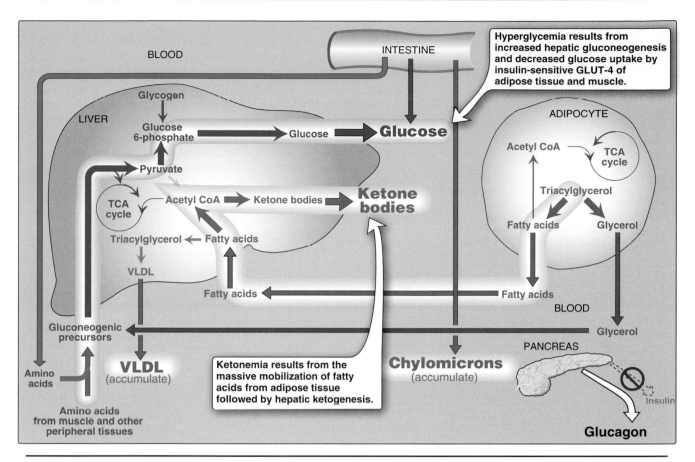

Figure 25.3
Intertissue relationships in type 1 diabetes. TCA = tricarboxylic acid; CoA = coenzyme A; VLDL = very-low-density lipoproteins; GLUT = glucose transporter.

B. Metabolic changes

The metabolic abnormalities of T1D result from a deficiency of insulin that profoundly affects metabolism in three tissues: liver, skeletal muscle, and white adipose (Fig. 25.3).

1. **Hyperglycemia and ketonemia:** Elevated levels of blood glucose and ketone bodies are the hallmarks of untreated T1D (see Fig. 25.3). Hyperglycemia is caused by increased hepatic production of glucose via gluconeogenesis, combined with diminished peripheral utilization (muscle and adipose tissue have the insulin-regulated glucose transporter GLUT-4; see p. 97). Ketonemia results from increased mobilization of fatty acids (FA) from triacylglycerol (TAG) in adipose tissue, combined with accelerated hepatic FA β-oxidation and synthesis of 3-hydroxybutyrate and acetoacetate (ketone bodies; see p. 196). [Note: Acetyl coenzyme A from β-oxidation is the substrate for ketogenesis and the allosteric activator of *pyruvate carboxylase*, a gluconeogenic enzyme.] Diabetic ketoacidosis (DKA), a type of metabolic acidosis caused by an imbalance between ketone body production and use, occurs in 25%–40% of those newly diagnosed with T1D and may recur if the patient becomes ill (most commonly with an infection) or does not comply with therapy. DKA is treated by replacing fluid and electrolytes and administering short-acting insulin to gradually correct hyperglycemia without precipitating hypoglycemia.

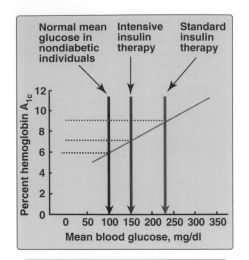

Figure 25.4
Correlation between mean blood glucose and percent hemoglobin A₁c in patients with type 1 diabetes receiving intensive or standard insulin therapy. [Note: Nondiabetic individuals are included for comparison.]

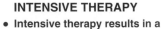
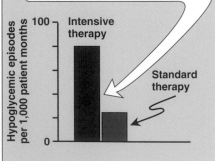

Figure 25.5
Effect of tight glucose control on hypoglycemic episodes in a population of patients on intensive therapy or standard therapy.

2. **Hypertriacylglycerolemia:** Not all of the FA flooding the liver can be disposed of through oxidation and ketone body synthesis. These excess FA are converted to TAG, which are packaged and secreted in very-low-density lipoproteins ([VLDL] see p. 230). Chylomicrons rich in dietary TAG are secreted by the intestinal mucosal cells following a meal (see p. 227). Because lipoprotein TAG degradation catalyzed by *lipoprotein lipase* in the capillary beds of adipose tissue (see p. 228) is low in diabetes (synthesis of the enzyme is decreased when insulin levels are low), the plasma chylomicron and VLDL levels are elevated, resulting in hypertriacylglycerolemia (see Fig. 25.3).

C. Treatment

Individuals with T1D must rely on exogenous insulin delivered subcutaneously (subq) either by periodic injection or by continuous pump-assisted infusion to control the hyperglycemia and ketonemia. Two types of therapeutic injection regimens are currently used, standard and intensive. [Note: Pump delivery is also considered intensive therapy.]

1. **Standard versus intensive treatment:** Standard treatment is typically two to three daily injections of recombinant human insulin. Mean blood glucose levels obtained are typically 225–275 mg/dl, with a glycated hemoglobin (HbA₁c) level (see p. 33) of 8%–9% of the total hemoglobin (blue arrow in Fig. 25.4). [Note: The rate of formation of HbA₁c is proportional to the average blood glucose concentration over the previous 3 months. Thus, HbA₁c provides a measure of how well treatment has normalized blood glucose over that time in a patient with diabetes.] In contrast to standard therapy, intensive treatment seeks to more closely normalize blood glucose through more frequent monitoring and subsequent injections of insulin, typically ≥4 times a day. Mean blood glucose levels of 150 mg/dl can be achieved, with HbA₁c ~7% of the total hemoglobin (see red arrow in Fig. 25.4). [Note: Normal mean blood glucose is ~100 mg/dl, and HbA₁c is ≤6% (see black arrow in Fig. 25.4).] Therefore, normalization of glucose values (euglycemia) is not achieved even in intensively treated patients. Nonetheless, patients on intensive therapy show a ≥50% reduction in the long-term microvascular complications of diabetes (that is, retinopathy, nephropathy, and neuropathy) compared with patients receiving standard care. This confirms that the complications of diabetes are related to an elevation of plasma glucose.

2. **Hypoglycemia:** One of the therapeutic goals in cases of diabetes is to decrease blood glucose levels in an effort to minimize the development of long-term complications of the disease (see p. 345 for a discussion of the chronic complications of diabetes). However, appropriate dosage of insulin is difficult to achieve. Hypoglycemia caused by excess insulin is the most common complication of insulin therapy, occurring in >90% of patients. The frequency of hypoglycemic episodes, seizures, and coma is particularly high with intensive treatment regimens designed to achieve tight control of blood glucose (Fig. 25.5). In normal individuals, hypoglycemia triggers a compensatory secretion of counterregulatory hormones, most notably glucagon and epinephrine, which promote hepatic production of glucose (see p. 315). However, patients with T1D also develop a deficiency of glucagon secretion. This defect

occurs early in the disease and is almost universally present 4 years after diagnosis. Therefore, these patients rely on epinephrine secretion to prevent severe hypoglycemia. However, as the disease progresses, T1D patients show diabetic autonomic neuropathy and impaired ability to secrete epinephrine in response to hypoglycemia. The combined deficiency of glucagon and epinephrine secretion creates a symptom-free condition sometimes called "hypoglycemia unawareness." Thus, patients with long-standing T1D are particularly vulnerable to hypoglycemia. Hypoglycemia can also be caused by strenuous exercise. Because exercise promotes glucose uptake into muscle and decreases the need for exogenous insulin, patients are advised to check blood glucose levels before or after intensive exercise to prevent or abort hypoglycemia.

3. **Contraindications for tight control:** Children are not put on a program of tight control of blood glucose before age 8 years because of the risk that episodes of hypoglycemia may adversely affect brain development. Elderly people typically do not go on tight control because hypoglycemia can cause strokes and heart attacks in this population. Also, the major goal of tight control is to prevent complications many years later. Tight control, then, is most worthwhile for otherwise healthy people who can expect to live at least 10 more years. [Note: For most nonpregnant adults with diabetes, the individual treatment strategies and goals are based on the duration of diabetes, age/life expectancy, and known comorbid conditions.]

III. TYPE 2

T2D is the most common form of the disease, afflicting >90% of the U.S. population with diabetes. [Note: American Indians, Alaskan Natives, Hispanic and Latino Americans, African Americans, and Asian Americans have the highest prevalence.] Typically, T2D develops gradually without obvious symptoms. The disease is often detected by routine screening tests. However, many individuals with T2D have symptoms of polyuria and polydipsia of several weeks' duration. Polyphagia may be present but is less common. Patients with T2D have a combination of insulin resistance and dysfunctional β cells (Fig. 25.6) but do not require insulin to sustain life. However, in >90% of these patients, insulin eventually will be required to control hyperglycemia and keep HbA$_{1c}$ <7%. The metabolic alterations observed in T2D are milder than those described for type 1, in part because insulin secretion in T2D, although inadequate, does restrain ketogenesis and blunts the development of DKA. [Note: Insulin suppresses the release of glucagon (see p. 314).] Diagnosis is based on the presence of hyperglycemia as described above. The pathogenesis does not involve viruses or autoimmune antibodies and is not completely understood. [Note: An acute complication of T2D in the elderly is a hyperosmolar hyperglycemic state characterized by severe hyperglycemia and dehydration and altered mental status.]

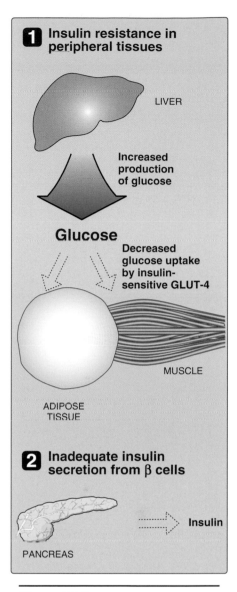

1 Insulin resistance in peripheral tissues

LIVER

Increased production of glucose

Glucose

Decreased glucose uptake by insulin-sensitive GLUT-4

MUSCLE

ADIPOSE TISSUE

2 Inadequate insulin secretion from β cells

Insulin

PANCREAS

Figure 25.6
Major factors contributing to hyperglycemia observed in type 2 diabetes. GLUT = glucose transporter.

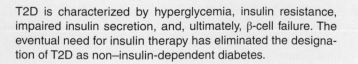

T2D is characterized by hyperglycemia, insulin resistance, impaired insulin secretion, and, ultimately, β-cell failure. The eventual need for insulin therapy has eliminated the designation of T2D as non–insulin-dependent diabetes.

A. Insulin resistance

Insulin resistance is the decreased ability of target tissues, such as the liver, white adipose, and skeletal muscle, to respond properly to normal (or elevated) circulating concentrations of insulin. For example, insulin resistance is characterized by increased hepatic glucose production, decreased glucose uptake by muscle and adipose tissue, and increased adipose lipolysis with production of free fatty acids (FFA).

1. **Insulin resistance and obesity:** Although obesity is the most common cause of insulin resistance and increases the risk of T2D, most people with obesity and insulin resistance do not develop diabetes. In the absence of a defect in β-cell function, obese individuals can compensate for insulin resistance with elevated levels of insulin. For example, Figure 25.7A shows that insulin secretion is two to three times higher in obese subjects than it is in lean individuals. This higher insulin concentration compensates for the diminished effect of the hormone (as a result of insulin resistance) and produces blood glucose levels similar to those observed in lean individuals (Fig. 25.7B).

2. **Insulin resistance and type 2 diabetes:** Insulin resistance alone will not lead to T2D. Rather, T2D develops in insulin-resistant individuals who also show impaired β-cell function. Insulin resistance and subsequent risk for the development of T2D is commonly observed in individuals who are obese, physically inactive, or elderly and in the 3%–5% of pregnant women who develop gestational diabetes. These patients are unable to sufficiently compensate for insulin resistance with increased insulin release. Figure 25.8 shows the time course for the development of hyperglycemia and the loss of β-cell function.

3. **Causes of insulin resistance:** Insulin resistance increases with weight gain and decreases with weight loss, and excess adipose tissue (particularly in the abdomen) is key in the development of insulin resistance. Adipose is not simply an energy storage tissue, but also a secretory tissue. With obesity, there are changes

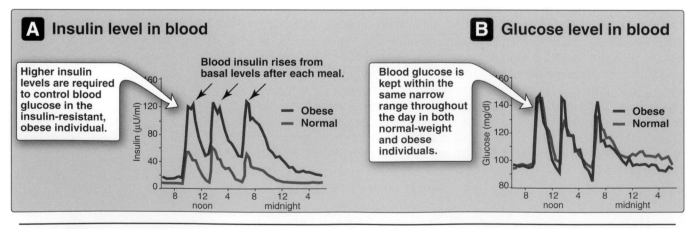

Figure 25.7
Blood insulin (A) and blood glucose levels (B) in normal-weight and obese subjects.

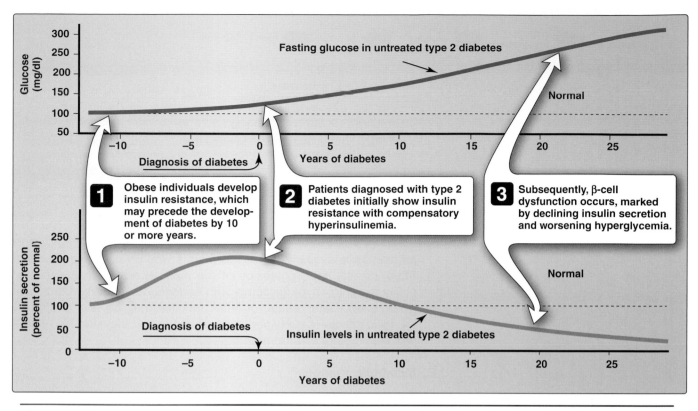

Figure 25.8
Progression of blood glucose and insulin levels in patients with type 2 diabetes.

in adipose secretions that result in insulin resistance (Fig. 25.9). These include secretion of proinflammatory cytokines such as interleukin 6 and tumor necrosis factor-α by activated macrophages (inflammation is associated with insulin resistance); increased synthesis of leptin, a protein with proinflammatory effects (see p. 353 for additional effects of leptin); and decreased secretion of adiponectin (see p. 350), a protein with anti-inflammatory effects. The net result is chronic, low-grade inflammation. One effect of insulin resistance is increased lipolysis and production of FFA (see Fig. 25.9). FFA availability decreases use of glucose, contributing to hyperglycemia, and increases ectopic deposition of TAG in liver (hepatic steatosis). [Note: Steatosis results in nonalcoholic fatty liver disease (NAFLD). If accompanied by inflammation, a more serious condition, nonalcoholic steatohepatitis (NASH), can develop.] FFA also have a proinflammatory effect. In the long term, FFA impair insulin signaling. [Note: Adiponectin increases FA β-oxidation (see p. 349). Consequently, a decrease in this adipocyte protein contributes to FFA availability.]

B. Dysfunctional β cells

In T2D, the pancreas initially retains β-cell capacity, resulting in insulin levels that vary from above normal to below normal. However, with time, the β cell becomes increasingly dysfunctional and fails to secrete enough insulin to correct the prevailing hyperglycemia. For example, insulin levels are high in typical, obese, T2D patients but not

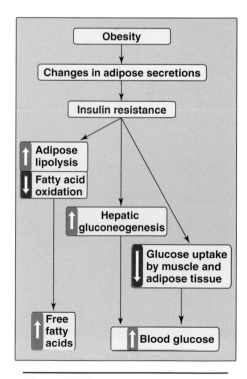

Figure 25.9
Obesity, insulin resistance, and hyperglycemia. [Note: Inflammation also is associated with insulin resistance.]

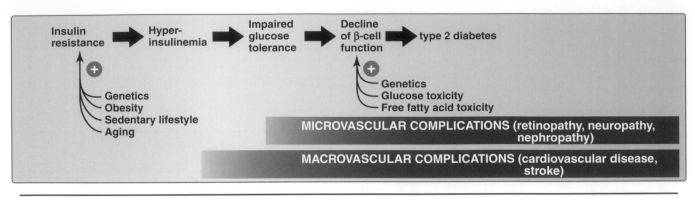

Figure 25.10
Typical progression of type 2 diabetes.

as high as in similarly obese individuals who do not have diabetes. Thus, the natural progression of the disease results in a declining ability to control hyperglycemia with endogenous secretion of insulin (Fig. 25.10). Deterioration of β-cell function may be accelerated by the toxic effects of sustained hyperglycemia and elevated FFA and a proinflammatory environment.

C. Metabolic changes

The abnormalities of glucose and TAG metabolism in T2D are the result of insulin resistance expressed primarily in liver, skeletal muscle, and white adipose tissue (Fig. 25.11).

1. **Hyperglycemia:** Hyperglycemia is caused by increased hepatic production of glucose, combined with diminished use of glucose by muscle and adipose tissues. Ketonemia is usually minimal or absent in patients with T2D because the presence of insulin, even in the presence of insulin resistance, restrains hepatic ketogenesis.

2. **Dyslipidemia:** In the liver, FFA are converted to TAG, which are packaged and secreted in VLDL. Dietary TAG–rich chylomicrons are synthesized and secreted by the intestinal mucosal cells following a meal. Because lipoprotein TAG degradation catalyzed by *lipoprotein lipase* in adipose tissue is low in diabetes, the plasma chylomicron and VLDL levels are elevated, resulting in hypertriacylglycerolemia (see Fig. 25.10). Low levels of high-density lipoproteins are also associated with T2D, likely as a result of increased degradation.

D. Treatment

The goal in treating T2D is to maintain blood glucose concentrations within normal limits and to prevent the development of long-term complications. Weight reduction, exercise, and medical nutrition therapy (dietary modifications) often correct the hyperglycemia of newly diagnosed T2D. Oral hypoglycemic agents, such as metformin (decreases hepatic gluconeogenesis), sulfonylureas (increase insulin secretion; see p. 310), thiazolidinediones (decrease FFA levels and increase peripheral insulin sensitivity), α-*glucosidase* inhibitors (decrease absorption of dietary carbohydrate), and SGLT inhibitors (decrease renal reabsorption of glucose), or subq insulin therapy

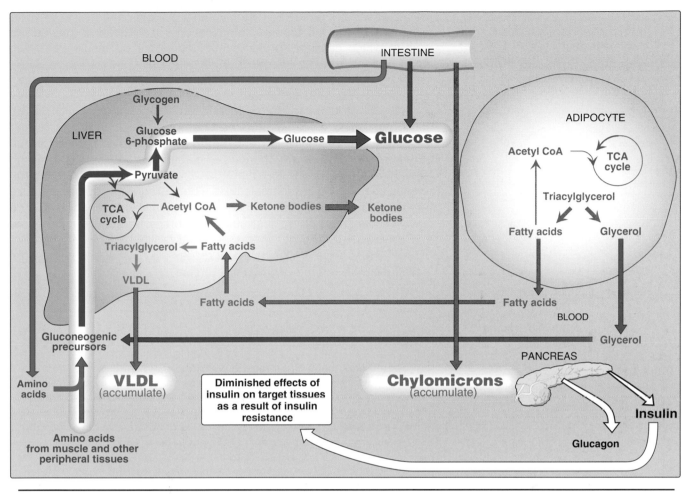

Figure 25.11
Intertissue relationships in type 2 diabetes. [Note: Ketogenesis is restrained as long as insulin action is adequate.] TCA = tricarboxylic acid; CoA = coenzyme A; VLDL = very-low-density lipoproteins.

may be required to achieve satisfactory plasma glucose levels. [Note: Bariatric surgery in morbidly obese individuals with T2D has been shown to result in disease remission in most patients. Remission may not be permanent.]

IV. CHRONIC EFFECTS AND PREVENTION

As noted previously, available therapies moderate the hyperglycemia of diabetes but fail to completely normalize metabolism. The long-standing elevation of blood glucose is associated with the chronic vascular complications of diabetes including cardiovascular disease (CVD) and stroke (macrovascular complications) as well as retinopathy, nephropathy, and neuropathy (microvascular). Intensive insulin treatment (see p. 340) delays the onset and slows the progression of some long-term complications. For example, the incidence of retinopathy decreases as control of blood glucose improves and HbA$_{1c}$ levels decrease (Fig. 25.12). [Note: Data concerning the effect of tight control on CVD in T2D are less clear.] The benefits of tight control of blood glucose outweigh

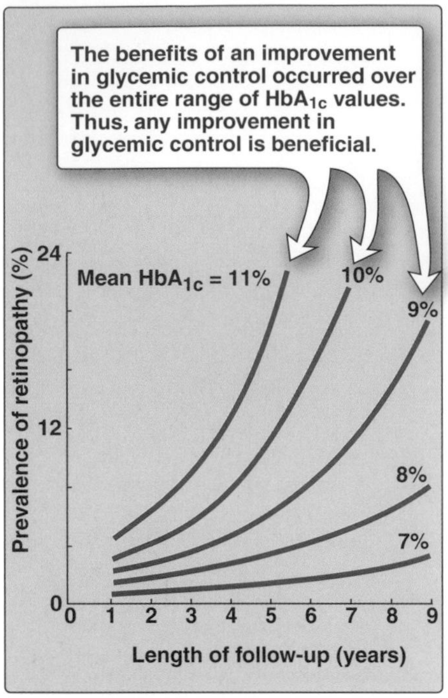

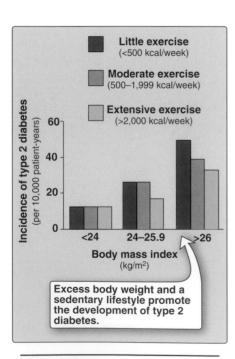

Figure 25.12
Relationship of glycemic control and diabetic retinopathy. HbA$_{1c}$ = glycated hemoglobin.

Figure 25.13
Effect of body mass index and exercise on the development of type 2 diabetes.

the increased risk of severe hypoglycemia in most patients. How hyperglycemia causes the chronic complications of diabetes is unclear. In cells in which glucose uptake is not dependent on insulin, elevated blood glucose leads to increased intracellular glucose and its metabolites. For example, increased intracellular sorbitol contributes to cataract formation (see p. 140) in diabetes. Additionally, hyperglycemia promotes glycation of cellular proteins in a reaction analogous to the formation of HbA$_{1c}$. These glycated proteins undergo additional reactions and become advanced glycation end products (AGE) that mediate some of the early microvascular changes of diabetes and can reduce wound healing. Some AGE bind to a membrane receptor (RAGE), causing the release of proinflammatory molecules. There is currently no preventative treatment for T1D. The risk for T2D can be significantly decreased by a combined regimen of medical nutrition therapy, weight loss, exercise, and aggressive control of hypertension and dyslipidemias. For example, Figure 25.13 shows the incidence of disease in normal and overweight individuals with varying degrees of exercise.

V. CHAPTER SUMMARY

Diabetes mellitus is a heterogeneous group of syndromes characterized by an **elevation** of **fasting blood glucose** that is caused by a relative or absolute deficiency of insulin (Fig. 25.14). Diabetes is the leading cause of **adult blindness** and **amputation** and a major cause of **renal failure**, **nerve damage**, **heart attacks**, and **stroke**. Diabetes can be classified into two groups, **type 1** (**T1D**) and **type 2** (**T2D**). T1D constitutes ~10% of >29 million cases of diabetes in the United States. The disease is characterized by an **absolute deficiency** of **insulin** caused by an **autoimmune attack** on the **pancreatic β cells**. This destruction requires an **environmental stimulus** (such as a viral infection) and a **genetic determinant** that causes the β cell to be mistakenly identified as "nonself." The **metabolic abnormalities** of T1D include **hyperglycemia**, **diabetic ketoacidosis** (**DKA**), and **hypertriacylglycerolemia** that result from a deficiency of insulin. Those with T1D must rely on **exogenous insulin** delivered subcutaneously to control hyperglycemia and ketoacidosis. **T2D** has a strong **genetic** component. It results from a combination of **insulin resistance** and **dysfunctional β cells**. Insulin resistance is the decreased ability of target tissues, such as liver, white adipose, and skeletal muscle, to respond properly to normal (or elevated) circulating concentrations of insulin. **Obesity** is the most common cause of insulin resistance. However, most people with obesity and insulin resistance do not develop diabetes. In the absence of a defect in β-cell function, obese individuals without diabetes can compensate for insulin resistance with elevated levels of insulin. Insulin resistance alone will not lead to T2D. Rather, T2D develops in insulin-resistant individuals who also show impaired β-cell function. The acute **metabolic alterations** observed in T2D are **milder** than those described for the insulin-dependent form of the disease, in part because insulin secretion in T2D, although inadequate, does restrain **ketogenesis** and blunts the development of DKA. Available treatments for diabetes moderate the hyperglycemia but fail to completely normalize metabolism. The long-standing elevation of blood glucose is associated with the **chronic complications** of diabetes including **cardiovascular disease** and **stroke** (**macrovascular**) as well as **retinopathy**, **nephropathy**, and **neuropathy** (**microvascular**).

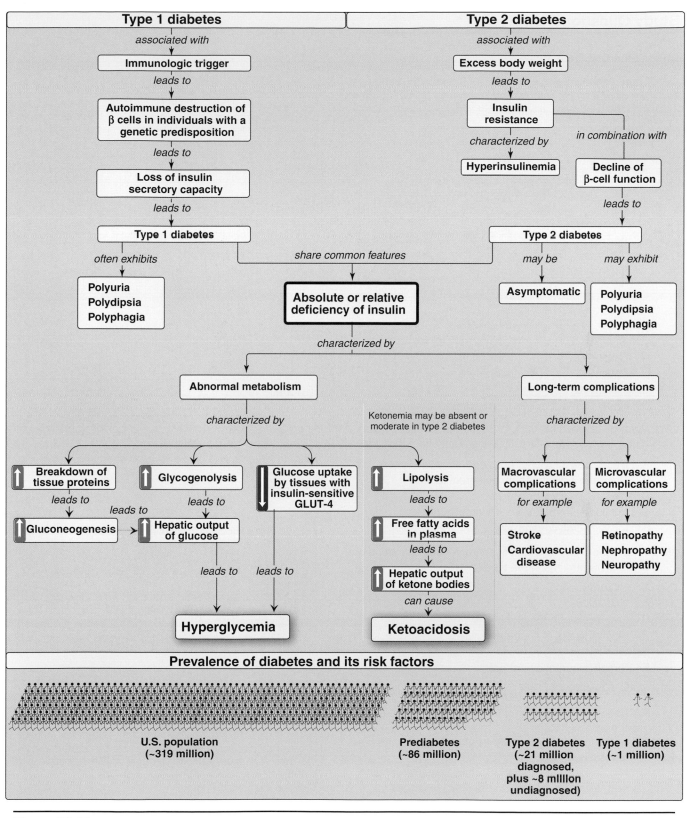

Figure 25.14
Key concept map for diabetes. [Note: Data are from 2014.] GLUT = glucose transporter.

Study Questions

Choose the ONE best answer.

25.1 Three patients being evaluated for gestational diabetes are given an oral glucose tolerance test. Based on the data shown below, which patient is prediabetic?

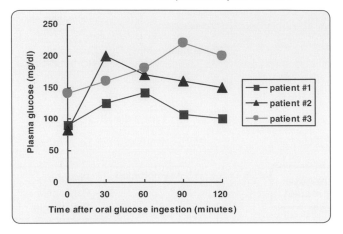

A. Patient #1
B. Patient #2
C. Patient #3
D. None

> Correct answer = B. Patient #2 has a normal fasting blood glucose (FBG) but an impaired glucose tolerance (GT) as reflected in her blood glucose level at 2 hours and, so, is described as prediabetic. Patient #1 has a normal FBG and GT, whereas patient #3 has diabetes.

25.2 Relative or absolute lack of insulin in humans would result in which one of the following reactions in the liver?

A. Decreased activity of hormone-sensitive lipase
B. Decreased gluconeogenesis from lactate
C. Decreased glycogenolysis
D. Increased formation of 3-hydroxybutyrate
E. Increased glycogenesis

> Correct answer = D. Low insulin levels favor the liver producing ketone bodies, using acetyl coenzyme A generated by β-oxidation of the fatty acids provided by hormone-sensitive lipase (HSL) in adipose tissue (not liver). Low insulin also causes activation of HSL, decreased glycogen synthesis, and increased gluconeogenesis and glycogenolysis.

25.3 Which one of the following is characteristic of untreated diabetes regardless of the type?

A. Hyperglycemia
B. Ketoacidosis
C. Low levels of hemoglobin A_{1c}
D. Normal levels of C-peptide
E. Obesity
F. Simple inheritance pattern

> Correct answer = A. Elevated blood glucose occurs in type 1 diabetes (T1D) as a result of a lack of insulin. In type 2 diabetes (T2D), hyperglycemia is due to a defect in β-cell function and insulin resistance. The hyperglycemia results in elevated hemoglobin A_{1c} levels. Ketoacidosis is rare in T2D, whereas obesity is rare in T1D. C (connecting)-peptide is a measure of insulin synthesis. It would be virtually absent in T1D and initially increased then decreased in T2D. Both forms of the disease show complex genetics.

25.4 An obese individual with type 2 diabetes typically:

A. benefits from receiving insulin about 6 hours after a meal.
B. has a lower plasma level of glucagon than does a normal individual.
C. has a lower plasma level of insulin than does a normal individual early in the disease process.
D. shows improvement in glucose tolerance if body weight is reduced.
E. shows sudden onset of symptoms.

> Correct answer = D. Many individuals with type 2 diabetes are obese, and almost all show some improvement in blood glucose with weight reduction. Symptoms usually develop gradually. These patients have elevated insulin levels and usually do not require insulin (certainly not 6 hours after a meal) until late in the disease. Glucagon levels are typically normal.

Obesity

26

I. OVERVIEW

Obesity is a disorder of body weight regulatory systems characterized by an accumulation of excess body fat. In primitive societies, in which daily life required a high level of physical activity and food was only available intermittently, a genetic tendency favoring storage of excess calories as fat may have had a survival value. Today, however, the sedentary lifestyle and abundance and wide variety of palatable, inexpensive foods in industrialized societies has undoubtedly contributed to an obesity epidemic. As adiposity has increased, so has the risk of developing associated diseases, such as type 2 diabetes (T2D), cardiovascular disease (CVD), hypertension, cancer, and arthritis. Particularly alarming is the explosion of obesity in children and adolescents, which has shown a threefold increase in prevalence over the last four decades. [Note: Approximately 17% of those age 2–19 years are obese.] In the United States, the lifetime risk of becoming overweight or obese is ~50% and 25%, respectively. Obesity has increased globally, and, by some estimates, there are more obese than undernourished individuals worldwide.

II. ASSESSMENT

Because the amount of body fat is difficult to measure directly, it is usually determined from an indirect measure, the body mass index (BMI), which has been shown to correlate with the amount of body fat in most individuals. [Note: Exceptions are athletes who have large amounts of lean muscle mass.] Measuring the waist size with a tape measure is also used to screen for obesity, because this measurement reflects the amount of fat in the central abdominal area of the body. The presence of excess central fat is associated with an increased risk for morbidity and mortality, independent of the BMI. [Note: A waist size ≥40 in (men) and ≥35 in (women) is considered a risk factor.]

A. Body mass index

The BMI (defined as weight in kg/[height in m]^2) provides a measure of relative weight, adjusted for height. This allows comparisons within and between populations. The healthy range for the BMI is between 18.5 and 24.9. Individuals with a BMI between 25 and 29.9 are considered overweight, those with a BMI ≥30 are defined as obese, and a BMI >40 is considered severely (morbidly) obese (Fig. 26.1). These cutoffs are based on studies examining the relationship of BMI to premature death and are similar in men and women. Nearly two thirds of

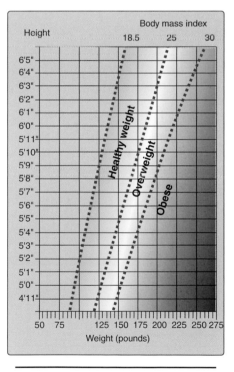

Figure 26.1
To use this body mass index (BMI) chart, find height in the left-hand column. Move across the row to weight. Height and weight intersect at the individual's BMI. [Note: To calculate BMI using pounds and inches, use BMI = weight in pounds/(height in inches)^2 × 703. Anyone >100 pounds overweight is considered morbidly obese.]

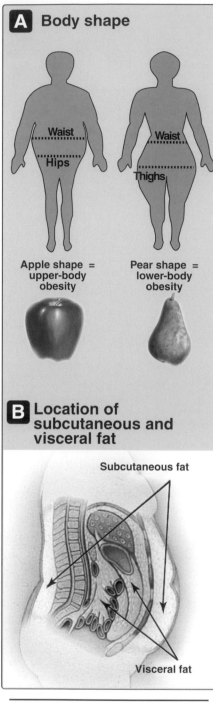

A Body shape

Waist

Hips

Waist

Thighs

Apple shape =
upper-body
obesity

Pear shape =
lower-body
obesity

B Location of
subcutaneous and
visceral fat

Subcutaneous fat

Visceral fat

Figure 26.2
A. Individuals with upper-body
obesity (left) have greater health
risks than individuals with lower-
body obesity (right). B. Visceral fat is
located inside the abdominal cavity,
packed in between the internal
organs. Subcutaneous fat is found
underneath the skin.

U.S. adults are overweight, and more than one third of those are obese. Children with a BMI-for-age above the 95th percentile are considered obese.

B. Anatomic differences in fat deposition

The anatomic distribution of body fat has a major influence on associated health risks. A waist/hip ratio (WHR) >0.8 for women and >1.0 for men is defined as android, apple-shaped, or upper-body obesity and is associated with more fat deposition in the trunk (Fig. 26.2A). In contrast, a lower WHR reflects a preponderance of fat distributed in the hips and thighs and is called gynoid, pear-shaped, or lower-body obesity. It is defined as a WHR of <0.8 for women and <1.0 for men. The pear shape, more commonly found in women, presents a much lower risk of metabolic disease, and some studies indicate that it may actually be protective. Thus, the clinician can use simple indices of body shape to identify those who may be at higher risk for metabolic diseases associated with obesity.

> About 80%–90% of human body fat is stored in subcutaneous (subq) depots in the abdominal (upper body) and the gluteal-femoral (lower body) regions. The remaining 10%–20% is in visceral depots located deep within the abdominal cavity (Fig. 26.2B). Excess fat in visceral and abdominal subq stores increases health risks associated with obesity.

C. Biochemical differences in regional fat depots

The regional types of fat described above are biochemically different. Subq adipocytes from the lower body, particularly in women, are larger, very efficient at fat (triacylglycerol [TAG]) deposition, and tend to mobilize fatty acids (FA) more slowly than subq adipocytes from the upper body. Visceral adipocytes are the most metabolically active. In obese individuals, both abdominal subcutaneous and visceral depots have high rates of lipolysis and contribute to increased availability of free fatty acids (FFA). These metabolic differences may contribute to the higher health risk found in individuals with upper body (abdominal) obesity. [Note: FFA impair insulin signaling and are proinflammatory (see p. 343).]

1. **Endocrine function:** White adipose tissue, once thought to be a passive reservoir of TAG, is now known to play an active role in body weight regulatory systems. For example, the adipocyte is an endocrine cell that secretes a number of protein regulators (adipokines), such as the hormones leptin and adiponectin. Leptin regulates appetite as well as metabolism (see p. 352). Adiponectin reduces FFA levels in the blood (by increasing FA oxidation in muscles) and has been associated with improved lipid profiles, increased insulin sensitivity resulting in better glycemic control, and reduced inflammation in patients with diabetes. [Note: Adiponectin levels decrease as body weight increases, whereas leptin levels increase.]

2. **Importance of portal circulation:** With obesity, there is increased release of FFA and secretion of proinflammatory cytokines, such as interleukin 6 (IL-6) and tumor necrosis factor-α (TNF-α), from adipose

tissue. [Note: Cytokines are small proteins that regulate the immune system.] One hypothesis for why abdominal adipose depots have such a large influence on metabolic dysfunction in obesity is that the FFA and cytokines released from these depots enter the portal vein and, therefore, have direct access to the liver. In the liver, they may lead to insulin resistance (see p. 343) and increased hepatic synthesis of TAG, which are released as components of very-low-density lipoprotein particles and contribute to the hypertriacylglycerolemia associated with obesity. By contrast, FFA from lower body subq adipose depots enter the general circulation, where they can be oxidized in muscle and, therefore, reach the liver in lower concentration.

D. Adipocyte size and number

As TAG are stored, adipocytes can expand to an average of two to three times their normal volume (Fig. 26.3). However, the ability of fat cells to expand is limited. With prolonged overnutrition, preadipocytes within adipose tissue are stimulated to proliferate and differentiate into mature fat cells, increasing the number of adipocytes. Thus, most obesity is due to a combination of increased fat cell size (hypertrophy) and number (hyperplasia). Obese individuals can have up to five times the normal number of adipocytes. [Note: Like other tissues, the adipose tissue undergoes continuous remodeling. Contrary to early dogma, we now know that adipocytes can die. The estimated average lifespan of an adipocyte is 10 years.] If excess calories cannot be accommodated within adipose tissue, the excess FA "spill over" into other tissues, such as muscle and the liver. The amount of this ectopic fat is strongly associated with insulin resistance. With weight loss in an obese individual, the size of the fat cells is reduced, but the number is not usually affected. Thus, a normal amount of body fat is achieved by decreasing the size of the fat cell below normal. However, small fat cells are very efficient at reaccumulating fat, and this may drive appetite and weight regain.

III. BODY WEIGHT REGULATION

The body weight of most individuals tends to be relatively stable over time. This observation prompted the hypothesis that each individual has a biologically predetermined "set point" for body weight. The body attempts to add to adipose stores when the body weight falls below the set point and to lose adipose from stores when the body weight rises above the set point. Thus, the body defends the set point. For example, with weight loss, appetite increases and energy expenditure falls, whereas with overfeeding, appetite falls and energy expenditure may slightly increase (Fig. 26.4). However, a strict set point model explains neither why some individuals fail to revert to their starting weight after a period of overeating nor the current epidemic of obesity.

A. Genetic contributions

It is now evident that genetic mechanisms play a major role in determining body weight.

1. **Biologic origin:** The importance of genetics as a determinant of obesity is indicated by the observation that children who are adopted usually show a body weight that correlates with their biologic rather

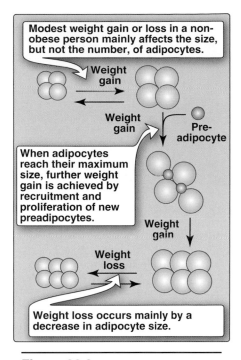

Figure 26.3
Hypertrophic (increased size) and hyperplastic (increased number) changes to adipocytes are thought to occur in severe obesity.

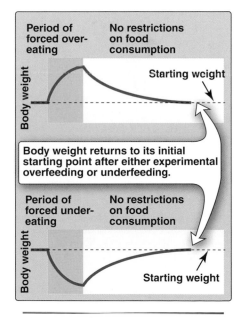

Figure 26.4
Weight changes following episodes of overfeeding or underfeeding followed by feeding with no restrictions.

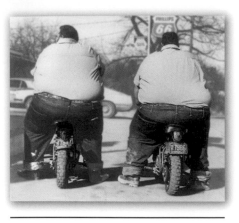

Figure 26.5
Identical twins with combined weight of 1,300 lb. Note similarity in body shape.

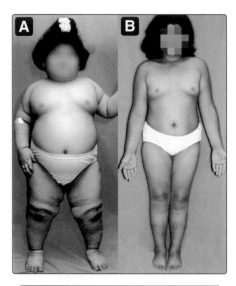

Figure 26.6
A. Patient with leptin deficiency before initiation of therapy at age 5 years. B. Patient at age 9 years after 48 months of therapy with subcutaneous injections of recombinant leptin.

than adoptive parents. Furthermore, identical twins have very similar BMI (Fig. 26.5), whether reared together or apart, and their BMI are more similar than those of nonidentical, dizygotic twins.

2. **Mutations:** Rare, single gene mutations can cause human obesity. For example, mutations in the gene for leptin (causing decreased production) or its receptor (decreased function) result in hyperphagia (increased appetite for and consumption of food) and severe obesity (Fig. 26.6), underscoring the importance of the leptin system in regulating human body weight (see IV below). [Note: Most obese humans have elevated leptin levels but are resistant to the appetite-regulating effects of this hormone.]

B. Environmental and behavioral contributions

The epidemic of obesity occurring over the last several decades cannot be simply explained by changes in genetic factors, which are stable on this short time scale. Clearly, environmental factors, such as the ready availability of palatable, energy-dense foods, play a role. Furthermore, sedentary lifestyles decrease physical activity and enhance the tendency to gain weight. Eating behaviors, such as portion size, variety of foods consumed, an individual's food preferences, and the number of people present during eating, also influence food consumption. However, it is important to note that many individuals in this same environment do not become obese. The susceptibility to obesity appears to be explained, at least in part, by an interaction of an individual's genes and his or her environment and can be influenced by additional factors such as maternal under- or overnutrition that may "set" the body regulatory systems to defend a higher or lower level of body fat. Thus, epigenetic changes (see p. 476) likely influence the risk for obesity.

IV. MOLECULAR INFLUENCES

The cause of obesity can be summarized in a deceptively simple application of the first law of thermodynamics: Obesity results when energy (caloric) intake exceeds energy expenditure. However, the mechanism underlying this imbalance involves a complex interaction of biochemical, neurologic, environmental, and psychologic factors. The basic neural and humoral pathways that regulate appetite, energy expenditure, and body weight involve systems that regulate short-term food intake (meal to meal), and signals for the long-term (day to day, week to week, year to year) regulation of body weight (Fig. 26.7).

A. Long-term signals

Long-term signals reflect the status of fat (TAG) stores.

1. **Leptin:** Leptin is an adipocyte peptide hormone that is made and secreted in proportion to the size of fat stores. It acts on the brain to regulate food intake and energy expenditure. When we consume more calories than we need, body fat increases, and leptin production by adipocytes increases. The body adapts by increasing energy use (increasing activity) and decreasing appetite (an anorexigenic effect). When body fat decreases, the opposite effects occur. Unfortunately, most obese individuals are leptin resistant, and the leptin system may be better at preventing weight loss than prevent-

ing weight gain. [Note: Leptin's effects are mediated through binding to receptors in the arcuate nucleus of the hypothalamus.]

2. **Insulin:** Obese individuals are also hyperinsulinemic. Like leptin, insulin acts on hypothalamic neurons to dampen appetite. (See Chapter 23 for the effects of insulin on metabolism.) [Note: Obesity is associated with insulin resistance (see p. 342).]

B. Short-term signals

Short-term signals from the gastrointestinal (GI) tract control hunger and satiety, which affect the size and number of meals over a time course of minutes to hours. In the absence of food intake (between meals), the stomach produces ghrelin, an orexigenic (appetite-stimulating) hormone that drives hunger. As food is consumed, GI hormones, including cholecystokinin and peptide YY, among others, induce satiety (an anorexigenic effect), thereby terminating eating, through actions on gastric emptying and neural signals to the hypothalamus. Within the hypothalamus, neuropeptides (such as orexigenic neuropeptide Y [NPY] and anorexigenic α-melanocyte–stimulating hormone [α-MSH]) and neurotransmitters (such as anorexigenic serotonin and dopamine) are important in regulating hunger and satiety. Long-term and short-term signals interact, insofar as leptin increases secretion of α-MSH and decreases secretion of NPY. Thus, there are many complex regulatory loops that control the size and number of meals in relationship to the status of body fat stores. [Note: α-MSH, a cleavage product of proopiomelanocortin, binds to the melanocortin-4 receptor (MC4R). Loss-of-function mutations to MC4R are associated with early-onset obesity.]

V. METABOLIC EFFECTS

The primary metabolic effects of obesity include dyslipidemias, glucose intolerance, and insulin resistance expressed primarily in the liver, skeletal muscle, and adipose tissue. These metabolic abnormalities reflect molecular signals originating from the increased mass of adipocytes (see Fig. 25.9, p. 343, and Fig. 26.7). [Note: About 30% of obese individuals do not show these metabolic abnormalities.]

A. Metabolic syndrome

Abdominal obesity is associated with a cluster of metabolic abnormalities (hyperglycemia, insulin resistance, hyperinsulinemia, dyslipidemia [low levels of high-density lipoprotein (HDL) and elevated TAG], and hypertension) that is referred to as the metabolic syndrome (Fig. 26.8). It is a risk factor for CVD and T2D. The low-grade, chronic, systemic inflammation seen with obesity contributes to the pathogenesis of insulin resistance and T2D and likely plays a role in metabolic syndrome. In obesity, adipocytes release proinflammatory mediators such as IL-6 and TNF-α. Additionally, levels of adiponectin, which normally dampens inflammation and sensitizes tissues to insulin, are low.

B. Nonalcoholic liver disease

Obesity is associated with ectopic deposition of TAG in the liver (hepatic steatosis) and results in increased risk for nonalcoholic fatty liver disease ([NAFLD], see p. 343).

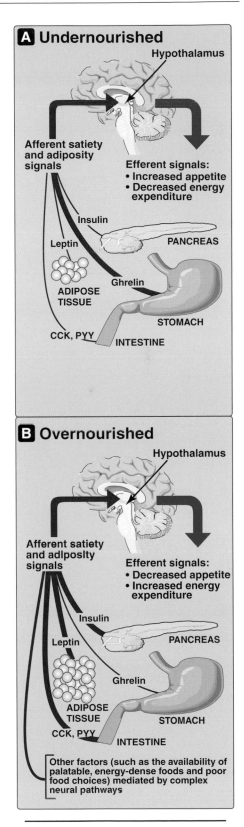

Figure 26.7
Some signals that influence appetite and satiety in undernourished (A) and overnourished (B) states. CCK = cholecystokinin; PYY = peptide YY.

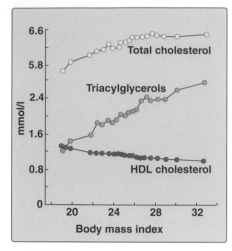

Figure 26.8
Body mass index and changes in blood lipids. HDL = high-density lipoprotein.

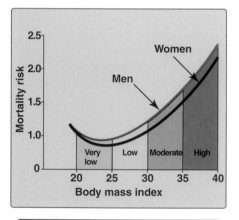

Figure 26.9
Body mass index and the relative risk of death.

VI. OBESITY AND HEALTH

Obesity is correlated with an increased risk of death (Fig. 26.9) and is a risk factor for a number of chronic conditions, including T2D, dyslipidemias, hypertension, CVD, some cancers, gallstones, arthritis, gout, pelvic floor disorders (for example, urinary incontinence), NAFLD, and sleep apnea. The relationship between obesity and associated morbidities is stronger among individuals age <55 years. After age 74 years, there is no longer an association between increased BMI and mortality. [Note: Obesity also has social consequences (for example, stigmatization and discrimination).] Weight loss in obese individuals leads to decreased blood pressure, plasma TAG, and blood glucose levels. HDL increase.

VII. WEIGHT REDUCTION

Weight reduction can help reduce the complications of obesity. To achieve weight reduction, the obese patient must decrease energy intake or increase energy expenditure, although decreasing energy intake is thought to contribute more to inducing weight loss. Typically, a plan for weight reduction combines dietary change; increased physical activity; and behavioral modification, which can include nutrition education and meal planning, recording food intake through food diaries, modifying factors that lead to overeating, and relearning cues to satiety. Medications or surgery may be recommended. Once weight loss is achieved, weight maintenance is a separate process that requires vigilance because the majority of patients regain weight after they stop their weight-loss efforts.

A. Caloric restriction

Dieting is the most commonly practiced approach to weight control. Because 1 lb of adipose tissue corresponds to ~3,500 kcal, the effect that caloric restriction will have on the amount of adipose tissue can be estimated. Weight loss on calorie-restricted diets is determined primarily by caloric intake and not nutrient composition. [Note: However, compositional aspects can affect glycemic control and the blood lipid profile.] Caloric restriction is ineffective over the long term for many individuals. Over 90% of people who attempt to lose weight regain the lost weight when dietary intervention is suspended. Nonetheless, although few individuals will reach their ideal weight with treatment, weight losses of 10% of body weight over a 6-month period often reduce blood pressure and lipid levels and enhance control of T2D.

B. Physical activity

An increase in physical activity can create an energy deficit. Although adding exercise to a hypocaloric regimen may not produce a greater weight loss initially, exercise is a key component of programs directed at maintaining weight loss. In addition, physical activity increases cardiopulmonary fitness and reduces the risk of CVD, independent of weight loss. Persons who combine caloric restriction and exercise with behavioral treatment may expect to lose ~5%–10% of initial body weight over a period of 4–6 months. Studies show that individuals who maintain their exercise program regain less weight after their initial weight loss.

C. Pharmacologic treatment

The U.S. Food and Drug Administration has approved several weight-loss medications for use in adults. They include orlistat (decreases absorption of dietary fat), lorcaserin and phentermine in combination with topiramate (promote satiety through serotonin signaling), lira-glutide (decreases appetite by activating the glucagon-like peptide 1 receptor), and buproprion in combination with naltrexone (increase metabolism by increasing norepinephrine). Their effects on weight reduction tend to be modest. [Note: Pharmacologic activation of brown adipocytes (see p. 79) is being explored.]

D. Surgical treatment

Gastric bypass and restriction surgeries are effective in causing weight loss in severely obese individuals. Through mechanisms that remain poorly understood, these operations greatly improve glycemic control in morbidly obese diabetic individuals. [Note: Implantation of a device that electrically stimulates the vagus nerve to decrease food intake has been approved.]

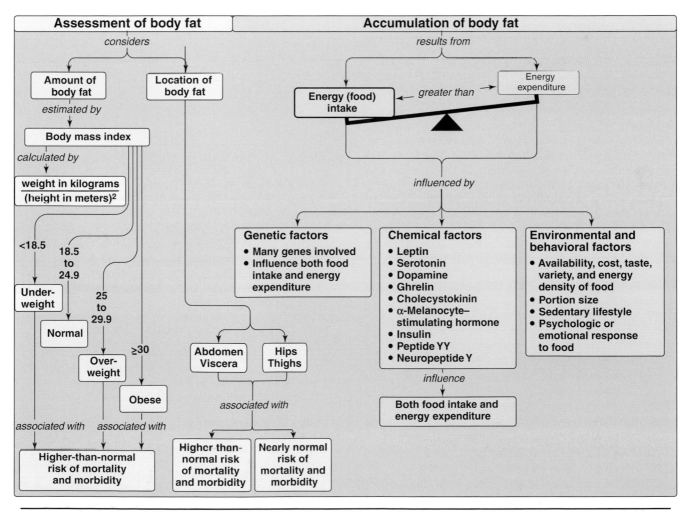

Figure 26.10
Key concept map for obesity. [Note: Body mass index may also be calculated by weight in pounds/(height in inches)^2 × 703.]

VIII. CHAPTER SUMMARY

Obesity, the accumulation of excess body fat, results when **energy (caloric) intake** exceeds **energy expenditure** (Fig. 26.10). Obesity is increasing in industrialized countries because of a reduction in daily energy expenditure and an increase in energy intake resulting from the increasing availability of palatable, inexpensive foods. The **body mass index (BMI)** is easy to determine and highly correlated to body fat. Nearly 69% of U.S. adults are **overweight** (BMI ≥25), and >33% of this group are **obese** (BMI ≥30). The anatomic distribution of body fat has a major influence on associated health risks. Excess fat located in the **abdomen** (upper body, apple shape), as reflected in **waist size**, is associated with greater risk for **hypertension**, **insulin resistance**, **diabetes**, **dyslipidemia**, and **coronary heart disease** as compared to fat located in the hips and thighs (lower body, pear shape). A person's weight is determined by genetic and environmental factors. **Appetite** is influenced by afferent, or incoming, signals (that is, neural signals, circulating hormones such as **leptin**, and metabolites) that are integrated by the **hypothalamus**. These diverse signals prompt release of hypothalamic peptides (such as **neuropeptide Y** and **α-melanocyte–stimulating hormone**) and activate outgoing, efferent neural signals. Obesity is correlated with an increased risk of **death** and is also a risk factor for a number of **chronic conditions**. **Weight reduction** is achieved best with **negative energy balance**, that is, by decreasing caloric intake and increasing physical activity. Virtually all diets that limit particular groups of foods or macronutrients lead to short-term weight loss. Long-term maintenance of weight loss is difficult to achieve. Modest reduction in food intake occurs with **pharmacologic treatment**. **Surgical procedures**, such as gastric bypass, designed to limit food intake are an option for the severely obese patient who has not responded to other treatments.

Study Questions

Choose the ONE best answer.

For Questions 26.1 and 26.2, use the following scenario.

A 40-year-old woman, 5 ft, 1 in (155 cm) tall and weighing 188 lb (85.5 kg), seeks your advice on how to lose weight. Her waist measured 41 in and her hips 39 in. The remainder of the physical examination and the blood laboratory data were all within the normal range. Her only child (who is age 14 years), her sister, and both of her parents are overweight. The patient recalls being overweight throughout her childhood and adolescence. Over the past 15 years, she had been on seven different diets for periods of 2 weeks to 3 months, losing from 5 to 25 lb each time. On discontinuation of the diets, she regained weight, returning to 185–190 lb.

26.1 Calculate and interpret the body mass index for the patient.

26.2 Which one of the following statements best describes the patient?

A. She has approximately the same number of adipocytes as an individual of normal weight, but each adipocyte is larger.
B. She shows an apple pattern of fat distribution.
C. She would be expected to show higher-than-normal levels of adiponectin.
D. She would be expected to show lower-than-normal levels of circulating leptin.
E. She would be expected to show lower-than-normal levels of circulating triacylglycerols.

Body mass index (BMI) = weight in kg/(height in m)^2 = $85.5/1.55^2$ = 35.6. Because her BMI is >30, the patient is classified as obese.

Correct answer = B. Her waist/hip ratio (WHR) is 1.05 (41/39). Apple shape is defined as a WHR of >0.8 for women and >1.0 for men. Therefore, she has an apple pattern of fat distribution, more commonly seen in males. Compared with other women of the same body weight who have a gynoid (pear-shaped) fat pattern, her android fat pattern places her at greater risk for diabetes, hypertension, dyslipidemia, and coronary heart disease. Individuals with marked obesity and a history dating to early childhood have a fat depot made up of too many adipocytes, each fully loaded with triacylglycerol (TAG). Plasma leptin levels are proportional to fat mass, suggesting that resistance to leptin, rather than its deficiency, occurs in human obesity. Adiponectin levels decrease with increasing fat mass. The elevated circulating free fatty acids characteristic of obesity are carried to the liver and converted to TAG. The TAG are released as components of very-low-density lipoproteins, resulting in elevated plasma TAG levels, or are stored in the liver, resulting in hepatic steatosis.

Nutrition: Overview and Macronutrients

27

I. OVERVIEW

Nutrients are the constituents of food necessary to sustain the normal functions of the body. All energy (calories) is provided by three classes of nutrients: fats, carbohydrates, and protein (Fig. 27.1). Because the intake of these energy-rich molecules is larger (g amounts) than that of the other dietary nutrients, they are called macronutrients. This chapter focuses on the kinds and amounts of macronutrients that are needed to maintain optimal health and prevent chronic disease. Those nutrients needed in lesser amounts (mg or μg), vitamins and minerals, are called micronutrients and are considered in Chapters 28 and 29.

II. DIETARY REFERENCE INTAKES

Committees of U.S. and Canadian experts organized by the Food and Nutrition Board of the Institute of Medicine of the National Academy of Sciences have compiled Dietary Reference Intakes (DRI), which are estimates of the amounts of nutrients required to prevent deficiencies and maintain optimal health and growth. The DRI expands on the Recommended Dietary Allowances (RDA), which have been published with periodic revisions since 1941. Unlike the RDA, the DRI establishes upper limits on the consumption of some nutrients and incorporates the role of nutrients in lifelong health, going beyond deficiency diseases. Both the DRI and the RDA refer to long-term average daily nutrient intakes, because it is not necessary to consume the full RDA every day.

A. Definition

The DRI consists of four dietary reference standards for the intake of nutrients designated for specific life stage (age) groups, physiologic states, and gender (Fig. 27.2).

1. **Estimated average requirement:** The average daily nutrient intake level estimated to meet the requirement of one half of the healthy individuals in a particular life stage and gender group is the

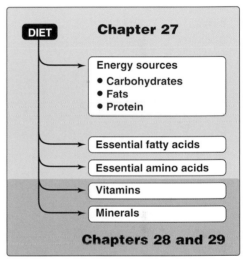

Figure 27.1
Essential nutrients obtained from the diet. [Note: Ethanol may provide a significant contribution to the daily caloric intake of some individuals.]

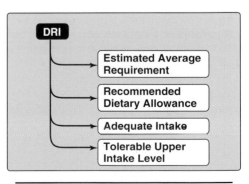

Figure 27.2
Components of the Dietary Reference Intakes (DRI).

357

MICRO-NUTRIENT	EAR, RDA, or AI	UL
Thiamine	EAR, RDA	—
Riboflavin	EAR, RDA	—
Niacin	EAR, RDA	UL
Vitamin B_6	EAR, RDA	UL
Folate	EAR, RDA	UL
Vitamin B_{12}	EAR, RDA	—
Pantothenic acid	AI	—
Biotin	AI	—
Choline	AI	UL
Vitamin C	EAR, RDA	UL
Vitamin A	EAR, RDA	UL
Vitamin D	EAR, RDA	UL
Vitamin E	EAR, RDA	UL
Vitamin K	AI	—
Boron	—	UL
Calcium	EAR, RDA	UL
Chromium	AI	—
Copper	EAR, RDA	UL
Fluoride	AI	UL
Iodine	EAR, RDA	UL
Iron	EAR, RDA	UL
Magnesium	EAR, RDA	UL
Manganese	AI	UL
Molybdenum	EAR, RDA	UL
Nickel	—	UL
Phosphorus	EAR, RDA	UL
Selenium	EAR, RDA	UL
Vanadium	—	UL
Zinc	EAR, RDA	UL

Figure 27.3
Dietary Reference Intakes for vitamins and minerals in individuals age 1 year and older. [Note: An RDA has been set for carbohydrate and protein (macronutrients) but not for fat.] EAR = Estimated Average Requirement; RDA = Recommended Dietary Allowance; AI = Adequate Intake; UL = Tolerable Upper Intake Level; — = no value established.

Estimated Average Requirement (EAR). It is useful in estimating the actual requirements in groups and individuals.

2. **Recommended dietary allowance:** The RDA is the average daily nutrient intake level that is sufficient to meet the requirements of nearly all (97%–98%) individuals in a particular life stage and gender group. The RDA is not the minimal requirement for healthy individuals, but it is intentionally set to provide a margin of safety for most individuals. The EAR serves as the foundation for setting the RDA. If the standard deviation (SD) of the EAR is available and the requirement for the nutrient is normally distributed, the RDA is set at 2 SD above the EAR (that is, RDA = EAR + 2 SD$_{EAR}$).

3. **Adequate intake:** An Adequate Intake (AI) is set instead of an RDA if sufficient scientific evidence is not available to calculate an EAR or RDA. The AI is based on estimates of nutrient intake by a group (or groups) of apparently healthy people. For example, the AI for young infants, for whom human milk is the recommended sole source of food for the first 6 months, is based on the estimated daily mean nutrient intake supplied by human milk for healthy, full-term infants who are exclusively breast-fed.

4. **Tolerable upper intake level:** The highest average daily nutrient intake level that is likely to pose no risk of adverse health effects to almost all individuals in the general population is the Tolerable Upper Intake Level (UL, or TUL). As intake increases above the UL, the potential risk of adverse effects may increase. The UL is useful because of the increased availability of fortified foods and the increased use of dietary supplements. For some nutrients, there may be insufficient data on which to develop a UL.

B. Using the dietary reference intakes

Most nutrients have a set of DRI (Fig. 27.3). Usually a nutrient has an EAR and a corresponding RDA. Most are set by age and gender and may be influenced by special factors, such as pregnancy and lactation in women (see p. 372). When the data are not sufficient to estimate an EAR (or an RDA), an AI is designated. Intakes below the EAR need to be improved because the probability of adequacy is ≤50% (Fig. 27.4). Intakes between the EAR and RDA likely need to be improved because the probability of adequacy is <98%, and intakes at or above the RDA can be considered adequate. Intakes above the AI can be considered adequate. Intakes between the UL and the RDA can be considered to have no risk for adverse effects. [Note: Because the DRI is designed to meet the nutritional needs of the healthy, it does not include any special needs of the sick.]

III. ENERGY REQUIREMENT IN HUMANS

The Estimated Energy Requirement (EER) is the average dietary energy intake predicted to maintain an energy balance (that is, the calories consumed are equal to the energy expended) in a healthy adult of a defined age, gender, and height whose weight and level of physical activity are consistent with good health. Differences in the genetics, body composition, metabolism, and behavior of individuals make it difficult to accurately

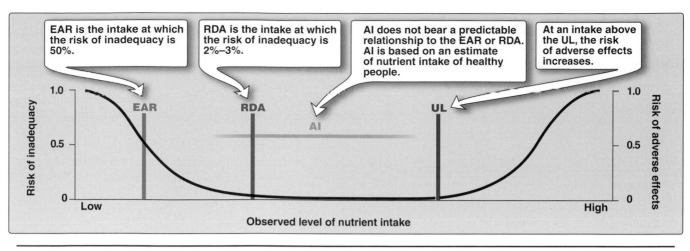

Figure 27.4
Comparison of the components of the Dietary Reference Intakes. EAR = estimated average requirement; RDA = recommended dietary allowance; AI = adequate intake; UL = tolerable upper intake level.

predict a person's caloric requirements. However, some simple approximations can provide useful estimates. For example, sedentary adults require ~30 kcal/kg/day to maintain body weight, moderately active adults require 35 kcal/kg/day, and very active adults require 40 kcal/kg/day.

A. Energy content of food

The energy content of food is calculated from the heat released by the total combustion of food in a calorimeter. It is expressed in kilocalories (kcal, or Cal). The standard conversion factors for determining the metabolic caloric value of fat, protein, and carbohydrate are shown in Figure 27.5. Note that the energy content of fat is more than twice that of carbohydrate or protein, whereas the energy content of ethanol is intermediate between those of fat and carbohydrate. [Note: The joule (J) is a unit of energy widely used in countries other than the United States. One cal = 4.2 J; 1 kcal (1 Cal, 1 food calorie) = 4.2 kJ. For uniformity, many scientists are promoting the use of joules rather than calories in the United States. However, kcal still predominates and is used throughout this text.]

B. Use of food energy in the body

The energy generated by metabolism of the macronutrients is used for three energy-requiring processes that occur in the body: resting metabolic rate (RMR), physical activity, and the thermic effect of food. The number of kcal expended by these processes in a 24-hour period is the total energy expenditure (TEE).

1. **Resting metabolic rate:** RMR is the energy expended by an individual in a resting, postabsorptive state. It represents the energy required to carry out the normal body functions, such as respiration, blood flow, and ion transport. RMR can be determined by measuring oxygen (O_2) consumed or carbon dioxide (CO_2) produced (indirect calorimetry). [Note: The ratio of CO_2 to O_2 is the respiratory quotient (RQ). It reflects the substrate being oxidized for energy (Fig. 27.6).] RMR also can be estimated using equations that include sex and age (RMR reflects lean muscle mass, which

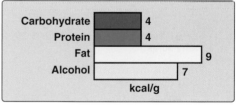

Figure 27.5
Average energy available from the macronutrients and alcohol.

SUBSTRATE	RQ
Carbohydrate	1.00
Protein	0.84
Fat	0.71

Figure 27.6
The respiratory quotient (RQ). [Note: For protein, the nitrogen is removed and excreted, and the α-keto acids are oxidized.]

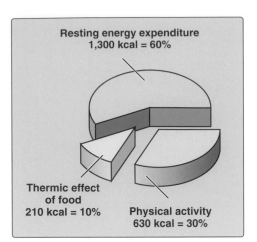

Figure 27.7
Estimated total energy expenditure in a healthy 20-year-old woman, 5 ft, 4 in (165 cm) tall, weighing 110 lb (50 kg), and engaged in light activity.

MACRONUTRIENT	AMDR (percent of energy)
Fat	20–35
ω–6 Polyunsaturated fatty acids	5–10
ω–3 Polyunsaturated fatty acids	0.6–1.2*
Approximately 10% of the total fat can come from longer-chain, ω–3 or ω–6 fatty acids.	
Carbohydrate	45–65
• RDA Men and women: 130 g/day	
No more than 10% of total calories should come from added sugars.	
Fiber	
• AI Men: 38 g/day; women: 25 g/day	
Protein	10–35
• RDA Men: 56 g/day; women: 46 g/day	

Figure 27.8
Acceptable Macronutrient Distribution Ranges (AMDR) in adults. [Note: *A growing body of evidence suggests that higher levels of ω-3 polyunsaturated fatty acids provide protection against coronary heart disease.] RDA = recommended dietary allowance; AI = adequate intake.

is highest in men and the young) as well as height and weight. A commonly used rough estimate is 1 kcal/kg/hour for men and 0.9 kcal/kg/hour for women. [Note: A basal metabolic rate (BMR) can be determined if more stringent environmental conditions are used, but it is not routinely done. RMR is ~10% higher than the BMR.] In an adult, the 24-hour RMR, known as the resting energy expenditure (REE), is ~1,800 kcal for men (70 kg) and 1,300 kcal for women (50 kg). From 60%–75% of the TEE in sedentary individuals is attributable to the REE (Fig. 27.7). [Note: Hospitalized individuals are commonly hypercatabolic, and the RMR is multiplied by an injury factor that ranges from 1.0 (mild infection) to 2.0 (severe burns) in calculating their TEE.]

2. **Physical activity:** Muscular activity provides the greatest variation in the TEE. The amount of energy consumed depends on the duration and intensity of the exercise. This energy cost is expressed as a multiple of the RMR (range is 1.1 to >8.0) that is referred to as the physical activity ratio (PAR) or the metabolic equivalent of the task (MET). In general, a lightly active person requires ~30%–50% more calories than the RMR (see Fig. 27.7), whereas a highly active individual may require ≥100% calories above the RMR.

3. **Thermic effect of food:** The production of heat by the body increases as much as 30% above the resting level during the digestion and absorption of food. This is called the thermic effect of food, or diet-induced thermogenesis. The thermic response to food intake may amount to 5%–10% of the TEE.

IV. ACCEPTABLE MACRONUTRIENT DISTRIBUTION RANGES

Acceptable Macronutrient Distribution Ranges (AMDR) are defined as a range of intakes for a particular macronutrient that is associated with reduced risk of chronic disease while providing adequate amounts of essential nutrients. The AMDR for adults is 45%–65% of their total calories from carbohydrates, 20%–35% from fat, and 10%–35% from protein (Fig. 27.8). The biologic properties of dietary fat, carbohydrate, and protein are described below.

V. DIETARY FATS

The incidence of a number of chronic diseases is significantly influenced by the kinds and amounts of nutrients consumed (Fig. 27.9). Dietary fats most strongly influence the incidence of coronary heart disease (CHD), but evidence linking dietary fat and the risk for cancer or obesity is much weaker.

> Earlier recommendations emphasized decreasing the total amount of dietary fat. Unfortunately, this resulted in increased consumption of refined grains and added sugars. Data now show that the type of fat is a more important risk factor than the total amount of fat.

A. Plasma lipids and coronary heart disease

Plasma cholesterol may arise from the diet or from endogenous biosynthesis. In either case, cholesterol is transported between the tissues in combination with protein and phospholipids as lipoproteins.

1. **Low-density and high-density lipoproteins:** The level of plasma cholesterol is not precisely regulated but, rather, varies in response to diet. Elevated levels of total cholesterol (hypercholesterolemia) result in an increased risk for CHD (Fig. 27.10). A much stronger correlation exists between CHD and the level of cholesterol in low-density lipoproteins ([LDL-C] see p. 234). As LDL-C increases, CHD increases. In contrast, elevated levels of high-density lipoprotein cholesterol (HDL-C) have been associated with a decreased risk for heart disease (see p. 235). [Note: Elevated plasma triacylglycerol (TAG) is associated with CHD, but a causative relationship has yet to be demonstrated.] Abnormal levels of plasma lipids (dyslipidemias) act in combination with smoking, obesity, sedentary lifestyle, insulin resistance, and other risk factors to increase the risk of CHD.

2. **Benefits of lowering plasma cholesterol:** Dietary or drug treatment of hypercholesterolemia has been shown to be effective in decreasing LDL-C, increasing HDL-C, and reducing the risk for cardiovascular events. The diet-induced changes in plasma cholesterol concentrations are modest, typically 10%–20%, whereas treatment with statin drugs decreases plasma cholesterol by 30%–60% (see p. 224). [Note: Dietary and drug treatment can also lower TAG.]

B. Dietary fats and plasma lipids

TAG are quantitatively the most important class of dietary fats. The influence of TAG on blood lipids is determined by the chemical nature of their constituent fatty acids. The absence or presence and number of double bonds (saturated versus mono- and polyunsaturated), the location of the double bonds (ω-6 versus ω-3), and the cis versus trans configuration of the unsaturated fatty acids are the most important structural features that influence blood lipids.

1. **Saturated fats:** TAG composed primarily of fatty acids whose hydrocarbon chains do not contain any double bonds are referred to as saturated fats. Consumption of saturated fats is positively associated with high levels of total plasma cholesterol and LDL-C and an increased risk of CHD. The main sources of saturated fatty acids are dairy and meat products and some vegetable oils, such as coconut and palm oils (a major source of fat in Latin America and Asia, although not in the United States). Many experts strongly advise limiting intake of saturated fats to <10% of total caloric intake and replacing them with unsaturated fats (and whole grains).

> Saturated fatty acids with carbon chain lengths of 14 (myristic) and 16 (palmitic) are most potent in increasing the plasma cholesterol level. Stearic acid (18 carbons, found in many foods including chocolate) has little effect on blood cholesterol.

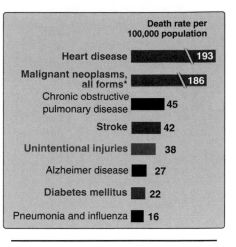

Figure 27.9
Influence of nutrition on some common causes of death in the United States in the year 2010. Red indicates causes of death in which the diet plays a significant role. Blue indicates causes of death in which excessive alcohol consumption plays a part. [Note: *Diet plays a role in only some forms of cancer.]

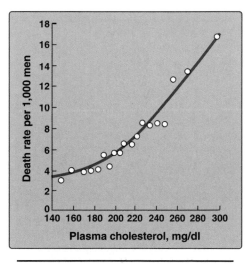

Figure 27.10
Correlation of the death rate from coronary heart disease with the concentration of plasma cholesterol. [Note: The data were obtained from a multiyear study of men with the death rate adjusted for age.]

2. Monounsaturated fats: TAG containing primarily fatty acids with one double bond are referred to as monounsaturated fats. Monounsaturated fatty acids (MUFA) are generally obtained from plant-based oils. When substituted for saturated fatty acids in the diet, MUFA lower both total plasma cholesterol and LDL-C and maintain or increase HDL-C. This ability of MUFA to favorably modify lipoprotein levels may explain, in part, the observation that Mediterranean cultures, with diets rich in olive oil (high in monounsaturated oleic acid), show a low incidence of CHD. [Note: Although there is no AMDR for MUFA, a common recommendation is 10%–20% of caloric intake.]

a. The Mediterranean diet: The Mediterranean diet is an example of a diet rich in MUFA (from olive oil) and polyunsaturated fatty acids or PUFA (from fish oils, plant oils, and some nuts) but low in saturated fat. For example, Figure 27.11 shows the composition of the Mediterranean diet in comparison with both a Western diet similar to that consumed in the United States and a typical low-fat diet. The Mediterranean diet contains seasonally fresh food, with an abundance of plant material, low amounts of red meat, and olive oil as the principal source of fat. The Mediterranean diet is associated with decreased plasma total cholesterol and LDL-C, decreased TAG, and increased HDL-C when compared with a typical Western diet higher in saturated fats.

3. Polyunsaturated fats: TAG containing primarily fatty acids with more than one double bond are referred to as polyunsaturated fats. The effects of PUFA on cardiovascular disease are influenced by the location of the double bonds within the molecule.

a. ω-6 Fatty acids: These are long-chain PUFA, with the first double bond beginning at the sixth bond position when starting from the methyl (ω) end of the fatty acid molecule. [Note: They are also called n-6 fatty acids (see p. 182).] Consumption of fats containing ω-6 PUFA, principally linoleic acid (18:2 [9,12]), obtained from vegetable oils, lowers plasma cholesterol when substituted for saturated fats. Plasma LDL-C is lowered, but HDL-C, which protects against CHD, is also lowered, partially offsetting the benefits of lowering LDL-C. Nuts, avocados, olives, soybeans, and various oils, including sunflower and corn oil, are common sources of these fatty acids. The AMDR for linoleic acid is 5%–10%. [Note: The lower recommendation for intake of PUFA relative to MUFA is because of concern that free radical–mediated oxidation (peroxidation) of PUFA may lead to deleterious products.]

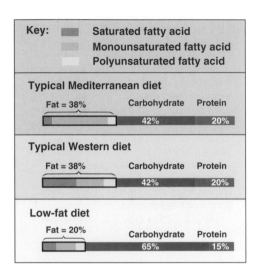

Figure 27.11
Composition of typical Mediterranean, Western, and low-fat diets.

Linoleic acid
(18:2, ω-6)

α-Linolenic acid
(18:3, ω-3)

b. ω-3 Fatty acids: These are long-chain PUFA, with the first double bond beginning at the third bond position from the methyl (ω) end. Dietary ω-3 PUFA suppress cardiac arrhythmias, reduce plasma TAG, decrease the tendency for thrombosis, lower blood pressure, and substantially reduce risk of cardiovascular mortality (Fig. 27.12), but they have little effect on LDL-C or HDL-C levels. Evidence suggests that they have anti-inflammatory effects. The ω-3 PUFA, principally α-linolenic acid, 18:3(9,12,15), are found in plant oils, such as flaxseed and canola, and some nuts, such as walnuts. The AMDR for α-linolenic acid is 0.6%–1.2%. Fish oil contains the long-chain ω-3 docosahexaenoic acid (DHA, 22:6) and eicosapentaenoic acid (EPA, 20:5). Two fatty fish (for example, salmon) meals per week are recommended. For patients with documented CHD, 1 g/day of fish oils is recommended, while 2–4 g/day is prescribed to lower TAG. [Note: DHA is included in infant formulas to promote brain development.] Linoleic and α-linolenic acids are essential fatty acids (EFA) required for membrane fluidity and synthesis of eicosanoids (see p. 213). EFA deficiency, caused primarily by fat malabsorption, is characterized by scaly dermatitis as a result of the depletion of skin ceramides with long-chain fatty acids (see p. 206).

4. Trans fatty acids: Trans fatty acids (Fig. 27.13) are chemically classified as unsaturated fatty acids but behave more like saturated fatty acids in the body because they elevate LDL-C and lower HDL-C, thereby increasing the risk of CHD. Trans fatty acids do not occur naturally in plants but occur in small amounts in animals. However, trans fatty acids are formed during the hydrogenation of vegetable oils (for example, in the manufacture of margarine and partially hydrogenated vegetable oil). Trans fatty acids are a major component of many commercial baked goods, such as cookies, and most deep-fried foods. Many manufacturers have reformulated their products to be free of trans fats. In 2006, the U.S. Food and Drug Administration required that Nutrition Facts labels (see p. 370) portray the trans fat content of packaged food. By 2018, virtually no industrial trans fatty acids will be permitted in food.

5. Dietary cholesterol: Cholesterol is found only in animal products. The effect of dietary cholesterol on plasma cholesterol (Fig. 27.14) is less important than the amount and types of fatty acids consumed. Many experts recommend ≤300 mg/day. However, having an upper limit has become controversial.

C. Other dietary factors affecting coronary heart disease

Moderate consumption of alcohol (up to 1 drink/day for women and up to 2 drinks/day for men) decreases the risk of CHD, because there is a positive correlation between moderate alcohol (ethanol) consumption and the plasma concentration of HDL-C. However, because of the potential dangers of alcohol abuse, health professionals are reluctant to recommend increased alcohol consumption to their patients. Red wine may provide cardioprotective benefits in addition to those resulting from its alcohol content (for example, red wine contains phenolic compounds that inhibit lipoprotein oxidation; see p. 235). [Note: These antioxidants are also present in raisins and grape juice.] Figure 27.15

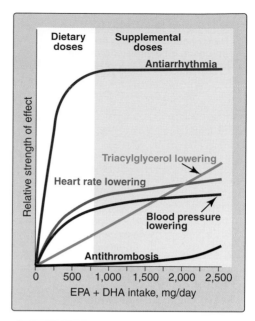

Figure 27.12
Dose responses of physiologic effects of fish oil (ω-3) intake. EPA = eicosapentaenoic acid (20:5); DHA = docosahexaenoic acid (22:6).

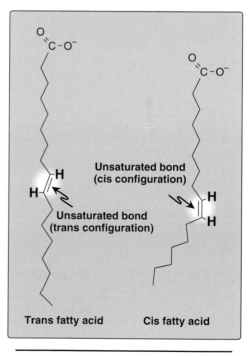

Figure 27.13
Structure of cis and trans fatty acids.

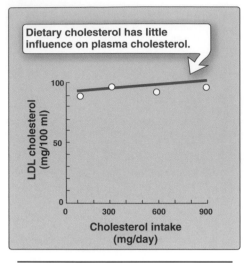

Figure 27.14
Response of plasma low-density lipoprotein (LDL) cholesterol concentrations to an increase in dietary cholesterol intake.

summarizes the effects of dietary fats. [Note: Recent studies (including meta-analyses) have raised questions concerning the current guidelines for dietary fat in the prevention of CHD.]

VI. DIETARY CARBOHYDRATES

The primary role of dietary carbohydrates is to provide energy. Although self-reported caloric intake in the United States peaked in 2003 and is now declining, the incidence of obesity has dramatically increased (see p. 349). During this same period, carbohydrate consumption has significantly increased (as fat consumption decreased), leading some observers to link obesity with carbohydrate consumption. However, obesity has also been related to increasingly inactive lifestyles and to calorie-dense foods served in expanded portion size. Carbohydrates are not inherently fattening.

A. Classification

Dietary carbohydrates are classified as simple sugars (monosaccharides and disaccharides), complex sugars (polysaccharides), and fiber.

1. **Monosaccharides:** Glucose and fructose are the principal monosaccharides found in food. Glucose is abundant in fruits, sweet corn, corn syrup, and honey. Free fructose is found together with free glucose in honey and fruits (for example, apples).

   a. **High-fructose corn syrup:** High-fructose corn syrups (HFCS) are corn syrups that have undergone enzymatic processing to convert their glucose into fructose and have then been mixed with pure corn syrup (100% glucose) to produce a desired sweetness. In the United States, HFCS 55 (containing 55%

TYPE OF FAT	METABOLIC EFFECTS		EFFECTS ON DISEASE PREVENTION
Trans fatty acid	⬆ LDL ⬇ HDL		⬆ Incidence of coronary heart disease
Saturated fatty acid	⬆ LDL Little effect on HDL		⬆ Incidence of coronary heart disease; may increase risk of prostate, colon cancer
Monounsaturated fatty acid	⬇ LDL Maintain or increase HDL		⬇ Incidence of coronary heart disease
Polyunsaturated ω–6 fatty acids such as linoleic acid	⬇ LDL ⬇ HDL **Provide arachidonic acid, which is an important precursor of prostaglandins and leukotrienes**		⬇ Incidence of coronary heart disease
Polyunsaturated ω–3 fatty acids such as DHA	Little effect on LDL Little effect on HDL **Suppress cardiac arrhythmias, reduce serum triacylglycerols, decrease the tendency for thrombosis, lower blood pressure, reduce inflammation**		⬇ Incidence of coronary heart disease ⬇ Risk of sudden cardiac death

Figure 27.15
Effects of dietary fats. LDL = low-density lipoprotein; HDL = high-density lipoprotein; DHA = docosahexaenoic acid.

fructose and 42% glucose) is commonly used as a substitute for sucrose in beverages, including soft drinks, with HFCS 42 used in processed foods. The composition and metabolism of HFCS and sucrose are similar, the major difference being that HFCS is ingested as a mixture of monosaccharides (Fig. 27.16). Most studies have shown no significant difference between sucrose and HFCS meals in either postprandial glucose or insulin responses. [Note: The rise in the use of HFCS parallels the rise in obesity, but a causal relationship has not been demonstrated.]

2. **Disaccharides:** The most abundant disaccharides are sucrose (glucose + fructose), lactose (glucose + galactose), and maltose (glucose + glucose). Sucrose is ordinary table sugar and is abundant in molasses and maple syrup. Lactose is the principal sugar found in milk. Maltose is a product of enzymic digestion of polysaccharides. It is also found in significant quantities in beer and malt liquors. The term "sugar" refers to monosaccharides and disaccharides. "Added sugars" are those sugars and syrups (such as HFCS) added to foods during processing or preparation.

3. **Polysaccharides:** Complex carbohydrates are polysaccharides (most often polymers of glucose) that do not have a sweet taste. Starch is an example of a complex carbohydrate that is found in abundance in plants. Common sources include wheat and other grains, potatoes, dried peas and beans (legumes), and vegetables.

4. **Fiber:** Dietary fiber is defined as the nondigestible, nonstarch carbohydrates and lignin (a noncarbohydrate polymer of aromatic alcohols) present intact in plants. Soluble fiber is the edible part of plants that is resistant to digestion and absorption in the human small intestine but is completely or partially fermented by bacteria to short-chain fatty acids in the large intestine. Insoluble fiber passes through the digestive track largely unchanged. Dietary fiber provides little energy but has several beneficial effects. First, it adds bulk to the diet (Fig. 27.17). Fiber can absorb 10–15 times its own weight in water, drawing fluid into the lumen of the intestine and increasing bowel motility and promoting bowel movements (laxation). Soluble fiber delays gastric emptying and can result in a sensation of fullness (satiety). This delayed emptying also results in reduced spikes in blood glucose following a meal. Second, consumption of soluble fiber has been shown to lower LDL-C levels by increasing fecal bile acid excretion and interfering with bile acid reabsorption (see p. 225). For example, diets rich (25–50 g/day) in the soluble fiber oat bran are associated with a modest, but significant, reduction in risk for CHD by lowering total cholesterol and LDL-C levels. Also, fiber-rich diets decrease the risk for constipation, hemorrhoids, and diverticulosis. The AI for dietary fiber is 25 g/day for women and 38 g/day for men. However, most American diets are far lower in fiber at ~15 g/day. [Note: "Functional fiber" is the term used for isolated fiber that has proven health benefits such as commercially available fiber supplements.]

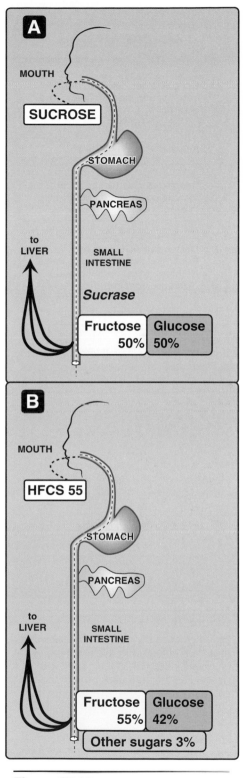

Figure 27.16
Digestion of sucrose (A) or high-fructose corn syrup (HFCS) 55 (B) leads to absorption of glucose plus fructose.

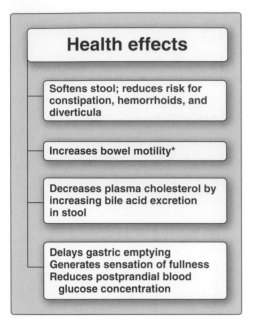

Figure 27.17
Actions of dietary fiber. [Note: *Increasing bowel motility decreases exposure time of the intestines to carcinogens.]

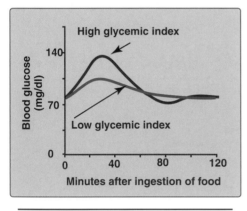

Figure 27.18
Blood glucose concentrations following ingestion of food with a low or high glycemic index (GI). [Note: The GI is defined as the area under the blood glucose curve.]

B. Dietary carbohydrate and blood glucose

Some carbohydrate-containing foods produce a rapid rise followed by a steep fall in blood glucose concentration, whereas others result in a gradual rise followed by a slow decline (Fig. 27.18). Thus, they differ in their glycemic response (GR). [Note: Fiber blunts the GR.] The glycemic index (GI) ranks carbohydrate-rich foods on a scale of 0–100 based on the GR they cause relative to the GR caused by the same amount (50 g) of carbohydrate eaten in the form of white bread or glucose. A low GI is <55, whereas a high GI is ≥70. Evidence suggests that a low-GI diet improves glycemic control in diabetic individuals. Food with a low GI tends to create a sense of satiety over a longer period of time and may be helpful in limiting caloric intake. [Note: How much a typical serving size of a food raises blood glucose is referred to as the glycemic load (GL). A food (for example, carrots) can have a high GI and a low GL.]

C. Carbohydrate requirements

Carbohydrates are not essential nutrients, because the carbon skeletons of most amino acids can be converted into glucose (see p. 261). However, the absence of dietary carbohydrate leads to ketogenesis (see p. 195) and degradation of body protein whose constituent amino acids provide carbon skeletons for gluconeogenesis (see p. 118). The RDA for carbohydrate is set at 130 g/day for adults and children, based on the amount of glucose used by carbohydrate-dependent tissues, such as the brain and erythrocytes. However, this level of intake is usually exceeded. Adults should consume 45%–65% of their total calories from carbohydrates. It is now recommended that added sugars represent no more than 10% of total energy intake because of concerns that they may displace nutrient-rich foods from the diet. [Note: Added sugars are associated with increased body weight and type 2 diabetes.]

D. Simple sugars and disease

There is no direct evidence that the consumption of simple sugars naturally present in food is harmful. Contrary to folklore, diets high in sucrose do not lead to diabetes or hypoglycemia. Also contrary to popular belief, carbohydrates are not inherently fattening. They yield 4 kcal/g (the same as protein and less than one half that of fat; see Fig. 27.5) and result in fat synthesis only when consumed in excess of the body's energy needs. However, there is an association between sucrose consumption and dental caries, particularly in the absence of fluoride treatment (see p. 405).

VII. DIETARY PROTEIN

The AMDR for protein is 10%–35%. Dietary protein provides the essential amino acids (see Fig. 20.2, p. 262). Nine of the 20 amino acids needed for the synthesis of body proteins are essential (that is, they cannot be synthesized in humans).

A. Protein quality

The quality of a dietary protein is a measure of its ability to provide the essential amino acids (EAA) required for tissue maintenance.

Most government agencies have adopted the Protein Digestibility–Corrected Amino Acid Score (PDCAAS) as the standard by which to evaluate protein quality. PDCAAS is based on the profile of EAA after correcting for the digestibility of the protein. The highest possible score under these guidelines is 1.00. This amino acid score provides a method to balance intakes of poorer-quality proteins with high-quality dietary proteins.

1. **Proteins from animal sources:** Proteins from animal sources (meat, poultry, milk, and fish) have a high quality because they contain all the EAA in proportions similar to those required for synthesis of human tissue proteins (Fig. 27.19), and they are more readily digested. [Note: Gelatin prepared from animal collagen is an exception. It has a low biologic value as a result of deficiencies in several EAA.]

2. **Proteins from plant sources:** Plant proteins have a lower quality than do animal proteins. However, proteins from different plant sources may be combined in such a way that the result is equivalent in nutritional value to animal protein. For example, wheat (lysine deficient but methionine rich) may be combined with kidney beans (methionine poor but lysine rich) to produce a higher biologic value than either of the component proteins (Fig. 27.20). [Note: Animal proteins can also complement the biologic value of plant proteins.]

B. Nitrogen balance

Nitrogen balance occurs when the amount of nitrogen consumed equals that of the nitrogen excreted in the urine (primarily as urinary urea nitrogen, or UUN), sweat, and feces. Most healthy adults are normally in nitrogen balance. [Note: There is, on average, 1 g nitrogen in 6.25 g protein.]

1. **Positive nitrogen balance:** This occurs when nitrogen intake exceeds nitrogen excretion. It is observed during situations in which tissue growth occurs, for example, in childhood, pregnancy, or during recovery from an emaciating illness.

2. **Negative nitrogen balance:** This occurs when nitrogen loss is greater than nitrogen intake. It is associated with inadequate dietary protein; lack of an essential amino acid; or during physiologic stresses, such as trauma, burns, illness, or surgery.

Source	PDCAAS value
Animal proteins	
Egg	1.00
Milk protein	1.00
Beef/poultry/fish	0.82–0.92
Gelatin	0.08
Plant proteins	
Soybean protein	1.00
Kidney beans	0.68
Whole wheat bread	0.40

Figure 27.19
Relative quality of some common dietary proteins. PDCAAS = Protein Digestibility–Corrected Amino Acid Score.

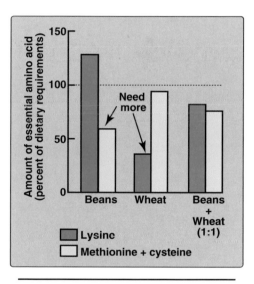

Figure 27.20
Combining two incomplete proteins that have complementary amino acid deficiencies results in a mixture with a higher biologic value.

Nitrogen (N) balance (g N_{in} − g N_{out}) in a 24-hour period can be determined by the formula, N balance = protein intake in g/6.25 − (UUN + 4 g), where 4 g accounts for urinary loss in forms other than UUN plus loss in skin and feces.

C. Protein requirements

The amount of dietary protein required in the diet varies with its biologic value. The greater the proportion of animal protein in the diet, the less protein is required. The RDA for protein is computed for proteins of mixed biologic value at 0.8 g/kg of body weight for adults, or ~56 g of protein for a 70-kg individual. People who exercise strenuously on a regular basis may benefit from extra protein to maintain muscle mass, and a daily intake of ~1 g/kg has been recommended for athletes. Women who are pregnant or lactating require up to 30 g/day in addition to their basal requirements. To support growth, infants should consume 2 g/kg/day. [Note: Disease states influence protein needs. Protein restriction may be needed in kidney disease, whereas burns require increased protein intake.]

1. **Consumption of excess protein:** There is no physiologic advantage to the consumption of more protein than the RDA. Protein consumed in excess of the body's needs is deaminated, and the resulting carbon skeletons are metabolized to provide energy or acetyl coenzyme A for fatty acid synthesis. When excess protein is eliminated from the body as urinary nitrogen, it is often accompanied by increased urinary calcium, thereby increasing the risk of nephrolithiasis (kidney stones) and osteoporosis.

2. **The protein-sparing effect of carbohydrates:** The dietary protein requirement is influenced by the carbohydrate content of the diet. When the intake of carbohydrates is low, amino acids are deaminated to provide carbon skeletons for the synthesis of glucose that is needed as a fuel by the central nervous system. If carbohydrate intake is <130 g/day, substantial amounts of protein are metabolized to provide precursors for gluconeogenesis. Therefore, carbohydrate is considered to be "protein-sparing," because it allows amino acids to be used for repair and maintenance of tissue protein rather than for gluconeogenesis.

D. Protein-energy (calorie) malnutrition

In developed countries, protein-energy malnutrition (PEM), also known as protein-energy undernutrition (PEU), is most commonly seen in patients with medical conditions that decrease appetite or alter how nutrients are digested or absorbed or in hospitalized patients with major trauma or infections. [Note: Such highly catabolic patients frequently require intravenous (IV, or parenteral) or tube-based (enteral) administration of nutrients.] PEM may also be seen in children or the elderly who are malnourished. In developing countries, an inadequate intake of protein and/or calories is the primary cause of PEM. Affected individuals show a variety of symptoms, including a depressed immune system with a reduced ability to resist infection. Death from secondary infection is common. PEM is a spectrum of degrees of malnutrition, and two extreme forms are kwashiorkor and marasmus (Fig. 27.21). [Note: Marasmic kwashiorkor has features of both forms.]

Type of PEM	Weight for age (% expected)	Weight for height	Edema	Muscle and fat content
Kwashiorkor	60–80	Normal or ↓	Present	↓
Marasmus	<60	Markedly ↓	Absent	Markedly ↓

Figure 27.21
Physical features of extreme protein-energy malnutrition (PEM) in children. [Note: The fatty liver and skin and hair changes of kwashiorkor are not seen in marasmus.]

1. **Kwashiorkor:** Kwashiorkor occurs when protein deprivation is relatively greater than the reduction in total calories. Protein deprivation is associated with severely decreased synthesis of visceral protein. Kwashiorkor is commonly seen in developing countries in children after weaning at about age 1 year, when their diet consists predominantly of carbohydrates. Typical symptoms include stunted growth, skin lesions, depigmented hair, anorexia, fatty liver, bilateral pitting edema, and decreased serum albumin concentration. Edema results from the lack of adequate blood proteins, primarily albumin, to maintain the distribution of water between blood and tissues. It may mask muscle and fat loss. Therefore, chronic malnutrition is reflected in the level of serum albumin. [Note: Because caloric intake from carbohydrates may be adequate, insulin levels suppress lipolysis and proteolysis. Kwashiorkor is, therefore, nonadapted malnutrition.]

> Cachexia, a wasting disorder characterized by loss of appetite and muscle atrophy (with or without increased lipolysis) that cannot be reversed by conventional nutritional support, is seen with a number of chronic diseases, such as cancer and chronic pulmonary and renal disease. It is associated with decreased treatment tolerance and response and decreased survival time.

2. **Marasmus:** Marasmus occurs when calorie deprivation is relatively greater than the reduction in protein. It usually occurs in developing countries in children younger than age 1 year when breast milk is supplemented or replaced with watery gruels of native cereals that are usually deficient in both protein and calories. Typical symptoms include arrested growth, extreme muscle wasting and depletion of subcutaneous fat (emaciation), weakness, and anemia (Fig. 27.22). Individuals with marasmus do not show the edema observed in kwashiorkor. [Note: Refeeding severely malnourished individuals can result in hypophosphatemia (see p. 400), because any available phosphate is used to phosphorylate carbohydrate intermediates. Milk is frequently given because it is rich in phosphate.]

VIII. NUTRITION TOOLS

A set of tools has been developed that gives consumers information about what (and how much) they should eat as well as the nutritional content of the foods they do eat. Additional tools allow medical professionals to assess whether or not the nutritional needs of an individual are being met.

A. MyPlate

MyPlate was designed by the U.S. Department of Agriculture (USDA) to graphically illustrate its recommendations as to what food groups and how much of each should be consumed daily. In MyPlate, the relative amounts of each of five food groups (vegetables, grains, protein, fruit, and dairy) are represented by the relative size of their section

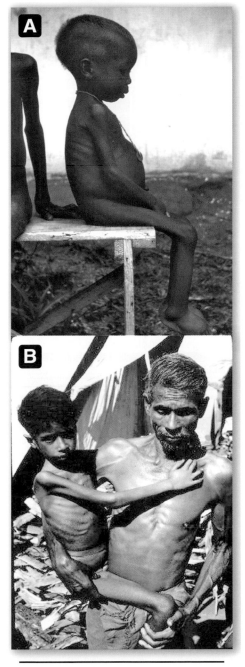

Figure 27.22
A. Listless child with kwashiorkor. Note the swollen belly and lower legs. B. Child suffering with marasmus.

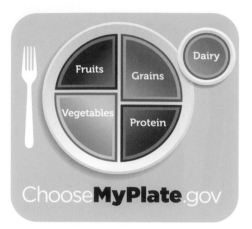

Figure 27.23
MyPlate.

Nutrition Facts

Serving Size 1 cup (228 g)
Servings Per Container about 2

Amount Per Serving

Calories 250 | Calories from Fat 110

	% Daily Value*
Total Fat 12 g	**18%**
Saturated Fat 3 g	**15%**
Trans Fat 3 g	
Cholesterol 30 mg	**10%**
Sodium 470 mg	**20%**
Total Carbohydrate 31 g	**10%**
Dietary Fiber 0 g	**0%**
Sugars 5 g	
Proteins 5 g	
Vitamin A	4%
Vitamin C	2%
Calcium	20%
Iron	4%

* Percent Daily Values are based on a 2,000 calorie diet.
Your Daily Values may be higher or lower depending on
your calorie needs:

	Calories:	2,000	2,500
Total Fat	Less than	65 g	80 g
Saturated Fat	Less than	20 g	25 g
Cholesterol	Less than	300 mg	300 mg
Sodium	Less than	2,400 mg	2,400 mg
Total Carbohydrate		300 g	375 g
Dietary Fiber		25 g	30 g

Figure 27.24
Nutrition Facts label (food label).

on the plate (Fig. 27.23). The number of servings depends on variables that include age and sex. [Note: MyPlate replaced MyPyramid in 2011.]

B. Nutrition facts label

Most types of packaged goods are required to have a Nutrition Facts label, or "food label" (Fig. 27.24), that includes the size of a single serving, the Cal it provides, and the number of servings per container. In addition, a percent daily value (%DV) is shown for most nutrients listed. [Note: The %DV is based on a 2,000-Cal diet for healthy adults.]

1. **Percent daily value:** The %DV compares the amount of a given nutrient in a single serving of a product to the recommended daily intake for that nutrient. For example, the %DV for the micronutrients listed, as well as for total carbohydrates and fiber, are based on their recommended minimum daily intake. Thus, if the label lists 20% for calcium, one serving provides 20% of the minimum recommended amount of calcium needed each day. In contrast, the %DV for saturated fat, cholesterol, and sodium are based on their recommended maximum daily intake, and the %DV reflects what percentage of this maximum a serving provides. There is no %DV for protein because the recommended intake depends on body weight (see p. 367). [Note: "Sugars" represents mono- and disaccharides. The remainder of the carbohydrate (total carbohydrate − [fiber + sugars]) is the oligo- and polysaccharides.]

2. **Proposed revisions:** In 2014, the USDA proposed the following changes to the Nutrition Facts label for implementation by 2018: Added sugars, vitamin D, and potassium are to be included; vitamins A and C, total fat, and Cal from fat are to be removed; and serving size is to be adjusted to reflect the amounts people are now consuming. Additionally, design changes to highlight key parts of the label were proposed (Fig. 27.25). [Note: The proposed addition/removal of certain micronutrients is based on newer data on the risk for underingestion.]

C. Nutrition assessment

Nutrition assessment evaluates nutritional status based on clinical information. It includes (but is not limited to) dietary history, anthropometric measures, and laboratory data. [Note: Assessment findings may result in medical nutrition therapy, which is the treatment of medical conditions through changes in diet (for example, replacement of long-chain TAG with medium-chain TAG in malabsorption disorders) and/or the method of intake (for example, enteral [tube] or parenteral [IV] feeding).]

1. **Dietary history:** This is a record of food intake over a period of time. For a food diary, the specific types and exact amounts of food eaten are recorded in "real time" (as soon as possible after eating) for a period of 3–7 days. Retrospective approaches include a food frequency questionnaire (for example, what fruits were eaten and how often they were eaten in a typical day, week, or month) and a 24-hour recall of the specific foods and the amounts eaten in the last 24 hours.

2. **Anthropometric measures:** These are physical measures of the body. They include (but are not limited to) weight, height, body mass index (an indicator of obesity, see p. 349), skin-fold thickness (an indicator of subcutaneous fat), and waist circumference (an indicator of abdominal fat, see p. 349). [Note: Ideal body weight can be calculated using the Hamwi method: 106 lb (for males) or 100 lb (for females) for the first 5 ft of height + 5 lb for every inch over 5 ft, with an adjustment of –10% for a small frame and + 10% for a large one.]

3. **Laboratory data:** These are obtained by tests performed on body fluids, tissues, and waste. They can include plasma LDL-C (for cardiovascular risk), fecal fat (for malabsorption), red cell indices (for vitamin deficiencies), and N balance and serum proteins (such as albumin and transthyretin [prealbumin]) for protein–energy status. [Note: These proteins are made in the liver and transport molecules such as fatty acids and thyroxine (see p. 406) through blood. Low albumin levels correlate with increased morbidity and mortality in hospitalized patients. The short half-life (2–3 days) of transthyretin as compared to that of albumin (20 days) has led to its use in monitoring the progress of hospitalized patients.]

> Nutritional insufficiency can be the result of inadequate nutrient intake (caused, for example, by an inability to eat, loss of appetite, or decreased availability), inadequate absorption, decreased utilization, increased excretion, or increased requirements.

IX. NUTRITION AND THE LIFE STAGES

Macronutrient energy sources, micronutrients, EFA, and EAA are required at every life stage. Additionally, each stage has specific nutrition needs.

A. Infancy, childhood, and adolescence

The rapid growth and development in infancy (birth to age 1 year) and childhood (age 1 year to adolescence) necessitate higher energy and protein needs relative to body size than are required in subsequent life stages. In adolescence, the marked increases in height and weight that occur increase nutritional needs. Growth charts (Fig. 27.26) are used to compare an individual's stature (height) and/or weight to the expected values for others of the same age (≤20 years) and sex. They are based on data from large numbers of normal individuals over time. [Note: Deviations from the expected growth curve, as reflected in the crossing of two or more percentile lines, raise concern.]

1. **Infants:** Ideal infant nutrition is based on human breast milk because it provides calories and most micronutrients in amounts appropriate for the human infant. Carbohydrates, protein, and fat are present in a 7:3:1 ratio. [Note: In addition to the disaccharide lactose, human milk contains nearly 200 unique oligosaccharides. About 90% of the microbiota (the population of

Nutrition Facts

8 servings per container

Serving size 2/3 cup (55 g)

Amount per 2/3 cup

Calories **230**

% DV*	
12%	**Total Fat** 8 g
5%	**Saturated Fat** 1 g
	Trans **Fat** 0 g
0%	**Cholesterol** 0 mg
7%	**Sodium** 160 mg
12%	**Total Carbs** 37 g
14%	**Dietary Fiber** 4 g
	Sugars 1 g
	Added Sugars 0 g
	Protein 3 g
10%	**Vitamin D** 2 mcg
20%	**Calcium** 260 mg
45%	**Iron** 8 mg
5%	**Potassium** 235 mg

* Footnote on Daily Values (DV) and calories reference to be inserted here.

Figure 27.25
Nutrition Facts label showing changes proposed in 2014 for implementation by 2018.

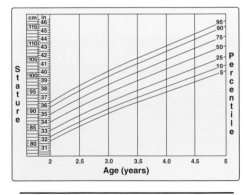

Figure 27.26
Clinical growth chart of stature-for-age for boys age 2–5 years from the Centers for Disease Control and Prevention (CDC) (see https://www.cdc.gov/growthcharts/). Charts for girls are pink.

microbes) in the breast-fed infant's intestine is represented by one type, <u>Bifidobacterium</u> <u>infantis</u>, which expresses all the enzymes needed to degrade these complex sugars. The sugars, in turn, act as prebiotics that support the growth of <u>B.</u> <u>infantis</u>, a probiotic (helpful bacteria).] Breast milk is low in vitamin D, however, and exclusively breast-fed babies require vitamin D supplementation. [Note: Human milk provides antibodies and other proteins that reduce the risk of infection.]

> The microbiota in and on the human body plus their genomes are referred to as the microbiome. It is acquired at birth from the environment and changes with the life stages. The gut microbiome influences host nutrition by facilitating processing of food consumed and is itself influenced by that food. Its relationship with undernutrition, obesity, and diabetes is under investigation.

2. **Children:** As with infants, children have increased need for calories and nutrients. The primary concerns in this stage, however, are deficiencies of iron and calcium.

3. **Adolescents:** In the teen years, the increases in height and weight increase the need for calories, protein, calcium, iron, and phosphorus. Eating patterns in this stage can result in overconsumption of fat, sodium, and sugar and underconsumption of vitamin A, thiamine, and folic acid. [Note: Eating disorders and obesity are concerns in this age group.]

B. Adulthood

Overnutrition is a concern in young adults, whereas malnutrition is a concern in older adults.

1. **Young adults:** Nutrition in young adults focuses on the maintenance of good health and the prevention of disease. The goal is a diet rich in plant-based foods (with a focus on fiber and whole grains), limited intake of saturated fat and trans fatty acids, and balanced intake of ω-3 and ω-6 PUFA.

2. **Pregnant or lactating women:** The requirements for calories, protein, and virtually all micronutrients increase in pregnancy and lactation. Supplementation with folic acid (to prevent neural tube defects [see p. 379]), vitamin D, calcium, iron, iodine, and DHA is typically recommended.

3. **Older adults:** Aging increases the risk of malnutrition. Decreased appetite resulting from a reduced sense of taste (dysgeusia) and smell (hyposmia) decreases nutrient intake. [Note: Physical limitations, including problems with dentition, and psychosocial factors, such as isolation, may also play a role in reduced intake.] Inadequate intake of protein, calcium, and vitamins D and B_{12} is common. B_{12} deficiency can result from decreased absorption caused by achlorhydria (reduced stomach acid, see p. 381). In aging, lean muscle mass decreases and fat increases, resulting in decreased RMR. [Note: Drug–nutrient interactions can occur at any life stage but are more common as the number of medications increases as in aging.]

Monoamine oxidase inhibitors (MAOI), used to treat depression (see p. 287) and early Parkinson disease, can interact with tyramine-containing foods. Tyramine is a monoamine derived from the decarboxylation of tyrosine during the curing, aging, or fermentation of food (Fig. 27.27). It causes the release of norepinephrine, increasing blood pressure and heart rate. Patients who take an MAOI and consume such foods are at risk for a hypertensive crisis.

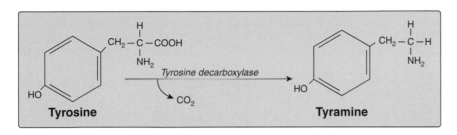

Figure 27.27
Decarboxylation of tyrosine to tyramine. CO_2 = carbon dioxide.

X. CHAPTER SUMMARY

The **Dietary Reference Intakes** (**DRI**) provide estimates of the amounts of nutrients required to prevent deficiencies and maintain optimal health and growth. They consist of the **Estimated Average Requirement** (**EAR**), the average daily nutrient intake level estimated to meet the requirement of 50% of the healthy individuals in a particular life stage (age) and gender group; the **Recommended Dietary Allowance** (**RDA**), the average daily dietary intake level that is sufficient to meet the nutrient requirements of nearly all (97%–98%) individuals in a life stage and gender group; the **Adequate Intake** (**AI**), which is set instead of an RDA if sufficient scientific evidence is not available to calculate the RDA; and the **Tolerable Upper Intake Level** (**UL**), the highest average daily nutrient intake level that is likely to pose no risk of adverse health effects to almost all individuals in the general population. The energy generated by the metabolism of the **macronutrients** (9 kcal/g of fat and 4 kcal/g of protein or carbohydrate) is used for three energy-requiring processes that occur in the body: **resting metabolic rate**, **physical activity**, and the **thermic effect of food**. **Acceptable Macronutrient Distribution Ranges** (**AMDR**) are defined as the ranges of intake for a particular macronutrient that are associated with reduced risk of chronic disease while providing adequate amounts of essential nutrients. Adults should consume **45%–65%** of their **total calories** from **carbohydrates, 20%–35%** from **fat**, and **10%–35%** from **protein** (Fig. 27.28). Elevated levels of cholesterol in low-density lipoproteins (LDL-C) result in increased risk for **coronary heart disease** (**CHD**). In contrast, elevated levels of cholesterol in high-density lipoproteins (HDL-C) have been associated with a decreased risk for CHD. Dietary or drug treatment of **hypercholesterolemia** is effective in decreasing LDL-C, increasing HDL-C, and reducing the risk for CHD. Consumption of **saturated fats** is strongly associated with high levels of total plasma and LDL-C. When substituted for saturated fatty acids in the diet, **monounsaturated fats** lower both total plasma cholesterol and LDL-C but maintain or increase HDL-C. Consumption of fats containing **ω-6 polyunsaturated fatty acids** lowers plasma LDL-C, but HDL-C, which protects against CHD, is also lowered. Dietary **ω-3 polyunsaturated fats** suppress cardiac arrhythmias and reduce plasma triacylglycerols, decrease the tendency for thrombosis, and substantially reduce the risk of cardiovascular mortality. **Carbohydrates** provide **energy** and **fiber** to the diet. When they are consumed as part of a diet in which caloric intake is equal to energy expenditure, they do not promote obesity. Dietary **protein** provides **essential amino acids**. **Protein quality** is a measure of its ability to provide the essential amino acids required for tissue maintenance. Proteins from animal sources, in general, have a higher-quality protein than that derived from plants. However, proteins from different plant sources may be combined in such a way that the result is equivalent in nutritional value to animal protein. **Positive nitrogen** (**N**) **balance** occurs when N intake exceeds N excretion. It is observed in situations in which tissue growth occurs, for example, in childhood, pregnancy, or during recovery from an emaciating illness. **Negative N balance** occurs when N losses are greater than N intake. It is associated with inadequate dietary protein; lack of an essential amino acid; or during physiologic stresses such as trauma, burns, illness, or surgery. **Kwashiorkor** occurs when protein deprivation is relatively greater than the reduction in total calories. It is characterized by edema. **Marasmus** occurs when calorie deprivation is relatively greater than the reduction in protein. No edema is seen. Both are extreme forms of **protein-energy malnutrition** (**PEM**). **Nutrition Facts labels** give consumers information about the nutritional content of packaged foods. Medical assessment of nutritional status includes **dietary history, anthropometric measures**, and **laboratory data**. Each life stage has specific nutrition needs. **Growth charts** are used to monitor the growth pattern of an individual from birth through adolescence. **Drug–nutrient interactions** are of concern, especially in older adults.

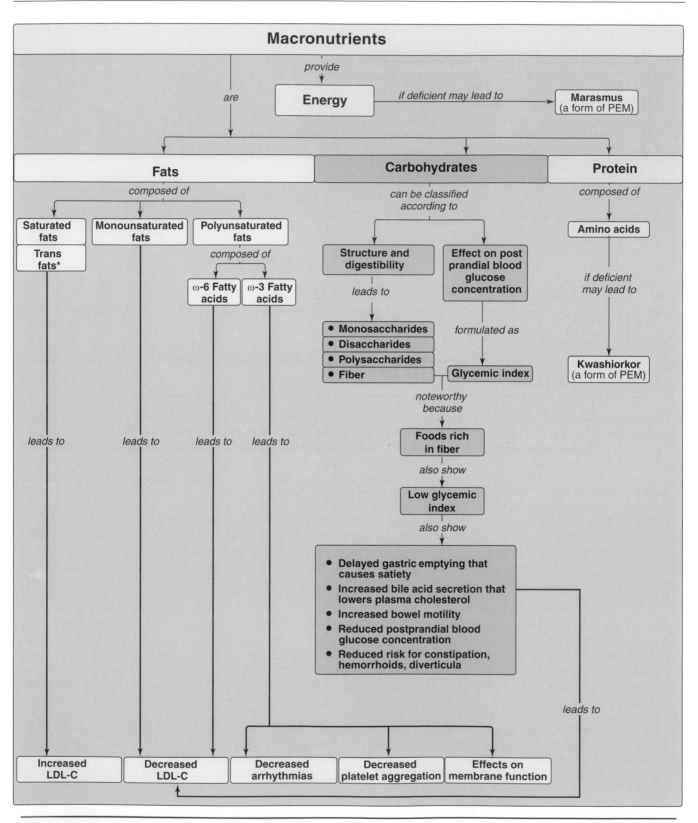

Figure 27.28

Key concept map for the macronutrients. [Note: *Trans fatty acids are chemically classified as unsaturated.] PEM = protein-energy malnutrition; LDL = low-density lipoprotein; C = cholesterol.

Study Questions

Choose the ONE best answer.

27.1 For the child shown at right, which of the statements would support a diagnosis of kwashiorkor? The child:

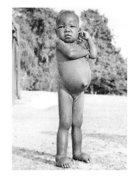

    A. appears plump due to increased deposition of fat in adipose tissue.

    B. displays abdominal and peripheral edema.

    C. has a serum albumin level above normal.

    D. has markedly decreased weight for height.

> The correct answer = B. Kwashiorkor is caused by inadequate protein intake in the presence of fair to good energy (calorie) intake. Typical findings in a patient with kwashiorkor include abdominal and peripheral edema (note the swollen belly and legs) caused largely by a decreased serum albumin concentration. Body fat stores are depleted, but weight for height can be normal because of edema. Treatment includes a diet adequate in calories and protein.

27.2 Which one of the following statements concerning dietary fat is correct?

    A. Coconut oil is rich in monounsaturated fats, and olive oil is rich in saturated fats.

    B. Fatty acids containing trans double bonds, unlike the naturally occurring cis isomers, raise high-density lipoprotein cholesterol levels.

    C. The polyunsaturated fatty acids linoleic and linolenic acids are required components.

    D. Triacylglycerols obtained from plants generally contain less unsaturated fatty acids than do those from animals.

> Correct answer = C. Humans are unable to make linoleic and linolenic fatty acids. Consequently, these fatty acids are essential in the diet. Coconut oil is rich in saturated fats, and olive oil is rich in monounsaturated fats. Trans fatty acids raise plasma levels of low-density lipoprotein cholesterol, not high-density lipoprotein cholesterol. Triacylglycerols obtained from plants generally contain more unsaturated fatty acids than do those from animals.

27.3 Given the information that a 70-kg man is consuming a daily average of 275 g of carbohydrate, 75 g of protein, and 65 g of fat, which one of the following conclusions can reasonably be drawn?

    A. About 20% of calories are derived from fats.

    B. The diet contains a sufficient amount of fiber.

    C. The individual is in nitrogen balance.

    D. The proportions of carbohydrate, protein, and fat in the diet conform to current recommendations.

    E. The total energy intake per day is about 3,000 kcal.

> Correct answer = D. The total energy intake is (275 g carbohydrate × 4 kcal/g) + (75 g protein × 4 kcal/g) + (65 g fat × 9 kcal/g) = 1,100 + 300 + 585 = 1,985 total kcal/day. The percentage of calories derived from carbohydrate is 1,100/1,985 = 55, from protein is 300/1,985 = 15, and from fat is 585/1,985 = 30. These are very close to current recommendations. The amount of fiber or nitrogen balance cannot be deduced from the data presented. If the protein is of low biologic value, a negative nitrogen balance is possible.

27.4 In chronic bronchitis, excessive mucus production causes airway obstruction that results in hypoxemia (low blood oxygen level), impaired expiration, and hypercapnia (carbon dioxide retention). Why might a high-fat, low-carbohydrate diet be recommended for a patient with chronic obstructive pulmonary disease caused by chronic bronchitis?

    A. Fat contains more oxygen atoms relative to carbon or hydrogen atoms than do carbohydrates.

    B. Fat is calorically less dense than carbohydrates.

    C. Fat metabolism generates less carbon dioxide.

    D. The respiratory quotient (RQ) for fat is higher than the RQ for carbohydrates.

> Correct answer = C. A treatment goal for the chronic obstructive pulmonary disease (COPD) caused by acute bronchitis is to insure appropriate nutrition without increasing the respiratory quotient (RQ), which is the ratio of carbon dioxide (CO_2) produced to oxygen consumed, thereby minimizing the production of CO_2. Less CO_2 is produced from the metabolism of fat (RQ = 0.7) than from the catabolism of carbohydrate (RQ =1.0). Fat contains fewer oxygen atoms. Fat is calorically denser than is carbohydrate. [Note: RQ is determined by indirect calorimetry.]

27.5 A 32-year-old man who was rescued from a house fire was admitted to the hospital with burns over 45% of his body (severe burns). The man weighs 154 lb (70 kg) and is 72 in (183 cm) tall. Which one of the following is the best rapid estimate of the immediate daily caloric needs of this patient?

A. 1,345 kcal

B. 1,680 kcal

C. 2,690 kcal

D. 3,360 kcal

Correct answer = D. A commonly used rough estimate of the total energy expenditure (TEE) for men is 1 kcal/1 kg body weight/24 hours. [Note: It is 0.8 kcal for women.] For this patient, that value is 1,680 kcal (1 kcal/kg/hour × 24 hours × 70 kg). In addition, an injury factor of 2 for severe burns must be included in the calculation: 1,680 kcal × 2 = 3,360 kcal.

27.6 Which one of the following is the best advice to give a patient who asks about the notation "%DV" (percent daily value) on the Nutrition Facts label?

A. Achieve 100% daily value for each nutrient each day.

B. Select foods that have the highest percent daily value for all nutrients.

C. Select foods with a low percent daily value for the micronutrients.

D. Select foods with a low percent daily value for saturated fat.

Correct answer = D. The percent daily value (%DV) compares the amount of a given nutrient in a single serving of a product to the recommended daily intake for that nutrient. The %DV for the micronutrients listed on the label, as well as for total carbohydrates and fiber, are based on their recommended minimum daily intake, whereas the %DV for saturated fat, cholesterol, and sodium are based on their recommended maximum daily intake.

For Questions 27.7 and 27.8, use the following case.

A sedentary 50-year-old man weighing 176 lb (80 kg) requests a physical. He denies any health problems. Routine blood analysis is unremarkable except for plasma total cholesterol of 295 mg/dl. (Reference value is <200 mg.) The man refuses drug therapy for his hypercholesterolemia. Analysis of a 1-day dietary recall showed the following:

Kilocalories	3,475 kcal	Cholesterol	822 mg
Protein	102 g	Saturated fat	69 g
Carbohydrate	383 g	Total fat	165 g
Fiber	6 g		

27.7 Decreasing which one of the following dietary components would have the greatest effect in lowering the patient's plasma cholesterol?

A. Carbohydrates

B. Cholesterol

C. Fiber

D. Monounsaturated fat

E. Polyunsaturated fat

F. Saturated fat

Correct answer = F. The intake of saturated fat most strongly influences plasma cholesterol in this diet. The patient is consuming a high-calorie, high-fat diet with 42% of the fat as saturated fat. The most important dietary recommendations are to lower total caloric intake, substitute monounsaturated and polyunsaturated fats for saturated fats, and increase dietary fiber. A decrease in dietary cholesterol would be helpful but is not a primary objective.

27.8 What information would be necessary to estimate the patient's total energy expenditure?

The daily basal energy expenditure (estimated resting metabolic rate/hour × 24 hours) and a physical activity ratio (PAR) based on the type and duration of physical activities are needed variables. An additional 10% would be added to account for the thermic effect of food. Note that if the patient were hospitalized, an injury factor (IF) would be included in the calculation, and the PAR would be modified. Tables of PAR and IF are available.

Micronutrients: Vitamins

28

I. OVERVIEW

Vitamins are chemically unrelated organic compounds that cannot be synthesized in adequate quantities by humans and, therefore, must be supplied by the diet. Nine vitamins (folic acid, cobalamin, ascorbic acid, pyridoxine, thiamine, niacin, riboflavin, biotin, and pantothenic acid) are classified as water soluble. Because they are readily excreted in the urine, toxicity is rare. However, deficiencies can occur quickly. Four vitamins (A, D, K, and E) are termed fat soluble (Fig. 28.1). They are released, absorbed, and transported (in chylomicrons, see p. 227) with dietary fat. They are not readily excreted, and significant quantities are stored in the liver and adipose tissue. In fact, consumption of vitamins A and D in excess of the Dietary Reference Intakes (see Chapter 27) can lead to accumulation of toxic quantities of these compounds. Vitamins are required to perform specific cellular functions. For example, many of the water-soluble vitamins are precursors of coenzymes for the enzymes of intermediary metabolism. In contrast to the water-soluble vitamins, only one fat-soluble vitamin (vitamin K) has a coenzyme function.

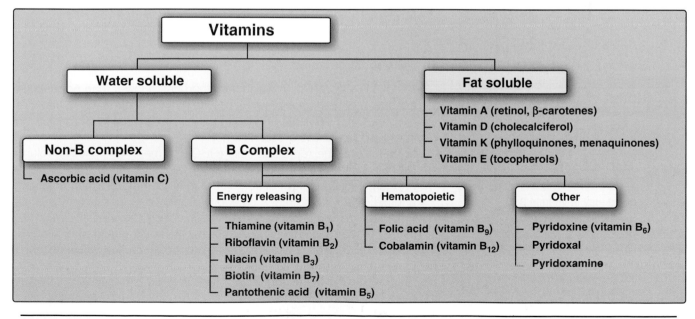

Figure 28.1
Classification of the vitamins. Because they are required in lesser amounts than the macronutrients (carbohydrate, protein, and lipid), vitamins are termed micronutrients.

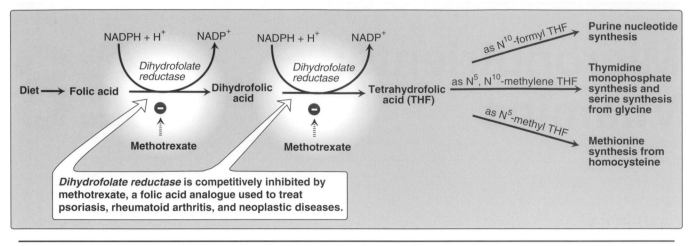

Figure 28.2
Production and use of tetrahydrofolate. NADP(H) = nicotinamide adenine dinucleotide phosphate.

II. FOLIC ACID (VITAMIN B$_9$)

Folic acid (or, folate), which plays a key role in one-carbon metabolism, is essential for the biosynthesis of several compounds. Folic acid deficiency is probably the most common vitamin deficiency in the United States, particularly among pregnant women and individuals with alcoholism. [Note: Leafy, dark-green vegetables are a good source of folic acid.]

A. Function

Tetrahydrofolate (THF), the reduced, coenzyme form of folate, receives one-carbon fragments from donors such as serine, glycine, and histidine and transfers them to intermediates in the synthesis of amino acids, purine nucleotides, and thymidine monophosphate (TMP), a pyrimidine nucleotide incorporated into DNA (Fig. 28.2).

B. Nutritional anemias

Anemia is a condition in which the blood has a lower than normal concentration of hemoglobin, which results in a reduced ability to transport oxygen (O_2). Nutritional anemias (that is, those caused by inadequate intake of one or more essential nutrients) can be classified according to the size of the red blood cells (RBC), or mean corpuscular volume (MCV), observed in the blood (Fig. 28.3). Microcytic anemia (MCV below normal), caused by lack of iron, is the most common form of nutritional anemia. The second major category of nutritional anemia, macrocytic (MCV above normal), results from a deficiency in folic acid or vitamin B$_{12}$. [Note: These macrocytic anemias are commonly called megaloblastic because a deficiency of either vitamin (or both) causes accumulation of large, immature RBC precursors, known as megaloblasts, in the bone marrow and the blood (Fig. 28.4). Hypersegmented neutrophils are also seen.]

1. **Folate and anemia:** Inadequate serum levels of folate can be caused by increased demand (for example, pregnancy and lactation; see p. 372), poor absorption caused by pathology of the small

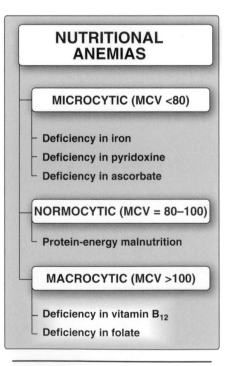

Figure 28.3
Classification of nutritional anemias by red cell size. The normal mean corpuscular volume (MCV) for people older than age 18 years is 80–100 µm^3. [Note: Microcytic anemia is also seen with heavy metal (for example, lead) poisoning.]

intestine, alcoholism, or treatment with drugs (for example, metho-trexate) that are *dihydrofolate reductase* inhibitors (see Fig. 28.2). A folate-free diet can cause a deficiency within a few weeks. A primary result of folic acid deficiency is megaloblastic anemia (see Fig. 28.4), caused by diminished synthesis of purine nucleotides and TMP, which leads to an inability of cells (including RBC precursors) to make DNA and, therefore, an inability to divide.

2. **Folate and neural tube defects:** Spina bifida and anencephaly, the most common neural tube defects (NTD), affect ~3,000 pregnancies in the United States annually. Folic acid supplementation before conception and during the first trimester has been shown to significantly reduce NTD. Therefore, all women of childbearing age are advised to consume 0.4 mg/day (400 µg/day) of folic acid to reduce the risk of having a pregnancy affected by NTD and ten times that amount if a previous pregnancy was affected. Adequate folate nutrition must occur at the time of conception because critical folate-dependent development occurs in the first weeks of fetal life, at a time when many women are not yet aware of their pregnancy. In 1998, the U.S. Food and Drug Administration authorized the addition of folic acid to wheat flour and enriched grain products, resulting in a dietary supplementation of ~0.1 mg/day. This supplementation allows ~50% of all reproductive-aged women to receive 0.4 mg of folate from all sources.

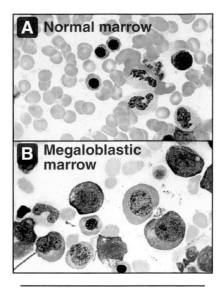

Figure 28.4
Bone marrow histology in normal (A) and folate-deficient (B) individuals.

III. COBALAMIN (VITAMIN B$_{12}$)

Vitamin B$_{12}$ is required in humans for two essential enzymatic reactions: the remethylation of homocysteine (Hcy) to methionine and the isomerization of methylmalonyl coenzyme A (CoA), which is produced during the degradation of some amino acids (isoleucine, valine, threonine, and methionine) and fatty acids (FA) with odd numbers of carbon atoms (Fig. 28.5). When cobalamin is deficient, unusual (branched) FA accumulate and become incorporated into cell membranes, including those of the central nervous system (CNS). This may account for some of the neurologic manifestations of vitamin B$_{12}$ deficiency. [Note: Folic acid (as N^5-methyl THF) is also required in the remethylation of Hcy. Therefore, deficiency of B$_{12}$ or folate results in elevated Hcy levels.]

A. Structure and coenzyme forms

Cobalamin contains a corrin ring system that resembles the porphyrin ring of heme (see p. 279), but differs in that two of the pyrrole rings are linked directly rather than through a methene bridge. Cobalt (see p. 407) is held in the center of the corrin ring by four coordination bonds with the nitrogens of the pyrrole groups. The remaining coordination bonds of the cobalt are with the nitrogen of 5,6-dimethylbenzimidazole and with cyanide in commercial preparations of the vitamin in the form of cyanocobalamin (Fig. 28.6). The physiologic coenzyme forms of cobalamin are 5′-deoxyadenosylcobalamin and methylcobalamin, in which cyanide is replaced with 5′-deoxyadenosine or a methyl group, respectively (see Fig. 28.6).

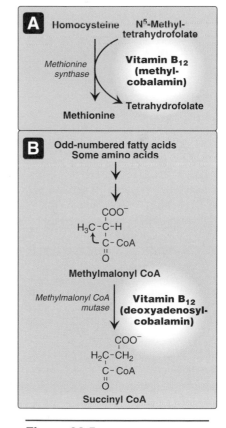

Figure 28.5
A, B. Reactions requiring coenzyme forms of vitamin B$_{12}$. CoA = coenzyme A.

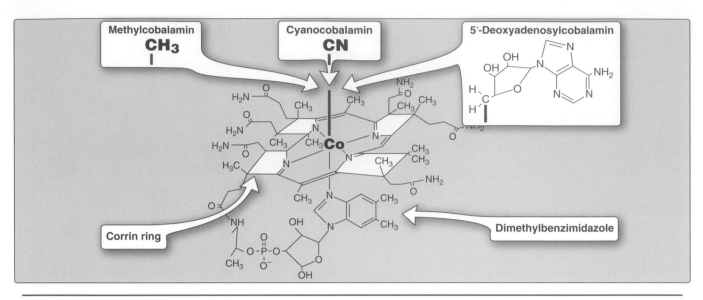

Figure 28.6
Structure of vitamin B_{12} (cyanocobalamin) and its coenzyme forms (methylcobalamin and 5′-deoxyadenosylcobalamin).

B. Distribution

Vitamin B_{12} is synthesized only by microorganisms, and it is not present in plants. Animals obtain the vitamin preformed from their intestinal microbiota (see p. 371) or by eating foods derived from other animals. Cobalamin is present in appreciable amounts in liver, red meat, fish, eggs, dairy products, and fortified cereals.

C. Folate trap hypothesis

The effects of cobalamin deficiency are most pronounced in rapidly dividing cells, such as the erythropoietic tissue of bone marrow and the mucosal cells of the intestine. Such tissues need both the N^5,N^{10}-methylene and N^{10}-formyl forms of THF for the synthesis of nucleotides required for DNA replication (see pp. 292 and 303). However, in vitamin B_{12} deficiency, the utilization of the N^5-methyl form of THF in the B_{12}-dependent methylation of Hcy to methionine is impaired. Because the methylated form cannot be converted directly to other forms of THF, folate is trapped in the N^5-methyl form, which accumulates. The levels of the other forms decrease. Thus, cobalamin deficiency leads to a deficiency of the THF forms needed in purine and TMP synthesis, resulting in the symptoms of megaloblastic anemia.

D. Clinical indications for cobalamin

In contrast to other water-soluble vitamins, significant amounts (2–5 mg) of vitamin B_{12} are stored in the body. As a result, it may take several years for the clinical symptoms of B_{12} deficiency to develop as a result of decreased intake of the vitamin. [Note: Deficiency happens much more quickly (in months) if absorption is impaired (see below). The Schilling test evaluates B_{12} absorption.] B_{12} deficiency can be determined by the level of methylmalonic acid in blood, which is elevated in individuals with low intake or decreased absorption of the vitamin.

1. **Pernicious anemia:** Vitamin B_{12} deficiency is most commonly seen in patients who fail to absorb the vitamin from the intestine (Fig. 28.7). B_{12} is released from food in the acidic environment of

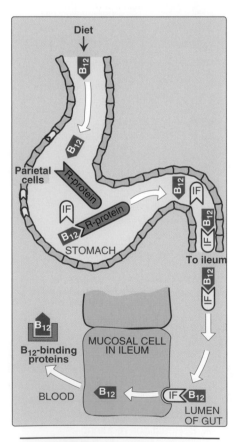

Figure 28.7
Absorption of vitamin B_{12}. [Note: Acid-dependent release of B_{12} from food is not shown.] IF = intrinsic factor.

the stomach. [Note: Malabsorption of cobalamin in the elderly is most often due to reduced secretion of gastric acid (achlorhydria).] Free B_{12} then binds a glycoprotein (R-protein or haptocorrin), and the complex moves into the intestine. B_{12} is released from the R-protein by pancreatic enzymes and binds another glycoprotein, intrinsic factor (IF). The cobalamin–IF complex travels through the intestine and binds to a receptor (cubilin) on the surface of mucosal cells in the ileum. The cobalamin is transported into the mucosal cell and, subsequently, into the general circulation, where it is carried by its binding protein (transcobalamin). B_{12} is taken up and stored in the liver, primarily. It is released into bile and efficiently reabsorbed in the ileum. Severe malabsorption of vitamin B_{12} leads to pernicious anemia. This disease is most commonly a result of an autoimmune destruction of the gastric parietal cells that are responsible for the synthesis of IF (lack of IF prevents B_{12} absorption). [Note: Patients who have had a partial or total gastrectomy become IF deficient and, therefore, B_{12} deficient.] Individuals with cobalamin deficiency are usually anemic (folate recycling is impaired), and they show neuropsychiatric symptoms as the disease develops. The CNS effects are irreversible. Pernicious anemia requires lifelong treatment with either high-dose oral B_{12} or intramuscular injection of cyanocobalamin. [Note: Supplementation works even in the absence of IF because ~1% of B_{12} uptake is by IF-independent diffusion.]

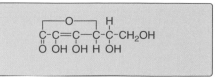

Figure 28.8
Structure of ascorbic acid.

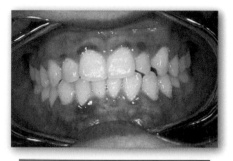

Figure 28.9
Oral manifestations in a patient with scurvy.

Folic acid supplementation can partially reverse the hematologic abnormalities of B_{12} deficiency and, therefore, can mask a cobalamin deficiency. Thus, to prevent the later CNS effects of B_{12} deficiency, therapy for megaloblastic anemia is initiated with both vitamin B_{12} and folic acid until the cause of the anemia can be determined.

IV. ASCORBIC ACID (VITAMIN C)

The active form of vitamin C is ascorbic acid (Fig. 28.8). Its main function is as a reducing agent. Vitamin C is a coenzyme in hydroxylation reactions (for example, hydroxylation of prolyl and lysyl residues in collagen; see p. 47), where its role is to keep the iron (Fe) of *hydroxylases* in the reduced, ferrous (Fe^{+2}) form. Thus, vitamin C is required for the maintenance of normal connective tissue as well as for wound healing. Vitamin C also facilitates the absorption of dietary nonheme iron from the intestine by reduction of the ferric form (Fe^{+3}) to Fe^{+2} (see p. 403).

A. Deficiency

Ascorbic acid deficiency results in scurvy, a disease characterized by sore and spongy gums, loose teeth, fragile blood vessels, hemorrhage, swollen joints, bone changes, and fatigue (Fig. 28.9). Many of the deficiency symptoms can be explained by the decreased hydroxylation of collagen, resulting in defective connective tissue. A microcytic anemia caused by decreased absorption of iron may also be seen.

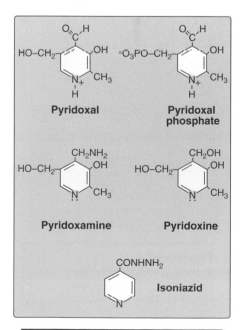

Figure 28.10
Structures of vitamin B_6 and the antituberculosis drug isoniazid.

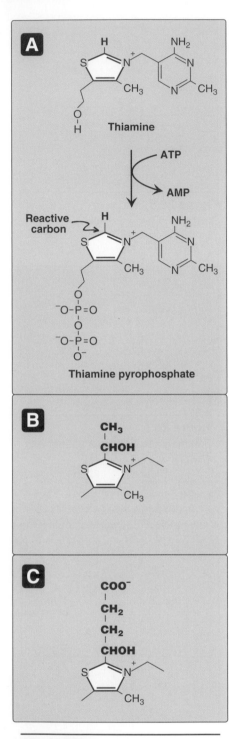

Figure 28.11
A. Structure of thiamine and
its coenzyme form, thiamine
pyrophosphate. B. Structure of
intermediate formed in the reaction
catalyzed by *pyruvate dehydrogenase*.
C. Structure of intermediate formed
in the reaction catalyzed by
α-ketoglutarate dehydrogenase.
AMP = adenosine monophosphate.

B. Chronic disease prevention

Vitamin C is one of a group of nutrients that includes vitamin E
(see p. 395) and β-carotene (see p. 386), which are known as antioxidants. [Note: Vitamin C regenerates the functional, reduced form of
vitamin E.] Consumption of diets rich in these compounds is associated with a decreased incidence of some chronic diseases, such as
cardiovascular disease (CVD) and certain cancers. However, clinical
trials involving supplementation with the isolated antioxidants have
failed to demonstrate any convincing preventive effects.

V. PYRIDOXINE (VITAMIN B₆)

Vitamin B$_6$ is a collective term for pyridoxine, pyridoxal, and pyridoxamine, all derivatives of pyridine. They differ only in the nature of the
functional group attached to the ring (Fig. 28.10). Pyridoxine occurs primarily in plants, whereas pyridoxal and pyridoxamine are found in foods
obtained from animals. All three compounds can serve as precursors of
the biologically active coenzyme, pyridoxal phosphate (PLP). PLP functions as a coenzyme for a large number of enzymes, particularly those
that catalyze reactions involving amino acids, for example, in the transsulfuration of Hcy to cysteine (see p. 264). [Note: PLP is also required by
glycogen phosphorylase (see p. 128).]

Reaction type	Example
Transamination	Oxaloacetate + glutamate $\rightleftarrows$ aspartate + α-ketoglutarate
Deamination	Serine → pyruvate + NH$_3$
Decarboxylation	Histidine → histamine + CO$_2$
Condensation	Glycine + succinyl CoA → δ-aminolevulinic acid

A. Clinical indications for pyridoxine

Isoniazid, a drug commonly used to treat tuberculosis, can induce a
vitamin B$_6$ deficiency by forming an inactive derivative with PLP. Thus,
dietary supplementation with B$_6$ is an adjunct to isoniazid treatment.
Otherwise, dietary deficiencies in pyridoxine are rare but have been
observed in newborn infants fed formulas low in B$_6$, in women taking
oral contraceptives, and in those with alcoholism.

B. Toxicity

Vitamin B$_6$ is the only water-soluble vitamin with significant toxicity.
Neurologic symptoms (sensory neuropathy) occur at intakes above
500 mg/day, an amount nearly 400 times the recommended dietary allowance (RDA) and over 5 times the tolerable upper limit (UL). (See Chapter
27 for a discussion of RDA and UL.) Substantial improvement, but not
complete recovery, occurs when the vitamin is discontinued.

VI. THIAMINE (VITAMIN B₁)

Thiamine pyrophosphate (TPP) is the biologically active form of the
vitamin, formed by the transfer of a pyrophosphate group from ATP to
thiamine (Fig. 28.11). TPP serves as a coenzyme in the formation or

degradation of α-ketols by *transketolase* (Fig. 28.12A) and in the oxidative decarboxylation of α-keto acids (Fig. 28.12B).

A. Clinical indications for thiamine

The oxidative decarboxylation of pyruvate and α-ketoglutarate, which plays a key role in energy metabolism of most cells, is particularly important in tissues of the CNS. In thiamine deficiency, the activity of these two *dehydrogenase*-catalyzed reactions is decreased, resulting in decreased production of ATP and, therefore, impaired cellular function. TPP is also required by *branched-chain α-keto acid dehydrogenase* of muscle (see p. 266). [Note: It is the *decarboxylase* of each of these *α-keto acid dehydrogenase* multienzyme complexes that requires TPP.] Thiamine deficiency is diagnosed by an increase in erythrocyte *transketolase* activity observed with addition of TPP.

1. **Beriberi:** This severe thiamine-deficiency syndrome is found in areas where polished rice is the major component of the diet. Adult beriberi is classified as dry (characterized by peripheral neuropathy, especially in the legs) or wet (characterized by edema because of dilated cardiomyopathy).

2. **Wernicke-Korsakoff syndrome:** In the United States, thiamine deficiency, which is seen primarily in association with chronic alcoholism, is due to dietary insufficiency or impaired intestinal absorption of the vitamin. Some individuals with alcoholism develop Wernicke-Korsakoff syndrome, a thiamine-deficiency state characterized by mental confusion, gait ataxia, nystagmus (a to-and-fro motion of the eyeballs), and ophthalmoplegia (weakness of eye muscles) with Wernicke encephalopathy as well as memory problems and hallucinations with Korsakoff dementia. The syndrome is treatable with thiamine supplementation, but recovery of memory is typically incomplete.

VII. NIACIN (VITAMIN B₃)

Niacin, or nicotinic acid, is a substituted pyridine derivative. The biologically active coenzyme forms are nicotinamide adenine dinucleotide

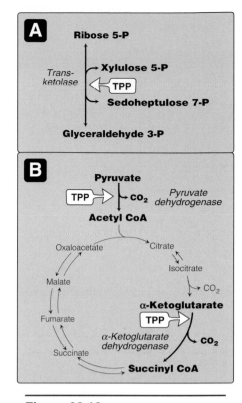

Figure 28.12
Reactions that use thiamine pyrophosphate (TPP) as coenzyme. A. *Transketolase.* B. *Pyruvate dehydrogenase* and *α-ketoglutarate dehydrogenase.* [Note: TPP is also used by *branched-chain α-keto acid dehydrogenase.*] P = phosphate; CoA = coenzyme A; CO₂ = carbon dioxide.

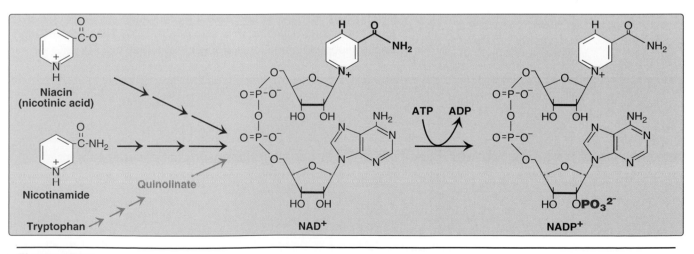

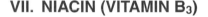

Figure 28.13
Structure and biosynthesis of oxidized nicotinamide adenine dinucleotide (NAD⁺) and nicotinamide adenine dinucleotide phosphate (NADP⁺). ADP = adenosine diphosphate.

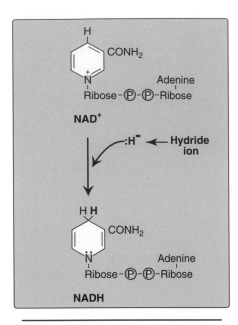

Figure 28.14
Reduction of oxidized nicotinamide adenine dinucleotide (NAD⁺) to NADH. [Note: The hydride ion consists of a hydrogen (H) atom plus an electron.] $\circleddash$ = phosphate.

(NAD⁺) and its phosphorylated derivative, nicotinamide adenine dinucleotide phosphate (NADP⁺), as shown in Figure 28.13. Nicotinamide, a derivative of nicotinic acid that contains an amide instead of a carboxyl group, also occurs in the diet. Nicotinamide is readily deaminated in the body and, therefore, is nutritionally equivalent to nicotinic acid. NAD⁺ and NADP⁺ serve as coenzymes in oxidation–reduction reactions in which the coenzyme undergoes reduction of the pyridine ring by accepting two electrons from a hydride ion, as shown in Figure 28.14. The reduced forms of NAD⁺ and NADP⁺ are NADH and NADPH, respectively. [Note: A metabolite of tryptophan, quinolinate, can be converted to NAD(P). In comparison, 60 mg of tryptophan = 1 mg of niacin.]

A. Distribution

Niacin is found in unrefined and enriched grains and cereal, milk, and lean meats (especially liver).

B. Clinical indications for niacin

1. **Deficiency:** A deficiency of niacin causes pellagra, a disease involving the skin, gastrointestinal tract, and CNS. The symptoms of pellagra progress through the three Ds: dermatitis (photosensitive), diarrhea, and dementia. If untreated, death (a fourth D) occurs. Hartnup disorder, characterized by defective absorption of tryptophan, can result in pellagra-like symptoms. [Note: Corn is low in both niacin and tryptophan. Corn-based diets can cause pellagra.]

2. **Hyperlipidemia treatment:** Niacin at doses of 1.5 g/day, or 100 times the RDA, strongly inhibits lipolysis in adipose tissue, the primary producer of circulating free fatty acids (FFA). The liver normally uses these circulating FFA as a major precursor for triacylglycerol (TAG) synthesis. Thus, niacin causes a decrease in liver TAG synthesis, which is required for very-low-density lipoprotein ([VLDL] see p. 230) production. Low-density lipoprotein (LDL, the cholesterol-rich lipoprotein) is derived from VLDL in the plasma. Thus, both plasma TAG (in VLDL) and cholesterol (in LDL) are lowered. Therefore, niacin is particularly useful in the treatment of type IIb hyperlipoproteinemia, in which both VLDL and LDL are elevated. The high doses of niacin required can cause acute, prostaglandin-mediated flushing. Aspirin can reduce this side effect by inhibiting prostaglandin synthesis (see p. 214). Itching may also occur. [Note: Niacin raises high-density lipoprotein and lowers Lp(a) levels (see p. 237).]

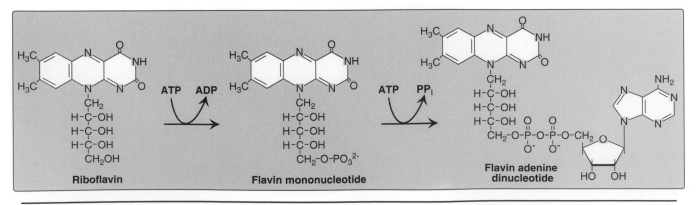

Figure 28.15
Structure and biosynthesis of the oxidized forms of flavin mononucleotide and flavin adenine dinucleotide. ADP = adenosine diphosphate; PPᵢ = pyrophosphate.

VIII. RIBOFLAVIN (VITAMIN B₂)

The two biologically active forms of B₂ are flavin mononucleotide (FMN) and flavin adenine dinucleotide (FAD), formed by the transfer of an adenosine monophosphate moiety from ATP to FMN (Fig. 28.15). FMN and FAD are each capable of reversibly accepting two hydrogen atoms, forming FMNH₂ or FADH₂, respectively. FMN and FAD are bound tightly, sometimes covalently, to flavoenzymes (for example, *NADH dehydrogenase* [FMN] and *succinate dehydrogenase* [FAD]) that catalyze the oxidation or reduction of a substrate. Riboflavin deficiency is not associated with a major human disease, although it frequently accompanies other vitamin deficiencies. Deficiency symptoms include dermatitis, cheilosis (fissuring at the corners of the mouth), and glossitis (the tongue appearing smooth and dark). [Note: Because riboflavin is light sensitive, phototherapy for hyperbilirubinemia (see p. 285) may require supplementation with the vitamin.]

IX. BIOTIN (VITAMIN B₇)

Biotin is a coenzyme in carboxylation reactions, in which it serves as a carrier of activated carbon dioxide (CO_2) (see Fig. 10.3, p. 119, for the mechanism of biotin-dependent carboxylations). Biotin is covalently bound to the ε-amino group of lysine residues in biotin-dependent enzymes (Fig. 28.16). Biotin deficiency does not occur naturally because the vitamin is widely distributed in food. Also, a large percentage of the biotin requirement in humans is supplied by intestinal bacteria. However, the addition of raw egg white to the diet as a source of protein can induce symptoms of biotin deficiency, namely, dermatitis, hair loss, loss of appetite, and nausea. Raw egg white contains the glycoprotein avidin, which tightly binds biotin and prevents its absorption from the intestine. With a normal diet, however, it has been estimated that 20 eggs/day would be required to induce a deficiency syndrome. [Note: Inclusion of raw eggs in the diet is not recommended because of the possibility of salmonellosis caused by infection with <u>Salmonella</u> <u>enterica</u>.]

|| Multiple carboxylase deficiency results from decreased ability to add biotin to *carboxylases* during their synthesis or to remove it during their degradation. Treatment is biotin supplementation.

X. PANTOTHENIC ACID (VITAMIN B₅)

Pantothenic acid is a component of CoA, which functions in the transfer of acyl groups (Fig. 28.17). CoA contains a thiol group that carries acyl compounds as activated thiol esters. Examples of such structures are succinyl CoA, fatty acyl CoA, and acetyl CoA. Pantothenic acid is also a component of the acyl carrier protein domain of *fatty acid synthase* (see p. 184). Eggs, liver, and yeast are the most important sources of pantothenic acid, although the vitamin is widely distributed. Pantothenic acid deficiency is not well characterized in humans, and no RDA has been established.

XI. VITAMIN A

Vitamin A is a fat-soluble vitamin that comes primarily from animal sources as retinol (preformed vitamin A), a retinoid. The retinoids, a

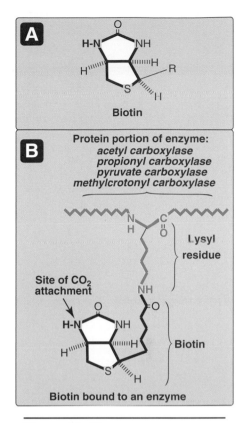

Figure 28.16
A. Structure of biotin. B. Biotin covalently bound to a lysyl residue of a biotin-dependent enzyme. CO_2 = carbon dioxide.

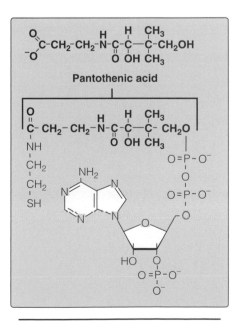

Figure 28.17
Structure of coenzyme A.

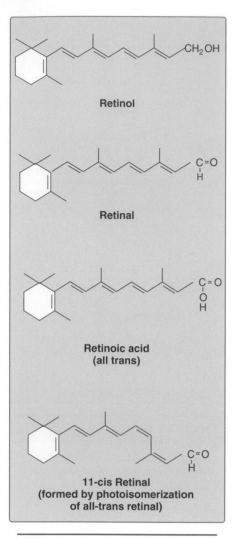

family of structurally related molecules, are essential for vision, reproduction, growth, and maintenance of epithelial tissues. They also play a
role in immune function. Retinoic acid, derived from oxidation of retinol,
mediates most of the actions of the retinoids, except for vision, which
depends on retinal, the aldehyde derivative of retinol.

A. Structure

The retinoids include the natural forms of vitamin A, retinol and its
metabolites (Fig. 28.18), and synthetic forms (drugs).

1. **Retinol:** A primary alcohol containing a β-ionone ring with an
   unsaturated side chain, retinol is found in animal tissues as a retinyl ester with long-chain FA. It is the storage form of vitamin A.

2. **Retinal:** This is the aldehyde derived from the oxidation of retinol.
   Retinal and retinol can readily be interconverted.

3. **Retinoic acid:** This is the acid derived from the oxidation of retinal. Retinoic acid cannot be reduced in the body and, therefore,
   cannot give rise to either retinal or retinol.

4. **β-Carotene:** Plant foods contain β-carotene (provitamin A), which
   can be oxidatively and symmetrically cleaved in the intestine to yield
   two molecules of retinal. In humans, the conversion is inefficient, and
   the vitamin A activity of β-carotene is only about 1/12 that of retinol.

B. Absorption and transport to the liver

Retinyl esters from the diet are hydrolyzed in the intestinal mucosa,
releasing retinol and FFA (Fig. 28.19). Retinol derived from esters
and from the reduction of retinal from β-carotene cleavage is
reesterified to long-chain FA within the enterocytes and secreted as a
component of chylomicrons into the lymphatic system. Retinyl esters
contained in chylomicron remnants are taken up by, and stored in, the
liver. [Note: All fat-soluble vitamins are carried in chylomicrons.]

C. Release from the liver

When needed, retinol is released from the liver and transported through
the blood to extrahepatic tissues by retinol-binding protein complexed
with transthyretin (see Fig. 28.19). The ternary complex binds to a
transport protein on the surface of the cells of peripheral tissues, permitting retinol to enter. An intracellular retinol-binding protein carries
retinol to sites in the nucleus where the vitamin regulates transcription
in a manner analogous to that of steroid hormones.

D. Retinoic acid mechanism of action

Retinol is oxidized to retinoic acid. Retinoic acid binds with high affinity to
specific receptor proteins (retinoic acid receptors [RAR]) present in the
nucleus of target tissues such as epithelial cells (Fig. 28.20). The activated retinoic acid–RAR complex binds to response elements on DNA
and recruits activators or repressors to regulate retinoid-specific RNA
synthesis, resulting in control of the production of specific proteins that
mediate several physiologic functions. For example, retinoids control the
expression of the gene for keratin in most epithelial tissues of the body.
[Note: The RAR proteins are part of the superfamily of transcriptional
regulators that includes the nuclear receptors for steroid and thyroid hormones and vitamin D, all of which function in a similar way (see p. 240).]

Figure 28.18
Structure of the retinoids.

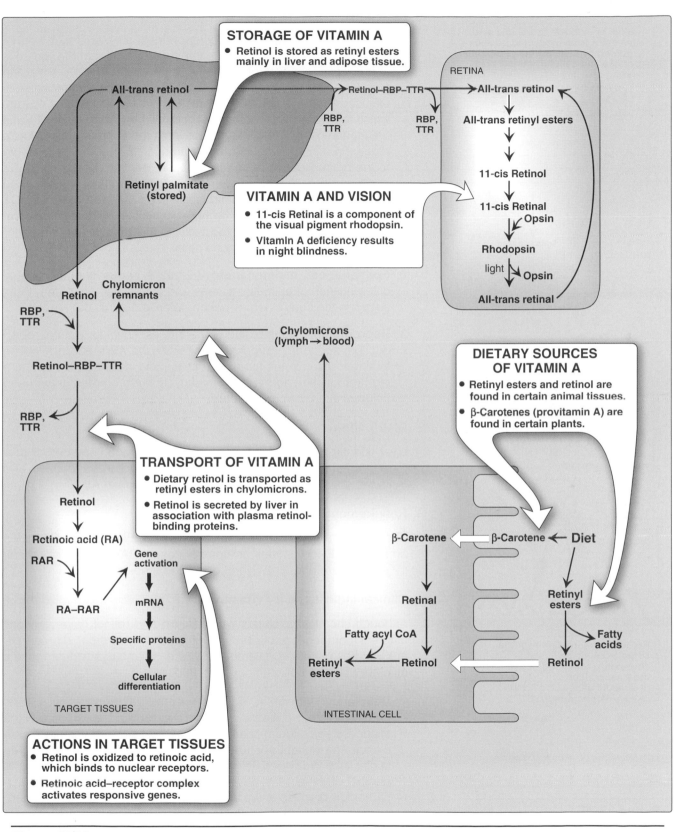

Figure 28.19

Absorption, transport, and storage of vitamin A and its derivatives. [Note: β-Carotene is a carotenoid, a plant pigment with antioxidant activity.] RBP = retinol binding protein; TTR = transthyretin; RAR = retinoic acid receptor; CoA = coenzyme A; mRNA = messenger RNA.

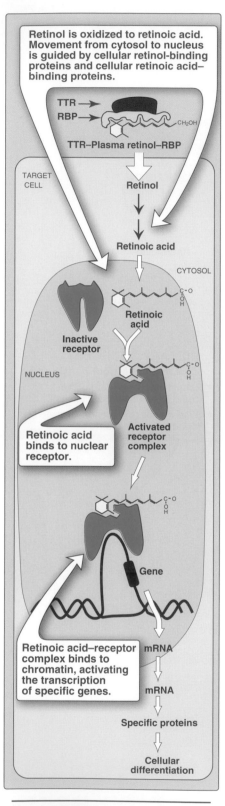

Figure 28.20

Action of the retinoids. [Note: Retinoic acid–receptor complex forms a dimer, but is shown as monomer for simplicity.] TTR = transthyretin; RBP = retinol-binding protein; mRNA = messenger RNA.

E. Functions

1. **Visual cycle:** Vitamin A is a component of the visual pigments of rod and cone cells. Rhodopsin, the visual pigment of the rod cells in the retina, consists of 11-cis retinal bound to the protein opsin (see Fig. 28.19). When rhodopsin, a G protein–coupled receptor, is exposed to light, a series of photochemical isomerizations occurs, which results in the bleaching of rhodopsin and release of all-trans retinal and opsin. This process activates the G protein transducin, triggering a nerve impulse that is transmitted by the optic nerve to the brain. Regeneration of rhodopsin requires isomerization of all-trans retinal back to 11-cis retinal. All-trans retinal is reduced to all-trans retinol, esterified, and isomerized to 11-cis retinol that is oxidized to 11-cis retinal. The latter combines with opsin to form rhodopsin, thus completing the cycle. Similar reactions are responsible for color vision in the cone cells.

2. **Epithelial cell maintenance:** Vitamin A is essential for normal differentiation of epithelial tissues and mucus secretion and, thus, supports the body's barrier-based defense against pathogens.

3. **Reproduction:** Retinol and retinal are essential for normal reproduction, supporting spermatogenesis in the male and preventing fetal resorption in the female. Retinoic acid is inactive in maintaining reproduction and in the visual cycle but promotes growth and differentiation of epithelial cells.

F. Distribution

Liver, kidney, cream, butter, and egg yolk are good sources of preformed vitamin A. Yellow, orange, and dark-green vegetables and fruits are good sources of the carotenes (provitamin A).

G. Requirement

The RDA for adults is 900 retinol activity equivalents (RAE) for males and 700 RAE for females. In comparison, 1 RAE = 1 μg of retinol, 12 μg of β-carotene, or 24 μg of other carotenoids.

H. Clinical indications for vitamin A

Although chemically related, retinoic acid and retinol have distinctly different therapeutic applications. Retinol and its carotenoid precursor are used as dietary supplements, whereas various forms of retinoic acid are useful in dermatology (Fig. 28.21).

1. **Deficiency:** Vitamin A, administered as retinol or retinyl esters, is used to treat patients who are deficient in the vitamin. Night blindness (nyctalopia) is one of the earliest signs of vitamin A deficiency. The visual threshold is increased, making it difficult to see in dim light. Prolonged deficiency leads to an irreversible loss in the number of visual cells. Severe deficiency leads to xerophthalmia, a pathologic dryness of the conjunctiva and cornea, caused, in part, by increased keratin synthesis. If untreated, xerophthalmia results in corneal ulceration and, ultimately, in blindness because of the formation of opaque scar tissue. The condition is most commonly seen in children in developing tropical countries. Over 500,000 children worldwide are blinded each year by xerophthalmia caused by insufficient vitamin A in the diet.

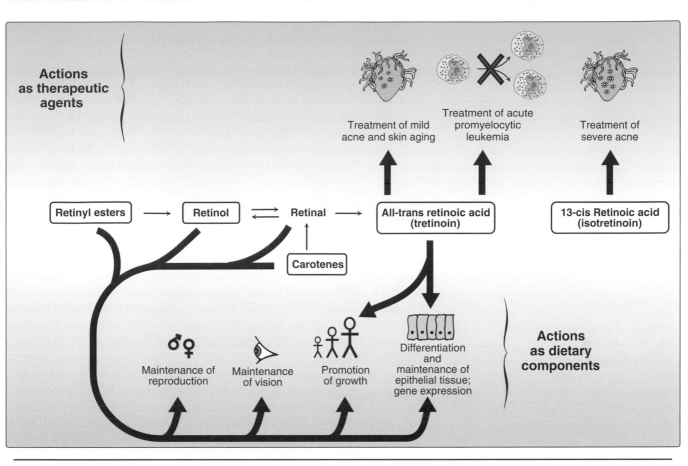

Figure 28.21
Summary of actions of retinoids. Compounds in ⎡boxes⎤ are available as dietary components or as pharmacologic agents.

2. **Skin conditions:** Dermatologic problems such as acne are effectively treated with retinoic acid or its derivatives (see Fig. 28.21). Mild cases of acne and skin aging are treated with tretinoin (all-trans retinoic acid). Tretinoin is too toxic for systemic (oral) administration in treating skin conditions and is confined to topical application. [Note: Oral tretinoin is used in treating acute promyelocytic leukemia.] In patients with severe cystic acne unresponsive to conventional therapies, isotretinoin (13-cis retinoic acid) is administered orally. An oral synthetic retinoid is used to treat psoriasis.

I. Retinoid toxicity

1. **Vitamin A:** Excessive intake of vitamin A (but not carotene) produces a toxic syndrome called hypervitaminosis A. Amounts exceeding 7.5 mg/day of retinol should be avoided. Early signs of chronic hypervitaminosis A are reflected in the skin, which becomes dry and pruritic (because of decreased keratin synthesis); in the liver, which becomes enlarged and can become cirrhotic; and in the CNS, where a rise in intracranial pressure may mimic the symptoms of a brain tumor. Pregnant women, in particular, should not ingest excessive quantities of vitamin A because of its potential for teratogenesis (causing congenital malformations in the developing fetus). UL is 3,000 μg preformed vitamin A/day. [Note: Vitamin A promotes bone growth. In

excess, however, it is associated with decreased bone mineral density and increased risk of fractures.]

2. **Isotretinoin:** The drug, an isomer of retinoic acid, is teratogenic and absolutely contraindicated in women with childbearing potential unless they have severe, disfiguring cystic acne that is unresponsive to standard therapies. Pregnancy must be excluded before treatment begins, and birth control must be used. Prolonged treatment with isotretinoin can result in an increase in TAG and cholesterol, providing some concern for an increased risk of CVD.

XII. VITAMIN D

The D vitamins are a group of sterols that have a hormone-like function. The active molecule, 1,25-dihydroxycholecalciferol ([1,25-diOH-D_3], or calcitriol), binds to intracellular receptor proteins. The 1,25-diOH-D_3–receptor complex interacts with response elements in the nuclear DNA of target cells in a manner similar to that of vitamin A (see Fig. 28.20) and either selectively stimulates or represses gene transcription. The most prominent actions of calcitriol are to regulate the serum levels of calcium and phosphorus.

A. Distribution

1. **Endogenous vitamin precursor:** 7-Dehydrocholesterol, an intermediate in cholesterol synthesis, is converted to cholecalciferol in the dermis and epidermis of humans exposed to sunlight and transported to liver bound to vitamin D–binding protein.

2. **Diet:** Ergocalciferol (vitamin D_2), found in plants, and cholecalciferol (vitamin D_3), found in animal tissues, are sources of preformed vitamin D activity (Fig. 28.22). Vitamin D_2 and vitamin D_3 differ chemically only in the presence of an additional double-bond and methyl group in the plant sterol. Dietary vitamin D is packaged into chylomicrons. [Note: Preformed vitamin D is a dietary requirement only in individuals with limited exposure to sunlight.]

B. Metabolism

1. **1,25-Dihydroxycholecalciferol formation:** Vitamins D_2 and D_3 are not biologically active but are converted <u>in</u> <u>vivo</u> to calcitriol, the active form of the D vitamin, by two sequential hydroxylation reactions (Fig. 28.23). The first hydroxylation occurs at the 25 position and is catalyzed by a specific *25-hydroxylase* in the liver. The product of the reaction, 25-hydroxycholecalciferol ([25-OH-D_3], calcidiol), is the predominant form of vitamin D in the serum and the major storage form. 25-OH-D_3 is further hydroxylated at the 1 position by *25-hydroxycholecalciferol 1-hydroxylase* found primarily in the kidney, resulting in the formation of 1,25-diOH-D_3 (calcitriol). [Note: Both *hydroxylases* are cytochrome P450 proteins (see p. 149).]

2. **Hydroxylation regulation:** Calcitriol is the most potent vitamin D metabolite. Its formation is tightly regulated by the level of serum phosphate (PO_4^{3-}) and calcium ions (Ca^{2+}) as shown in

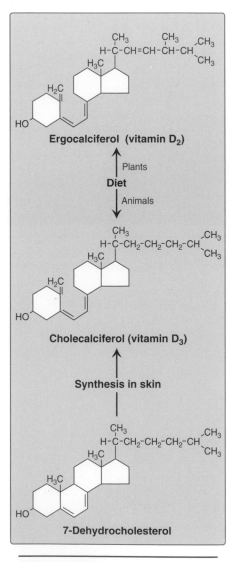

Figure 28.22
Sources of vitamin D. Vitamins D_2 and D_3 are first converted to calcidiol and then to calcitriol (active vitamin D). [Note: 7-Dehydrocholesterol (provitamin D_3) is decreased in the skin of older adults.]

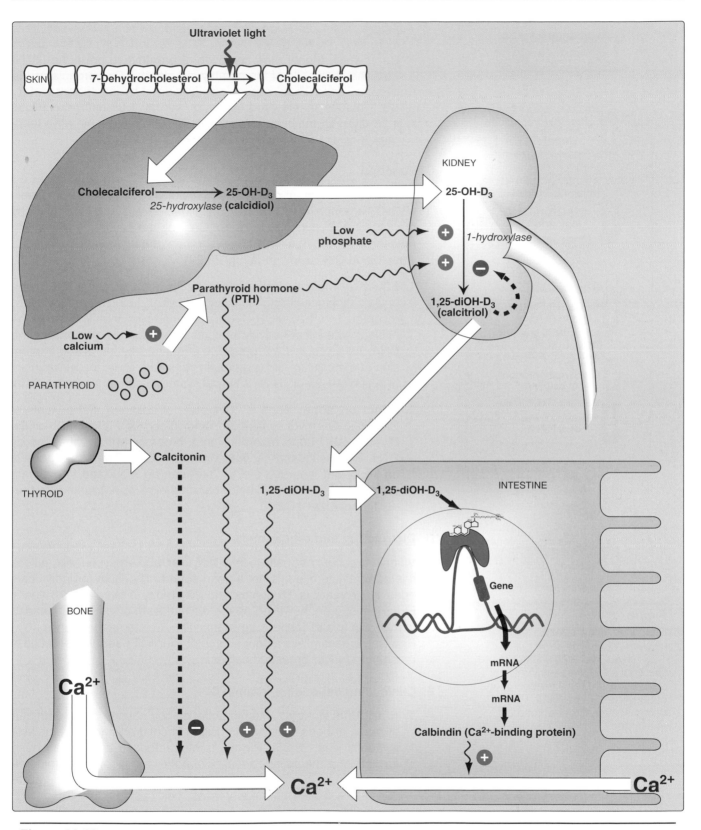

Figure 28.23
Metabolism and actions of vitamin D. [Note: Calcitonin, a thyroid hormone, decreases blood calcium (Ca^{2+}) by inhibiting mobilization from bone, absorption from the intestine, and reabsorption by the kidney. It opposes the actions of PTH.] mRNA = messenger RNA; 25-OH-D$_3$ = 25-hydroxycholecalciferol; 1,25-diOH-D$_3$ = 1,25-dihydroxycholecalciferol.

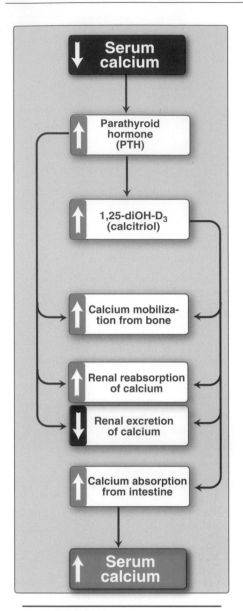

Figure 28.24

Response to low serum
calcium. 1,25-diOH-D$_3$ =
1,25-dihydroxycholecalciferol. [Note:
Calcitriol also increases intestinal
absorption and renal reabsorption
of phosphate. In contrast, PTH
decreases renal reabsorption of
phosphate.]

Figure 28.24. *25-Hydroxycholecalciferol 1-hydroxylase* activity is increased directly by low serum PO_4^{3-} or indirectly by low serum Ca^{2+}, which triggers the secretion of parathyroid hormone (PTH) from the chief cells of the parathyroid gland. PTH upregulates the *1-hydroxylase*. Thus, hypocalcemia caused by insufficient dietary Ca^{2+} results in elevated levels of serum 1,25-diOH-D$_3$. [Note: 1,25-diOH-D$_3$ inhibits expression of PTH, forming a negative feedback loop. It also inhibits activity of the *1-hydroxylase*.]

C. Function

The overall function of calcitriol is to maintain adequate serum levels of Ca^{2+}. It performs this function by 1) increasing uptake of Ca^{2+} by the intestine, 2) minimizing loss of Ca^{2+} by the kidney by increasing reabsorption, and 3) stimulating resorption (demineralization) of bone when blood Ca^{2+} is low (see Fig. 28.23).

1. **Effect on the intestine:** Calcitriol stimulates intestinal absorption of Ca^{2+} by first entering the intestinal cell and binding to a cytosolic receptor. The 1,25-diOH-D$_3$–receptor complex then moves to the nucleus where it selectively interacts with response elements on the DNA. As a result, Ca^{2+} uptake is enhanced by increased expression of the calcium-binding protein calbindin. Thus, the mechanism of action of 1,25-diOH-D$_3$ is typical of steroid hormones (see p. 240).

2. **Effect on bone:** Bone is composed of collagen and crystals of $Ca_5(PO_4)_3OH$ (hydroxylapatite). When blood Ca^{2+} is low, 1,25-diOH-D$_3$ stimulates bone resorption by a process that is enhanced by PTH. The result is an increase in serum Ca^{2+}. Therefore, bone is an important reservoir of Ca^{2+} that can be mobilized to maintain serum levels. [Note: PTH and calcitriol also work together to prevent renal loss of Ca^{2+}.]

D. Distribution and requirement

Vitamin D occurs naturally in fatty fish, liver, and egg yolk. Milk, unless it is artificially fortified, is not a good source. The RDA for individuals ages 1–70 years is 15 µg/day and 20 µg/day if over age 70 years. Experts disagree, however, on the optimal level of vitamin D needed to maintain health. [Note: 1 µg vitamin D = 40 international units (IU).] Because breast milk is a poor source of vitamin D, supplementation is recommended for breastfed babies.

E. Clinical indications for vitamin D

1. **Nutritional rickets:** Vitamin D deficiency causes a net demineralization of bone, resulting in rickets in children and osteomalacia in adults (Fig. 28.25). Rickets is characterized by the continued formation of the collagen matrix of bone, but incomplete mineralization results in soft, pliable bones. In osteomalacia, demineralization of preexisting bones increases their susceptibility to fracture. Insufficient exposure to daylight and/or deficiencies in vitamin D consumption occur predominantly in infants and the elderly. Vitamin D deficiency is more common in the northern latitudes, because less vitamin D synthesis occurs in the skin as a result of reduced exposure to ultraviolet light. [Note: Loss-of-function mutations in the vitamin D receptor result in hereditary vitamin D–deficient rickets.]

2. **Renal osteodystrophy:** Chronic kidney disease causes decreased ability to form active vitamin D as well as increased retention of PO_4^{3-}, resulting in hyperphosphatemia and hypocalcemia. The low blood Ca^{2+} causes a rise in PTH and associated bone demineralization with release of Ca^{2+} and PO_4^{3-}. Supplementation with vitamin D is an effective therapy. However, supplementation must be accompanied by PO_4^{3-} reduction therapy to prevent further bone loss and precipitation of calcium phosphate crystals.

3. **Hypoparathyroidism:** Lack of PTH causes hypocalcemia and hyperphosphatemia. [Note: PTH increases phosphate excretion.] Patients may be treated with vitamin D and calcium supplementation.

F. Toxicity

Like all fat-soluble vitamins, vitamin D can be stored in the body and is only slowly metabolized. High doses (100,000 IU for weeks or months) can cause loss of appetite, nausea, thirst, and weakness. Enhanced Ca^{2+} absorption and bone resorption results in hypercalcemia, which can lead to deposition of calcium salts in soft tissue (metastatic calcification). The UL is 100 µg/day (4,000 IU/day) for individuals ages 9 years or older, with a lower level for those under age 9 years. [Note: Toxicity is only seen with use of supplements. Excess vitamin D produced in the skin is converted to inactive forms.]

XIII. VITAMIN K

The principal role of vitamin K is in the posttranslational modification of a number of proteins (most of which are involved with blood clotting), in which it serves as a coenzyme in the carboxylation of certain glutamic acid residues in these proteins. Vitamin K exists in several active forms, for example, in plants as phylloquinone (or vitamin K_1), and in intestinal bacteria as menaquinone (or vitamin K_2). A synthetic form of vitamin K, menadione, is able to be converted to K_2.

A. Function

1. **γ-Carboxyglutamate formation:** Vitamin K is required in the hepatic synthesis of the blood clotting proteins, prothrombin (factor [F]II) and FVII, FIX, and FX. (See online Chapter 35.) Formation of the functional clotting factors requires the vitamin K–dependent carboxylation of several glutamic acid residues to γ-carboxyglutamate (Gla) residues (Fig. 28.26). The carboxylation reaction requires *γ-glutamyl carboxylase*, O_2, CO_2, and the hydroquinone form of vitamin K (which gets oxidized to the epoxide form). The formation of Gla residues is sensitive to inhibition by warfarin, a synthetic analog of vitamin K that inhibits *vitamin K epoxide reductase* (*VKOR*), the enzyme required to regenerate the functional hydroquinone form of vitamin K.

2. **Prothrombin interaction with membranes:** The Gla residues are good chelators of positively charged calcium ions, because of their two adjacent, negatively charged carboxylate groups. With prothrombin, for example, the prothrombin–calcium complex is able to bind to negatively charged membrane phospholipids on the surface of damaged endothelium and platelets. Attachment to

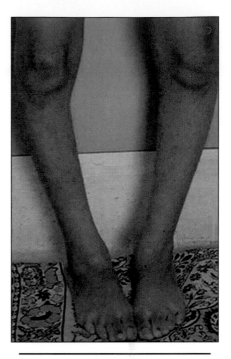

Figure 28.25
Bowed legs of middle-aged man with osteomalacia, a nutritional vitamin D deficiency that results in demineralization of the skeleton.

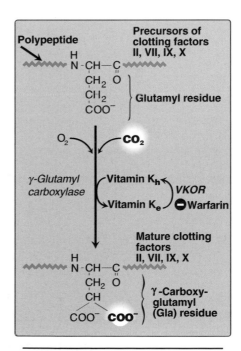

Figure 28.26
Carboxylation of glutamate to form γ-carboxyglutamate. h = hydroquinone; e = epoxide; *VKOR = vitamin K epoxide reductase.*

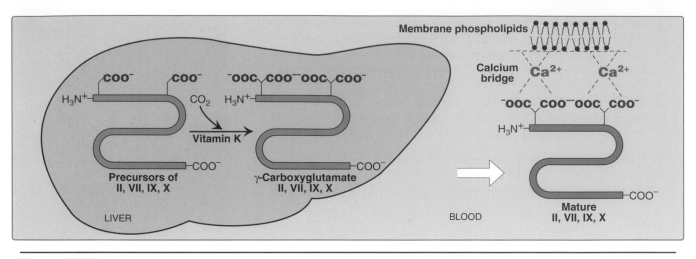

Figure 28.27
Role of vitamin K in blood coagulation. CO_2 = carbon dioxide.

membrane increases the rate at which the proteolytic conversion of prothrombin to thrombin can occur (Fig. 28.27).

3. **γ-Carboxyglutamate residues in other proteins:** Gla residues are also present in proteins other than those involved in forming a blood clot. For example, osteocalcin and matrix Gla protein of bone and proteins C and S (involved in limiting the formation of blood clots) also undergo γ-carboxylation.

B. Distribution and requirement

Vitamin K is found in cabbage, kale, spinach, egg yolk, and liver. The adequate intake for vitamin K is 120 μg/day for adult males and 90 μg for adult females. There is also synthesis of the vitamin by the gut microbiota.

C. Clinical indications for vitamin K

1. **Deficiency:** A true vitamin K deficiency is unusual because adequate amounts are generally obtained from the diet and produced by intestinal bacteria. If the bacterial population in the gut is decreased (for example, by antibiotics), the amount of endogenously formed vitamin is decreased, and this can lead to hypoprothrombinemia in the marginally malnourished individual (for example, a debilitated geriatric patient). This condition may require supplementation with vitamin K to correct the bleeding tendency. In addition, certain cephalosporin antibiotics (for example, cefamandole) cause hypoprothrombinemia, apparently by a warfarin-like mechanism that inhibits *VKOR*. Consequently, their use in treatment is usually supplemented with vitamin K. Deficiency can also affect bone health.

2. **Deficiency in the newborn:** Because newborns have sterile intestines, they initially lack the bacteria that synthesize vitamin K. Because human milk provides only about one fifth of the daily requirement for vitamin K, it is recommended that all newborns receive a single intramuscular dose of vitamin K as prophylaxis against hemorrhagic disease of the newborn.

D. Toxicity

Prolonged administration of large doses of menadione can produce hemolytic anemia and jaundice in the infant, because of toxic effects on the RBC membrane. Therefore, it is no longer used to treat vitamin K deficiency. No UL for the natural form has been set.

XIV. VITAMIN E

The E vitamins consist of eight naturally occurring tocopherols, of which α-tocopherol is the most active (Fig. 28.28). Vitamin E functions as an antioxidant in prevention of nonenzymic oxidations (for example, oxidation of LDL (see p. 232) and peroxidation of polyunsaturated FA by O_2 and free radicals). [Note: Vitamin C regenerates active vitamin E.]

A. Distribution and requirements

Vegetable oils are rich sources of vitamin E, whereas liver and eggs contain moderate amounts. The RDA for α-tocopherol is 15 mg/day for adults. The vitamin E requirement increases as the intake of polyunsaturated FA increases to limit FA peroxidation.

B. Deficiency

Newborns have low reserves of vitamin E, but breast milk (and formulas) contain the vitamin. Very-low-birth-weight infants may be given supplements to prevent the hemolysis and retinopathy associated with vitamin E deficiency. When observed in adults, deficiency is usually associated with defective lipid absorption or transport. [Note: Abetalipoproteinemia, caused by a defect in the formation of chylomicrons (and VLDL), results in vitamin E deficiency (see p. 231).]

C. Clinical indications for vitamin E

Vitamin E is not recommended for the prevention of chronic disease, such as CVD or cancer. Clinical trials using vitamin E supplementation have been uniformly disappointing. For example, subjects in the Alpha-Tocopherol, Beta-Carotene Cancer Prevention Study trial who received high doses of vitamin E not only lacked cardiovascular benefit but also had an increased incidence of stroke. [Note: Vitamins E and C are used to slow the progression of age-related macular degeneration.]

D. Toxicity

Vitamin E is the least toxic of the fat-soluble vitamins, and no toxicity has been observed at doses of 300 mg/day (UL = 1,000 mg/day).

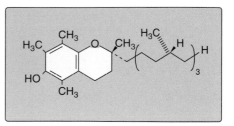

Figure 28.28
Structure of vitamin E (α-tocopherol).

> Populations consuming diets high in fruits and vegetables show decreased incidence of some chronic diseases. However, clinical trials have failed to show a definitive benefit from supplements of folic acid; vitamins A, C, or E; or antioxidant combinations for the prevention of cancer or CVD.

XV. CHAPTER SUMMARY

The vitamins are summarized in Figure 28.29 on pp. 396–397.

VITAMIN	OTHER NAMES	ACTIVE FORM	FUNCTION
Vitamin B_9	Folic acid	Tetrahydro-folic acid	Transfer one-carbon units; synthesis of methionine, serine, purine nucleotides, and thymidine monophosphate
Vitamin B_{12}	Cobalamin	Methylcobalamin Deoxyadenosyl cobalamin	Coenzyme for reactions: Homocysteine → methionine Methylmalonyl CoA → succinyl CoA
Vitamin C	Ascorbic acid	Ascorbic acid	Antioxidant Coenzyme for hydroxylation reactions, for example: In procollagen: Proline → hydroxyproline Lysine → hydroxylysine
Vitamin B_6	Pyridoxine Pyridoxamine Pyridoxal	Pyridoxal phosphate	Coenzyme for enzymes, particularly in amino acid metabolism
Vitamin B_1	Thiamine	Thiamine pyrophosphate	Coenzyme of enzymes catalyzing: Pyruvate → acetyl CoA α-Ketoglutarate → Succinyl CoA Ribose 5-P + xylulose 5-P → Sedoheptulose 7-P + Glyceraldehyde 3-P Branched-chain α-keto acid oxidation
Vitamin B_3	Niacin Nicotinic acid	NAD^+, $NADP^+$	Electron transfer
Vitamin B_2	Riboflavin	FMN, FAD	Electron transfer
Vitamin B_7	Biotin	Enzyme-bound biotin	Carboxylation reactions
Vitamin B_5	Pantothenic acid	Coenzyme A	Acyl carrier

WATER SOLUBLE

FAT SOLUBLE

Vitamin A	Retinol Retinal Retinoic acid β-Carotene	Retinol Retinal Retinoic acid	Maintenance of reproduction Vision Promotion of growth Differentiation and maintenance of epithelial tissues Gene expression
Vitamin D	Cholecalciferol Ergocalciferol	1,25-Dihydroxy-cholecalciferol	Calcium uptake Gene expression
Vitamin K	Menadione Menaquinone Phylloquinone	Menadione Menaquinone Phylloquinone	γ-Carboxylation of glutamate residues in clotting and other proteins
Vitamin E	α-Tocopherol	Any of several tocopherol derivatives	Antioxidant

Figure 28.29 (continued on next page)
Summary of vitamins. [Note: Choline, like vitamin D, is considered an essential micronutrient in humans even though we are able to synthesize it.] P = phosphate; NAD(P) = nicotinamide adenine dinucleotide (phosphate); FMN = flavin mononucleotide; FAD = flavin adenine dinucleotide; CoA = coenzyme A.

DEFICIENCY	SIGNS AND SYMPTOMS	TOXICITY	NOTES
Megaloblastic anemia Neural tube defects	Anemia Birth defects	None	Administration of high levels of folate can mask vitamin B_{12} deficiency
Pernicious anemia Dementia Spinal degeneration	Megaloblastic anemia Neuropsychiatric symptoms	None	Pernicious anemia is treated with intramuscular or high-dose oral vitamin B_{12}
Scurvy	Sore, spongy gums Loose teeth Poor wound healing Bleeding	None	Benefits of supplementation not established in controlled trials
Rare	Glossitis Neuropathy	Yes	Deficiency can be induced by isoniazid Sensory neuropathy occurs at high doses
Beriberi Wernicke-Korsakoff syndrome (most common in alcoholism)	Peripheral neuropathy (dry form), edema and cardiomyopathy (wet form) Confusion, ataxia, memory loss, hallucinations, dysregulated eye movements	None	—
Pellagra	Dermatitis Diarrhea Dementia	None	High doses of niacin used to treat hyperlipidemia
Rare	Dermatitis Angular stomatitis	None	—
Rare	Dermatitis	None	Consumption of large amounts of raw egg whites (which contains a protein, avidin, that binds biotin) can induce a biotin deficiency
Rare	—	None	—
			WATER SOLUBLE
			FAT SOLUBLE
Night blindness Xerophthalmia Infertility Growth retardation	Increased visual threshold Dryness of cornea	Yes	β-Carotene not acutely toxic, but supplementation is not recommended Excess vitamin A can increase incidence of fractures
Rickets (in children) Osteomalacia (in adults)	Soft, pliable bones	Yes	Vitamin D is not a true vitamin because it can be synthesized in skin; application of sunscreen lotions or presence of dark skin color decreases this synthesis.
Newborn Rare in adults	Bleeding	Rare	Vitamin K produced by intestinal bacteria. Vitamin K deficiency common in newborns Intramuscular treatment with vitamin K is recommended at birth
Rare	Red blood cell fragility leads to hemolytic anemia	None	Benefits of supplementation for disease prevention not established in controlled trials

Figure 28.29 (continued from previous page)
Summary of vitamins.

Study Questions

Choose the ONE best answer.

For Questions 28.1–28.5, match the vitamin deficiency to the clinical consequence.

A. Folic acid	E. Vitamin C
B. Niacin	F. Vitamin D
C. Vitamin A	G. Vitamin E
D. Vitamin B_{12}	H. Vitamin K

28.1 Bleeding

28.2 Diarrhea and dermatitis

28.3 Neural tube defects

28.4 Night blindness (nyctalopia)

28.5 Sore, spongy gums and loose teeth

28.6 A 52-year-old woman presents with fatigue of several months' duration. Blood studies reveal a macrocytic anemia, reduced levels of hemoglobin, elevated levels of homocysteine, and normal levels of methylmalonic acid. Which of the following is most likely deficient in this woman?

A. Folic acid
B. Folic acid and vitamin B_{12}
C. Iron
D. Vitamin C

28.7 A 10-month-old African American girl, whose family recently located from Maine to Virginia, is being evaluated for the bowed appearance of her legs. The parents report that the baby is still being breastfed and takes no supplements. Radiologic studies confirm the suspicion of rickets caused by vitamin D deficiency. Which one of the following statements concerning vitamin D is correct?

A. A deficiency results in an increased secretion of calbindin.
B. Chronic kidney disease results in overproduction of 1,25-dihydroxycholecalciferol (calcitriol).
C. 25-Hydroxycholecalciferol (calcidiol) is the active form of the vitamin.
D. It is required in the diet of individuals with limited exposure to sunlight.
E. Its actions are mediated through binding to G protein–coupled receptors.
F. It opposes the effect of parathyroid hormone.

28.8 Why might a deficiency of vitamin B_6 result in a fasting hypoglycemia? Deficiency of what other vitamin could also result in hypoglycemia?

Correct answers = H, B, A, C, E. Vitamin K is required for formation of the γ-carboxyglutamate residues in several proteins required for blood clotting. Consequently, a deficiency of vitamin K results in a tendency to bleed. Niacin deficiency is characterized by the three Ds: diarrhea, dermatitis, and dementia (and death, a fourth D, if untreated). Folic acid deficiency can result in neural tube defects in the developing fetus. Night blindness is one of the first signs of vitamin A deficiency. Rod cells in the retina detect white and black images and work best in low light, for example, at night. Rhodopsin, the visual pigment of the rod cells, consists of 11-cis retinal bound to the protein opsin. Vitamin C is required for the hydroxylation of proline and lysine during collagen synthesis. Severe vitamin C deficiency (scurvy) results in defective connective tissue, characterized by sore and spongy gums, loose teeth, capillary fragility, anemia, and fatigue.

Correct answer = A. Macrocytic anemia is seen with deficiencies of folic acid, vitamin B_{12}, or both. Vitamin B_{12} is utilized in only two reactions in the body: the remethylation of homocysteine (Hcy) to methionine, which also requires folic acid (as tetrahydrofolate [THF]), and the isomerization of methylmalonyl coenzyme A to succinyl coenzyme A, which does not require THF. The elevated Hcy and normal methylmalonic acid levels in the patient's blood reflect a deficiency of folic acid as the cause of the macrocytic anemia. Iron deficiency causes microcytic anemia, as can vitamin C deficiency.

Correct answer = D. Vitamin D is required in the diet of individuals with limited exposure to sunlight, such as those living at northern latitudes like Maine and those with dark skin. Note that breast milk is low in vitamin D, and the lack of supplementation increases the risk of a deficiency. Vitamin D deficiency results in decreased synthesis of calbindin. Chronic kidney disease decreases production of calcitriol (1,25-dihydroxycholecalciferol), the active form of the vitamin. Vitamin D binds to nuclear receptors and alters gene transcription. Its effects are synergistic with parathyroid hormone.

Vitamin B_6 is required for glycogen degradation by glycogen phosphorylase. A deficiency would result in fasting hypoglycemia. Additionally, a deficiency of biotin (required by pyruvate carboxylase of gluconeogenesis) would also result in fasting hypoglycemia.

Micronutrients: Minerals

29

I. OVERVIEW

Minerals are inorganic substances (elements) required in small amounts by the body. They function in a number of processes including formation of bones and teeth, fluid balance, nerve conduction, muscle contraction, signaling, and catalysis. [Note: Several minerals are essential enzyme cofactors.] Like the organic vitamins (see Chapter 28), minerals are micronutrients required in mg or μg amounts. Those required by adults in the largest amounts (>100 mg/day) are referred to as the macrominerals. Minerals required in amounts between 1 and 100 mg/day are the microminerals (trace minerals). Ultratrace minerals are required in amounts <1 mg/day (Fig. 29.1). [Note: The classification of specific minerals into these categories can vary among sources.] Mineral concentrations in the body are influenced by their rates of absorption and excretion.

II. MACROMINERALS

The macrominerals include calcium (Ca^{2+}), phosphorus ([P] as inorganic phosphate [P_i, or PO_4^{3-}]), magnesium (Mg^{2+}), sodium (Na^+), chloride (Cl^-), and potassium (K^+). [Note: The free ionic forms are electrolytes.]

A. Calcium and phosphorus

These macrominerals are considered together because they are components of hydroxylapatite ($Ca_5[PO_4]_3OH$), which makes up bones and teeth.

1. **Calcium:** Ca^{2+} is the most abundant mineral in the body, with ~98% being found in bones. The remainder is involved in a number of processes such as signaling, muscle contraction, and blood clotting. Ca^{2+} binds to a variety of proteins including calmodulin (see p. 133), *phospholipase A_2* (see p. 213), and *protein kinase C* (see p. 205) and alters their activity. [Note: Calbindin is a vitamin D–induced intracellular Ca^{2+}-binding protein involved in Ca^{2+} absorption in the intestine (see p. 392).] Dairy products, many green vegetables (for example, broccoli, but not spinach), and fortified orange juice are good dietary sources. Although dietary deficiency syndromes are unknown, average Ca^{2+} intake in the United States is insufficient for optimal bone health. Toxicity is seen only

MINERAL CLASSIFICATIONS	RDA (OR AI*) FOR ADULTS
MACROMINERALS	
Calcium (Ca)	1,000–2000 mg
Chloride (Cl)	1,800–2,300 mg*
Magnesium (Mg)	310–420 mg
Phosphorus (P)	700 mg
Potassium (K)	4,700 mg*
Sodium (Na)	1,500 mg*
MICROMINERALS (TRACE)	
Chromium (Cr)	30–35 mg
Copper (Cu)	900 μg
Fluorine (as fluoride [F^-])	3–4 mg
Iron (Fe)	8–18 mg
Manganese (Mn)	1.8–2.3 mg*
Zinc (Zn)	8–11 mg
MICROMINERALS (ULTRATRACE)	
Iodine (I)	150 μg
Molybdenum (Mo)	45 μg
Selenium (Se)	55 μg

Figure 29.1

Classification of minerals and recommended amounts to be consumed/day by adults. [Note: *An adequate intake (AI) is set if insufficient scientific evidence is available to calculate a Recommended Dietary Allowance (RDA).]

with supplements (tolerable upper limit [UL] = 2,500 mg/day for adults). Hypercalcemia (elevated serum Ca^{2+}) can result from overproduction of parathyroid hormone (PTH). This may cause constipation and kidney stones. Hypocalcemia (low serum Ca^{2+}) can result from a deficiency of PTH or vitamin D. It can lead to bone demineralization (resorption). [Note: The hormonal regulation of serum Ca^{2+} levels was presented in the vitamin D section of Chapter 28 and is reviewed in 3. below.]

> Bone mass increases from infancy through the early reproductive years and then shows an age-related loss in both men and women that increases the risk for fracture. This loss is greatest in postmenopausal Caucasian women. Some studies have shown that supplementation with Ca^{2+} and vitamin D decreases this risk.

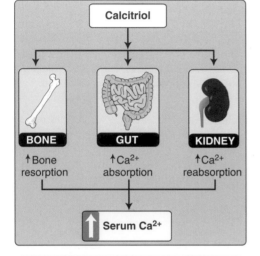

Figure 29.2
Effect of calcitriol on serum calcium (Ca^{2+}).

2. **Phosphorus:** Free phosphate (P_i) is the most abundant intracellular anion. However, 85% of the body's phosphorus is in the form of inorganic hydroxylapatite, with most of the remainder in intracellular organic compounds such as phospholipids, nucleic acids, ATP, and creatine phosphate. Phosphate is supplied as ATP for *kinases* and as P_i for *phosphorylases* (for example, *glycogen phosphorylase*, see p. 128). [Note: Its addition (by *kinases*) or removal (by *phosphatases*) is an important means of covalent regulation of enzymes (see Chapter 24).] Phosphorus is widely distributed in food (milk is a good source), and dietary deficiency is rare. Hypophosphatemia can be caused by refeeding carbohydrates to malnourished patients (refeeding syndrome, see p. 369), overuse of aluminum-containing antacids (aluminum chelates P_i), and increased urinary loss in response to increased production of PTH (see below). Muscle weakness is a common symptom. Hyperphosphatemia is caused primarily by decreased PTH levels. The excess P_i can combine with Ca^{2+} and form crystals that deposit in soft tissue (metastatic calcification). [Note: The Ca^{2+}/P_i ratio is important for bone formation (the ratio is ~2/1 in bone), and some experts are concerned that replacement of Ca^{2+}-rich milk by Ca^{2+}-poor, P_i-rich soft drinks can affect bone health.]

3. **Hormonal regulation:** Serum levels of Ca^{2+} and P_i are primarily controlled by calcitriol (1,25-dihydroxycholecalciferol, the active form of vitamin D) and PTH, both of which respond to a decrease in serum Ca^{2+}. Calcitriol, produced by the kidneys, increases serum Ca^{2+} and P_i by increasing bone resorption and intestinal absorption and renal reabsorption of Ca^{2+} and P_i (Fig. 29.2). PTH (from the parathyroid glands) increases serum Ca^{2+} by increasing bone resorption, increasing renal reabsorption of Ca^{2+}, and activating the renal *1-hydroxylase* that produces calcitriol from calcidiol (see p. 390) (Fig. 29.3). In contrast to calcitriol, PTH decreases P_i reabsorption in the kidneys, lowering serum P_i. [Note: High serum P_i increases PTH and decreases calcitriol.] A third hormone, calcitonin (from the C cells of the thyroid gland), responds to elevated serum Ca^{2+} levels by promoting bone mineralization and increasing renal excretion of Ca^{2+} (and P_i).

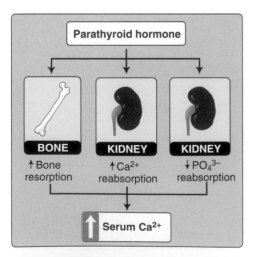

Figure 29.3
Effect of parathyroid hormone on serum calcium (Ca^{2+}). PO_4^{3-} = phosphate.

B. Magnesium

About 60% of the body's Mg^{2+} is in bone, but it accounts for just 1% of the bone mass. The mineral is required by a variety of enzymatic reactions, including phosphorylation by *kinases* (Mg^{2+} binds the ATP cosubstrate) and phosphodiester bond formation by *DNA and RNA polymerases*. Mg^{2+} is widely distributed in foods, but the average intake in the United States is below the recommended level. Hypomagnesemia can result from decreased absorption or increased excretion of Mg^{2+}. Symptoms include hyperexcitability of skeletal muscles and nerves and cardiac arrhythmias. With hypermagnesemia, hypotension is seen. [Note: Magnesium sulfate is used in the treatment of preeclampsia, a hypertensive disorder of pregnancy.]

C. Sodium, chloride, and potassium

These macrominerals are considered together because they play important roles in several physiologic processes. For example, they maintain water balance, osmotic equilibrium, acid–base balance (pH), and the electrical gradients across cell membranes (membrane potential) that are essential for the functioning of neurons and myocytes. [Note: These processes are discussed in Lippincott's Illustrated Reviews: Physiology.]

1. **Sodium and chloride:** Na^+ and Cl^- are primarily extracellular electrolytes. They are readily absorbed from foods containing salt (NaCl), much of which comes from processed foods. [Note: Na^+ is required for the intestinal absorption (and renal reabsorption) of glucose and galactose (see p. 87) and free amino acids (see p. 249) by Na^+-linked transporters. Cl^- is used to form hydrochloric acid required for digestion (see p. 248).] In the United States, the average daily consumption of NaCl is 1.5–3 times the adequate intake (AI) of 3.8 mg/day (UL = 5.8 g/day). Dietary deficiency is rare.

   a. **Hypertension:** Na^+ intake is related to blood pressure (BP). Ingestion of Na^+ stimulates thirst centers in the brain and secretion of antidiuretic hormone from the pituitary, leading to water retention. This results in an increase in plasma volume and, consequently, an increase in BP. Chronic hypertension can damage the heart, kidneys, and blood vessels. Modest reductions in Na^+ intake have been shown to result in modest reductions in BP. [Note: Some populations (for example, African Americans) are "salt sensitive" and have larger responses to Na^+.]

   b. **Hyper- and hyponatremia:** Hypernatremia, typically caused by excess water loss, and hyponatremia, typically caused by decreased ability to excrete water, can result in severe brain damage. [Note: Chronic hyponatremia increases Ca^{2+} excretion and can result in osteoporosis (low bone mass).]

2. **Potassium:** In contrast to Na^+, K^+ is primarily an intracellular electrolyte. [Note: The concentration differential of Na^+ and K^+ across the cell membrane is maintained by the *Na^+/K^+ ATPase* (Fig. 29.4).] In contrast to Na^+ and Cl^-, K^+ (like Mg^{2+}) is underingested in Western diets because its primary sources, fruits and vegetables, are underingested. [Note: Increasing dietary K^+ decreases BP

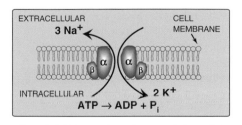

Figure 29.4
Na^+/K^+ ATPase. Na^+ = sodium; K^+ = potassium; ADP = adenosine diphosphate; P_i = phosphate.

by increasing Na$^+$ excretion.] There is a narrow range for normal serum K$^+$ levels, and even modest changes (up or down, resulting in hyper- or hypokalemia) can result in cardiac arrhythmias and skeletal muscle weakness. [Note: Hypokalemia can result from the inappropriate use of laxatives to lose weight.] No UL for K$^+$ has been established.

Cu-REQUIRING ENZYME	FUNCTION
Cytochrome c oxidase	Transfers electrons from cytochrome c to oxygen in the ETC (see p. 75)
Dopamine β-hydroxylase	Hydroxylates dopamine to norepinephrine (see p. 286)
Ferroxidases	Oxidize iron (see. p. 403)
Lysyl oxidase	Forms cross-links in collagen and elastin (see pp. 48–49)
Tyrosinase	Synthesizes melanin (see p. 288)
Superoxide dismutase (nonmitochondrial form; also requires zinc)	Converts superoxide to hydrogen peroxide (see p. 148)

Figure 29.5
Examples of enzymes that require copper (Cu). ETC = electron transport chain.

VARIABLE	MENKES	WILSON
Whole-body Cu	Low	High
Free serum Cu	Low	High
Urinary Cu	Low	High
Inheritance	X-linked	AR
Cu-transporting ATPase affected	*ATP7A*	*ATP7B*

Figure 29.6
Comparison of Menkes syndrome and Wilson disease. Cu = copper; AR = autosomal recessive.

III. MICROMINERALS (TRACE MINERALS)

The trace minerals include copper (Cu), iron (Fe), manganese (Mn), and zinc (Zn). They are required by adults in amounts between 1 and 100 mg/day.

A. Copper

Cu is a key component of several enzymes that play critical functions in the body (Fig. 29.5). These include *ferroxidases* such as the *ceruloplasmin* and *hephaestin* involved in the oxidation of ferrous iron (Fe^{2+}) to the ferric form (Fe^{3+}) that is required for its intracellular storage or transport through blood (see B.1. below). Meat, shellfish, nuts, and whole grains are good dietary sources of Cu. Dietary deficiency is uncommon. If a deficiency does develop, anemia may be seen because of the effect on Fe metabolism. Toxicity from dietary sources is rare (UL = 10 mg/day). Menkes syndrome and Wilson disease are genetic causes of Cu deficiency and Cu overload, respectively.

1. **Menkes syndrome:** In Menkes syndrome ("kinky hair" disease), a rare X-linked (1:140,000 males) disorder, efflux of dietary Cu out of intestinal enterocytes into the circulation by a Cu-transporting ATPase (*ATP7A*) is impaired. This results in systemic Cu deficiency. Consequently, urinary and serum free (unbound) Cu are low, as is the concentration of *ceruloplasmin*, which carries over 90% of the Cu in the circulation (Fig. 29.6). Progressive neurologic degeneration and connective tissue disorders are seen, as are changes to hair. Parenteral administration of Cu has been used as a treatment with varying success. [Note: The mildest form of Menkes syndrome is called occipital horn syndrome.]

2. **Wilson disease:** In Wilson disease, an autosomal-recessive (AR) disorder affecting 1:35,000 live births, efflux of excess Cu from the liver by *ATP7B* is impaired. Cu accumulates in the liver; leaks into the blood; and is deposited in the brain, eyes, kidneys, and skin. In contrast to Menkes syndrome, urinary and serum free Cu are high (see Fig. 29.6). Hepatic dysfunction and neurologic and psychiatric symptoms are seen. Kayser-Fleischer rings (corneal deposits of Cu) may be present (Fig. 29.7). Life-long use of Cu-chelating agents, such as penicillamine, is the treatment.

> The bioavailability (percent of the amount ingested that is able to be absorbed) of a mineral can be influenced by other minerals. For example, excess Zn decreases the absorption of Cu, and Cu is needed for the absorption of Fe.

B. Iron

The adult body typically contains 3–4 g of Fe. It is a component of many proteins, both catalytic (for example, *hydroxylases* such as *prolyl hydroxylase*, see p. 47) and noncatalytic. Iron can be linked to sulfur (S) as seen in the Fe–S proteins of the electron transport chain (see p. 75), or it can be part of the heme prosthetic group (see p. 25) in proteins such as hemoglobin (~70% of all Fe), myoglobin, and the cytochromes. [Note: Free ionic Fe is toxic because it can cause production of the hydroxyl radical, a reactive oxygen species (ROS).] Dietary Fe is available as Fe^{2+} in heme (animal sources) and Fe^{3+} in nonheme sources (plants). Heme iron is less abundant, but it is better absorbed. Meat, poultry, some shellfish, ready-to-eat cereals, lentils, and molasses are good dietary sources of Fe. About 10% of ingested Fe is absorbed. This amount, ~1–2 mg/day, is sufficient to replace Fe lost from the body primarily by the sloughing of cells.

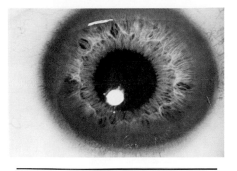

Figure 29.7
Kaiser-Fleischer rings.

1. **Absorption, storage, and transport:** Intestinal uptake of heme is by a heme carrier protein (Fig. 29.8). Within the enterocytes, *heme oxygenase* releases Fe^{2+} from heme (see p. 282). Nonheme Fe is taken up via the apical membrane protein divalent metal ion transporter-1 (DMT-1). [Note: Vitamin C enhances absorption of nonheme Fe because it is the coenzyme for *duodenal cytochrome b (Dcytb)*, a *ferrireductase* that reduces Fe^{3+} to Fe^{2+}.] Absorbed Fe^{2+} from heme and nonheme sources has two possible fates: It can be 1) oxidized to Fe^{3+} and stored by the intracellular protein ferritin (up to 4,500 Fe^{3+}/ferritin) or 2) transported out of the enterocyte by the basolateral membrane protein ferroportin, oxidized by the Cu-containing membrane protein *hephaestin*, and taken up by the plasma transport protein transferrin (2 Fe^{3+}/transferrin), as

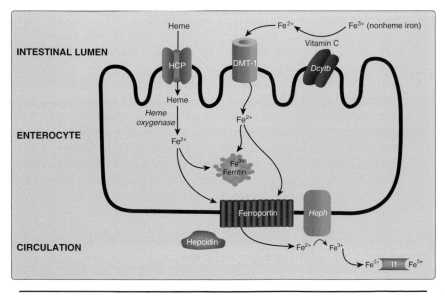

Figure 29.8
Absorption, storage, and transport of dietary iron (Fe). HCP = heme carrier protein; DMT = divalent metal ion transporter; *Dcytb = duodenal cytochrome b* (a *ferrireductase*); *Heph = hephaestin*; Tf = transferrin.

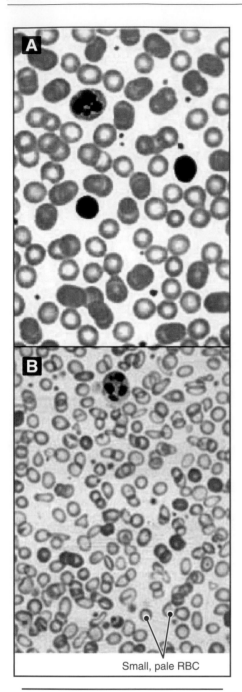

Figure 29.9
A. Normal red blood cells (RBC).
B. Small (microcytic), pale
(hypochromic) RBC in microcytic
anemia.

shown in Figure 29.8. [Note: Cells other than enterocytes use the Cu-containing plasma protein *ceruloplasmin* in place of *hephaestin*.] In normal individuals, transferrin (Tf) is about one third saturated with Fe^{3+}. Ferroportin, the only known exporter of Fe from cells to the blood in humans, is regulated by the hepatic peptide hepcidin that induces internalization and lysosomal degradation of ferroportin. Therefore, hepcidin is the central molecule in Fe homeostasis. [Note: Transcription of hepcidin is suppressed when Fe is deficient.]

2. **Recycling:** Macrophages phagocytose old and/or damaged red blood cells (RBC), freeing heme Fe that is sent out of the cells via ferroportin, oxidized by *ceruloplasmin*, and transported by Tf as described above. This recycled Fe meets ~90% of our daily need, which is predominantly for erythropoiesis.

3. **Uptake:** Tf-bound Fe^{3+} from enterocytes and macrophages binds to receptors (TfR) on erythroblasts and other Fe-requiring cells and is taken up by receptor-mediated endocytosis. The Fe^{3+} is released from Tf for use (or stored on ferritin), and the TfR (and Tf) is recycled in a process similar to the receptor-mediated endocytosis seen with low-density lipoprotein particles (see p. 231). [Note: Regulation of the translation of the messenger RNA for ferritin and the TfR by iron regulatory proteins and iron-responsive elements is discussed on p. 474.]

4. **Deficiency:** Fe deficiency can result in a microcytic, hypochromic anemia (Fig. 29.9), the most common anemia in the United States, as a result of decreased hemoglobin synthesis and, consequently, decreased RBC size. Treatment is the administration of Fe.

5. **Excess:** Fe overload can occur with accidental ingestion. [Note: Acute Fe poisoning is the most common cause of poisoning deaths of children age <6 years (UL = 40 mg/day for children, 45 mg/day for adults).] Treatment is use of an Fe chelator. Overload can also occur with genetic defects. An example is hereditary hemochromatosis (HH), an AR disorder of Fe overload found primarily in those of Northern European ancestry. It is most commonly caused by mutations to the HFE (high iron) gene. Hyperpigmentation with hyperglycemia ("bronze diabetes") and damage to the liver (a major storage site for Fe), pancreas, and heart may be seen. In HH, serum Fe and Tf saturation are elevated. Treatment is phlebotomy or use of Fe chelators. [Note: Fe overload is seen with mutations to proteins of Fe metabolism that result in inappropriately low levels of hepcidin. It can result in hemosiderosis (the deposition of hemosiderin, an intracellular, insoluble storage form of Fe).]

C. Manganese

Mn is important for the function of several enzymes (Fig. 29.10). Whole grains, legumes (for example, beans and peas), nuts, and tea (especially green tea) are good sources of the mineral. Consequently, Mn deficiency in humans is rare. Toxicity from foods and/or supplements is also rare (UL = 11 mg/day for adults).

D. Zinc

Zn plays important structural and catalytic functions in the body. Zinc fingers are supersecondary structures (motifs, see p. 18) in proteins (for example, transcription factors) that bind to DNA and regulate gene expression (Fig. 29.11). Hundreds of enzymes require Zn for activity. Examples include *alcohol dehydrogenase*, which oxidizes ethanol to acetaldehyde (see p. 317); *carbonic anhydrase*, which is important in the bicarbonate buffer system (see p. 30); *porphobilinogen synthase* of heme synthesis, which is inhibited by lead (lead replaces the zinc; see p. 279); and the nonmitochondrial isoform of *superoxide dismutase* (*SOD*), which also requires Cu (see Fig. 29.5). Dietary sources of Zn include meat, fish, eggs, and dairy products. Phytates (phosphate storage molecules in some plant products) irreversibly bind Zn in the intestine, decreasing its absorption, and can result in a deficiency. [Note: Phytates may also bind Ca^{2+} and nonheme Fe.] Several drugs (for example, penicillamine) chelate metals, and their use may cause Zn deficiency. [Note: Severe deficiency is seen with a defect in the intestinal transporter for Zn that results in the malabsorption disorder acrodermatitis enteropathica. Symptoms include rashes, slowed growth and development, diarrhea, and immune deficiencies. Vision problems may also occur because Zn is needed in the metabolism of vitamin A.]

> Eukaryotic cells infected with bacteria can restrict availability of the essential micronutrients Fe, Mn, and Zn to the pathogens. This decreases the intracellular survival of the pathogen and is known as "nutritional immunity."

E. Other microminerals

Chromium (Cr) and fluorine (F) also play roles in the body. Cr potentiates the action of insulin by an unknown mechanism. It is found in fruits, vegetables, dairy products, and meat. F (as fluoride [F^-]) is added to water in many parts of the world to reduce the incidence of dental caries (Fig. 29.12). F^- replaces the hydroxyl group of hydroxylapatite, forming fluoroapatite that is more resistant to the enamel-dissolving acid produced by mouth bacteria.

IV. ULTRATRACE MINERALS

The ultratrace minerals include iodine (I), selenium (Se), and molybdenum (Mo). They are required by adults in amounts <1 mg/day.

A. Iodine

I is utilized in the synthesis of the thyroid hormones triiodothyronine (T_3) and thyroxine (T_4) that are required for development, growth, and metabolism. Circulating iodide (I^-) is taken up ("trapped") and concentrated in the epithelial follicular cells of the thyroid gland. It then is sent into the colloid of the follicular lumen where it is oxidized to iodine (I_2) by *thyroperoxidase* (*TPO*), as shown in Figure 29.13.

Mn-REQUIRING ENZYME	FUNCTION
Arginase-I	Hydrolyzes arginine to urea plus ornithine in the urea cycle (see p. 255)
Glycosyltransferases	Transfer sugars in proteoglycan synthesis (see p. 158)
Pyruvate carboxylase	Carboxylates pyruvate to OAA in gluconeogenesis (see p. 118)
Superoxide dismutase (mitochondrial form)	Converts superoxide to hydrogen peroxide (see p. 148)

Figure 29.10
Examples of enzymes that require manganese (Mn). OAA = oxaloacetate.

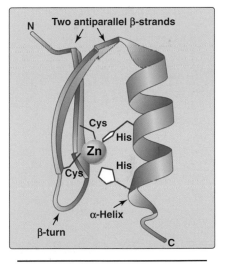

Figure 29.11
Zinc (Zn) finger is a common motif in proteins that bind DNA. Cys = cysteine; His = histidine.

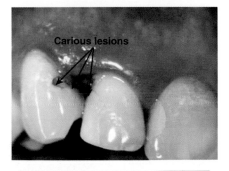

Figure 29.12
Dental caries (cavities).

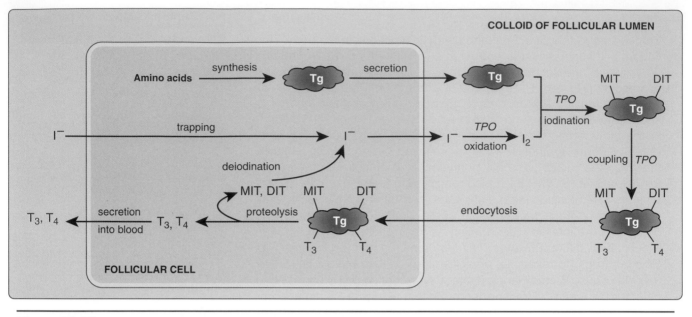

Figure 29.13

Thyroid hormone synthesis. Tg = thyroglobulin; I^- = iodide; I_2 = iodine; *TPO = thyroperoxidase*; MIT = monoiodinated tyrosine; DIT = diiodinated tyrosine; T_3 = triiodothyronine; T_4 = thyroxine.

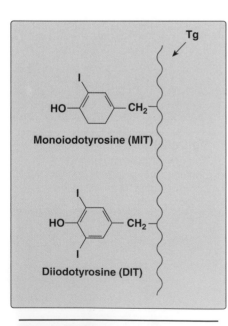

Figure 29.14

Iodination of thyroglobulin (Tg) with production of MIT and DIT.

TPO then uses I_2 to iodinate selected tyrosine residues in thyroglobulin (Tg), forming monoiodinated tyrosine (MIT) and diiodinated tyrosine (DIT), as shown in Figure 29.14. [Note: Tg is synthesized and secreted into colloid by follicular cells.] The coupling of two DIT on Tg gives T_4, whereas coupling one MIT and one DIT gives T_3. The iodinated Tg is endocytosed and stored in follicular cells until needed, at which time it is proteolytically digested to release T_3 and T_4, which are secreted into the circulation (see Fig. 29.13). Under normal conditions, ~90% of secreted thyroid hormone is T_4 that is carried by transthyretin. In target tissues (for example, the liver and developing brain), T_4 is converted to T_3 (the more active form) by Se-containing *deiodinases*. T_3 binds to a nuclear receptor that binds DNA at thyroid response elements and functions as a transcription factor. [Note: Thyroid hormone production is controlled by thyrotropin (thyroid-stimulating hormone ([TSH]) from the anterior pituitary. TSH secretion is itself controlled by thyrotropin-releasing hormone (TRH) from the hypothalamus.]

1. **Hypothyroidism:** Underingestion of I can result in goiter (enlargement of the thyroid in response to excessive stimulation by TSH), as shown in Figure 29.15. More severe deficiency results in hypothyroidism that is characterized by fatigue, weight gain, decreased thermogenesis, and decreased metabolic rate (see p. 359). If hormone deficiency occurs during fetal and infant development (congenital hypothyroidism), irreversible intellectual disability (formerly called "cretinism"), hearing loss, spasticity, and short stature can result. In the United States, dairy products, seafood, and meat are the primary sources of I. The use of iodized salt has greatly reduced

dietary I deficiency. [Note: Autoimmune destruction of *TPO* is a cause of Hashimoto thyroiditis (a primary hypothyroidism).]

2. **Hyperthyroidism:** This condition is the result of overproduction of thyroid hormone. Although it can be caused by overingestion of I-containing supplements (UL = 1.1 g/day for adults), the most common cause of hyperthyroidism is Graves disease, in which an antibody that mimics the effect of TSH is produced, resulting in dysregulated production of thyroid hormone. This can cause nervousness, weight loss, increased perspiration and heart rate, protruding eyes (exophthalmos, Fig. 29.16), and goiter.

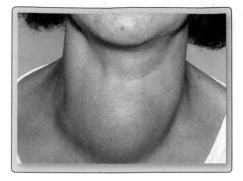

Figure 29.15
Goiter.

B. Selenium

Se is present in ~25 human proteins (selenoproteins) as a constituent of the amino acid selenocysteine, which is derived from serine (see p. 268). Selenoproteins include *glutathione peroxidase* that oxidizes glutathione in the reduction of hydrogen peroxide, a ROS, to water (see p. 148); *thioredoxin reductase* that reduces thioredoxin, a coenzyme of *ribonucleotide reductase* (see p. 297); and *deiodinases* that remove I from thyroid hormones. Meat, dairy products, and grains are important dietary sources. Keshan disease, first identified in China, is a cardiomyopathy caused by eating foods produced from Se-deficient soil. Toxicity (selenosis) caused by overingestion of supplements causes brittle nails and hair. Cutaneous and neurologic effects may also be seen (UL = 400 μg in adults).

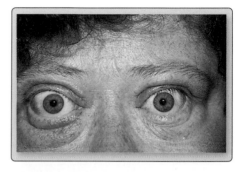

Figure 29.16
Exophthalmos.

C. Molybdenum

Mo functions as a cofactor for a small number of mammalian *oxidases* (Fig. 29.17). Legumes are important dietary sources. No dietary deficiency syndromes are known. Mo has low toxicity in humans (UL = 2 mg/day in adults).

> Cobalt (Co), an ultratrace mineral, is a component of vitamin B$_{12}$ (cobalamin, see p. 379), which is required as methylcobalamin in the remethylation of homocysteine to methionine (see p. 264) or adenosylcobalamin in the isomerization of methylmalonyl coenzyme A (CoA) to succinyl CoA (see p. 194). No Recommended Dietary Allowance or Daily Reference Intake (see p. 358) has been established for Co.

Mo-REQUIRING ENZYME	FUNCTION
Aldehyde oxidase	Metabolizes drugs
Sulfite oxidase	Converts sulfite to sulfate in metabolism of the sulfur-containing amino acids methionine and cysteine (see pp. 263–264)
Xanthine oxidase	Oxidizes hypoxanthine to xanthine and xanthine to uric acid in purine degradation (see p. 299)

Figure 29.17
Enzymes (*oxidases*) that require molybdenum (Mo).

V. CHAPTER SUMMARY

The minerals are summarized in Figure 29.18 on p. 408.

CLASSIFICATION	FUNCTION(S)	NOTES
Macrominerals: **>100 mg/day for adults**		
Calcium (Ca)	Component of hydroxylapatite ($Ca_5[PO_4]_3OH$) of bone and teeth, muscle contraction, signaling, blood clotting	Dietary deficiencies unknown; toxicity from supplements; hypocalcemia with PTH or vitamin D deficiency causes kidney stones; hypercalcemia with increased PTH causes bone resorption
Chloride (Cl)	Fluid balance (along with Na, K), digestion	Dietary deficiency rare; overingested as NaCl
Magnesium (Mg)	Component (minor) of bone; regulates enzyme activity (binds substrate or enzyme)	Average U.S. intake is below recommended level; hyperexcitability and arrhythmias seen with hypomagnesemia; hypotension with hypermagnesemia
Phosphorus (P)	Component of hydroxylapatite of bone and teeth, energy storage, membrane structure, regulation	Dietary deficiency rare; hypophosphatemia with muscle weakness in refeeding syndrome, increased PTH, and use of aluminum-containing antacids; hyperphosphatemia with metastatic calcification in PTH deficiency
Potassium (K)	Membrane potential, blood pressure	Average U.S. intake is below recommended level; modest changes up or down in serum level result in arrhythmias and muscle weakness
Sodium (Na)	Membrane potential; blood volume and pressure; uptake of glucose, galactose, and amino acids	Dietary deficiency rare; overingested as NaCl; hyponatremia seen with excess water loss; hypernatremia with water retention
Microminerals (Trace): **1–100 mg/day**		
Chromium (Cr)	Potentiates insulin action	Mechanism unknown
Copper (Cu)	Enzyme cofactor	Dietary deficiency rare; Menkes (genetic systemic Cu deficiency) and Wilson (genetic systemic Cu overload)
Fluorine (as fluoride [F^-])	Increases resistance to enamel-dissolving acid of mouth bacteria	Deficiency results in dental caries
Iron (Fe)	Enzyme cofactor, oxygen binding, Fe-S proteins	Dietary deficiency results in microcytic anemia; hereditary hemochromatosis, a genetic disease of Fe overload, with "bronze diabetes" (hyperglycemia, hyperpigmentation)
Manganese (Mn)	Enzyme cofactor	Dietary deficiency rare
Zinc (Zn)	Enzyme cofactor, protein structure (Zn finger)	Phytates and some drugs decrease absorption; severe deficiency (acrodermatitis enteropathica) with transporter defect
Microminerals (Ultratrace): **<1 mg/day**		
Iodine (I)	Thyroid hormone (T_3, T_4) synthesis	Underingestion causes goiter, hypothyroidism with fatigue, weight gain, and decreased metabolic rate; neurologic damage in congenital deficiency; hyperthyroidism (overproduction of T_3, T_4) in Graves disease
Molybdenum (Mo)	Enzyme cofactor	Dietary deficiency unknown
Selenium (Se)	Found (as selenocysteine) in selenoproteins	Dietary deficiency rare (Keshan disease with Se-deficient soil), toxicity from supplements

Figure 29.18

Summary of minerals. PTH = parathyroid hormone; Cl^- = chloride; S = sulfur; T_3 = triiodothyronine; T_4 = thyroxine.

Study Questions

For Questions 29.1–29.7, match the mineral to the most appropriate description.

A. Calcium
B. Chloride
C. Copper
D. Iodine
E. Iron
F. Magnesium
G. Manganese
H. Molybdenum
I. Phosphorus
J. Potassium
K. Selenium
L. Sodium
M. Zinc

29.1 Elevated levels of which mineral may result in hypertension in certain populations?

29.2 Which mineral is the major extracellular anion?

29.3 A decrease of which mineral is seen in refeeding syndrome and with overuse of aluminum-containing antacids?

29.4 Which mineral is a constituent of some amino acids found in proteins involved in antioxidant defense, thyroid hormone metabolism, and redox reactions?

29.5 Which mineral is required for the formation of a supersecondary protein structure that allows binding to DNA? (Its deficiency can result in a dermatitis.)

29.6 Deficiency of which mineral can cause bone pain, tetany (intermittent muscle spasms), paresthesia (a "pins and needles" sensation), and an increased tendency to bleed?

29.7 Deficiency of which mineral can result in goiter and a decreased metabolic rate?

Correct answers = L, B, I, K, M, A, D. Hypernatremia (elevation of serum sodium) can lead to water retention that can cause hypertension in salt-sensitive populations (for example, African Americans). Chloride is the major extracellular anion. [Note: Sodium is the major extracellular cation, potassium is the major intracellular cation, and phosphate is the major intracellular anion. The concentration differential across the membrane is maintained by active transport.] Carbohydrate metabolism involves the generation of phosphorylated intermediates. Refeeding severely malnourished individuals traps phosphate and results in hypophosphatemia. Muscle weakness is a common symptom. Selenocysteine, an amino acid formed from serine and selenium, is found in proteins (selenoproteins) such as glutathione peroxidase, deiodinases, and thioredoxin reductase. Zinc fingers are a type of structural motif found in proteins (for example, transcription factors) that bind to DNA. Severe deficiency of zinc as a result of mutations to its intestinal transporter can result in acrodermatitis enteropathica, which is characterized by dermatitis, diarrhea, and alopecia. Calcium is required for bone mineralization, muscle contraction, nerve conduction, and blood clotting. Its deficiency will affect all of these processes. Thyroid hormones are iodinated tyrosines released by proteolytic digestion of thyroglobulin. Underingestion of iodine causes enlargement of the thyroid in an attempt to increase hormone synthesis. [Note: Goiter can also result if too much hormone is made, as in Graves disease, or if too little is made, as in Hashimoto disease. Both are autoimmune diseases.] Thyroid hormone increases the resting metabolic rate.

29.8 DiGeorge syndrome is a congenital condition that results in structural anomalies and failure of the thymus and parathyroid glands to develop. Clinical manifestations include recurrent infections as a consequence of a deficiency in T cells. Which one of the following is an expected clinical consequence of the deficiency in parathyroid hormone?

A. Increased bone resorption
B. Increased calcium reabsorption in the kidney
C. Increased serum calcitriol
D. Increased serum phosphate

Correct answer = D. Parathyroid hormone (PTH) increases bone resorption (demineralization) resulting in the release of calcium and phosphate. It also increases the renal reabsorption of calcium, because PTH activates the renal hydroxylase that converts calcidiol to calcitriol. PTH also increases the renal excretion of phosphate. With the hypoparathyroidism of DiGeorge syndrome, all of these activities of PTH are impaired. Consequently, hypocalcemia and hyperphosphatemia are seen.

For questions 29.9 and 29.10, match the signs and symptoms to the pathology.

A. Graves disease
B. Hereditary hemochromatosis
C. Hypercalcemia
D. Hyperphosphatemia
E. Keshan disease
F. Menkes syndrome
G. Selenosis
H. Wilson disease

29.9 A 28-year-old male is seen for complaints of recent, severe, upper-right-quadrant pain. He also reports some difficulty with fine motor tasks. No jaundice is observed on physical examination. Laboratory tests were remarkable for elevated liver function tests (serum aspartate and alanine aminotransferases) and elevated urinary calcium and phosphate. Ophthalmology consult revealed Kayser-Fleischer rings in the cornea. The patient was started on penicillamine and zinc.

Correct answer = H. The patient has Wilson disease, an autosomal-recessive disorder that decreases copper efflux from the liver because of mutations to the hepatic copper transport protein ATP7B. Some copper leaks into the blood and is deposited in the brain, eyes, kidney, and skin. This results in liver and kidney damage, neurologic effects, and corneal changes caused by the excess copper. Administration of the metal chelator penicillamine is the treatment. [Note: Because zinc is also chelated, supplementation with zinc is common.] Graves disease results in hyperthyroidism. Hereditary hemochromatosis is a disorder of iron overload. Keshan disease is the result of selenium deficiency, whereas selenosis is caused by selenium excess. Menkes syndrome is the result of a systemic deficiency in copper as a result of mutations to ATP7A, an intestinal copper transport protein.

29.10 A 52-year-old female is seen because of unplanned changes in the pigmentation of her skin that give her a tanned appearance. Physical examination shows hyperpigmentation, hepatomegaly, and mild scleral icterus. Laboratory tests are remarkable for elevated serum transaminases (liver function tests) and fasting blood glucose. Results of other tests are pending.

Correct answer = B. The patient has hereditary hemochromatosis, a disease of iron overload that results from inappropriately low levels of hepcidin caused primarily by mutations to the HFE (high iron) gene. Hepcidin regulates ferroportin, the only known iron export protein in humans, by increasing its degradation. The increase in iron with hepcidin deficiency causes hyperpigmentation and hyperglycemia ("bronze diabetes"). Phlebotomy or use of iron chelators is the treatment. [Note: Pending lab tests would show an increase in serum iron and transferrin saturation.]

DNA Structure, Replication, and Repair

30

I. OVERVIEW

Nucleic acids are required for the storage and expression of genetic information. There are two chemically distinct types of nucleic acids: deoxyribonucleic acid (DNA) and ribonucleic acid ([RNA] see Chapter 31). DNA, the repository of genetic information (or, genome), is present not only in chromosomes in the nucleus of eukaryotic organisms, but also in mitochondria and the chloroplasts of plants. Prokaryotic cells, which lack nuclei, have a single chromosome but may also contain nonchromosomal DNA in the form of plasmids. The genetic information found in DNA is copied and transmitted to daughter cells through DNA replication. The DNA contained in a fertilized egg encodes the information that directs the development of an organism. This development may involve the production of billions of cells. Each cell is specialized, expressing only those functions that are required for it to perform its role in maintaining the organism. Therefore, DNA must be able not only to replicate precisely each time a cell divides, but also to have the information that it contains be selectively expressed. Transcription (RNA synthesis) is the first stage in the expression of genetic information (see Chapter 31). Next, the code contained in the nucleotide sequence of messenger RNA molecules is translated (protein synthesis; see Chapter 32), thus completing gene expression. The regulation of gene expression is discussed in Chapter 33.

 The flow of information from DNA to RNA to protein is termed the "central dogma" of molecular biology (Fig. 30.1) and is descriptive of all organisms, with the exception of some viruses that have RNA as the repository of their genetic information.

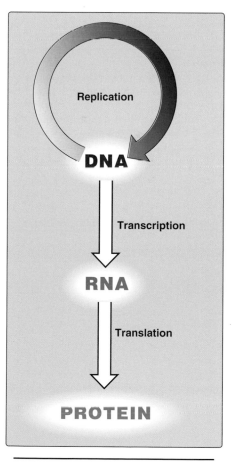

Figure 30.1
The "central dogma" of molecular biology.

411

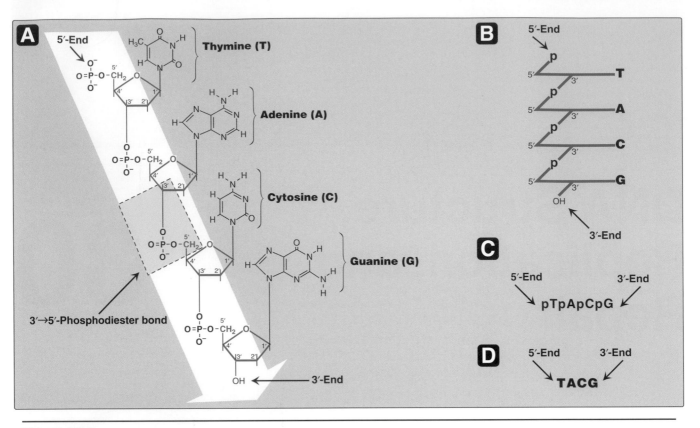

Figure 30.2
A. DNA with the nucleotide sequence shown written in the 5′→3′ direction. A 3′→5′-phosphodiester bond is shown highlighted in the blue box, and the deoxyribose-phosphate backbone is shaded in yellow. B. DNA written in a more stylized form, emphasizing the deoxyribose-phosphate (p) backbone. C. A simpler representation of the nucleotide sequence. D. The simplest (and most common) representation. [Note: The nucleotide base sequence is assumed to be written in the 5′→3′ direction unless otherwise indicated.]

II. DNA STRUCTURE

DNA is a polymer of deoxyribonucleoside monophosphates (dNMP) covalently linked by 3′→5′-phosphodiester bonds. With the exception of a few viruses that contain single-stranded DNA (ssDNA), DNA exists as a double-stranded molecule (dsDNA), in which the two strands wind around each other, forming a double helix. [Note: The sequence of the linked dNMP is primary structure, whereas the double helix is secondary structure.] In eukaryotic cells, DNA is found associated with various types of proteins (known collectively as nucleoprotein) present in the nucleus, whereas the protein–DNA complex is present in a non–membrane-bound region known as the nucleoid in prokaryotes.

A. 3′→5′-Phosphodiester bonds

Phosphodiester bonds join the 3′-hydroxyl group of the deoxypentose of one nucleotide to the 5′-hydroxyl group of the deoxypentose of an adjacent nucleotide through a phosphoryl group (Fig. 30.2). The resulting long, unbranched chain has polarity, with both a 5′-end (the end with the free phosphate) and a 3′-end (the end with the free hydroxyl) that are not attached to other nucleotides. By convention, the bases located along the resulting deoxyribose-phosphate backbone are always written in sequence from the 5′-end of the chain to the 3′-end. For example, the sequence of bases in the DNA shown in Figure 30.2D (5′-TACG-3′) is read "thymine, adenine, cytosine, guanine." Phosphodiester linkages between nucleotides can be hydrolyzed enzymatically by a family of *nucleases*, *deoxyribonucleases* for DNA and *ribonucleases* for RNA, or cleaved hydrolytically by chemicals. [Note: Only RNA is cleaved by alkali.]

B. Double helix

In the double helix, the two chains are coiled around a common axis called the helical axis. The chains are paired in an antiparallel manner (that is, the 5′-end of one strand is paired with the 3′-end of the other strand), as shown in Figure 30.3. In the DNA helix, the hydrophilic deoxyribose-phosphate backbone of each chain is on the outside of the molecule, whereas the hydrophobic bases are stacked inside. The overall structure resembles a twisted ladder. The spatial relationship between the two strands in the helix creates a major (wide) groove and a minor (narrow) groove. These grooves provide access for the binding of regulatory proteins to their specific recognition sequences along the DNA chain. [Note: Certain anticancer drugs, such as dactinomycin (actinomycin D), exert their cytotoxic effect by intercalating into the narrow groove of the DNA double helix, thereby interfering with DNA (and RNA) synthesis.]

1. **Base-pairing:** The bases of one strand of DNA are paired with the bases of the second strand, so that an adenine (A) is always paired with a thymine (T), and a cytosine (C) is always paired with a guanine (G). [Note: The base pairs are perpendicular to the helical axis (see Fig. 30.3).] Therefore, one polynucleotide chain of the DNA double helix is always the complement of the other. Given the sequence of bases on one chain, the sequence of bases on the complementary chain can be determined (Fig. 30.4). [Note: The specific base-pairing in DNA leads to the Chargaff rule, which states that in any sample of dsDNA, the amount of A equals the amount of T, the amount of G equals the amount of C, and the total amount of purines (A + G) equals the total amount of pyrimidines (T + C).] The base pairs are held together by hydrogen bonds: two between A and T and three between G and C (Fig. 30.5). These hydrogen bonds, plus the hydrophobic interactions between the stacked bases, stabilize the structure of the double helix.

2. **DNA strand separation:** The two strands of the double helix separate when hydrogen bonds between the paired bases are disrupted. Disruption can occur in the laboratory if the pH of the DNA solution is altered so that the nucleotide bases ionize, or if the solution is heated. [Note: Covalent phosphodiester bonds are not broken by such treatment.] When DNA is heated, the temperature at which one half of the helical structure is lost is defined as the melting temperature (T_m). The loss of helical structure in DNA, called denaturation, can be monitored by measuring its absorbance at 260 nm. [Note: ssDNA has a higher relative absorbance at this wavelength than does dsDNA.] Because there are three hydrogen bonds between G and C but only two between

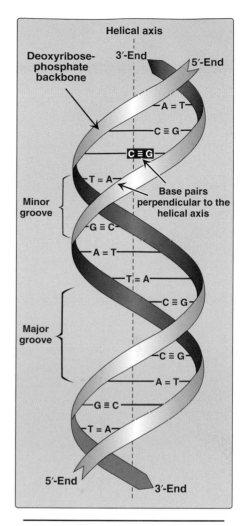

Figure 30.3
DNA double helix, illustrating some of its major structural features.

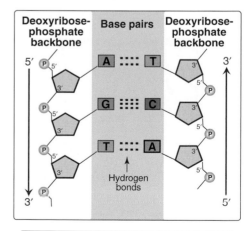

Figure 30.4
Two complementary DNA sequences. T = thymine; A = adenine; C = cytosine; G = guanine.

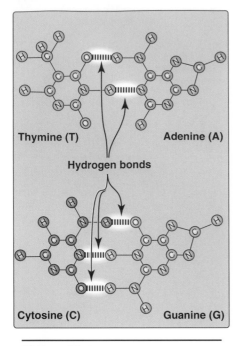

Figure 30.5
Hydrogen bonds between complementary bases.

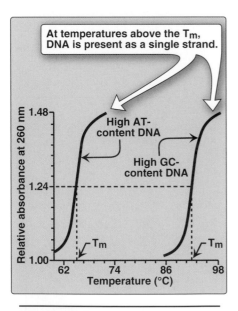

Figure 30.6
Melting temperatures (T$_m$) of DNA molecules with different nucleotide compositions. A = adenine; T = thymine; G = guanine; C = cytosine.

A and T, DNA that contains high concentrations of A and T denatures at a lower temperature than does G- and C-rich DNA (Fig. 30.6). Under appropriate conditions, complementary DNA strands can reform the double helix by the process called renaturation (or, reannealing). [Note: Separation of the two strands over short regions occurs during both DNA and RNA synthesis.]

3. **Structural forms:** There are three major structural forms of DNA: the B form (described by Watson and Crick in 1953), the A form, and the Z form. The B form is a right-handed helix with 10 base pairs (bp) per 360° turn (or twist) of the helix, and with the planes of the bases perpendicular to the helical axis. Chromosomal DNA is thought to consist primarily of B-DNA (Fig. 30.7 shows a space-filling model of B-DNA). The A form is produced by moderately dehydrating the B form. It is also a right-handed helix, but there are 11 bp per turn, and the planes of the base pairs are tilted 20° away from the perpendicular to the helical axis. The conformation found in DNA–RNA hybrids (see p. 418) or RNA–RNA double-stranded regions is probably very close to the A form. Z-DNA is a left-handed helix that contains 12 bp per turn (see Fig. 30.7). [Note: The deoxyribose-phosphate backbone zigzags, hence, the name Z-DNA.] Stretches of Z-DNA can occur naturally in regions of DNA that have a sequence of alternating purines and pyrimidines (for example, poly GC). Transitions between the B and Z helical forms of DNA may play a role in regulating gene expression.

C. **Linear and circular DNA molecules**

Each chromosome in the nucleus of a eukaryote consists of one long, linear molecule of dsDNA, which is bound by a complex mixture of proteins (histone and nonhistone, see p. 425) to form chromatin. Eukaryotes have closed, circular, dsDNA molecules in their mitochondria, as do plant chloroplasts. A prokaryotic organism typically contains a single, circular, dsDNA molecule. [Note: Circular DNA is "supercoiled," that is, the double helix crosses over on itself one or more times. Supercoiling can result in overwinding (positive supercoiling) or underwinding (negative supercoiling) of DNA. Supercoiling, a type of tertiary structure, compacts DNA.] Each prokaryotic chromosome is associated with nonhistone proteins that help compact the DNA to form a nucleoid. In addition, most species of bacteria also contain small, circular, extrachromosomal DNA molecules called plasmids. Plasmid DNA carries genetic information and undergoes replication that may or may not be synchronized to chromosomal division. [Note: The use of plasmids as vectors in recombinant DNA technology is described in Chapter 34.]

Plasmids may carry genes that convey antibiotic resistance to the host bacterium and may facilitate the transfer of genetic information from one bacterium to another.

III. STEPS IN PROKARYOTIC DNA REPLICATION

When the two strands of dsDNA are separated, each can serve as a template for the replication (synthesis) of a new complementary strand. This produces two daughter molecules, each of which contains two DNA strands (one old, one new) in an antiparallel orientation (see Fig. 30.3). This process is called semiconservative replication because, although the parental duplex is separated into two halves (and, therefore, is not conserved as an entity), each of the parental strands remains intact in one of the two new duplexes (Fig. 30.8). The enzymes involved in DNA replication are template-directed, magnesium (Mg^{2+})-requiring *polymerases* that can synthesize the complementary sequence of each strand with extraordinary fidelity. The reactions described in this section were first known from studies of the bacterium <u>Escherichia coli</u> (<u>E. coli</u>), and the description given below refers to the process in prokaryotes. DNA synthesis in higher organisms is more complex but involves the same types of mechanisms. In either case, initiation of DNA replication commits the cell to continue the process until the entire genome has been replicated.

A. Complementary strand separation

In order for the two complementary strands of the parental dsDNA to be replicated, they must first separate (or "melt") over a small region, because the *polymerases* use only ssDNA as a template. In prokaryotic organisms, DNA replication begins at a single, unique nucleotide sequence, a site called the origin of replication, or ori (oriC in <u>E. coli</u>), as shown in Figure 30.9A. [Note: This sequence is referred to as a consensus sequence, because the order of nucleotides is essentially the same at each site.] The ori includes short, AT-rich segments that facilitate melting. In eukaryotes, replication begins at multiple sites along the DNA helix (Fig. 30.9B). Having multiple origins of replication provides a mechanism for rapidly replicating the great length of eukaryotic DNA molecules.

B. Replication fork formation

As the two strands unwind and separate, synthesis occurs at two replication forks that move away from the origin in opposite directions (bidirectionally), generating a replication bubble (see Fig. 30.9). [Note: The term "replication fork" derives from the Y-shaped structure in which the tines of the fork represent the separated strands (Fig. 30.10).]

1. **Required proteins:** Initiation of DNA replication requires the recognition of the origin (start site) by a group of proteins that form the prepriming complex. These proteins are responsible for melting at the ori, maintaining the separation of the parental strands, and unwinding the double helix ahead of the advancing replication fork. In <u>E. coli</u>, these proteins include the following.

   a. **DnaA protein:** *DnaA* protein initiates replication by binding to specific nucleotide sequences (*DnaA* boxes) within oriC. Binding causes an AT-rich region (the DNA unwinding element) in the origin to melt. Melting (strand separation) results in a short, localized region of ssDNA.

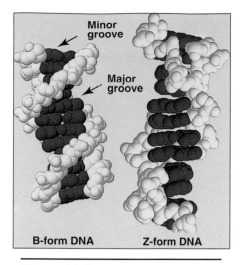

Figure 30.7
Structures of B-DNA and Z-DNA.

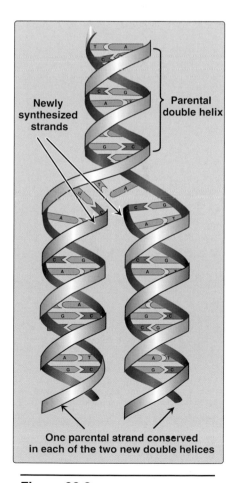

Figure 30.8
Semiconservative replication of DNA. T = thymine; A = adenine; C = cytosine; G = guanine.

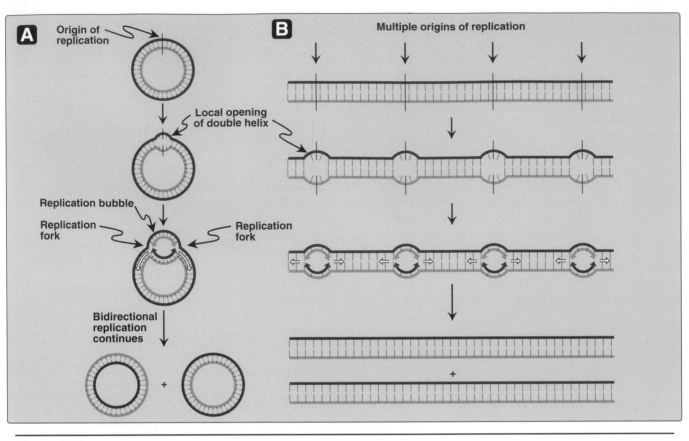

Figure 30.9
Replication of DNA: origins and replication forks. A. Small, circular prokaryotic DNA. B. Long, linear eukaryotic DNA.

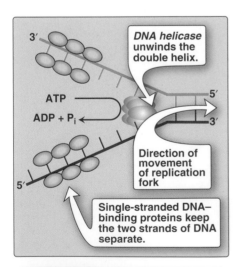

Figure 30.10
Proteins responsible for maintaining the separation of the parental strands and unwinding the double helix ahead of the advancing replication fork (➤). ADP = adenosine diphosphate; P$_i$ = inorganic phosphate.

b. DNA helicases: These enzymes bind to ssDNA near the replication fork and then move into the neighboring double-stranded region, forcing the strands apart (in effect, unwinding the double helix). *Helicases* require energy provided by ATP hydrolysis (see Fig. 30.10). Unwinding at the replication fork causes supercoiling in other regions of the DNA molecule. [Note: *DnaB* is the principal *helicase* of replication in E. coli. Binding of this hexameric protein to DNA requires *DnaC*.]

c. Single-stranded DNA–binding protein: This protein binds to the ssDNA generated by *helicases* (see Fig. 30.10). Binding is cooperative (that is, the binding of one molecule of single-stranded binding [SSB] protein makes it easier for additional molecules of SSB protein to bind tightly to the DNA strand). The SSB proteins are not enzymes, but rather serve to shift the equilibrium between dsDNA and ssDNA in the direction of the single-stranded forms. These proteins not only keep the two strands of DNA separated in the area of the replication origin, thus providing the single-stranded template required by *polymerases*, but also protect the DNA from *nucleases* that degrade ssDNA.

2. Solving the problem of supercoils: As the two strands of the double helix are separated, a problem is encountered, namely, the appearance of positive supercoils in the region of DNA ahead of the replication fork as a result of overwinding (Fig. 30.11) and negative supercoils in the region behind the fork. The accumulating positive supercoils interfere with further unwinding of the double helix. [Note: Supercoiling can be demonstrated by tightly grasping one end of a helical telephone cord while twisting the other end. If the cord is twisted in the direction of tightening the coils, the cord will wrap around itself in space to form positive supercoils. If the cord is twisted in the direction of loosening the coils, the cord will wrap around itself in the opposite direction to form negative supercoils.] To solve this problem, there is a group of enzymes called *DNA topoisomerases*, which are responsible for removing supercoils in the helix by transiently cleaving one or both of the DNA strands.

a. **Type I DNA topoisomerases:** These enzymes reversibly cleave one strand of the double helix. They have both strand-cutting and strand-resealing activities. They do not require ATP, but rather appear to store the energy from the phosphodiester bond they cleave, reusing the energy to reseal the strand (Fig. 30.12). Each time a transient nick is created in one DNA strand, the intact DNA strand is passed through the break before it is resealed, thus relieving (relaxing) accumulated supercoils. *Type I topoisomerases* relax negative supercoils (that is, those that contain fewer turns of the helix than does relaxed DNA) in E. coli and both negative and positive supercoils (that is, those that contain fewer or more turns of the helix than does relaxed DNA) in many prokaryotic cells (but not E. coli) and in eukaryotic cells.

b. **Type II DNA topoisomerases:** These enzymes bind tightly to the DNA double helix and make transient breaks in both strands. The enzyme then causes a second stretch of the DNA double helix to pass through the break and, finally, reseals the break (Fig. 30.13). As a result, both negative and positive supercoils can be relieved by this ATP-requiring process. *DNA gyrase*, a *type II topoisomerase* found in bacteria and plants, has the unusual property of being able to introduce negative supercoils into circular DNA using energy from the hydrolysis of ATP. This facilitates the replication of DNA because the negative supercoils neutralize the positive supercoils introduced during opening of the double helix. It also aids in the transient strand separation required during transcription (see p. 436).

Anticancer agents, such as the camptothecins, target human *type I topoisomerases*, whereas etoposide targets human *type II topoisomerases*. Bacterial *DNA gyrase* is a unique target of a group of antimicrobial agents called fluoroquinolones (for example, ciprofloxacin).

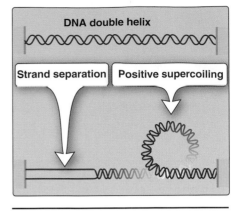

Figure 30.11
Positive supercoiling resulting from DNA strand separation.

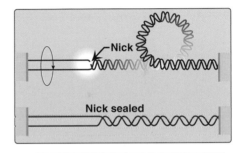

Figure 30.12
Action of *type I DNA topoisomerases*.

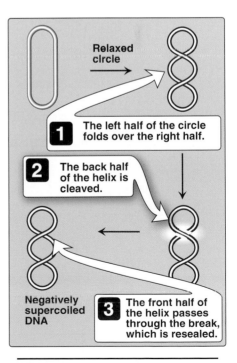

Figure 30.13
Action of *type II DNA topoisomerase*.

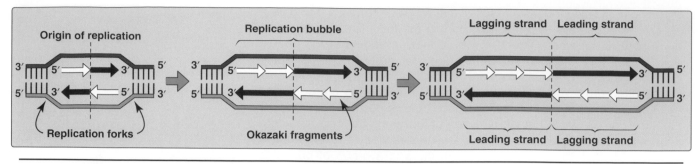

Figure 30.14
Semidiscontinuous synthesis of DNA. Black arrows = continuous synthesis; white arrows = discontinuous.

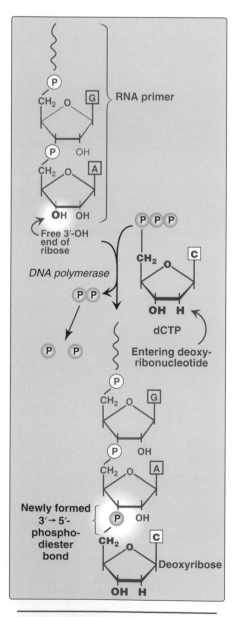

Figure 30.15
Use of an RNA primer to initiate DNA synthesis. (P) and (P) = phosphate; dCTP = deoxycytidine triphosphate.

C. Direction of DNA replication

The *DNA polymerases* (*DNA pols*) responsible for copying the DNA templates are only able to read the parental nucleotide sequences in the 3'→5' direction, and they synthesize the new DNA strands only in the 5'→3' (antiparallel) direction. Therefore, beginning with one parental double helix, the two newly synthesized stretches of nucleotide chains must grow in opposite directions, one in the 5'→3' direction toward the replication fork and one in the 5'→3' direction away from the replication fork (Fig. 30.14). This feat is accomplished by a slightly different mechanism on each strand.

1. **Leading strand:** The strand that is being copied in the direction of the advancing replication fork is synthesized continuously and is called the leading strand.

2. **Lagging strand:** The strand that is being copied in the direction away from the replication fork is synthesized discontinuously, with small fragments of DNA being copied near the replication fork. These short stretches of discontinuous DNA, termed Okazaki fragments, are eventually joined (ligated) by *ligase* to become a single, continuous strand. The new strand of DNA produced by this mechanism is termed the lagging strand.

D. RNA primer

DNA pols cannot initiate synthesis of a complementary strand of DNA on a totally single-stranded template. Rather, they require an RNA primer, which is a short piece of RNA base-paired to the DNA template, thereby forming a double-stranded DNA–RNA hybrid. The free hydroxyl group on the 3'-end of the RNA primer serves as the first acceptor of a deoxynucleotide by action of a *DNA pol* (Fig. 30.15). [Note: Recall that *glycogen synthase* also requires a primer (see p. 126).]

1. **Primase:** A specific *RNA polymerase*, called *primase* (*DnaG*), synthesizes the short stretches of RNA (~10 nucleotides long) that are complementary and antiparallel to the DNA template. In the resulting hybrid duplex, the U (uracil) in RNA pairs with A in DNA. As shown in Figure 30.16, these short RNA sequences are constantly being synthesized at the replication fork on the lagging strand, but only one RNA sequence at the origin of replication is required on the leading strand. The substrates for this process are 5'-ribonucleoside triphosphates, and pyrophosphate is released

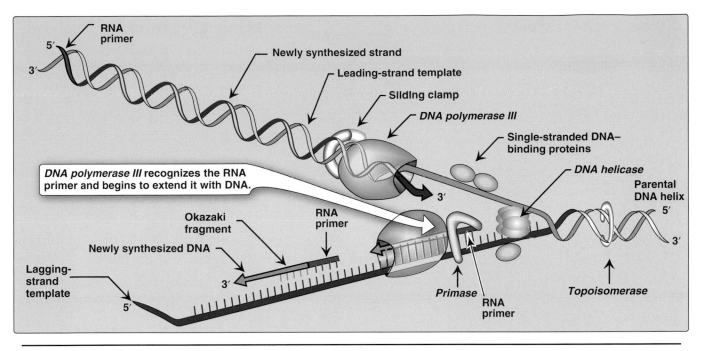

Figure 30.16
Elongation of the leading and lagging strands. [Note: The DNA sliding clamp is not shown for the lagging strand.]

as each ribonucleoside monophosphate is added through formation of a $3' \rightarrow 5'$-phosphodiester bond. [Note: The RNA primer is later removed, as described in F. below.]

2. **Primosome:** The addition of *primase* converts the prepriming complex of proteins required for DNA strand separation (see p. 415) to a primosome. The primosome makes the RNA primer required for leading-strand synthesis and initiates Okazaki fragment formation in discontinuous lagging-strand synthesis. As with DNA synthesis, the direction of synthesis of the primer is $5' \rightarrow 3'$.

E. Chain elongation

Prokaryotic (and eukaryotic) *DNA pols* elongate a new DNA strand by adding deoxyribonucleotides, one at a time, to the 3'-end of the growing chain (see Fig. 30.16). The sequence of nucleotides that are added is dictated by the base sequence of the template strand with which the incoming nucleotides are paired.

1. **DNA polymerase III:** DNA chain elongation is catalyzed by the multisubunit enzyme, *DNA pol III*. Using the 3'-hydroxyl group of the RNA primer as the acceptor of the first deoxyribonucleotide, *DNA pol III* begins to add nucleotides along the single-stranded template that specifies the sequence of bases in the newly synthesized chain. *DNA pol III* is a highly processive enzyme (that is, it remains bound to the template strand as it moves along and does not diffuse away and then rebind before adding each new nucleotide). The processivity of *DNA pol III* is the result of the β subunits of the holoenzyme forming a ring that encircles and moves along the template strand of the DNA, thus serving as a sliding DNA clamp. [Note: Clamp formation is facilitated by a protein complex,

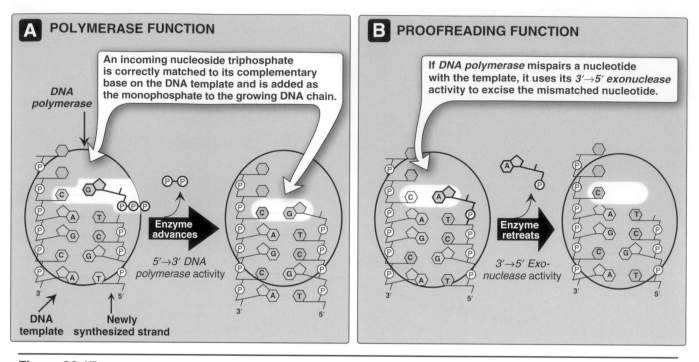

Figure 30.17
3′→5′ Exonuclease activity enables *DNA polymerase III* to proofread the newly synthesized DNA strand.

the clamp loader, and ATP hydrolysis.] The new (daughter) strand grows in the 5′→3′ direction, antiparallel to the parental strand (see Fig. 30.16). The nucleotide substrates are 5′-deoxyribonucleoside triphosphates. Pyrophosphate (PP$_i$) is released when each new deoxynucleoside monophosphate is added to the free 3′-hydroxyl group of the growing chain through a 3′→5′-phosphodiester bond (see Fig. 30.15). Hydrolysis of PP$_i$ to 2 P$_i$ by *pyrophosphatase* means that a total of two high-energy bonds are used to drive the addition of each deoxynucleotide.

> The production of PP$_i$ with subsequent hydrolysis to 2 P$_i$ is a common theme in biochemistry. Removal of the PP$_i$ product drives a reaction in the forward direction, making it essentially irreversible.

All four substrates (deoxyadenosine triphosphate [dATP], deoxythymidine triphosphate [dTTP], deoxycytidine triphosphate [dCTP], and deoxyguanosine triphosphate [dGTP]) must be present for DNA elongation to occur. If one of the four is in short supply, DNA synthesis stops when that nucleotide is depleted.

2. **Proofreading newly synthesized DNA:** It is highly important for the survival of an organism that the nucleotide sequence of DNA be replicated with as few errors as possible. Misreading of the template sequence could result in deleterious, perhaps lethal, mutations. To insure replication fidelity, *DNA pol III* has a proofreading activity (*3′→5′ exonuclease*, Fig. 30.17) in addition to its 5′→3′

polymerase activity. As each nucleotide is added to the chain, *DNA pol III* checks to make certain the base of the newly added nucleotide is, in fact, the complement of the base on the template strand. If it is not, the *3′→5′ exonuclease* activity removes the error in the direction opposite to polymerization. [Note: Because the enzyme requires an improperly base-paired 3′-hydroxy terminus, it does not degrade correctly paired nucleotide sequences.] For example, if the template base is C and the enzyme inserts an A instead of a G into the new chain, the *3′→5′ exonuclease* activity hydrolytically removes the misplaced nucleotide. The *5′→3′ polymerase* activity then replaces it with the correct nucleotide containing G (see Fig. 30.17). [Note: The *5′→3′ polymerase* and *3′→5′ exonuclease* domains are located on different subunits of *DNA pol III*.]

F. RNA primer excision and replacement by DNA

DNA pol III continues to synthesize DNA on the lagging strand until it is blocked by proximity to an RNA primer. When this occurs, the RNA is excised and the gap filled by *DNA pol I.*

1. **5′→3′ Exonuclease activity:** In addition to having the *5′→3′ polymerase* activity that synthesizes DNA and the *3′→5′ exonuclease* activity that proofreads the newly synthesized DNA like *DNA pol III*, monomeric *DNA pol I* also has a *5′→3′ exonuclease* activity that is able to hydrolytically remove the RNA primer. [Note: *Exonucleases* remove nucleotides from the end of the DNA chain, rather than cleaving the chain internally as do *endonucleases* (Fig. 30.18).] First, *DNA pol I* locates the space (nick) between the 3′-end of the DNA newly synthesized by *DNA pol III* and the 5′-end of the adjacent RNA primer. Next, *DNA pol I* hydrolytically removes the RNA nucleotides ahead of itself, moving in the 5′→3′ direction (*5′→3′ exonuclease* activity). As it removes ribonucleotides, *DNA pol I* replaces them with deoxyribonucleotides, synthesizing DNA in the 5′→3′ direction (*5′→3′ polymerase* activity). As it synthesizes the DNA, it also proofreads using its *3′→5′ exonuclease* activity to remove errors. This removal/synthesis/proofreading continues until the RNA primer is totally degraded, and the gap is filled with DNA (Fig. 30.19). [Note: *DNA pol I* uses its *5′→3′ polymerase* activity to fill in gaps generated during most types of DNA repair (see p. 428).]

2. **Comparison of 5′→3′ and 3′→5′ exonuclease activities:** The *5′→3′ exonuclease* activity of *DNA pol I* allows the *polymerase*, moving 5′→3′, to hydrolytically remove one or more nucleotides at a time from the 5′-end of the ~10 nucleotide–long RNA primer. In contrast, the *3′→5′ exonuclease* activity of *DNA pol I* and *pol III* allows these *polymerases*, moving 3′→5′, to hydrolytically remove one misplaced nucleotide at a time from the 3′-end of a growing DNA strand, increasing the fidelity of replication such that newly replicated DNA has one error per 10^7 nucleotides.

G. DNA ligase

The final phosphodiester linkage between the 5′-phosphate group on the DNA synthesized by *DNA pol III* and the 3′-hydroxyl group on the DNA made by *DNA pol I* is catalyzed by *DNA ligase* (Fig. 30.20). The

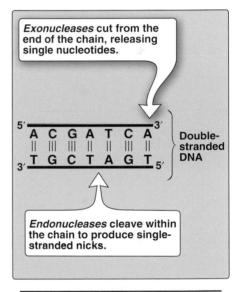

Figure 30.18
Endonuclease versus *exonuclease* activity. [Note: *Restriction endonucleases* (see p. 481) cleave both strands.] T = thymine; A = adenine; C = cytosine; G = guanine.

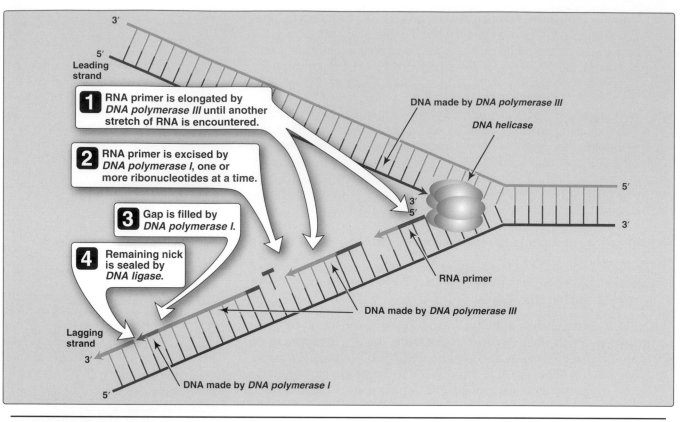

Figure 30.19
Removal of RNA primer and filling of the resulting gaps by *DNA polymerase I*.

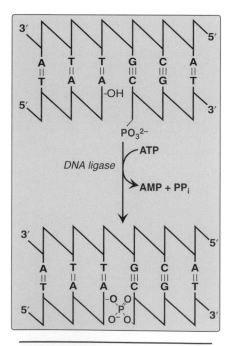

Figure 30.20
Formation of a phosphodiester bond by *DNA ligase*. [Note: Adenosine monophosphate (AMP) is first linked to *ligase*, then to the 5′-phosphate, and then released.]

joining of these two stretches of DNA requires energy, which in most organisms is provided by the cleavage of ATP to adenosine monophosphate + PP$_i$.

H. Termination

Replication termination in E. coli is mediated by sequence-specific binding of the protein Tus (terminus utilization substance) to replication termination (ter) sites on the DNA, stopping the movement of the replication fork.

IV. EUKARYOTIC DNA REPLICATION

The process of eukaryotic DNA replication closely follows that of prokaryotic DNA synthesis. Some differences, such as the multiple origins of replication in eukaryotic cells versus single origins of replication in prokaryotes, have already been noted. Eukaryotic origin recognition proteins, ssDNA-binding proteins, and ATP-dependent *DNA helicases* have been identified, and their functions are analogous to those of the prokaryotic proteins previously discussed. In contrast, RNA primers are removed by *RNase H* and *flap endonuclease 1* (*FEN1*) rather than by a *DNA pol* (Fig. 30.21).

A. Eukaryotic cell cycle

The events surrounding eukaryotic DNA replication and cell division (mitosis) are coordinated to produce the cell cycle (Fig. 30.22). The period preceding replication is called the G_1 phase (Gap 1). DNA replication occurs during the S (synthesis) phase. Following DNA synthesis, there is another phase (G_2, or Gap 2) before mitosis (M). Cells that have stopped dividing, such as mature T lymphocytes, are said to have gone out of the cell cycle into the G_0 phase. Such quiescent cells can be stimulated to reenter the G_1 phase to resume division. [Note: The cell cycle is controlled at a series of checkpoints that prevent entry into the next phase of the cycle until the preceding phase has been completed. Two key classes of proteins that control the progress of a cell through the cell cycle are the cyclins and *cyclin-dependent kinases* (*Cdk*).]

B. Eukaryotic DNA polymerases

At least five high-fidelity eukaryotic *DNA pols* have been identified and categorized on the basis of molecular weight, cellular location, sensitivity to inhibitors, and the templates or substrates on which they act. They are designated by Greek letters rather than by Roman numerals (Fig. 30.23).

1. **Pol α:** *Pol α* is a multisubunit enzyme. One subunit has *primase* activity, which initiates strand synthesis on the leading strand and at the beginning of each Okazaki fragment on the lagging strand. The *primase* subunit synthesizes a short RNA primer that is extended by the $5' {\rightarrow} 3'$ *polymerase* activity of *pol α*, generating a short piece of DNA. [Note: *Pol α* is also referred to as *pol α/primase*.]

2. **Pol ε and pol δ:** *Pol ε* is recruited to complete DNA synthesis on the leading strand, whereas *pol δ* elongates the Okazaki fragments of the lagging strand, each using $3' {\rightarrow} 5'$ *exonuclease* activity to proofread the newly synthesized DNA. [Note: *DNA pol ε* associates with proliferating cell nuclear antigen (PCNA), a protein that serves as a sliding DNA clamp in much the same way the β subunits of *DNA pol III* do in E. coli, thus insuring high processivity.]

3. **Pol β and pol γ:** *Pol β* is involved in gap filling in DNA repair. *Pol γ* replicates mitochondrial DNA.

C. Telomeres

Telomeres are complexes of DNA plus proteins (collectively known as shelterin) located at the ends of linear chromosomes. They maintain the structural integrity of the chromosome, preventing attack by *nucleases*, and allow repair systems to distinguish a true end from a break in dsDNA. In humans, telomeric DNA consists of several thousand tandem repeats of a noncoding hexameric sequence, AGGGTT, base-paired to a complementary region containing C and A. The G-rich strand is longer than its C-rich complement, leaving ssDNA a few hundred nucleotides in length at the 3'-end. The single-stranded region is thought to fold back on itself, forming a loop structure that is stabilized by protein.

1. **Telomere shortening:** Eukaryotic cells face a special problem in replicating the ends of their linear DNA molecules. Following

FUNCTION	PROTEIN(S)
Origin recognition	ORC
Helicase activity	*MCM*
ssDNA protection	RPA
Primer synthesis	*Pol a/primase*
Sliding clamp	PCNA
Primer removal	*RNase H, FEN1*

Figure 30.21
Proteins and their function in eukaryotic replication. ORC = origin recognition complex; *MCM = minichromosome maintenance (complex)*; RPA = replication protein A; PCNA = proliferating cell nuclear antigen; *FEN = flap endonuclease.*

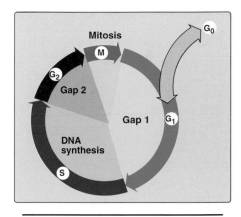

Figure 30.22
The eukaryotic cell cycle. [Note: Cells can leave the cell cycle and enter a reversible quiescent state called G_0.]

POLY-MERASE	FUNCTION	PROOF-READING*
Pol α (alpha)	• Contains *primase* • Initiates DNA synthesis	–
Pol β (beta)	• Repair	–
Pol δ (delta)	• Elongates Okazaki fragments of the lagging strand	+
Pol ε (epsilon)	• Elongates the leading strand	+
Pol γ (gamma)	• Replicates mitochondrial DNA	+

Figure 30.23
Activities of eukaryotic *DNA polymerases* (*pol*). [Note: The asterisk (*) denotes $3' {\rightarrow} 5'$ *exonuclease* activity.]

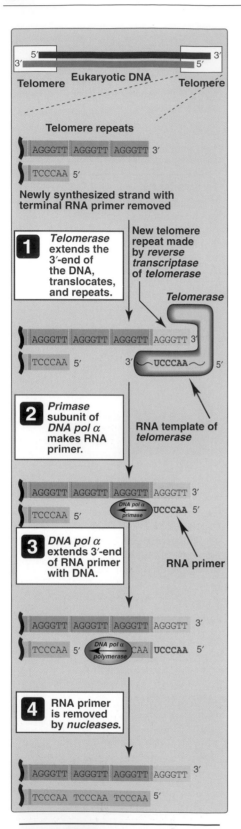

Figure 30.24
Mechanism of action of *telomerase*, a ribonucleoprotein. T = thymine; A = adenine; C = cytosine; G = guanine; *pol = polymerase*.

removal of the RNA primer from the extreme 5′-end of the lagging strand, there is no way to fill in the remaining gap with DNA. Consequently, in most normal human somatic cells, telomeres shorten with each successive cell division. Once telomeres are shortened beyond some critical length, the cell is no longer able to divide and is said to be senescent. In germ cells and stem cells, as well as in cancer cells, telomeres do not shorten and the cells do not senesce. This is a result of the ribonucleoprotein *telomerase*, which maintains telomeric length in these cells.

2. **Telomerase:** This complex contains a protein (Tert) that acts as a *reverse transcriptase* and a short piece of RNA (Terc) that acts as a template. The C-rich RNA template base-pairs with the G-rich, single-stranded 3′-end of telomeric DNA (Fig. 30.24). The *reverse transcriptase* uses the RNA template to synthesize DNA in the usual 5′→3′ direction, extending the already longer 3′-end. *Telomerase* then translocates to the newly synthesized end, and the process is repeated. Once the G-rich strand has been lengthened, *primase* activity of *DNA pol α* can use it as a template to synthesize an RNA primer. The primer is extended by *DNA pol α* and then removed by *nucleases*.

> Telomeres may be viewed as mitotic clocks in that their length in most cells is inversely related to the number of times the cells have divided. The study of telomeres provides insight into the biology of normal aging, diseases of premature aging (the progerias), and cancer.

D. Reverse transcriptases

As seen with *telomerase, reverse transcriptases* are RNA-directed *DNA pols*. A *reverse transcriptase* is involved in the replication of retroviruses, such as human immunodeficiency virus (HIV). These viruses carry their genome in the form of ssRNA molecules. Following infection of a host cell, the viral enzyme *reverse transcriptase* uses the viral RNA as a template for the 5′→3′ synthesis of viral DNA, which then becomes integrated into host chromosomes. *Reverse transcriptase* activity is also seen with transposons, DNA elements that can move about the genome (see p. 477). In eukaryotes, most transposons are transcribed to RNA, the RNA is used as a template for DNA synthesis by a *reverse transcriptase* encoded by the transposon, and the DNA is randomly inserted into the genome. [Note: Transposons that involve an RNA intermediate are called retrotransposons or retroposons.]

E. DNA replication inhibition by nucleoside analogs

DNA chain growth can be blocked by the incorporation of certain nucleoside analogs that have been modified on the sugar portion (Fig. 30.25). For example, removal of the hydroxyl group from the 3′-carbon of the deoxyribose ring as in 2′,3′-dideoxyinosine ([ddI] also known as didanosine), or conversion of the deoxyribose to another sugar, such as arabinose, prevents further chain elongation. By blocking DNA replication, these compounds slow the division of rapidly growing cells and viruses. Cytosine arabinoside (cytarabine, or araC) has been used in anticancer chemotherapy, whereas adenine arabinoside (vidarabine, or araA) is an antiviral agent. Substitution on the sugar moiety, as seen in azidothymidine (AZT), also called zidovudine (ZDV), also terminates DNA chain elongation. [Note: These drugs are generally supplied as nucleosides, which are then converted to nucleotides by cellular *kinases*.]

V. EUKARYOTIC DNA ORGANIZATION

A typical (diploid) human somatic cell contains 46 chromosomes, whose total DNA is ~2 m long! It is difficult to imagine how such a large amount of genetic material can be effectively packaged into a volume the size of a cell nucleus so that it can be efficiently replicated and its genetic information expressed. To do so requires the interaction of DNA with a large number of proteins, each of which performs a specific function in the ordered packaging of these long molecules of DNA. Eukaryotic DNA is associated with tightly bound basic proteins, called histones. These serve to order the DNA into fundamental structural units, called nucleosomes, which resemble beads on a string. Nucleosomes are further arranged into increasingly more complex structures that organize and condense the long DNA molecules into chromosomes that can be segregated during cell division. [Note: The complex of DNA and protein found inside the nuclei of eukaryotic cells is called chromatin.]

A. Histones and nucleosome formation

There are five classes of histones, designated H1, H2A, H2B, H3, and H4. These small, evolutionarily conserved proteins are positively charged at physiologic pH as a result of their high content of lysine and arginine. Because of their positive charge, they form ionic bonds with negatively charged DNA. Histones, along with ions such as Mg^{2+}, help neutralize the negatively charged DNA phosphate groups.

1. **Nucleosomes:** Two molecules each of H2A, H2B, H3, and H4 form the octameric core of the individual nucleosome "beads." Around this structural core, a segment of dsDNA is wound nearly twice (Fig. 30.26). Winding eliminates a helical turn, causing negative supercoiling. [Note: The N-terminal ends of these histones can be acetylated, methylated, or phosphorylated. These reversible covalent modifications influence how tightly the histones bind to the DNA, thereby affecting the expression of specific genes. Histone modification is an example of epigenetics, or heritable changes in gene expression caused without alteration of the nucleotide sequence.] Neighboring nucleosomes are joined by linker DNA ~50 bp long. H1 is not found in the nucleosome core, but instead binds to the linker DNA chain between the nucleosome beads. H1 is the most tissue specific and species specific of the histones. It facilitates the packing of nucleosomes into more compact structures.

2. **Higher levels of organization:** Nucleosomes can be packed more tightly (stacked) to form a nucleofilament. This structure assumes the shape of a coil, often referred to as a 30-nm fiber. The fiber

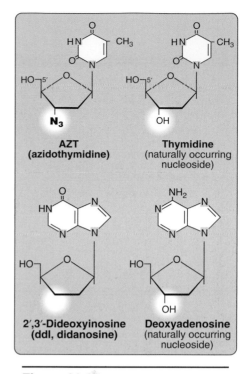

Figure 30.25
Examples of nucleoside analogs that lack a 3′-hydroxyl group. [Note: The ddI is converted to its active form (dideoxy ATP).]

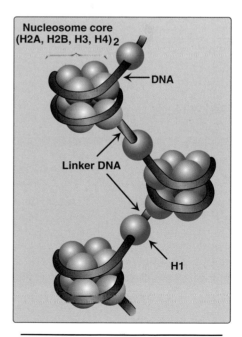

Figure 30.26
Organization of human DNA, illustrating the structure of nucleosomes. H = histone.

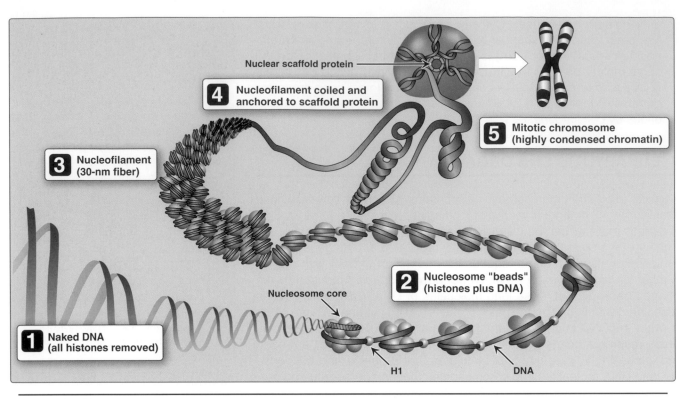

Figure 30.27
Structural organization of eukaryotic DNA. [Note: A 10^4 linear compaction is seen from 1–5.] H = histone.

is organized into loops that are anchored by a nuclear scaffold containing several proteins. Additional levels of organization lead to the final chromosomal structure (Fig. 30.27).

B. Nucleosome fate during DNA replication

Parental nucleosomes are disassembled to allow access to DNA during replication. Once DNA is synthesized, nucleosomes form rapidly. Their histone proteins come both from <u>de novo</u> synthesis and from the transfer of parental histones.

@ VI. DNA REPAIR

Despite the elaborate proofreading system employed during DNA synthesis, errors (including incorrect base-pairing or insertion of one to a few extra nucleotides) can occur. In addition, DNA is constantly being subjected to environmental insults that cause the alteration or removal of nucleotide bases. The damaging agents can be either chemicals (for example, nitrous acid, which can deaminate bases) or radiation (for example, nonionizing ultraviolet [UV] radiation, which can fuse two pyrimidines adjacent to each other in the DNA, and high-energy ionizing radiation, which can cause double-strand breaks). Bases are also altered or lost spontaneously from mammalian DNA at a rate of many thousands per cell per day. If the damage is not repaired, a permanent change (mutation) is introduced that can result in any of a number of deleterious effects, including loss of control over the proliferation of the mutated cell, leading to cancer. Luckily, cells are remarkably efficient at repairing damage done to their DNA. Most of the repair systems involve recognition of the damage (lesion) on the DNA, removal or excision of the damage, replacement or filling the gap left by excision using the sister strand as a template for DNA synthesis, and ligation. These excision repair systems remove one to tens of nucleotides. [Note: Repair synthesis of DNA can occur outside of the S phase.]

A. Mismatch repair

Sometimes replication errors escape the proofreading activity during DNA synthesis, causing a mismatch of one to several bases. In E. coli, mismatch repair (MMR) is mediated by a group of proteins known as the Mut proteins (Fig. 30.28). Homologous proteins are present in humans. [Note: MMR occurs within minutes of replication and reduces the error rate of replication from 1 in 10^7 to 1 in 10^9 nucleotides.]

1. **Mismatched strand identification:** When a mismatch occurs, the Mut proteins that identify the mispaired nucleotide(s) must be able to discriminate between the correct strand and the strand with the mismatch. In prokaryotes, discrimination is based on the degree of methylation. GATC sequences, which are found once every thousand nucleotides, are methylated on the adenine (A) residue by *DNA adenine methylase (DAM)*. This methylation is not done immediately after synthesis, so the DNA is hemimethylated (that is, the parental strand is methylated, but the daughter strand is not). The methylated parental strand is assumed to be correct, and it is the daughter strand that gets repaired. [Note: The exact mechanism by which the daughter strand is identified in eukaryotes is not yet known, but likely involves recognition of nicks in the newly synthesized strand.]

2. **Repair procedure:** When the strand containing the mismatch is identified, an *endonuclease* nicks the strand, and the mismatched nucleotide(s) is/are removed by an *exonuclease*. Additional nucleotides at the 5'- and 3'-ends of the mismatch are also removed. The gap left by removal of the nucleotides is filled, using the sister strand as a template, by a *DNA pol*, typically *DNA pol III*. The 3'-hydroxyl of the newly synthesized DNA is joined to the 5'-phosphate of the remaining stretch of the original DNA strand by *DNA ligase*.

Mutation to the proteins involved in MMR in humans is associated with hereditary nonpolyposis colorectal cancer (HNPCC), also known as Lynch syndrome. Although HNPCC confers an increased risk for developing colon cancer (as well as other cancers), only about 5% of all colon cancer is the result of mutations in MMR.

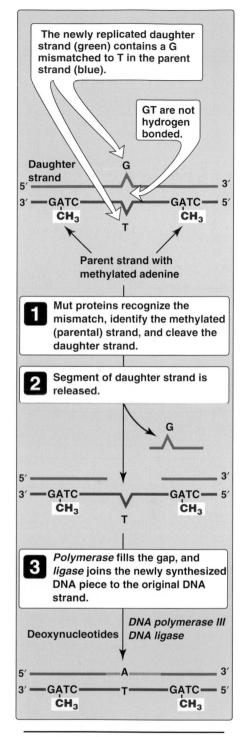

Figure 30.28
Methyl-directed mismatch repair in Escherichia coli. [Note: Mut S protein recognizes the mismatch and recruits Mut L. The complex activates Mut H, which cleaves the unmethylated (daughter) strand.] A = adenine; C = cytosine; G = guanine; T = thymine.

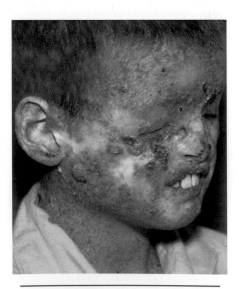

Figure 30.29

Nucleotide excision repair of pyrimidine dimers in <u>Escherichia coli</u> DNA. UV = ultraviolet.

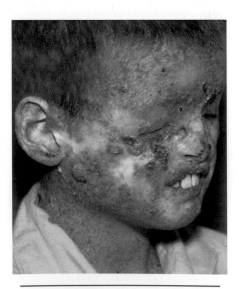

Figure 30.30

Patient with xeroderma pigmentosum.

B. Nucleotide excision repair

Exposure of a cell to UV radiation can result in the covalent joining of two adjacent pyrimidines (usually thymines), producing a dimer. These intrastrand cross-links prevent *DNA pol* from replicating the DNA strand beyond the site of dimer formation. Thymine dimers are excised in bacteria by UvrABC proteins in a process known as nucleotide excision repair (NER), as illustrated in Figure 30.29. A related pathway is present in humans (see 2. below). [Note: Transcription-coupled repair, a type of NER, fixes DNA lesions encountered during RNA synthesis.]

1. **Recognition and excision of UV-induced dimers:** A *UV-specific endonuclease* (called *uvrABC excinuclease*) recognizes the bulky dimer and cleaves the damaged strand on both the 5′-side and 3′-side of the lesion. A short oligonucleotide containing the dimer is excised, leaving a gap in the DNA strand. This gap is filled in using a *DNA pol I* and *DNA ligase*. NER occurs throughout the cell cycle.

2. **UV radiation and cancer:** Pyrimidine dimers can be formed in the skin cells of humans exposed to UV radiation in unfiltered sunlight. In the rare genetic disease xeroderma pigmentosum (XP), the cells cannot repair the damaged DNA, resulting in extensive accumulation of mutations and, consequently, early and numerous skin cancers (Fig. 30.30). XP can be caused by defects in any of the several genes that code for the XP proteins required for NER of UV damage in humans.

C. Base excision repair

DNA bases can be altered, either spontaneously, as is the case with cytosine, which slowly undergoes deamination (the loss of its amino group) to form uracil, or by the action of deaminating or alkylating compounds. For example, nitrous acid, which is formed by the cell from precursors such as the nitrates, deaminates cytosine, adenine (to hypoxanthine), and guanine (to xanthine). Dimethyl sulfate can alkylate (methylate) adenine. Bases can also be lost spontaneously. For example, ~10,000 purine bases are lost this way per cell per day. Lesions involving base alterations or loss can be corrected by base excision repair ([BER], Fig. 30.31).

1. **Abnormal base removal:** In BER, abnormal bases, such as uracil, which can occur in DNA by either deamination of cytosine or improper use of dUTP instead of dTTP during DNA synthesis, are recognized by specific *DNA glycosylases* that hydrolytically cleave them from the deoxyribose-phosphate backbone of the strand. This leaves an apyrimidinic site, or apurinic if a purine was removed, both referred to as AP sites.

2. **AP site recognition and repair:** Specific *AP endonucleases* recognize that a base is missing and initiate the process of excision and gap filling by making an endonucleolytic cut just to the 5′-side of the AP site. A *deoxyribose phosphate lyase* removes the single, base-free, sugar phosphate residue. *DNA pol I* and *DNA ligase* complete the repair process.

D. Double-strand break repair

Ionizing radiation, chemotherapeutic agents such as doxorubicin, and oxidative free radicals (see p. 148) can cause double-strand breaks in DNA that can be lethal to the cell. [Note: Such breaks also occur naturally during genetic recombination.] dsDNA breaks cannot be corrected by the previously described strategy of excising the damage on one strand and using the undamaged strand as a template for replacing the missing nucleotide(s). Instead, they are repaired by one of two systems. The first is nonhomologous end joining (NHEJ), in which a group of proteins mediates the recognition, processing, and ligation of the ends of two DNA fragments. However, some DNA is lost in the process. Consequently, NHEJ is error prone and mutagenic. Defects in NHEJ are associated with a predisposition to cancer and immunodeficiency syndromes. The second repair system, homologous recombination (HR), uses the enzymes that normally perform genetic recombination between homologous chromosomes during meiosis. This system is much less error prone ("error-free") than NHEJ because any DNA that was lost is replaced using homologous DNA as a template. HR occurs in late S and G$_2$ of the cell cycle, whereas NHEJ can occur anytime. [Note: Mutations to the proteins BRCA1 or BRCA2 (breast cancer 1 or 2), which are involved in HR, increase the risk for developing breast and ovarian cancer.]

VII. CHAPTER SUMMARY

DNA is a polymer of deoxynucleoside monophosphates covalently linked by **3′→5′-phosphodiester bonds** (Fig. 30.32). The resulting long, unbranched chain has **polarity**, with both a 5′-end (free phosphate) and a 3′-end (free hydroxyl). The sequence of nucleotides is read 5′→3′. DNA exists as a **double-stranded** molecule, in which the two chains are paired in an **antiparallel** manner and wind around each other, forming a **double helix**. **Adenine** pairs with **thymine**, and **cytosine** pairs with **guanine**. Each strand of the double helix serves as a **template** for constructing a **complementary** daughter strand (**semiconservative replication**). DNA replication occurs in the **S phase** of the **cell cycle** and begins at an **origin of replication**. As the two strands unwind and separate, synthesis occurs at two **replication forks** that move away from the origin in opposite directions (bidirectionally). **Helicase** unwinds the double helix. As the two strands of the double helix are separated, positive **supercoils** are produced in the region of DNA ahead of the replication fork and negative supercoils behind the fork. **DNA topoisomerases** types **I** and **II** remove supercoils. **DNA polymerases** (**pols**) synthesize new DNA strands only in the **5′→3′** direction. Therefore, one of the newly synthesized stretches of nucleotide chains must grow in the 5′→3′ direction toward the replication fork (**leading strand**) and one in the 5′→3′ direction away from the replication fork (**lagging strand**). DNA pols require a **primer**, a short stretch of RNA synthesized by **primase**. Leading-strand synthesis needs only one RNA primer (**continuous** synthesis), whereas the lagging strand needs many (**discontinuous** synthesis involving **Okazaki fragments**). In Escherichia coli (E. coli), DNA chain elongation is catalyzed by **DNA pol III**, using **5′-deoxyribonucleoside triphosphates** as substrates. The enzyme **proofreads** the newly synthesized DNA, removing

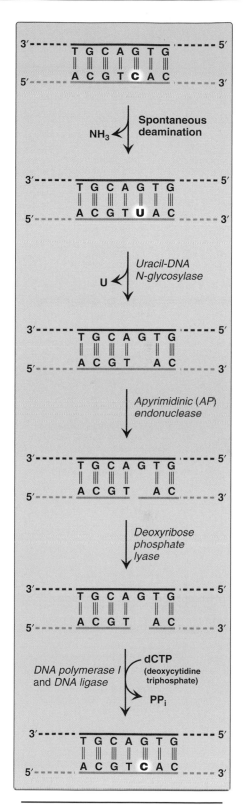

Figure 30.31
Correction of base alterations by base excision repair. C = cytosine; U = uracil; NH$_3$ = ammonia; PP$_i$ = pyrophosphate.

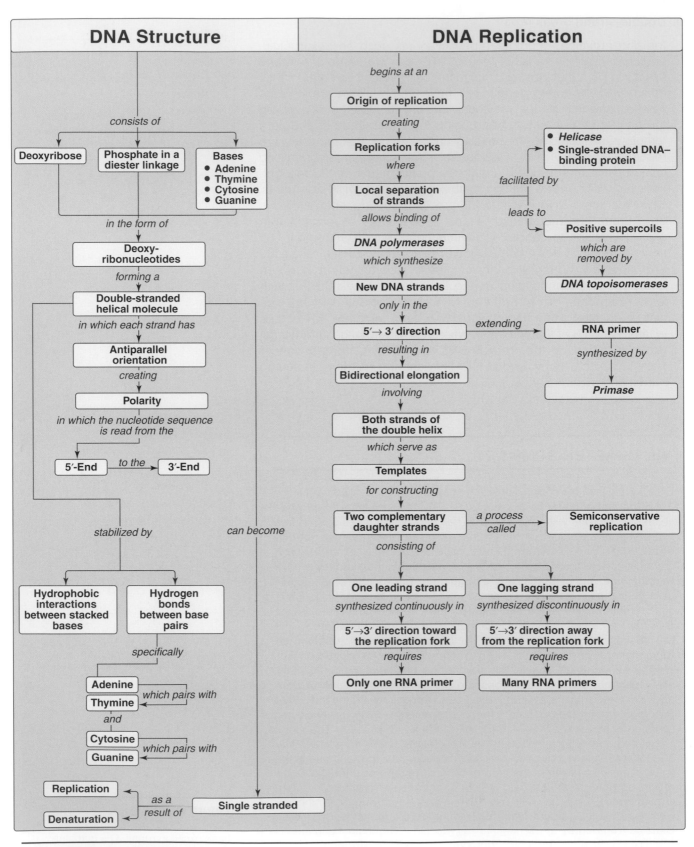

Figure 30.32 (continued on next page)
Key concept map for DNA structure, replication, and repair.

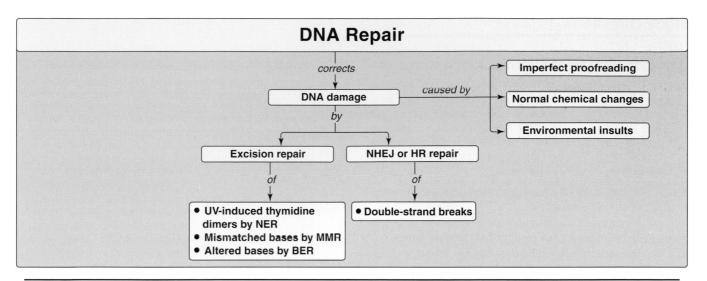

Figure 30.32 (continued from previous page)
Key concept map for DNA structure, replication, and repair. NHEJ = nonhomologous end joining; HR = homologous recombination; UV = ultraviolet; NER = nucleotide excision repair; MMR = mismatch repair; BER = base excision repair.

terminal mismatched nucleotides with its *3′→5′ exonuclease* activity. RNA primers are removed by ***DNA pol I***, using its *5′→3′ exonuclease* activity. This enzyme fills the gaps with DNA, proofreading as it synthesizes. The final phosphodiester linkage is catalyzed by ***DNA ligase***. There are at least five high-fidelity **eukaryotic DNA pols**. **Pol** α is a multisubunit enzyme, one subunit of which is a ***primase***. Pol α *5′→3′ polymerase* activity adds a short piece of DNA to the RNA primer. ***Pol*** ε completes DNA synthesis on the leading strand, whereas ***pol*** δ elongates each lagging strand fragment. **Pol** β is involved with DNA repair, and ***pol*** γ replicates mitochondrial DNA. *Pols* ε, δ, and γ use *3′→5′ exonuclease* activity to proofread. **Nucleoside analogs** containing modified sugars can be used to block DNA chain growth. They are useful in anticancer and antiviral chemotherapy. **Telomeres** are stretches of **highly repetitive DNA** complexed with protein that protect the **ends** of linear chromosomes. As most cells divide and age, these sequences are shortened, contributing to senescence. In cells that do not senesce (for example, germline and cancer cells), the ribonucleoprotein **telomerase** employs its protein component ***reverse transcriptase*** to extend the telomeres, using its **RNA** component as a **template**. There are five classes of **positively charged histone (H) proteins**. Two of each of histones H2A, H2B, H3, and H4 form an octameric structural core around which DNA is wrapped, creating a **nucleosome**. The DNA connecting the nucleosomes, called **linker DNA**, is bound to H1. Nucleosomes can be packed more tightly to form a nucleofilament. Additional levels of organization create a chromosome. Most DNA damage can be corrected by **excision repair** involving recognition and removal of the damage by repair proteins, followed by replacement by *DNA pols* and joining by *ligase*. **Ultraviolet radiation** can cause **thymine dimers** that are recognized and removed in E. coli by **uvrABC proteins** of **nucleotide excision repair**. Defects in the **XP proteins** needed for nucleotide excision repair of thymine dimers in humans result in **xeroderma pigmentosum**. **Mismatched** bases are repaired by a similar process of recognition and removal by **Mut proteins** in E. coli. The extent of **methylation** is used for strand identification in prokaryotes. Defective mismatch repair by homologous proteins in humans is associated with **hereditary nonpolyposis colorectal cancer**. Abnormal bases (such as uracil) are removed by ***DNA N-glycosylases*** in **base excision repair**, and the sugar phosphate at the apyrimidinic or apurinic site is cut out. Double-strand breaks in DNA are repaired by **nonhomologous end joining** (error prone) and template-requiring **homologous recombination** ("error-free").

Study Questions

Choose the ONE best answer.

30.1 A 10-year-old girl is brought by her parents to the dermatologist. She has many freckles on her face, neck, arms, and hands, and the parents report that she is unusually sensitive to sunlight. Two basal cell carcinomas are identified on her face. Based on the clinical picture, which of the following processes is most likely to be defective in this patient?

A. Repair of double-strand breaks by error-prone homologous recombination

B. Removal of mismatched bases from the 3′-end of Okazaki fragments by a methyl-directed process

C. Removal of pyrimidine dimers from DNA by nucleotide excision repair

D. Removal of uracil from DNA by base excision repair

Correct answer = C. The sensitivity to sunlight, extensive freckling on parts of the body exposed to the sun, and presence of skin cancer at a young age indicate that the patient most likely suffers from xeroderma pigmentosum (XP). These patients are deficient in any one of several XP proteins required for nucleotide excision repair of pyrimidine dimers in ultraviolet radiation–damaged DNA. Double-strand breaks are repaired by nonhomologous end joining (error prone) or homologous recombination ("error free"). Methylation is not used for strand discrimination in eukaryotic mismatch repair. Uracil is removed from DNA molecules by a specific glycosylase in base excision repair, but a defect in this process does not cause XP.

30.2 Telomeres are complexes of DNA and protein that protect the ends of linear chromosomes. In most normal human somatic cells, telomeres shorten with each division. In stem cells and in cancer cells, however, telomeric length is maintained. In the synthesis of telomeres:

A. telomerase, a ribonucleoprotein, provides both the RNA and the protein needed for synthesis.

B. the RNA of telomerase serves as a primer.

C. the RNA of telomerase is a ribozyme.

D. the protein of telomerase is a DNA-directed DNA polymerase.

E. the shorter 3′→5′ strand gets extended.

F. the direction of synthesis is 3′→5′.

Correct answer = A. Telomerase is a ribonucleoprotein particle required for telomere maintenance. Telomerase contains an RNA that serves as the template, not the primer, for the synthesis of telomeric DNA by the reverse transcriptase of telomerase. Telomeric RNA has no catalytic activity. As a reverse transcriptase, telomerase synthesizes DNA using its RNA template and so is an RNA-directed DNA polymerase. The direction of synthesis, as with all DNA synthesis, is 5′→3′, and it is the 3′-end of the already longer 5′→3′ strand that gets extended.

30.3 While studying the structure of a small gene that was sequenced during the Human Genome Project, an investigator notices that one strand of the DNA molecule contains 20 A, 25 G, 30 C, and 22 T. How many of each base is found in the complete double-stranded molecule?

A. A = 40, G = 50, C = 60, T = 44

B. A = 42, G = 55, C = 55, T = 42

C. A = 44, G = 60, C = 50, T = 40

D. A = 45, G = 45, C = 52, T = 52

E. A = 50, G = 47, C = 50, T = 47

Correct answer = B. The two DNA strands are complementary to each other, with A base-paired with T and G base-paired with C. So, for example, the 20 A on the first strand would be paired with 20 T on the second strand, the 25 G on the first strand would be paired with 25 C on the second strand, and so forth. When these are all added together, the correct numbers of each base are indicated in choice B. Notice that, in the correct answer, A = T and G = C.

30.4 List the order in which the following enzymes participate in prokaryotic replication.

A. Ligase

B. Polymerase I (3′→5′ exonuclease activity)

C. Polymerase I (5′→3′ exonuclease activity)

D. Polymerase I (5′→3′ polymerase activity)

E. Polymerase III

F. Primase

Correct answer: F, E, C, D, B, A. Primase makes the RNA primer; polymerase (pol) III extends the primer with DNA (and proofreads); pol I removes the primer with its 5′→3′ exonuclease activity, fills in the gap with its 5′→3′ polymerase activity, and removes errors with its 3′→5′ exonuclease activity; and ligase makes the 5′→3′-phosphodiester bond that links the DNA made by pols I and III.

30.5 Dideoxynucleotides lack a 3′-hydroxyl group. Why would incorporation of a dideoxynucleotide into DNA stop replication?

The lack of the 3′-OH group prevents formation of the 3′-hydroxyl → 5′-phosphate bond that links one nucleotide to the next in DNA.

RNA Structure, Synthesis, and Processing

31

I. OVERVIEW

The genetic master plan of an organism is contained in the sequence of deoxyribonucleotides in its DNA. However, it is through ribonucleic acid (RNA), the "working copies" of DNA, that the master plan is expressed (Fig. 31.1). The copying process, during which a DNA strand serves as a template for the synthesis of RNA, is called transcription. Transcription produces messenger RNA (mRNA), which are translated into sequences of amino acids (proteins), and ribosomal RNA (rRNA), transfer RNA (tRNA), and additional RNA molecules that perform specialized structural, catalytic, and regulatory functions and are not translated. That is, they are noncoding RNA (ncRNA). Therefore, the final product of gene expression can be RNA or protein, depending upon the gene. [Note: Only ~2% of the genome encodes proteins.] A central feature of transcription is that it is highly selective. For example, many transcripts are made of some regions of the DNA. In other regions, few or no transcripts are made. This selectivity is due, at least in part, to signals embedded in the nucleotide sequence of the DNA. These signals instruct the *RNA polymerase* where to start, how often to start, and where to stop transcription. Several regulatory proteins are also involved in this selection process. The biochemical differentiation of an organism's tissues is ultimately a result of the selectivity of the transcription process. [Note: This selectivity of transcription is in contrast to the "all-or-none" nature of genomic replication.] Another important feature of transcription is that many RNA transcripts that initially are faithful copies of one of the two DNA strands may undergo various modifications, such as terminal additions, base modifications, trimming, and internal segment removal, which convert the inactive primary transcript into a functional molecule. The transcriptome is the complete set of RNA transcripts expressed by a genome.

II. RNA STRUCTURE

There are three major types of RNA that participate in the process of protein synthesis: rRNA, tRNA, and mRNA. Like DNA, these RNA are unbranched polymeric molecules composed of nucleoside monophosphates joined together by $3' \rightarrow 5'$-phosphodiester bonds (see p. 412). However, they differ from DNA in several ways. For example, they are considerably smaller than DNA, contain ribose instead of deoxyribose

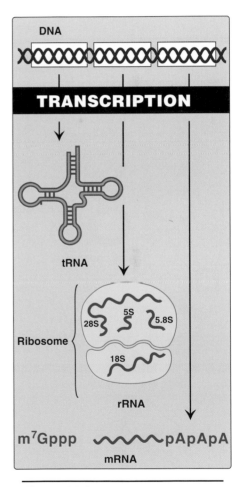

Figure 31.1
Expression of genetic information by transcription. [Note: RNA shown are eukaryotic.] tRNA = transfer RNA; rRNA = ribosomal RNA; mRNA = messenger RNA; m⁷Gppp = 7-methylguanosine-triphosphate cap; pApApA = poly-A tail; p = phosphate.

433

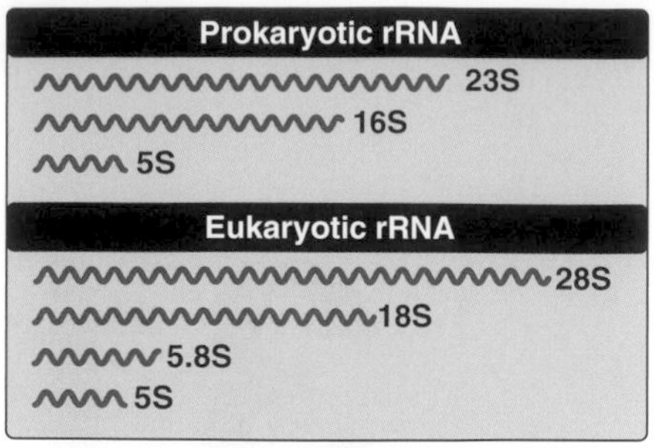

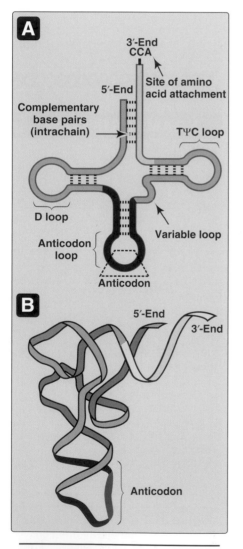

Figure 31.2

Prokaryotic and eukaryotic ribosomal RNA (rRNA). S = Svedberg unit.

Figure 31.3

A. Characteristic transfer RNA (tRNA) secondary structure (cloverleaf). B. Folded (tertiary) tRNA structure found in cells. D = dihydrouracil; Ψ = pseudouracil; T = thymine; C = cytosine; A = adenine.

and uracil instead of thymine, and exist as single strands that are capable of folding into complex structures. The three major types of RNA also differ from each other in size, function, and special structural modifications. [Note: In eukaryotes, additional small ncRNA molecules found in the nucleolus (snoRNA), nucleus (snRNA), and cytoplasm (microRNA [miRNA]) perform specialized functions as described on pp. 441, 442, and 475.]

A. Ribosomal RNA

rRNA are found in association with several proteins as components of the ribosomes, the complex structures that serve as the sites for protein synthesis (see p. 451). Prokaryotic cells contain three distinct size species of rRNA (23S, 16S, and 5S, where S is the Svedberg unit for sedimentation rate that is determined by the size and shape of the particle), as shown in Figure 31.2. Eukaryotic cells contain four rRNA species (28S, 18S, 5.8S, and 5S). Together, rRNA make up ~80% of the total RNA in the cell. [Note: Some RNA function as catalysts, for example, an rRNA in protein synthesis (see p. 455). RNA with catalytic activity is termed a ribozyme.]

B. Transfer RNA

tRNA are the smallest (4S) of the three major types of RNA molecules. There is at least one specific type of tRNA molecule for each of the 20 amino acids commonly found in proteins. Together, tRNA make up ~15% of the total RNA in the cell. The tRNA molecules contain a high percentage of unusual (modified) bases, for example, dihydrouracil (see Fig. 22.2, p. 292), and have extensive intrachain base-pairing (Fig. 31.3) that leads to characteristic secondary and tertiary structure. Each tRNA serves as an adaptor molecule that carries its specific amino acid, covalently attached to its 3′-end, to the site of protein synthesis. There, it recognizes the genetic code sequence on an mRNA, which specifies the addition of that amino acid to the growing peptide chain (see p. 447).

C. Messenger RNA

mRNA comprises only ~5% of the RNA in a cell, yet is by far the most heterogeneous type of RNA in size and base sequence. mRNA is coding RNA in that it carries genetic information from DNA for use in protein synthesis. In eukaryotes, this involves transport of mRNA out of the nucleus and into the cytosol. An mRNA carrying information from more than one gene is polycistronic (cistron = gene). Polycistronic mRNA is characteristic of prokaryotes. An mRNA carrying information from only one gene is monocistronic and is characteristic of eukaryotes. In addition to the protein-coding regions that can be translated, mRNA contains untranslated regions at its 5′- and 3′-ends (Fig. 31.4). Special structural characteristics of eukaryotic (but not prokaryotic) mRNA include a long sequence of adenine nucleotides (a poly-A tail) on the 3′-end of the RNA, plus a cap on the 5′-end consisting of a molecule of 7-methylguanosine attached through an unusual (5′→5′) triphosphate linkage. The mechanisms for modifying mRNA to create these special structural characteristics are discussed on pp. 441–442.

III. PROKARYOTIC GENE TRANSCRIPTION

The structure of magnesium-requiring *RNA polymerase* (*RNA pol*), the signals that control transcription, and the varieties of modification that RNA transcripts can undergo differ among organisms, particularly from prokaryotes to eukaryotes. Therefore, the discussions of prokaryotic and eukaryotic transcription are presented separately.

A. Prokaryotic RNA polymerase

In bacteria, one species of *RNA pol* synthesizes all of the RNA except for the short RNA primers needed for DNA replication [Note: RNA primers are synthesized by the specialized, monomeric enzyme *primase* (see p. 418).] *RNA pol* is a multisubunit enzyme that recognizes a nucleotide sequence (the promoter region) at the beginning of a length of DNA that is to be transcribed. It next makes a complementary RNA copy of the DNA template strand and then recognizes the end of the DNA sequence to be transcribed (the termination region). RNA is synthesized from its 5′-end to its 3′-end, antiparallel to its DNA template strand (see p. 415). The template is copied as it is in DNA synthesis, in which a guanine (G) on the DNA specifies a cytosine (C) in the RNA, a C specifies a G, a thymine (T) specifies an adenine (A), but an A specifies a uracil (U) instead of a T (Fig. 31.5). The RNA, then, is complementary to the DNA template (antisense, minus) strand and identical to the coding (sense, plus) strand, with U replacing T. Within the DNA molecule, regions of both strands can serve as templates for transcription. For a given gene, however, only one of the two DNA strands can be the template. Which strand is used is determined by the location of the promoter for that gene. Transcription by *RNA pol* involves a core enzyme and several auxiliary proteins.

1. **Core enzyme:** Five of the enzyme's peptide subunits, 2 α, 1 β, 1 β′, and 1 Ω, are required for enzyme assembly (α, Ω), template binding (β′), and the *5′→3′ polymerase* activity (β) and together are referred to as the core enzyme (Fig. 31.6). However, this enzyme lacks specificity (that is, it cannot recognize the promoter region on the DNA template).

2. **Holoenzyme:** The σ subunit (sigma factor) enables *RNA pol* to recognize promoter regions on the DNA. The σ subunit plus the core enzyme make up the holoenzyme. [Note: Different σ factors recognize different groups of genes, with σ^{70} predominating.]

B. Steps in RNA synthesis

The process of transcription of a typical gene of Escherichia coli (E. coli) can be divided into three phases: initiation, elongation, and termination. A transcription unit extends from the promoter to the termination region, and the initial product of transcription by *RNA pol* is termed the primary transcript.

1. **Initiation:** Transcription begins with the binding of the *RNA pol* holoenzyme to a region of the DNA known as the promoter, which is not transcribed. The prokaryotic promoter contains characteristic consensus sequences (Fig. 31.7). [Note: Consensus sequences

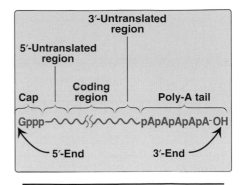

Figure 31.4
Structure of eukaryotic messenger RNA. G = guanine; A = adenine.

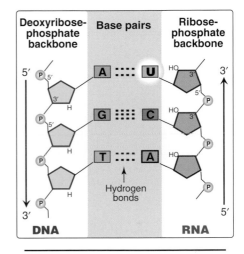

Figure 31.5
Antiparallel, complementary base pairs between DNA and RNA.
T = thymine; A = adenine;
C = cytosine; G = guanine; U = uracil.

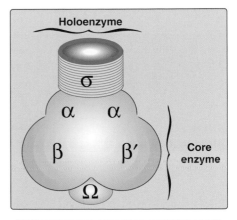

Figure 31.6
Components of prokaryotic *RNA polymerase*.

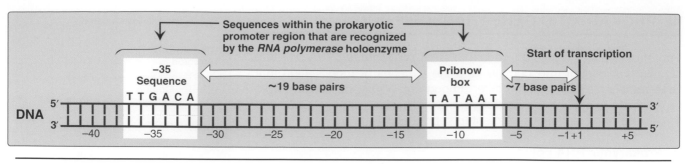

Figure 31.7
Structure of the prokaryotic promoter region. T = thymine; G = guanine; A = adenine; C = cytosine.

are idealized sequences in which the base shown at each position is the base most frequently (but not necessarily always) encountered at that position.] Those that are recognized by prokaryotic *RNA pol* σ factors include the following.

a. **−35 Sequence:** A consensus sequence (5′-TTGACA-3′), centered about 35 bases to the left of the transcription start site (see Fig. 31.7), is the initial point of contact for the holoenzyme, and a closed complex is formed. [Note: By convention, the regulatory sequences that control transcription are designated by the 5′→3′ nucleotide sequence on the coding strand. A base in the promoter region is assigned a negative number if it occurs prior to (to the left of, toward the 5′-end of, or "upstream" of) the transcription start site. Therefore, the TTGACA sequence is centered at approximately base −35. The first base at the transcription start site is assigned a position of +1. There is no base designated "0".]

b. **Pribnow box:** The holoenzyme moves and covers a second consensus sequence (5′-TATAAT-3′), centered at about −10 (see Fig. 31.7), which is the site of melting (unwinding) of a short stretch (~14 base pairs) of DNA. This initial melting converts the closed initiation complex to an open complex known as a transcription bubble. [Note: A mutation in either the −10 or the −35 sequence can affect the transcription of the gene controlled by the mutant promoter.]

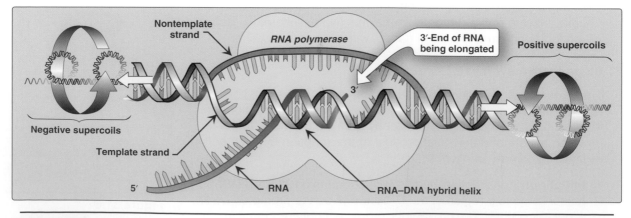

Figure 31.8
Local unwinding of DNA by *RNA polymerase* and formation of an open initiation complex (transcription bubble).

2. **Elongation:** Once the promoter has been recognized and bound by the holoenzyme, local unwinding of the DNA helix continues (Fig. 31.8), mediated by the *polymerase*. [Note: Unwinding generates supercoils in the DNA that can be relieved by *DNA topoisomerases* (see p. 417).] *RNA pol* begins to synthesize a transcript of the DNA sequence, and several short pieces of RNA are made and discarded. The elongation phase begins when the transcript (typically starting with a purine) exceeds 10 nucleotides in length. Sigma is then released, and the core enzyme is able to leave (clear) the promoter and move along the template strand in a processive manner, serving as its own sliding clamp. During transcription, a short DNA–RNA hybrid helix is formed (see Fig. 31.8). Like *DNA pol*, *RNA pol* uses nucleoside triphosphates as substrates and releases pyrophosphate each time a nucleoside monophosphate is added to the growing chain. As with replication, transcription is always in the $5' \rightarrow 3'$ direction. In contrast to *DNA pol*, *RNA pol* does not require a primer and does not have a $3' \rightarrow 5'$ exonuclease domain for proofreading. [Note: Misincorporation of a ribonucleotide causes *RNA pol* to pause, backtrack, cleave the transcript, and restart. Nonetheless, transcription has a higher error rate than does replication.]

3. **Termination:** The elongation of the single-stranded RNA chain continues until a termination signal is reached. Termination can be intrinsic (occur without additional proteins) or dependent upon the participation of a protein known as the ρ (rho) factor.

   a. **ρ-Independent:** Seen with most prokaryotic genes, this requires that a sequence in the DNA template generates a sequence in the nascent (newly made) RNA that is self-complementary (Fig. 31.9). This allows the RNA to fold back on itself, forming a GC-rich stem (stabilized by hydrogen bonds) plus a loop. This structure is known as a "hairpin." Additionally, just beyond the hairpin, the RNA transcript contains a string of Us at the 3'-end. The bonding of these Us to the complementary As of the DNA template is weak. This facilitates the separation of the newly synthesized RNA from its DNA template, as the double helix "zips up" behind the *RNA pol*.

   b. **ρ-Dependent:** This requires the participation of the additional protein rho, which is a hexameric *ATPase* with *helicase* activity. Rho binds a C-rich rho utilization (rut) site near the 5'-end of the nascent RNA and, using its *ATPase* activity, moves along the RNA until it reaches the *RNA pol* paused at the termination site. The ATP-dependent *helicase* activity of rho separates the RNA–DNA hybrid helix, causing the release of the RNA.

4. **Antibiotics:** Some antibiotics prevent bacterial cell growth by inhibiting RNA synthesis. For example, rifampin (rifampicin) inhibits transcription initiation by binding to the β subunit of prokaryotic *RNA pol* and preventing chain growth beyond three nucleotides (Fig. 31.10). Rifampin is important in the treatment of tuberculosis. Dactinomycin (actinomycin D) was the first antibiotic to find therapeutic application in tumor chemotherapy. It inserts (intercalates) between the DNA bases and inhibits transcription initiation and elongation.

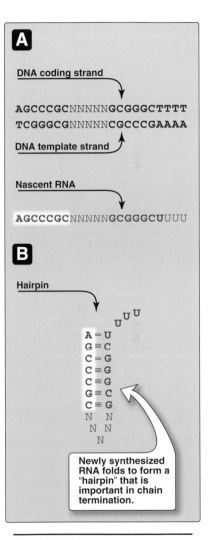

A

DNA coding strand

AGCCCGCNNNNNGCGGGCTTTT
TCGGGCGNNNNNCGCCCGAAAA

DNA template strand

Nascent RNA

AGCCCGCNNNNNGCGGGCUUUU

B

Hairpin

A	= U
G	≡ C
C	≡ G
C	≡ G
C	≡ G
G	≡ C
C	≡ G
N	N
N	N
N	

U U U

Newly synthesized RNA folds to form a "hairpin" that is important in chain termination.

Figure 31.9

Rho-independent termination of prokaryotic transcription. A. DNA template sequence generates a self-complementary sequence in the nascent RNA. B. Hairpin structure formed by the RNA. N represents a noncomplementary base; A = adenine, T = thymine; G = guanine; C = cytosine; U = uracil.

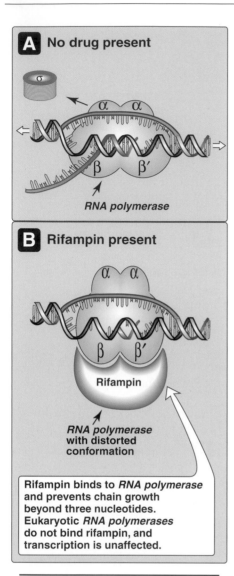

A No drug present

RNA polymerase

B Rifampin present

Rifampin

RNA polymerase
**with distorted
conformation**

**Rifampin binds to *RNA polymerase*
and prevents chain growth
beyond three nucleotides.
Eukaryotic *RNA polymerases*
do not bind rifampin, and
transcription is unaffected.**

Figure 31.10
Inhibition of prokaryotic *RNA
polymerase* by rifampin (rifampicin).

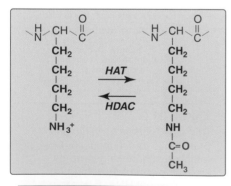

Figure 31.11
Acetylation/deacetylation of a lysine
residue in a histone. Acetyl coenzyme
A provides the acetyl group. *HAT =
histone acetyltransferase*; *HDAC =
histone deacetylase*.

IV. EUKARYOTIC GENE TRANSCRIPTION

The transcription of eukaryotic genes is a far more complicated process than transcription in prokaryotes. Eukaryotic transcription involves separate *polymerases* for the synthesis of rRNA, tRNA, and mRNA. In addition, a large number of proteins called transcription factors (TF) are involved. TF bind to distinct sites on the DNA within the core promoter region, close (proximal) to it, or some distance away (distal). They are required for both the assembly of a transcription initiation complex at the promoter and the determination of which genes are to be transcribed. [Note: Each eukaryotic *RNA pol* has its own promoters and TF that bind core promoter sequences.] For TF to recognize and bind to their specific DNA sequences, the chromatin structure in that region must be decondensed (relaxed) to allow access to the DNA. The role of transcription in the regulation of gene expression is discussed in Chapter 33.

A. Chromatin structure and gene expression

The association of DNA with histones to form nucleosomes (see p. 425) affects the ability of the transcription machinery to access the DNA to be transcribed. Most actively transcribed genes are found in a relatively decondensed form of chromatin called euchromatin, whereas most inactive segments of DNA are found in highly condensed heterochromatin. The interconversion of these forms is called chromatin remodeling. A major component of chromatin remodeling is the covalent modification of histones (for example, the acetylation of lysine residues at the amino terminus of histone proteins), as shown in Figure 31.11. Acetylation, mediated by *histone acetyltransferases* (*HAT*), eliminates the positive charge on the lysine, thereby decreasing the interaction of the histone with the negatively charged DNA. Removal of the acetyl group by *histone deacetylases* (*HDAC*) restores the positive charge and fosters stronger interactions between histones and DNA. [Note: The ATP-dependent repositioning of nucleosomes is also required to access DNA.]

B. Nuclear RNA polymerases

There are three distinct types of *RNA pol* in the nucleus of eukaryotic cells. All are large enzymes with multiple subunits. Each type of *RNA pol* recognizes particular genes. [Note: Mitochondria contain a single *RNA pol* that resembles the bacterial enzyme.]

1. **RNA polymerase I:** This enzyme synthesizes the precursor of the 28S, 18S, and 5.8S rRNA in the nucleolus.

2. **RNA polymerase II:** This enzyme synthesizes the nuclear precursors of mRNA that are processed and then translated to proteins. *RNA pol II* also synthesizes certain small ncRNA, such as snoRNA, snRNA, and miRNA.

   a. **Promoters for RNA polymerase II:** In some genes transcribed by *RNA pol II*, a sequence of nucleotides (TATAAA) that is nearly identical to that of the Pribnow box (see p. 436) is found centered ~25 nucleotides upstream of the transcription start site. This core promoter consensus sequence is called the TATA, or Hogness, box. In the majority of genes, however, no TATA box is present. Instead, different core promoter elements

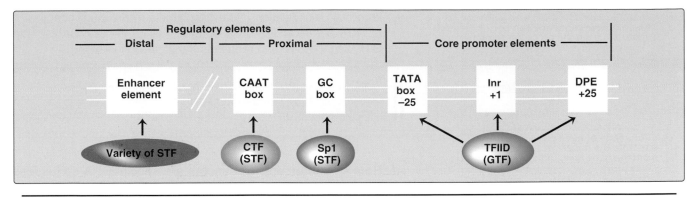

Figure 31.12
Eukaryotic gene cis-acting promoter and regulatory elements and their trans-acting general and specific transcription factors (GTF and STF, respectively). Inr = initiator; DPE = downstream promoter element.

such as Inr (initiator) or DPE (downstream promoter element) are present (Fig. 31.12). [Note: No one consensus sequence is found in all core promoters.] Because these sequences are on the same molecule of DNA as the gene being transcribed, they are cis-acting. The sequences serve as binding sites for proteins known as general transcription factors (GTF), which in turn interact with each other and with *RNA pol II*.

b. **General transcription factors:** GTF are the minimal requirements for recognition of the promoter, recruitment of *RNA pol II* to the promoter, formation of the preinitiation complex, and initiation of transcription at a basal level (Fig. 31.13A). GTF are encoded by different genes, synthesized in the cytosol, and diffuse (transit) to their sites of action, and so are trans-acting. [Note: In contrast to the prokaryotic holoenzyme, eukaryotic *RNA pol II* does not itself recognize and bind the promoter. Instead, TFIID, a GTF containing TATA-binding protein and TATA-associated factors, recognizes and binds the TATA box (and other core promoter elements). TFIIF, another GTF, brings the *polymerase* to the promoter. The *helicase* activity of TFIIH melts the DNA, and its *kinase* activity phosphorylates *polymerase*, allowing it to clear the promoter.]

c. **Regulatory elements and transcriptional activators:** Additional consensus sequences lie upstream of the core promoter (see Fig. 31.12). Those close to the core promoter (within ~200 nucleotides) are the proximal regulatory elements, such as the CAAT and GC boxes. Those farther away are the distal regulatory elements such as enhancers (see d. below). Proteins known as transcriptional activators or specific transcription factors (STF) bind these regulatory elements. STF bind to promoter proximal elements to regulate the frequency of transcription initiation and to distal elements to mediate the response to signals such as hormones (see p. 472) and regulate which genes are expressed at a given point in time. A typical protein-coding eukaryotic gene has binding sites for many such factors. STF have two binding domains. One is a DNA-binding domain, the other is a transcription activation domain that recruits the GTF to the core promoter as well as coactivator proteins such as the *HAT* enzymes involved in

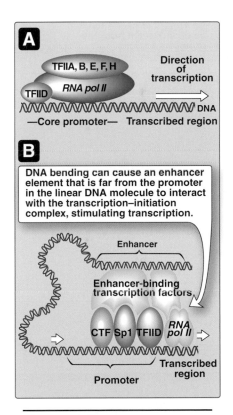

Figure 31.13
A. Association of the general transcription factors (TFII) and *RNA polymerase II (RNA pol II)* at the core promoter. [Note: The Roman numeral II denotes a TF for *RNA pol II*.] B. Enhancer stimulation of transcription. CTF = CAAT box transcription factor; Sp1 = specificity factor-1.

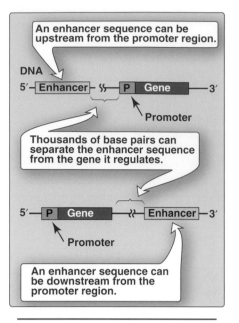

Figure 31.14
Some possible locations of enhancer sequences.

chromatin modification. [Note: Mediator, a multisubunit coactivator of *RNA pol II*–catalyzed transcription, binds the *polymerase*, the GTF, and the STF and regulates transcription initiation.]

 Transcriptional activators bind DNA through a variety of motifs, such as the helix-loop-helix, zinc finger, and leucine zipper (see p. 18).

    d. Role of enhancers: Enhancers are special DNA sequences that increase the rate of initiation of transcription by *RNA pol II*. Enhancers are typically on the same chromosome as the gene whose transcription they stimulate (Fig. 31.13B). However, they can 1) be located upstream (to the 5′-side) or downstream (to the 3′-side) of the transcription start site, 2) be close to or thousands of base pairs away from the promoter (Fig. 31.14), and 3) occur on either strand of the DNA. Enhancers contain DNA sequences called response elements that bind STF. By bending or looping the DNA, STF can interact with other TF bound to a promoter and with *RNA pol II*, thereby stimulating transcription (see Fig. 31.13B). Mediator also binds enhancers. [Note: Although silencers are similar to enhancers in that they also can act over long distances, they reduce gene expression.]

    e. RNA polymerase II inhibitor: α-Amanitin, a potent toxin produced by the poisonous mushroom <u>Amanita</u> <u>phalloides</u> (sometimes called the "death cap"), binds *RNA pol II* tightly and slows its movement, thereby inhibiting mRNA synthesis.

  3. RNA polymerase III: This enzyme synthesizes tRNA, 5S rRNA, and some snRNA and snoRNA.

V. POSTTRANSCRIPTIONAL MODIFICATION OF RNA

A primary transcript is the initial, linear, RNA copy of a transcription unit (the segment of DNA between specific initiation and termination sequences). The primary transcripts of both prokaryotic and eukaryotic tRNA and rRNA are posttranscriptionally modified by cleavage of the original transcripts by *ribonucleases*. tRNA are further modified to help give each species its unique identity. In contrast, prokaryotic mRNA is generally identical to its primary transcript, whereas eukaryotic mRNA is extensively modified both co- and posttranscriptionally.

A. Ribosomal RNA

rRNA of both prokaryotic and eukaryotic cells are generated from long precursor molecules called pre-rRNA. The 23S, 16S, and 5S rRNA of prokaryotes are produced from a single pre-rRNA molecule, as are the 28S, 18S, and 5.8S rRNA of eukaryotes (Fig. 31.15). [Note: Eukaryotic 5S rRNA is synthesized by *RNA pol III* and modified separately.] The pre-rRNA are cleaved by *ribonucleases* to yield intermediate-sized pieces of rRNA, which are further processed (trimmed by *exonucleases* and modified at some bases and

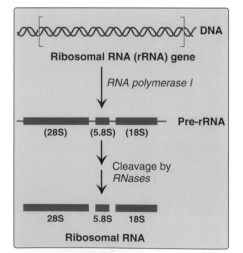

Figure 31.15
Posttranscriptional processing of eukaryotic ribosomal RNA by *ribonucleases* (*RNases*). S = Svedberg unit.

riboses) to produce the required RNA species. [Note: In eukaryotes, rRNA genes are found in long, tandem arrays. rRNA synthesis and processing occur in the nucleolus, with base and sugar modifications facilitated by snoRNA.]

B. Transfer RNA

Both eukaryotic and prokaryotic tRNA are also made from longer precursor molecules that must be modified (Fig. 31.16). Sequences at both ends of the molecule are removed, and, if present, an intron is removed from the anticodon loop by *nucleases*. Other posttranscriptional modifications include addition of a –CCA sequence by *nucleotidyltransferase* to the 3′-terminal end of tRNA and modification of bases at specific positions to produce the unusual bases characteristic of tRNA (see p. 291).

C. Eukaryotic messenger RNA

The collection of all the primary transcripts synthesized in the nucleus by *RNA pol II* is known as heterogeneous nuclear RNA (hnRNA). The pre-mRNA components of hnRNA undergo extensive co- and posttranscriptional modification in the nucleus and become mature mRNA. These modifications usually include the following. [Note: *Pol II* itself recruits the proteins required for the modifications.]

1. **Addition of a 5′-cap:** This is the first of the processing reactions for pre-mRNA (Fig. 31.17). The cap is a 7-methylguanosine attached to the 5′-terminal end of the mRNA through an unusual 5′→5′-triphosphate linkage that is resistant to most *nucleases*. Creation of the cap requires removal of the γ phosphoryl group

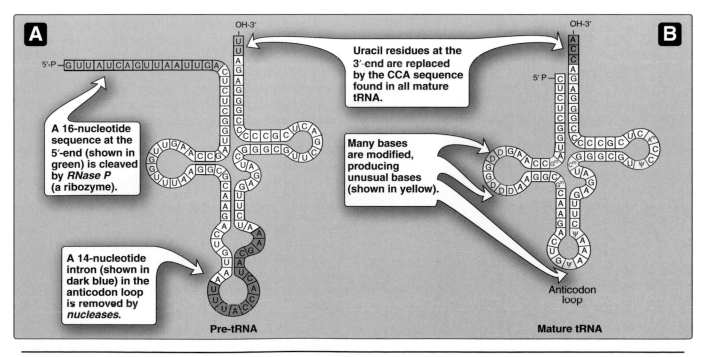

Figure 31.16
A. Precursor transfer RNA (pre-tRNA) transcript. B. Mature (functional) tRNA after posttranscriptional modification. Modified bases include D (dihydrouracil), ψ (pseudouracil), and ^{m}, which means that the base has been methylated.

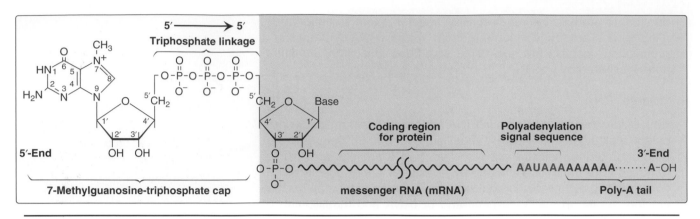

Figure 31.17
Posttranscriptional modification of mRNA showing the 7-methylguanosine cap and polyadenylate (poly-A) tail.

from the 5′-triphosphate of the pre-mRNA, followed by addition of guanosine monophosphate (from guanosine triphosphate) by the nuclear enzyme *guanylyltransferase*. Methylation of this terminal guanine occurs in the cytosol and is catalyzed by *guanine-7-methyltransferase*. S-Adenosylmethionine is the source of the methyl group (see p. 263). Additional methylation steps may occur. The addition of this 7-methylguanosine cap helps stabilize the mRNA and permits efficient initiation of translation (see p. 455).

2. **Addition of a 3′-poly-A tail:** Most eukaryotic mRNA (with several exceptions, including those for the histones) have a chain of 40–250 adenylates (adenosine monophosphates) attached to the 3′-end (see Fig. 31.17). This poly-A tail is not transcribed from the DNA but rather is added by the nuclear enzyme, *polyadenylate polymerase*, using ATP as the substrate. The pre-mRNA is cleaved downstream of a consensus sequence, called the polyadenylation signal sequence (AAUAAA), found near the 3′-end of the RNA, and the poly-A tail is added to the new 3′-end. Tailing terminates eukaryotic transcription. Tails help stabilize the mRNA, facilitate its exit from the nucleus, and aid in translation. After the mRNA enters the cytosol, the poly-A tail is gradually shortened.

3. **Splicing:** Maturation of eukaryotic mRNA usually involves removal from the primary transcript of RNA sequences (introns or intervening sequences) that do not code for protein. The remaining coding (expressed) sequences, the exons, are joined together to form the mature mRNA. The process of removing introns and joining exons is called splicing. The molecular complex that accomplishes these tasks is known as the spliceosome. A few eukaryotic primary transcripts contain no introns (for example, those from histone genes). Others contain a few introns, whereas some, such as the primary transcripts for the α chains of collagen, contain >50 introns that must be removed.

   a. **Role of small nuclear RNA:** In association with multiple proteins, uracil-rich snRNA form five small nuclear ribonucleoprotein particles (snRNP, or "snurp") designated as U1, U2, U4, U5, and U6 that mediate splicing. They facilitate the removal of introns by forming base pairs with the consensus sequences at each end of the intron (Fig. 31.18). [Note: In systemic lupus erythematosus, an autoimmune disease, patients produce antibodies against their own nuclear proteins such as snRNP.]

b. **Mechanism:** The binding of snRNP brings the sequences of neighboring exons into the correct alignment for splicing, allowing two transesterification reactions (catalyzed by the RNA of U2, U5, and U6) to occur. The 2'-OH group of an adenine nucleotide (known as the branch site A) in the intron attacks the phosphate at the 5'-end of the intron (splice-donor site), forming an unusual 2'→5'-phosphodiester bond and creating a "lariat" structure (see Fig. 31.18). The newly freed 3'-OH of exon 1 attacks the 5'-phosphate at the splice-acceptor site, forming a phosphodiester bond that joins exons 1 and 2. The excised intron is released as a lariat, which is typically degraded but may be a precursor for ncRNA such as snoRNA. [Note: The GU and AG sequences at the beginning and end, respectively, of introns are invariant. However, additional sequences are critical for splice-site recognition.] After introns have been removed and exons joined, the mature mRNA molecules pass into the cytosol through pores in the nuclear membrane. [Note: The introns in tRNA (see Fig. 31.16) are removed by a different mechanism.]

c. **Effect of splice site mutations:** Mutations at splice sites can lead to improper splicing and the production of aberrant proteins. It is estimated that at least 20% of all genetic diseases are a result of mutations that affect RNA splicing. For example, mutations that cause the incorrect splicing of β-globin mRNA are responsible for some cases of β-thalassemia, a disease in which the production of the β-globin protein is defective (see p. 38). Splice site mutations can result in exons being skipped (removed) or introns retained. They can also activate cryptic splice sites, which are sites that contain the 5' or 3' consensus sequence but are not normally used.

4. **Alternative splicing:** The pre-mRNA molecules from >90% of human genes can be spliced in alternative ways in different tissues. Because this produces multiple variations of the mRNA and, therefore, of its protein product (Fig. 31.19), it is a mechanism for producing a large, diverse set of proteins from a limited set of genes. For example, the mRNA for tropomyosin (TM), an actin filament–binding protein of the cytoskeleton (and of the contractile apparatus in muscle cells), undergoes extensive tissue-specific alternative splicing with production of multiple isoforms of the TM protein.

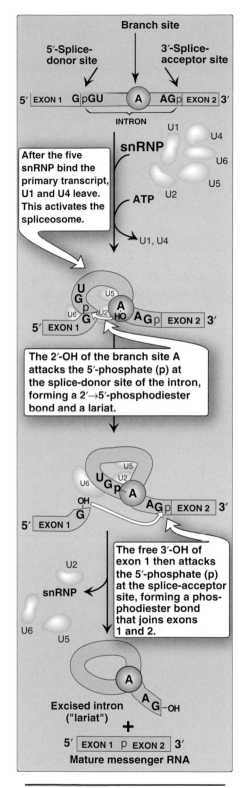

Figure 31.18

Splicing. [Note: U1 binds the 5'-donor site, and U2 binds the branch A and the 3'-acceptor site. Addition of U4–U6 completes the complex.] snRNP = small nuclear ribonucleoprotein particle.

VI. CHAPTER SUMMARY

Three major types of RNA participate in the process of protein synthesis: **ribosomal RNA (rRNA)**, **transfer RNA (tRNA)**, and **messenger RNA (mRNA)**, as shown in Figure 31.20. They are unbranched polymers of

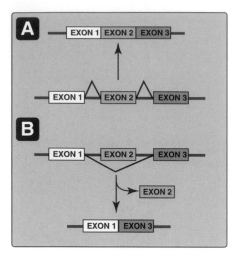

Figure 31.19
Alternative splicing patterns in eukaryotic messenger RNA (mRNA). The removal (skipping) of exon 2 from the mRNA in panel B results in a protein product that is different than the one made from the mRNA in panel A.

nucleotides but differ from DNA by containing **ribose** instead of deoxyribose and **uracil** instead of thymine. **rRNA** is a component of the **ribosomes**. **tRNA** serves as an **adaptor** molecule that carries a specific amino acid to the site of protein synthesis. **mRNA** (coding RNA) carries genetic information from DNA for use in protein synthesis. The process of RNA synthesis is called **transcription**, and the substrates are **ribonucleoside triphosphates**. The enzyme that synthesizes RNA is *RNA polymerase* (*RNA pol*). In **prokaryotic** cells, the **core enzyme** has five subunits (2α, 1β, $1 \beta'$, and 1Ω) and possesses $5' \rightarrow 3'$ *polymerase* activity needed for transcription. The core enzyme requires an additional subunit, **sigma (σ) factor**, to recognize the nucleotide sequence (**promoter** region) at the beginning of the DNA to be transcribed. This region contains **consensus sequences** that are highly conserved and include the **−10 Pribnow box** and the **−35 sequence**. Another protein, **rho (ρ)**, is required for **termination** of transcription of some genes. There are three distinct types of *RNA pol* in the nucleus of **eukaryotic** cells. *RNA pol I* synthesizes the precursor of rRNA in the nucleolus. In the nucleoplasm, *RNA pol II* synthesizes the precursors for mRNA and some noncoding RNA, and *RNA pol III* synthesizes the precursors of tRNA and 5S rRNA. In both prokaryotes and eukaryotes, *RNA pol* does not require a primer. Proofreading involves the *polymerase* backtracking and cleaving the transcript. Core **promoters** for genes transcribed by *RNA pol II* contain **cis-acting** consensus sequences, such as the **TATA (Hogness) box**, which serve as binding sites for **trans-acting general transcription factors**. Upstream of these are **proximal** regulatory elements, such as the CAAT and GC boxes, and **distal** regulatory elements, such as **enhancers**. **Specific transcription factors** (transcriptional activators) and **Mediator complex** bind these elements and regulate the frequency of transcription initiation, the response to signals such as hormones, and which genes are expressed at any given time. Eukaryotic transcription requires that the **chromatin** be relaxed (decondensed) in a process known as **chromatin remodeling**. **A primary transcript** is a linear copy of a **transcription unit**, the segment of DNA between specific initiation and termination sequences. The primary transcripts of both prokaryotic and eukaryotic tRNA and rRNA are **posttranscriptionally modified**. The rRNA are synthesized from long precursor molecules called **pre-rRNA**. These precursors are cleaved and trimmed by *ribonucleases*, producing the three largest rRNA, and bases and sugars are modified. Eukaryotic 5S rRNA is synthesized by *RNA pol III* and is modified separately. Prokaryotic and eukaryotic tRNA are also made from longer precursor molecules (**pre-tRNA**). If present, an intron is removed by *nucleases*, and both ends of the molecule are trimmed by *ribonucleases*. A **3'-CCA** sequence is added, and bases at specific positions are modified. Prokaryotic mRNA is generally identical to its primary transcript, whereas eukaryotic **pre-mRNA** is extensively modified co- and posttranscriptionally. For example, a **7-methylguanosine cap** is attached to the 5'-end of the mRNA through a $5' \rightarrow 5'$ linkage. A **long poly-A tail**, not transcribed from the DNA, is attached by *polyadenylate polymerase* to the 3'-end of most mRNA. Most eukaryotic mRNA also contains **intervening sequences** (**introns**) that must be removed for the mRNA to be functional. Their removal, as well as the joining of **expressed sequences** (**exons**), requires a **spliceosome** composed of **small nuclear ribonucleoprotein particles** ("snurps") that mediate the process of **splicing**. Eukaryotic mRNA is **monocistronic**, containing information from just one gene, whereas prokaryotic mRNA is **polycistronic**.

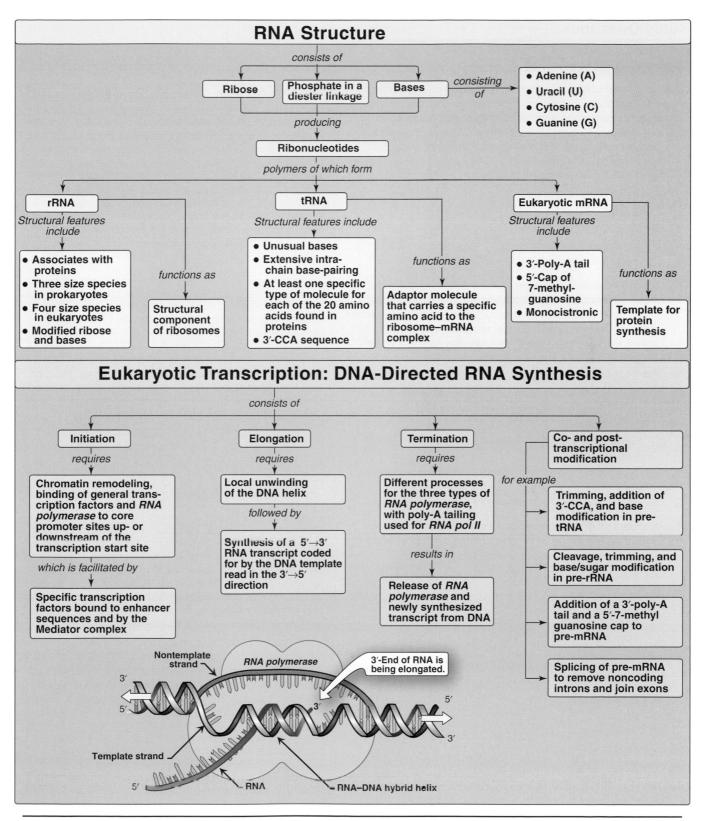

Figure 31.20
Key concept map for RNA structure and synthesis. rRNA = ribosomal RNA; tRNA = transfer RNA; mRNA = messenger RNA.

Study Questions

Choose the ONE best answer.

31.1 An 8-month-old male with severe anemia is found to have β-thalassemia. Genetic analysis shows that one of his β-globin genes has a mutation that creates a new splice-acceptor site 19 nucleotides upstream of the normal splice-acceptor site of the first intron. Which of the following best describes the new messenger RNA molecule that can be produced from this mutant gene?

A. Exon 1 will be too short.
B. Exon 1 will be too long.
C. Exon 2 will be too short.
D. Exon 2 will be too long.
E. Exon 2 will be missing.

Correct answer = D. Because the mutation creates an additional splice-acceptor site (the 3′-end) upstream of the normal acceptor site of intron 1, the 19 nucleotides that are usually found at the 3′-end of the excised intron 1 lariat can remain behind as part of exon 2. The presence of these extra nucleotides in the coding region of the mutant messenger RNA (mRNA) molecule will prevent the ribosome from translating the message into a normal β-globin protein molecule. Those mRNA for which the normal splice site is used to remove the first intron will be normal, and their translation will produce normal β-globin protein.

31.2 A 4-year-old child who easily tires and has trouble walking is diagnosed with Duchenne muscular dystrophy, an X-linked recessive disorder. Genetic analysis shows that the patient's gene for the muscle protein dystrophin contains a mutation in its promoter region. Of the choices listed, which would be the most likely effect of this mutation?

A. Initiation of dystrophin transcription will be defective.
B. Termination of dystrophin transcription will be defective.
C. Capping of dystrophin messenger RNA will be defective.
D. Splicing of dystrophin messenger RNA will be defective.
E. Tailing of dystrophin messenger RNA will be defective.

Correct answer = A. Mutations in the promoter typically prevent formation of the RNA polymerase II transcription initiation complex, resulting in a decrease in the initiation of messenger RNA (mRNA) synthesis. A deficiency of dystrophin mRNA will result in a deficiency in the production of the dystrophin protein. Capping, splicing, and tailing defects are not a consequence of promoter mutations. They can, however, result in mRNA with decreased stability (capping and tailing defects) or an mRNA in which exons have been skipped (lost) or introns retained (splicing defects).

31.3 A mutation to this sequence in eukaryotic messenger RNA (mRNA) will affect the process by which the 3′-end polyadenylate (poly-A) tail is added to the mRNA.

A. AAUAAA
B. CAAT
C. CCA
D. GU... A ... AG
E. TATAAA

Correct answer = A. An endonuclease cleaves mRNA just downstream of this polyadenylation signal, creating a new 3′-end to which polyadenylate polymerase adds the poly-A tail using ATP as the substrate in a template-independent process. CAAT and TATAAA are sequences found in promoters for RNA polymerase II. CCA is added to the 3′-end of pre-transfer RNA by nucleotidyltransferase. GU...A...AG denotes an intron in eukaryotic pre-mRNA.

31.4 This protein factor identifies the promoter of protein-coding genes in eukaryotes.

A. Pribnow box
B. Rho
C. Sigma
D. TFIID
E. U1

Correct answer = D. The general transcription factor TFIID recognizes and binds core promoter elements such as the TATA-like box in eukaryotic protein-coding genes. These genes are transcribed by RNA polymerase II. The Pribnow box is a cis-acting element in prokaryotic promoters. Rho is involved in the termination of prokaryotic transcription. Sigma is the subunit of prokaryotic RNA polymerase that recognizes and binds the prokaryotic promoter. U1 is a ribonucleoprotein involved in splicing of eukaryotic pre-mRNA.

31.5 What is the sequence (conventionally written) of the RNA product of the DNA template sequence, GATCTAC, also conventionally written?

Correct answer = 5′-GUAGAUC-3′. Nucleic acid sequences are conventionally written 5′ to 3′. The template strand (5′-GATCTAC-3′) is used as 3′-CATCTAG-5′. The RNA product is complementary to the template strand (and identical to the coding strand), with U replacing T.

Protein Synthesis

32

I. OVERVIEW

Genetic information, stored in the chromosomes and transmitted to daughter cells through DNA replication, is expressed through transcription to RNA and, in the case of messenger RNA (mRNA), subsequent translation into proteins (polypeptides) as shown in Figure 32.1. [Note: The proteome is the complete set of proteins expressed in a cell.] The process of protein synthesis is called translation because the "language" of the nucleotide sequence on the mRNA is translated into the language of an amino acid sequence. Translation requires a genetic code, through which the information contained in the nucleotide sequence is expressed to produce a specific amino acid sequence. Any alteration in the nucleotide sequence may result in an incorrect amino acid being inserted into the protein, potentially causing disease or even death of the organism. Newly made immature (nascent) proteins undergo a number of processes to achieve their functional form. They must fold properly, and misfolding can result in aggregation or degradation of the protein. Many proteins are covalently modified to alter their activities. Lastly, proteins are targeted to their final intra- or extracellular destinations by signals present in the proteins themselves.

II. THE GENETIC CODE

The genetic code is a "dictionary" that identifies the correspondence between a sequence of nucleotide bases and a sequence of amino acids. Each individual "word" in the code is composed of three nucleotide bases. These genetic words are called codons.

A. Codons

Codons are presented in the mRNA language of adenine (A), guanine (G), cytosine (C), and uracil (U). Their nucleotide sequences are always written from the 5′-end to the 3′-end. The four nucleotide bases are used to produce the three-base codons. Therefore, 64 different combinations of bases exist, taken three at a time (a triplet code), as shown in the table in Figure 32.2.

1. **How to translate a codon:** This table can be used to translate any codon and, thus, to determine which amino acids are coded for by an mRNA sequence. For example, the codon AUG codes for

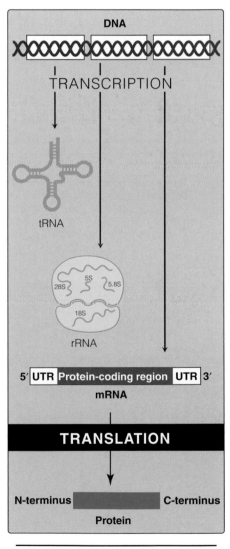

Figure 32.1
Protein synthesis or translation. tRNA = transfer RNA; rRNA = ribosomal RNA; mRNA = messenger RNA; UTR = untranslated region.

447

5'-BASE		MIDDLE BASE			3'-BASE
	U	**C**	**A**	**G**	
U	Phe	Ser	Tyr	Cys	U
	Phe	Ser	Tyr	Cys	C
	Leu	Ser	Stop	Stop	A
	Leu	Ser	Stop	Trp	G
C	Leu	Pro	His	Arg	U
	Leu	Pro	His	Arg	C
	Leu	Pro	Gln	Arg	A
	Leu	Pro	Gln	Arg	G
A	Ile	Thr	Asn	Ser	U
	Ile	Thr	Asn	Ser	C
	Ile	Thr	Lys	Arg	A
	Met	Thr	Lys	Arg	G
G	Val	Ala	Asp	Gly	U
	Val	Ala	Asp	Gly	C
	Val	Ala	Glu	Gly	A
	Val	Ala	Glu	Gly	G

1 These four rows show 16 amino acids whose codons begin (5') with A.

3 These four, separated rows show 16 amino acids whose codons end (3') with G.

2 This column shows 16 amino acids whose codons have the middle base U.

4 The codon AUG designates methionine (Met).

Figure 32.2
Use of the genetic code table to translate the codon AUG. A = adenine; G = guanine; C = cytosine; U = uracil. The three-letter abbreviations for many common amino acids are shown as examples.

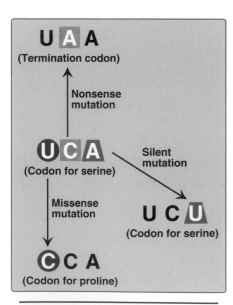

Figure 32.3
Possible effects of changing a single nucleotide base in the coding region of a messenger RNA. A = adenine; C = cytosine; U = uracil.

methionine ([Met] see Fig. 32.2). [Note: AUG is the initiation (start) codon for translation.] Sixty-one of the 64 codons code for the 20 standard amino acids (see p. 1).

2. **Termination codons:** Three of the codons, UAA, UAG, and UGA, do not code for amino acids but, rather, are termination (also called stop, or nonsense) codons. When one of these codons appears in an mRNA sequence, synthesis of the polypeptide coded for by that mRNA stops.

B. Characteristics

Usage of the genetic code is remarkably consistent throughout all living organisms. It is assumed that once the standard genetic code evolved in primitive organisms, any mutation (a permanent change in DNA sequence) that altered its meaning would have caused the alteration of most, if not all, protein sequences, resulting in lethality. Characteristics of the genetic code include the following.

1. **Specificity:** The genetic code is specific (unambiguous), because a particular codon always codes for the same amino acid.

2. **Universality:** The genetic code is virtually universal insofar as its specificity has been conserved from very early stages of evolution, with only slight differences in the manner in which the code is translated. [Note: An exception occurs in mitochondria, in

which a few codons have meanings different than those shown in Figure 32.2. For example, UGA codes for tryptophan (Trp).]

3. **Degeneracy:** The genetic code is degenerate (sometimes called redundant). Although each codon corresponds to a single amino acid, a given amino acid may have more than one triplet coding for it. For example, arginine (Arg) is specified by six different codons (see Fig. 32.2). Only Met and Trp have just one coding triplet.

4. **Nonoverlapping and commaless:** The genetic code is nonoverlapping and commaless, meaning that the code is read from a fixed starting point as a continuous sequence of bases, taken three at a time without any punctuation between codons. For example, AGCUGGAUACAU is read as AGC UGG AUA CAU.

C. Consequences of altering the nucleotide sequence

Changing a single nucleotide base (a point mutation) in the coding region of an mRNA can lead to any one of three results (Fig. 32.3).

1. **Silent mutation:** The codon containing the changed base may code for the same amino acid. For example, if the serine (Ser) codon UCA is changed at the third base and becomes UCU, it still codes for Ser. This is termed a silent mutation.

2. **Missense mutation:** The codon containing the changed base may code for a different amino acid. For example, if the Ser codon UCA is changed at the first base and becomes CCA, it will code for a different amino acid (in this case, proline [Pro]). This is termed a missense mutation.

3. **Nonsense mutation:** The codon containing the changed base may become a termination codon. For example, if the Ser codon UCA is changed at the second base and becomes UAA, the new codon causes premature termination of translation at that point and the production of a shortened (truncated) protein. This is termed a nonsense mutation. [Note: The nonsense-mediated degradation pathway can degrade mRNA containing premature stops.]

4. **Other mutations:** These can alter the amount or structure of the protein produced by translation.

    a. **Trinucleotide repeat expansion:** Occasionally, a sequence of three bases that is repeated in tandem will become amplified in number so that too many copies of the triplet occur. If this happens within the coding region of a gene, the protein will contain many extra copies of one amino acid. For example, expansion of the CAG codon in exon 1 of the gene for huntingtin protein leads to the insertion of many extra glutamine residues in the protein, causing the neurodegenerative disorder Huntington disease (Fig. 32.4). The additional glutamines result in an abnormally long protein that is cleaved, producing toxic fragments that aggregate in neurons. If the trinucleotide repeat expansion occurs in an untranslated region (UTR) of a gene, the result can be a decrease in the amount of protein produced, as seen in fragile X syndrome and myotonic dystrophy.

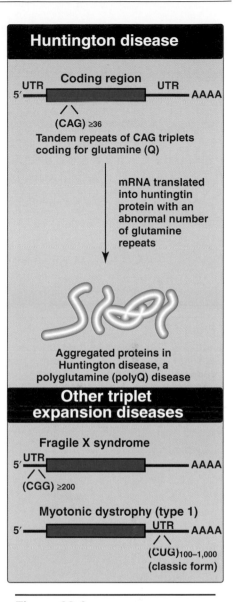

Figure 32.4
Tandem triplet repeats in messenger RNA (mRNA) causing Huntington disease and other triplet expansion diseases. [Note: In unaffected individuals, the number of repeats in the huntingtin protein is <27; in fragile X mental retardation protein, it is 5–44; and in *myotonic dystrophy protein kinase*, it is 5–34.] UTR = untranslated region; A = adenine; C = cytosine; G = guanine; U = uracil; Q = single-letter abbreviation for glutamine.

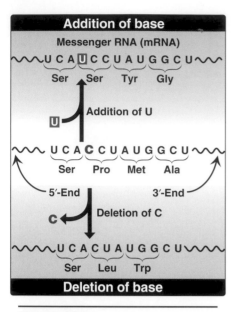

Figure 32.5
Frameshift mutations as a result of addition or deletion of a base can cause an alteration in the reading frame of mRNA. A = adenine; C = cytosine; G = guanine; U = uracil.

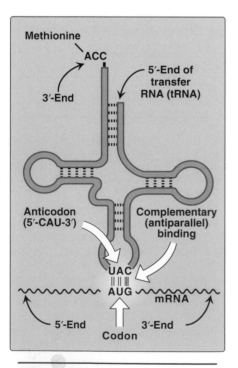

Figure 32.6
Complementary, antiparallel binding of the anticodon for methionyl-tRNA (CAU) to the messenger RNA (mRNA) codon for methionine (AUG), the initiation codon for translation.

Over 20 triplet expansion diseases are known. [Note: In fragile X syndrome, the most common cause of intellectual disability in males, the expansion results in gene silencing through DNA hypermethylation (see p. 476).]

b. **Splice site mutations:** Mutations at splice sites (see p. 443) can alter the way in which introns are removed from pre-mRNA molecules, producing aberrant proteins. [Note: In myotonic dystrophy, a muscle disorder, gene silencing is the result of splicing alterations due to triplet expansion.]

c. **Frameshift mutations:** If one or two nucleotides are either deleted from or added to the coding region of an mRNA, a frameshift mutation occurs, altering the reading frame. This can result in a product with a radically different amino acid sequence or a truncated product due to the eventual creation of a termination codon (Fig. 32.5). If three nucleotides are added, a new amino acid is added to the peptide. If three are deleted, an amino acid is lost. Loss of three nucleotides maintains the reading frame but can result in serious pathology. For example, cystic fibrosis (CF), a chronic, progressive, inherited disease that primarily affects the pulmonary and digestive systems, is most commonly caused by deletion of three nucleotides from the coding region of a gene, resulting in the loss of phenylalanine (Phe, or F; see p. 5) at the 508th position (ΔF508) in the CF transmembrane conductance regulator (CFTR) protein encoded by that gene. This ΔF508 mutation prevents normal folding of CFTR, leading to its destruction by the proteasome (see p. 247). CFTR normally functions as a chloride channel in epithelial cells, and its loss results in the production of thick, sticky secretions in the lungs and pancreas, leading to lung damage and digestive deficiencies (see p. 174). The incidence of CF is highest (1 in 3,300) in those of Northern European origin. In >70% of individuals with CF, the ΔF508 mutation is the cause of the disease.

III. COMPONENTS REQUIRED FOR TRANSLATION

A large number of components are required for the synthesis of a protein. These include all the amino acids that are found in the finished product, the mRNA to be translated, transfer RNA (tRNA) for each of the amino acids, functional ribosomes, energy sources, and enzymes as well as noncatalytic protein factors needed for the initiation, elongation, and termination steps of polypeptide chain synthesis.

A. Amino acids

All the amino acids that eventually appear in the finished protein must be present at the time of protein synthesis. If one amino acid is missing, translation stops at the codon specifying that amino acid. [Note: This demonstrates the importance of having all the essential amino acids (see p. 262) in sufficient quantities in the diet to insure continued protein synthesis.]

B. Transfer RNA

At least one specific type of tRNA is required for each amino acid. In humans, there are at least 50 species of tRNA, whereas bacteria contain at least 30 species. Because there are only 20 different amino acids commonly carried by tRNA, some amino acids have more than one specific tRNA molecule. This is particularly true of those amino acids that are coded for by several codons.

1. **Amino acid attachment site:** Each tRNA molecule has an attachment site for a specific (cognate) amino acid at its 3′-end (Fig. 32.6). The carboxyl group of the amino acid is in an ester linkage with the 3′-hydroxyl of the ribose portion of the A nucleotide in the –CCA sequence at the 3′-end of the tRNA. [Note: A tRNA with a covalently attached (activated) amino acid is charged. Without an attached amino acid, it is uncharged.]

2. **Anticodon:** Each tRNA molecule also contains a three-base nucleotide sequence, the anticodon, which pairs with a specific codon on the mRNA (see Fig. 32.6). This codon specifies the insertion into the growing polypeptide chain of the amino acid carried by that tRNA.

C. Aminoacyl-tRNA synthetases

This family of 20 different enzymes is required for attachment of amino acids to their corresponding tRNA. Each member of this family recognizes a specific amino acid and all the tRNA that correspond to that amino acid (isoaccepting tRNA, up to five per amino acid). *Aminoacyl-tRNA synthetases* catalyze a two-step reaction that results in the covalent attachment of the α-carboxyl group of an amino acid to the A in the –CCA sequence at the 3′-end of its corresponding tRNA. The overall reaction requires ATP, which is cleaved to adenosine monophosphate and inorganic pyrophosphate (PP$_i$), as shown in Figure 32.7. The extreme specificity of the *synthetases* in recognizing both the amino acid and its cognate tRNA contributes to the high fidelity of translation of the genetic message. In addition to their synthetic activity, the *aminoacyl-tRNA synthetases* have a proofreading, or editing activity that can remove an incorrect amino acid from the enzyme or the tRNA molecule.

D. Messenger RNA

The specific mRNA required as a template for the synthesis of the desired polypeptide must be present. [Note: In eukaryotes, mRNA is circularized for use in translation.]

E. Functionally competent ribosomes

As shown in Figure 32.8, ribosomes are large complexes of protein and ribosomal RNA (rRNA), in which rRNA predominates. They consist of two subunits (one large and one small) whose relative sizes are given in terms of their sedimentation coefficients, or S (Svedberg) values. [Note: Because the S values are determined by both shape and size, their numeric values are not strictly additive.

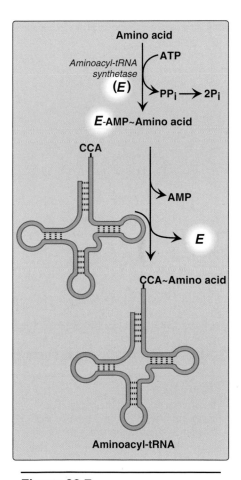

Figure 32.7
Attachment of a specific amino acid to its corresponding transfer RNA (tRNA) by an *aminoacyl-tRNA synthetase*. PP$_i$ = pyrophosphate; P$_i$ = inorganic phosphate; A = adenine; C = cytosine; AMP = adenosine monophosphate; ~ = high-energy bond.

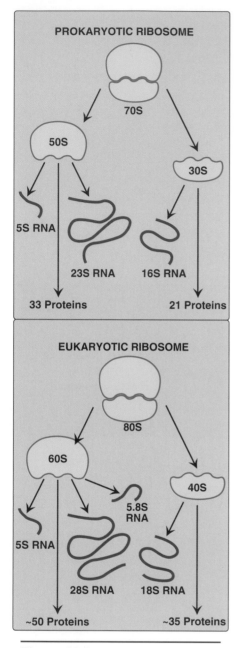

PROKARYOTIC RIBOSOME

70S

50S

30S

5S RNA

23S RNA   16S RNA

33 Proteins   21 Proteins

EUKARYOTIC RIBOSOME

80S

60S

40S

5.8S RNA

5S RNA

28S RNA   18S RNA

~50 Proteins   ~35 Proteins

Figure 32.8
Ribosomal composition. [Note: The number of proteins in the eukaryotic ribosomal subunits varies somewhat from species to species.] S = Svedberg unit.

For example, the prokaryotic 50S and 30S ribosomal subunits together form a 70S ribosome. The eukaryotic 60S and 40S subunits form an 80S ribosome.] Prokaryotic and eukaryotic ribosomes are similar in structure and serve the same function, namely, as the macromolecular complexes in which the synthesis of proteins occurs.

> The small ribosomal subunit binds mRNA and determines the accuracy of translation by insuring correct base-pairing between the mRNA codon and the tRNA anticodon. The large ribosomal subunit catalyzes formation of the peptide bonds that link amino acid residues in a protein.

1. **Ribosomal RNA:** As discussed on p. 434, prokaryotic ribosomes contain three size species of rRNA, whereas eukaryotic ribosomes contain four (see Fig. 32.8). The rRNA are generated from a single pre-rRNA by the action of *ribonucleases*, and some bases and riboses are modified.

2. **Ribosomal proteins:** Ribosomal proteins are present in greater numbers in eukaryotic ribosomes than in prokaryotic ribosomes. These proteins play a variety of roles in the structure and function of the ribosome and its interactions with other components of the translation system.

3. **A, P, and E sites:** The ribosome has three binding sites for tRNA molecules: the A, P, and E sites, each of which extends over both subunits. Together, they cover three neighboring codons. During translation, the A site binds an incoming aminoacyl-tRNA as directed by the codon currently occupying this site. This codon specifies the next amino acid to be added to the growing peptide chain. The P site is occupied by peptidyl-tRNA. This tRNA carries the chain of amino acids that has already been synthesized. The E site is occupied by the empty tRNA as it is about to exit the ribosome. (See Fig. 32.13 for an illustration of the role of the A, P, and E sites in translation.)

4. **Cellular location:** In eukaryotic cells, the ribosomes either are free in the cytosol or are in close association with the endoplasmic reticulum (which is then known as the rough endoplasmic reticulum, or RER). RER-associated ribosomes are responsible for synthesizing proteins (including glycoproteins; see p. 166) that are to be exported from the cell, incorporated into membranes, or imported into lysosomes (see p. 169 for an overview of the latter process). Cytosolic ribosomes synthesize proteins required in the cytosol itself or destined for the nucleus, mitochondria, or peroxisomes. [Note: Mitochondria contain their own ribosomes (55S) and their own unique, circular DNA. Most mitochondrial proteins, however, are encoded by nuclear DNA, synthesized completely in the cytosol, and then targeted to mitochondria.]

F. Protein factors

Initiation, elongation, and termination (or, release) factors are required for polypeptide synthesis. Some of these protein factors perform a catalytic function, whereas others appear to stabilize the synthetic machinery. [Note: A number of the factors are small, cytosolic G proteins and thus are active when bound to guanosine triphosphate (GTP) and inactive when bound to guanosine diphosphate (GDP). See p. 95 for a discussion of the membrane-associated G proteins.]

G. Energy sources

Cleavage of four high-energy bonds (see p. 73) is required for the addition of one amino acid to the growing polypeptide chain: two from ATP in the *aminoacyl-tRNA synthetase* reaction, one in the removal of PP_i and one in the subsequent hydrolysis of the PP_i, to two P_i by *pyrophosphatase*, and two from GTP, one for binding the aminoacyl-tRNA to the A site and one for the translocation step (see Fig. 32.13, p. 457). [Note: Additional ATP and GTP molecules are required for initiation in eukaryotes, whereas an additional GTP molecule is required for termination in both eukaryotes and prokaryotes.] Translation, then, is a major consumer of energy.

IV. CODON RECOGNITION BY TRANSFER RNA

Correct pairing of the codon in the mRNA with the anticodon of the tRNA is essential for accurate translation (see Fig. 32.6). Most tRNA (isoaccepting tRNA) recognize more than one codon for a given amino acid.

A. Antiparallel binding between codon and anticodon

Binding of the tRNA anticodon to the mRNA codon follows the rules of complementary and antiparallel binding, that is, the mRNA codon is read 5′→3′ by an anticodon pairing in the opposite (3′→5′) orientation (Fig. 32.9). [Note: Nucleotide sequences are always written in the 5′ to 3′ direction unless otherwise noted. Two nucleotide sequences orient in an antiparallel manner.]

B. Wobble hypothesis

The mechanism by which a tRNA can recognize more than one codon for a specific amino acid is described by the wobble hypothesis, which states that codon–anticodon pairing follows the traditional Watson-Crick rules (G pairs with C and A pairs with U) for the first two bases of the codon but can be less stringent for the last base. The base at the 5′-end of the anticodon (the first base of the anticodon) is not as spatially defined as the other two bases. Movement of that first base allows nontraditional base-pairing with the 3′-base of the codon (the last base of the codon). This movement is called wobble and allows a single tRNA to recognize more than one codon. Examples of these flexible pairings are shown in Figure 32.9. The result of wobble is that 61 tRNA species are not required to read the 61 codons that code for amino acids.

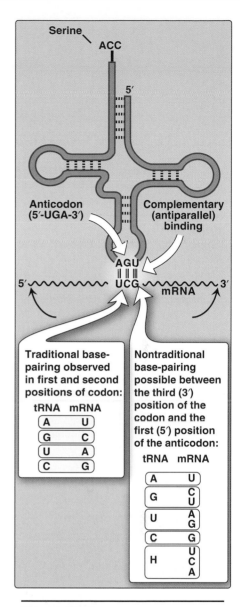

Figure 32.9

Wobble: Nontraditional base-pairing between the 5′-nucleotide (first nucleotide) of the anticodon and the 3′-nucleotide (last nucleotide) of the codon. Hypoxanthine (H) is the product of adenine deamination and the base in the nucleotide inosine monophosphate (IMP). A = adenine; G = guanine; C = cytosine; U = uracil; tRNA = transfer RNA; mRNA = messenger RNA.

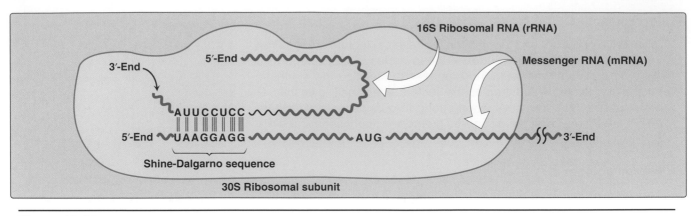

Figure 32.10
Complementary binding between prokaryotic mRNA Shine-Dalgarno sequence and 16S rRNA. S = Svedberg unit.

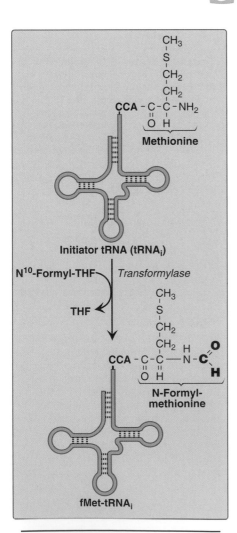

Figure 32.11
Generation of the initiator
N-formylmethionyl-transfer RNA
(fMet-tRNA$_i$). THF = tetrahydrofolate;
C = cytosine; A = adenine.

V. STEPS IN TRANSLATION

The process of protein synthesis translates the 3-letter alphabet of nucleotide sequences on mRNA into the 20-letter alphabet of amino acids that constitute proteins. The mRNA is translated from its 5′-end to its 3′-end, producing a protein synthesized from its amino (N)-terminal end to its carboxyl (C)-terminal end. Prokaryotic mRNA often have several coding regions (that is, they are polycistronic; see p. 434). Each coding region has its own initiation and termination codon and produces a separate species of polypeptide. In contrast, each eukaryotic mRNA has only one coding region (that is, it is monocistronic). The process of translation is divided into three separate steps: initiation, elongation, and termination. Eukaryotic translation resembles that of prokaryotes in most aspects. Individual differences are noted in the text.

> One important difference is that translation and transcription are temporally linked in prokaryotes, with translation starting before transcription is completed as a consequence of the lack of a nuclear membrane in prokaryotes.

A. Initiation

Initiation of protein synthesis involves the assembly of the components of the translation system before peptide-bond formation occurs. These components include the two ribosomal subunits, the mRNA to be translated, the aminoacyl-tRNA specified by the first codon in the message, GTP, and initiation factors that facilitate the assembly of this initiation complex (see Fig. 32.13). [Note: In prokaryotes, three initiation factors are known (IF-1, IF-2, and IF-3), whereas in eukaryotes, there are many (designated eIF to indicate eukaryotic origin). Eukaryotes also require ATP for initiation.] The following are two mechanisms by which the ribosome recognizes the nucleotide sequence (AUG) that initiates translation.

1. **Shine-Dalgarno sequence:** In Escherichia coli (E. coli), a purine-rich sequence of nucleotide bases, known as the Shine-Dalgarno (SD) sequence, is located six to ten bases upstream of the initiating AUG codon on the mRNA molecule (that is, near its 5′-end). The

16S rRNA component of the small (30S) ribosomal subunit has a nucleotide sequence near its 3′-end that is complementary to all or part of the SD sequence. Therefore, the 5′-end of the mRNA and the 3′-end of the 16S rRNA can form complementary base pairs, facilitating the positioning of the 30S subunit on the mRNA in close proximity to the initiating AUG codon (Fig. 32.10).

2. **5′-Cap:** Eukaryotic mRNA do not have SD sequences. In eukaryotes, the small (40S) ribosomal subunit (aided by members of the eIF-4 family of proteins) binds close to the cap structure at the 5′-end of the mRNA and moves 5′→3′ along the mRNA until it encounters the initiator AUG. This scanning process requires ATP. Cap-independent initiation can occur if the 40S subunit binds to an internal ribosome entry site close to the start codon. [Note: Interactions between the cap-binding eIF-4 proteins and the poly-A tail–binding proteins on eukaryotic mRNA mediate circularization of the mRNA and likely prevent the use of incompletely processed mRNA in translation.]

3. **Initiation codon:** The initiating AUG is recognized by a special initiator tRNA (tRNA$_i$). Recognition is facilitated by IF-2-GTP in prokaryotes and eIF-2-GTP (plus additional eIF) in eukaryotes. The charged tRNA$_i$ is the only tRNA recognized by (e)IF-2 and the only tRNA to go directly to the P site on the small subunit. [Note: Base modifications distinguish tRNA$_i$ from the tRNA used for internal AUG codons.] In bacteria and mitochondria, tRNA$_i$ carries an N-formylated methionine (fMet), as shown in Figure 32.11. After Met is attached to tRNA$_i$, the formyl group is added by the enzyme *transformylase*, which uses N^{10}-formyl tetrahydrofolate (see p. 267) as the carbon donor. In eukaryotes, tRNA$_i$ carries a Met that is not formylated. In both prokaryotic and eukaryotic cells, this N-terminal Met is usually removed before translation is completed. The large ribosomal subunit then joins the complex, and a functional ribosome is formed with the charged tRNA$_i$ in the P site. The A site is empty. [Note: Specific (e)IF function as anti-association factors and prevent premature addition of the large subunit.] The GTP on (e)IF-2 gets hydrolyzed to GDP. In eukaryotes, the guanine nucleotide exchange factor eIF-2B facilitates the reactivation of eIF-2-GDP through replacement of GDP by GTP.

B. Elongation

Elongation of the polypeptide involves the addition of amino acids to the carboxyl end of the growing chain. Delivery of the aminoacyl-tRNA whose codon appears next on the mRNA template in the ribosomal A site (a process known as decoding) is facilitated in E. coli by elongation factors EF-Tu-GTP and EF-Ts and requires GTP hydrolysis. [Note: In eukaryotes, comparable elongation factors are EF-1α-GTP and EF-1βγ. Both EF-Ts and EF-1βγ function in guanine nucleotide exchange.] Peptide-bond formation between the α-carboxyl group of the amino acid in the P site and the α-amino group of the amino acid in the A site is catalyzed by *peptidyltransferase*, an activity intrinsic to an rRNA of the large subunit (Fig. 32.12). [Note: Because this rRNA catalyzes the reaction, it is a ribozyme (see p. 54).] After the peptide bond has been formed, the peptide on the tRNA at the P site is transferred to the amino acid on the tRNA at the A site, a process known as transpeptidation. The ribosome then advances three nucleotides

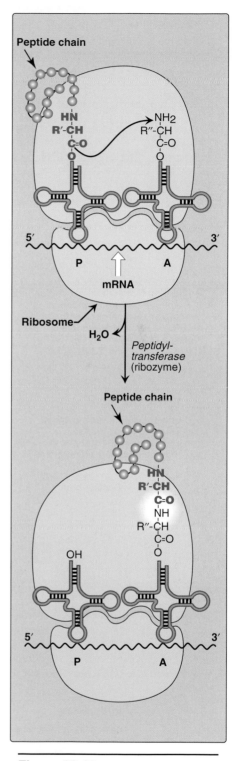

Figure 32.12
Formation of a peptide bond. Peptide-bond formation results in transfer of the peptide on the transfer RNA (tRNA) in the P site to the amino acid on the tRNA in the A site (transpeptidation). mRNA = messenger RNA; R′, R″ = different amino acid side chains.

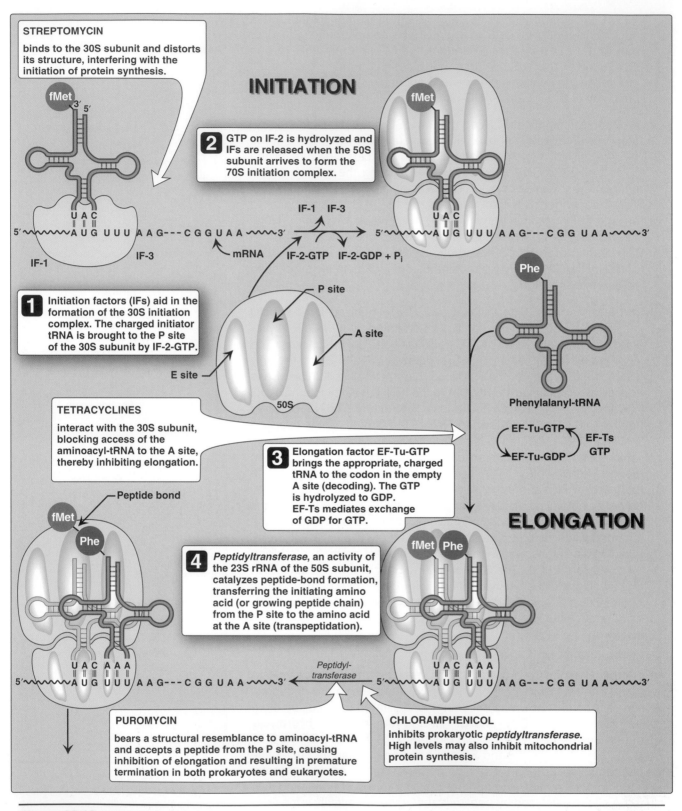

Figure 32.13 (continued on next page)

Steps in prokaryotic protein synthesis (translation), and their inhibition by antibiotics. [Note: EF-Ts is a guanine nucleotide exchange factor. It facilitates the removal of guanosine diphosphate (GDP) from EF-Tu, allowing its replacement by guanosine triphosphate (GTP). The eukaryotic equivalent is EF-1βγ.] fMet = formylated methionine; S = Svedberg unit; Phe = phenylalanine; Lys = lysine; Arg = arginine; tRNA = transfer RNA; mRNA = messenger RNA.

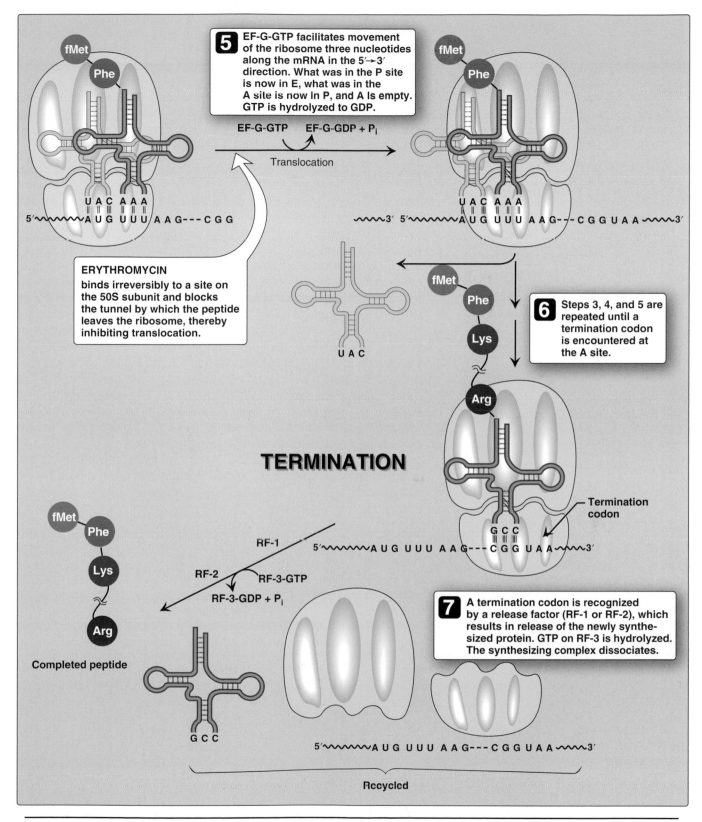

Figure 32.13 (continued from previous page)

[Note: In eukaryotes, diphtheria toxin inactivates EF-2, thereby inhibiting the translocation phase of elongation. Ricin, a toxin from castor beans, removes a specific A from the 28S ribosomal RNA (rRNA) in the large subunit of eukaryotic ribosomes, thereby inhibiting ribosomal function.]

Cell	Factor	Function
Initiation		
P E	IF-2-GTP eIF-2-GTP	Bring charged initiating tRNA to P site
P E	IF-3 eIF-3	Prevent association of subunits
Elongation		
P E	EF-Tu-GTP EF1α-GTP	Bring all other charged tRNA to A site
P E	EF-Ts EF-1βγ	Guanine nucleotide exchange factors
P E	EF-G-GTP EF-2-GTP	Translocation
Termination		
P E	RF-1, 2 eRF	Recognize stop codons
P E	RF-3-GTP eRF-3-GTP	Release of other RF

Figure 32.14

Protein factors in the three stages of translation. **P** = prokaryotes; **E** = eukaryotes; tRNA = transfer RNA; IF = initiation factor; EF = elongation factor; RF = release factor; GTP = guanosine triphosphate.

toward the 3′-end of the mRNA. This process is known as translocation and, in prokaryotes, requires the participation of EF-G-GTP (eukaryotes use EF-2-GTP) and GTP hydrolysis. Translocation causes movement of the uncharged tRNA from the P to the E site for release and movement of the peptidyl-tRNA from the A to the P site. The process is repeated until a termination codon is encountered. [Note: Because of the length of most mRNA, more than one ribosome at a time can translate a message. Such a complex of one mRNA and a number of ribosomes is called a polysome, or polyribosome.]

C. Termination

Termination occurs when one of the three termination codons moves into the A site. These codons are recognized in E. coli by release factors: RF-1, which recognizes UAA and UAG, and RF-2, which recognizes UGA and UAA. The binding of these release factors results in hydrolysis of the bond linking the peptide to the tRNA at the P site, causing the nascent protein to be released from the ribosome. A third release factor, RF-3-GTP, then causes the release of RF-1 or RF-2 as GTP is hydrolyzed (see Fig. 32.13). [Note: Eukaryotes have a single release factor, eRF, which recognizes all three termination codons. A second factor, eRF-3, functions like the prokaryotic RF-3. See Figure 32.14 for a summary of the factors used in translation.] The steps in prokaryotic protein synthesis, as well as some antibiotic inhibitors of the process, are summarized in Figure 32.13. The newly synthesized polypeptide may undergo further modification as described below, and the ribosomal subunits, mRNA, tRNA, and protein factors can be recycled and used to synthesize another polypeptide. [Note: In prokaryotes, ribosome recycling factors mediate separation of the subunits. In eukaryotes, eRF and ATP hydrolysis are required.]

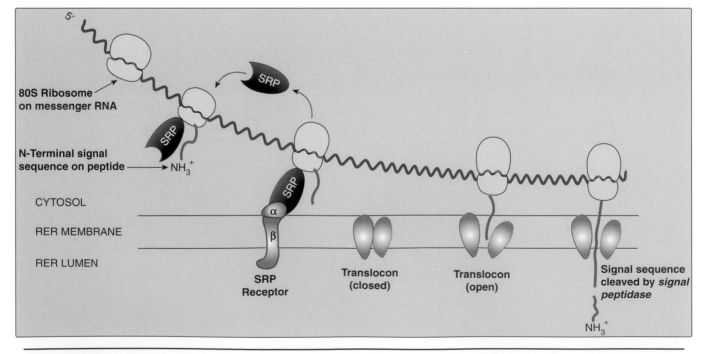

Figure 32.15

Cotranslational targeting of proteins to the rough endoplasmic reticulum (RER). SRP = signal recognition particle.

D. Translation regulation

Gene expression is most commonly regulated at the transcriptional level, but translation may also be regulated. An important mechanism by which this is achieved in eukaryotes is by covalent modification of eIF-2: Phosphorylated eIF-2 is inactive (see p. 476). In both eukaryotes and prokaryotes, regulation can also be achieved through proteins that bind mRNA and inhibit its use by blocking translation.

E. Protein folding

Proteins must fold to assume their functional, native state. Folding can be spontaneous (as a result of the primary structure) or facilitated by proteins known as chaperones (see p. 20).

F. Protein targeting

Although most protein synthesis in eukaryotes is initiated in the cytoplasm, many proteins perform their functions within subcellular organelles or outside of the cell. Such proteins normally contain amino acid sequences that direct the proteins to their final locations. For example, secreted proteins are targeted during synthesis (cotranslational targeting) to the RER by the presence of an N-terminal hydrophobic signal sequence. The sequence is recognized by the signal recognition particle (SRP), a ribonucleoprotein that binds the ribosome, halts elongation, and delivers the ribosome–peptide complex to an RER membrane channel (the translocon) via interaction with the SRP receptor. Translation resumes, the protein enters the RER lumen, and its signal sequence is cleaved (Fig. 32.15). The protein moves through the RER and the Golgi, is processed, packaged into vesicles, and secreted. Proteins targeted after synthesis (posttranslational) include nuclear proteins that contain an internal, short, basic nuclear localization signal; mitochondrial matrix proteins that contain an N-terminal, amphipathic, α-helical mitochondrial entry sequence; and peroxisomal proteins that contain a C-terminal tripeptide signal.

VI. CO- AND POSTTRANSLATIONAL MODIFICATIONS

Many polypeptides are covalently modified, either while they are still attached to the ribosome (cotranslational) or after their synthesis has been completed (posttranslational). These modifications may include removal of part of the translated sequence or the covalent addition of one or more chemical groups required for protein activity.

A. Trimming

Many proteins destined for secretion are initially made as large, precursor molecules that are not functionally active. Portions of the protein must be removed by specialized *endoproteases*, resulting in the release of an active molecule. The cellular site of the cleavage reaction depends on the protein to be modified. Some precursor proteins are cleaved in the RER or the Golgi; others are cleaved in developing secretory vesicles (for example, insulin; see Fig. 23.4, p. 309); and still others, such as collagen (see p. 47), are cleaved after secretion.

B. Covalent attachments

Protein function can be affected by the covalent attachment of a variety of chemical groups (Fig. 32.16). Examples include the following.

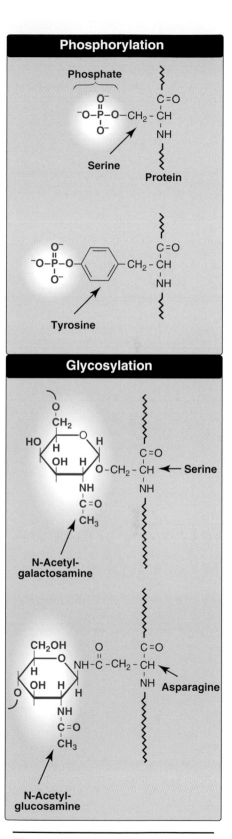

Figure 32.16 (continued on next page)

Covalent modification of some amino acid residues.

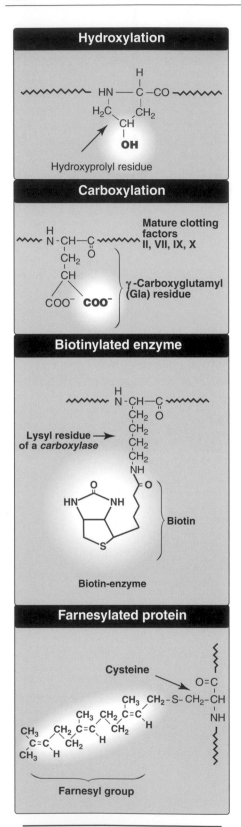

Figure 32.16 (continued from previous page) Covalent modification of some amino acid residues.

1. **Phosphorylation:** Phosphorylation occurs on the hydroxyl groups of serine, threonine, or, less frequently, tyrosine residues in a protein. It is catalyzed by one of a family of *protein kinases* and may be reversed by the action of *protein phosphatases.* The phosphorylation may increase or decrease the functional activity of the protein. Several examples of phosphorylation reactions have been previously discussed (for example, see Chapter 11, p. 132, for the regulation of glycogen synthesis and degradation).

2. **Glycosylation:** Many of the proteins that are destined to become part of a membrane or to be secreted from a cell have carbohydrate chains added en bloc to the amide nitrogen of an asparagine (N-linked) or built sequentially on the hydroxyl groups of a serine, threonine, or hydroxylysine (O-linked). N-glycosylation occurs in the RER and O-glycosylation in the Golgi. (The process of producing such glycoproteins was discussed on p. 165.) N-glycosylated *acid hydrolases* are targeted to the matrix of lysosomes by the phosphorylation of mannose residues at carbon 6 (see p. 169).

3. **Hydroxylation:** Proline and lysine residues of the α chains of collagen are extensively hydroxylated by vitamin C–dependent *hydroxylases* in the RER (see p. 47).

4. **Other covalent modifications:** These may be required for the functional activity of a protein. For example, additional carboxyl groups can be added to glutamate residues by vitamin K–dependent carboxylation (see p. 393). The resulting γ-carboxyglutamate (Gla) residues are essential for the activity of several of the blood-clotting proteins. (See online Chapter 35.) Biotin is covalently bound to the ε-amino groups of lysine residues of biotin-dependent enzymes that catalyze carboxylation reactions such as *pyruvate carboxylase* (see Fig. 10.3 on p. 119). Attachment of lipids, such as farnesyl groups, can help anchor proteins to membranes (see p. 221). Many eukaryotic proteins are cotranslationally acetylated at the N-end. [Note: Reversible acetylation of histone proteins influences gene expression (see p. 476).]

C. Protein degradation

Proteins that are defective (for example, misfolded) or destined for rapid turnover are often marked for destruction by ubiquitination, the covalent attachment of chains of a small, highly conserved protein called ubiquitin (see Fig. 19.3 on p. 247). Proteins marked in this way are rapidly degraded by the proteasome, which is a macromolecular, ATP-dependent, proteolytic system located in the cytosol. For example, misfolding of the CFTR protein (see p. 450) results in its proteasomal degradation. [Note: If folding is impeded, unfolded proteins accumulate in the RER causing stress that triggers the unfolded protein response, in which the expression of chaperones is increased; global translation is decreased by eIF-2 phosphorylation; and the unfolded proteins are sent to the cytosol, ubiquitinated, and degraded in the proteasome by a process called ER-associated degradation.]

VII. CHAPTER SUMMARY

Codons are composed of three nucleotide bases presented in the messenger RNA (mRNA) language of **adenine (A)**, **guanine (G)**, **cytosine (C)**, and **uracil (U)**. They are always written **5′→3′**. Of the 64 possible three-base combinations, 61 code for the 20 standard amino acids and 3 signal termination of protein synthesis (**translation**). Altering the nucleotide sequence in a codon can cause **silent mutations** (the altered codon codes for the original amino acid), **missense mutations** (the altered codon codes for a different amino acid), or **nonsense mutations** (the altered codon is a termination codon). Characteristics of the genetic code include **specificity**, **universality**, and **degeneracy**, and it is **nonoverlapping** and **commaless** (Fig. 32.17). Requirements for protein synthesis include all the **amino acids** that eventually appear in the finished protein; at least one specific type of **transfer RNA (tRNA)** for each amino acid; one *aminoacyl-tRNA synthetase* for each amino acid; the **mRNA** coding for the protein to be synthesized; fully competent **ribosomes** (70S in prokaryotes, 80S in eukaryotes); **protein factors** needed for initiation, elongation, and termination of protein synthesis; and **ATP** and **guanosine triphosphate (GTP)** as energy sources. tRNA has an attachment site for a specific amino acid at its 3′-end and an anticodon region that can recognize the codon specifying the amino acid the tRNA is carrying. Ribosomes are large complexes of **protein** and **ribosomal RNA (rRNA)**. They consist of **two subunits**, 30S and 50S in prokaryotes and 40S and 60S in eukaryotes. Each ribosome has three binding sites for tRNA molecules: the A, P, and E sites that cover three neighboring codons. The **A site** binds an **incoming aminoacyl-tRNA**, the **P site** is occupied by **peptidyl-tRNA**, and the **E site** is occupied by the **empty tRNA** as it is about to exit the ribosome. Recognition of an mRNA codon is accomplished by the tRNA **anticodon**, which binds to the codon following the rules of **complementarity** and **antiparallel** binding. The **wobble hypothesis** states that the first (5′) base of the anticodon is not as spatially defined as the other two bases. Movement of that first base allows nontraditional base-pairing with the last (3′) base of the codon, thus allowing a single tRNA to recognize more than one codon for a specific amino acid. For **initiation** of protein synthesis, the components of the translation system are assembled, and mRNA associates with the small ribosomal subunit. The process requires **initiation factors (IF)**. In **prokaryotes**, a purine-rich region of the mRNA (the **Shine-Dalgarno sequence**) base-pairs with a complementary sequence on 16S rRNA, resulting in the positioning of the small subunit on the mRNA so that translation can begin. The **5′-cap** (bound by proteins of the eIF-4 family) on **eukaryotic mRNA** is used to position the small subunit on the mRNA. The **initiation codon** is **AUG**, and **N-formylmethionine** is the initiating amino acid in prokaryotes, whereas **methionine** is used in eukaryotes. The charged initiating tRNA (tRNA$_i$) is brought to the P site by **(e)IF-2**. In **elongation**, the polypeptide chain is lengthened by the addition of amino acids to the carboxyl end of its growing chain. The process requires **elongation factors** that facilitate the binding of the aminoacyl-tRNA to the A site as well as the movement of the ribosome along the mRNA. The formation of the peptide bond is catalyzed by *peptidyltransferase*, which is an activity intrinsic to the rRNA of the large subunit and, therefore, is a **ribozyme**. Following peptide-bond formation, the ribosome advances along the mRNA in the **5′→3′ direction** to the next codon (**translocation**). Because of the length of most mRNA, more than one ribosome at a time can translate a message, forming a **polysome**. **Termination** begins when one of the three termination codons moves into the A site. These codons are recognized by **release factors**. The newly synthesized protein is released from the ribosomal complex, and the ribosome is dissociated from the mRNA. **Initiation**, **elongation**, and **termination** are driven by the hydrolysis of GTP. Initiation in eukaryotes also requires ATP for **scanning**. Numerous **antibiotics** interfere with the process of protein synthesis. Many polypeptide chains are covalently modified during or after translation. Such modifications include amino acid **removal**; **phosphorylation,** which may activate or inactivate the protein; **glycosylation**, which plays a role in **protein targeting**; and **hydroxylation** such as that seen in collagen. Protein targeting can be either **cotranslational** (as with secreted proteins) or **posttranslational** (as with mitochondrial matrix proteins). Proteins must **fold** to achieve their functional form. Folding can be spontaneous or facilitated by **chaperones**. Proteins that are defective (for example, misfolded) or destined for rapid turnover are marked for destruction by the attachment of chains of a small, highly conserved protein called **ubiquitin**. Ubiquitinated proteins are rapidly degraded by a cytosolic complex known as the **proteasome**.

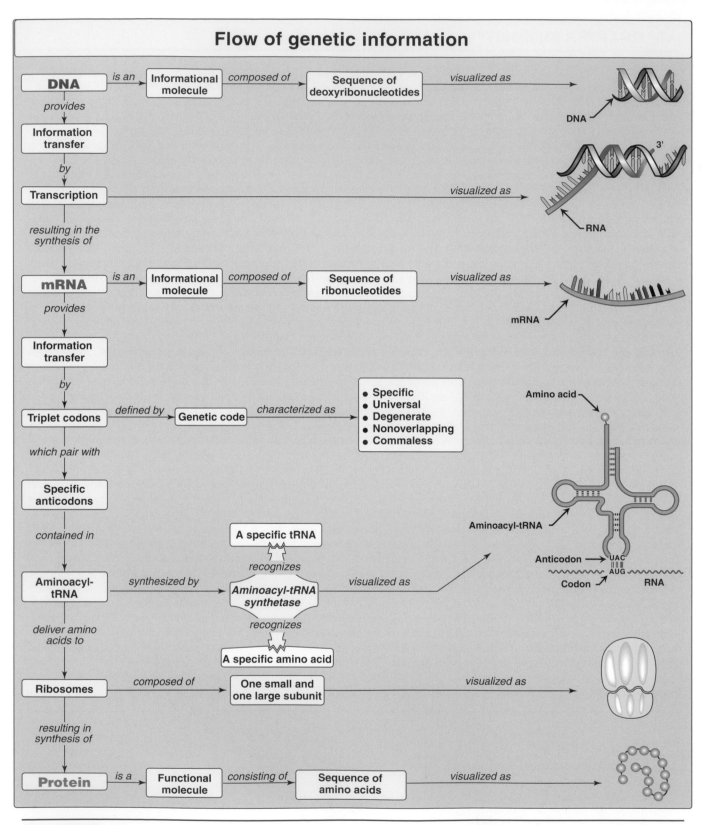

Flow of genetic information

DNA *is an* **Informational molecule** *composed of* **Sequence of deoxyribonucleotides** *visualized as*

DNA

provides

Information transfer

by

Transcription *visualized as*

RNA

resulting in the synthesis of

mRNA *is an* **Informational molecule** *composed of* **Sequence of ribonucleotides** *visualized as*

mRNA

provides

Information transfer

by

Triplet codons *defined by* **Genetic code** *characterized as*
- **Specific**
- **Universal**
- **Degenerate**
- **Nonoverlapping**
- **Commaless**

Amino acid

which pair with

Specific anticodons

Aminoacyl-tRNA

contained in

A specific tRNA

recognizes

Anticodon → UAC
AUG
Codon — RNA

Aminoacyl-tRNA *synthesized by* ***Aminoacyl-tRNA synthetase*** *visualized as*

recognizes

A specific amino acid

deliver amino acids to

Ribosomes *composed of* **One small and one large subunit** *visualized as*

resulting in synthesis of

Protein *is a* **Functional molecule** *consisting of* **Sequence of amino acids** *visualized as*

Figure 32.17

Key concept map for protein synthesis. mRNA = messenger RNA; tRNA = transfer RNA; A = adenine; G = guanine; C = cytosine; U = uracil.

Study Questions

Choose the ONE best answer.

32.1 A 20-year-old man with a microcytic anemia is found to have an abnormal form of β-globin (Hemoglobin Constant Spring) that is 172 amino acids long, rather than the 141 found in the normal protein. Which of the following point mutations is consistent with this abnormality? Use Figure 32.2 to answer the question.

    A. CGA → UGA

    B. GAU → GAC

    C. GCA → GAA

    D. UAA → CAA

    E. UAA → UAG

Correct answer = D. Mutating the normal termination (stop) codon from UAA to CAA in β-globin messenger RNA causes the ribosome to insert a glutamine at that point. It will continue extending the protein chain until it comes upon the next stop codon farther down the message, resulting in an abnormally long protein. The replacement of CGA (arginine) with UGA (stop) would cause the protein to be too short. GAU and GAC both code for aspartate and would cause no change in the protein. Changing GCA (alanine) to GAA (glutamate) would not change the size of the protein product. A change from UAA to UAG would simply change one termination codon for another and would have no effect on the protein.

32.2 A pharmaceutical company is studying a new antibiotic that inhibits bacterial protein synthesis. When this antibiotic is added to an in vitro protein synthesis system that is translating the messenger RNA sequence AUGUUUUUUUAG, the only product formed is the dipeptide fMet-Phe. What step in protein synthesis is most likely inhibited by the antibiotic?

    A. Initiation

    B. Binding of a charged transfer RNA to the ribosomal A site

    C. Peptidyltransferase activity

    D. Ribosomal translocation

    E. Termination

Correct answer = D. Because fMet-Phe (formylated methionyl-phenylalanine) is made, the ribosomes must be able to complete initiation, bind Phe-tRNA to the A site, and use peptidyltransferase activity to form the first peptide bond. Because the ribosome is not able to proceed any further, ribosomal movement (translocation) is most likely the inhibited step. Therefore, the ribosome is stopped before it reaches the termination codon of this message.

32.3 A transfer RNA (tRNA) molecule that is supposed to carry cysteine (tRNA^{cys}) is mischarged, so that it actually carries alanine (ala-tRNA^{cys}). Assuming no correction occurs, what will be the fate of this alanine residue during protein synthesis? It will:

    A. be incorporated into a protein in response to a codon for alanine.

    B. be incorporated into a protein in response to a codon for cysteine.

    C. be incorporated randomly at any codon.

    D. remain attached to the tRNA because it cannot be used for protein synthesis.

    E. be chemically converted to cysteine by cellular enzymes.

Correct answer = B. Once an amino acid is attached to a tRNA molecule, only the anticodon of that tRNA determines the specificity of incorporation. Therefore, the incorrectly activated alanine will be incorporated into the protein at a position determined by a cysteine codon.

32.4 In a patient with cystic fibrosis (CF) caused by the ΔF508 mutation, the mutant CF transmembrane conductance regulator (CFTR) protein folds incorrectly. The patient's cells modify this abnormal protein by attaching ubiquitin molecules to it. What is the fate of this modified CFTR protein?

    A. It performs its normal function because the ubiquitin largely corrects for the effect of the mutation.

    B. It is degraded by the proteasome.

    C. It is placed into storage vesicles.

    D. It is repaired by cellular enzymes.

    E. It is secreted from the cell.

Correct answer = B. Ubiquitination usually marks old, damaged, or misfolded proteins for destruction by the cytosolic proteasome. There is no known cellular mechanism for repair of damaged proteins.

32.5 Many antimicrobials inhibit translation. Which of the following antimicrobials is correctly paired with its mechanism of action?

    A. Erythromycin binds to the 60S ribosomal subunit.

    B. Puromycin inactivates elongation factor-2.

    C. Streptomycin binds to the 30S ribosomal subunit.

    D. Tetracyclines inhibit peptidyltransferase.

Correct answer = C. Streptomycin binds the 30S subunit and inhibits translation initiation. Erythromycin binds the 50S ribosomal subunit (60S denotes a eukaryote) and blocks the tunnel through which the peptide leaves the ribosome. Puromycin has structural similarity to aminoacyl-transfer RNA. It is incorporated into the growing chain, inhibits elongation, and results in premature termination in both prokaryotes and eukaryotes. Tetracyclines bind the 30S ribosomal subunit and block access to the A site, inhibiting elongation.

32.6 Translation of a synthetic polyribonucleotide containing the repeating sequence CAA in a cell-free protein-synthesizing system produces three homopolypeptides: polyglutamine, polyasparagine, and polythreonine. If the codons for glutamine and asparagine are CAA and AAC, respectively, which of the following triplets is the codon for threonine?

    A. AAC

    B. ACA

    C. CAA

    D. CAC

    E. CCA

Correct answer = B. The synthetic polynucleotide sequence of CAACAACAACAA … could be read by the in vitro protein-synthesizing system starting at the first C, the first A, or the second A (that is, in any one of three reading frames). In the first case, the first triplet codon would be CAA, which codes glutamine; in the second case, the first triplet codon would be AAC, which codes for asparagine; in the last case, the first triplet codon would be ACA, which codes for threonine.

32.7 Which of the following is required for both prokaryotic and eukaryotic protein synthesis?

    A. Binding of the small ribosomal subunit to the Shine-Dalgarno sequence

    B. Formylated methionyl-transfer (t)RNA

    C. Movement of the messenger RNA out of the nucleus and into the cytoplasm

    D. Recognition of the 5′-cap by initiation factors

    E. Translocation of the peptidyl-tRNA from the A site to the P site

Correct answer = E. In both prokaryotes and eukaryotes, continued translation (elongation) requires movement of the peptidyl-tRNA from the A to the P site to allow the next aminoacyl-tRNA to enter the A site. Only prokaryotes have a Shine-Dalgarno sequence and use formylated methionine and only eukaryotes have a nucleus and co- and posttranscriptionally process their mRNA.

32.8 α1-Antitrypsin (AAT) deficiency can result in emphysema, a lung pathology, because the action of elastase, a serine protease, is unopposed. Deficiency of AAT in the lungs is the consequence of impaired secretion from the liver, the site of its synthesis. Proteins such as AAT that are destined to be secreted are best characterized by which of the following statements?

    A. Their synthesis is initiated on the smooth endoplasmic reticulum.

    B. They contain a mannose 6-phosphate targeting signal.

    C. They always contain methionine as the N-terminal amino acid.

    D. They are produced from translation products that have an N-terminal hydrophobic signal sequence.

    E. They contain no sugars with O-glycosidic linkages because their synthesis does not involve the Golgi.

Correct answer = D. Synthesis of secreted proteins is begun on free (cytosolic) ribosomes. As the N-terminal signal sequence of the peptide emerges from the ribosome, it is bound by the signal recognition particle, taken to the rough endoplasmic reticulum (RER), threaded into the lumen, and cleaved as translation continues. The proteins move through the RER and the Golgi and undergo processing such as N-glycosylation (RER) and O-glycosylation (Golgi). In the Golgi, they are packaged in secretory vesicles and released from the cell. The smooth endoplasmic reticulum is associated with synthesis of lipids, not proteins, and has no ribosomes attached. Phosphorylation at carbon 6 of terminal mannose residues in glycoproteins targets these proteins (acid hydrolases) to lysosomes. The N-terminal methionine is removed from most proteins during processing.

32.9 Why is the genetic code described as both degenerate and unambiguous?

A given amino acid can be coded for by more than one codon (degenerate code), but a given codon codes for just one particular amino acid (unambiguous code).

Regulation of Gene Expression

33

I. OVERVIEW

Gene expression refers to the multistep process that ultimately results in the production of a functional gene product, either ribonucleic acid (RNA) or protein. The first step in gene expression, the use of deoxyribonucleic acid (DNA) for the synthesis of RNA (transcription), is the primary site of regulation in both prokaryotes and eukaryotes. In eukaryotes, however, gene expression also involves extensive posttranscriptional and posttranslational processes as well as actions that influence access to particular regions of the DNA. Each of these steps can be regulated to provide additional control over the kinds and amounts of functional products that are produced.

Not all genes are tightly regulated. For example, genes described as constitutive encode products required for basic cellular functions and so are expressed at essentially a constant level. They are also known as "housekeeping" genes. Regulated genes, however, are expressed only under certain conditions. They may be expressed in all cells or in only a subset of cells, for example, hepatocytes. The ability to regulate gene expression (that is, to determine if, how much, and when particular gene products will be made) gives the cell control over structure and function. It is the basis for cellular differentiation, morphogenesis, and adaptability of any organism. Control of gene expression is best understood in prokaryotes, but many themes are repeated in eukaryotes. Figure 33.1 shows some of the sites where gene expression can be controlled.

II. REGULATORY SEQUENCES AND MOLECULES

Regulation of transcription, the initial step in all gene expression, is controlled by regulatory sequences of DNA that are usually embedded in the noncoding regions of the genome. The interaction between these DNA sequences and regulatory molecules, such as transcription factors, can induce or repress the transcriptional machinery, influencing the kinds and amounts of products that are produced. The regulatory DNA sequences are called cis-acting because they influence expression of genes on the same chromosome as the regulatory sequence (see p. 439). The

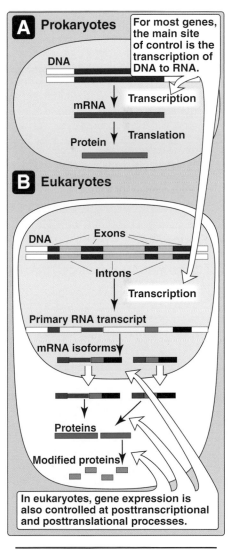

Figure 33.1
Control of gene expression. mRNA = messenger RNA.

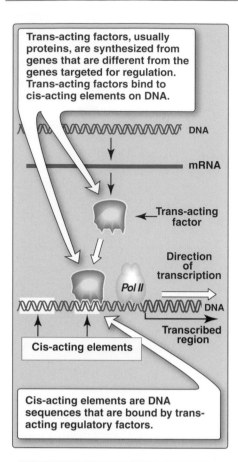

Trans-acting factors, usually proteins, are synthesized from genes that are different from the genes targeted for regulation. Trans-acting factors bind to cis-acting elements on DNA.

DNA

mRNA

Trans-acting factor

Direction of transcription

Pol II

DNA

Transcribed region

Cis-acting elements

Cis-acting elements are DNA sequences that are bound by trans-acting regulatory factors.

Figure 33.2
Cis-acting elements and trans-acting factors. mRNA = messenger RNA; *Pol II = RNA polymerase II.*

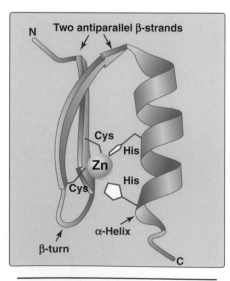

N

Two antiparallel β-strands

Cys
His
Zn
His
Cys

α-Helix

β-turn

C

Figure 33.3
Zinc (Zn) finger is a common motif in proteins that bind DNA. Cys = cysteine; His = histidine.

regulatory molecules are called trans-acting because they can diffuse (transit) through the cell from their site of synthesis to their DNA-binding sites (Fig. 33.2). For example, a protein transcription factor (a trans-acting molecule) that regulates a gene on chromosome 6 might itself have been produced from a gene on chromosome 11. The binding of proteins to DNA is through structural motifs such as the zinc finger (Fig. 33.3), leucine zipper, or helix-turn-helix in the protein.

III. REGULATION OF PROKARYOTIC GENE EXPRESSION

In prokaryotes such as the bacterium Escherichia coli (E. coli), regulation of gene expression occurs primarily at the level of transcription and, in general, is mediated by the binding of trans-acting proteins to cis-acting regulatory elements on their single DNA molecule (chromosome). [Note: Regulating the first step in the expression of a gene is an efficient approach, insofar as energy is not wasted making unneeded gene products.] Transcriptional control in prokaryotes can involve the initiation or premature termination of transcription.

A. Messenger RNA transcription from bacterial operons

In bacteria, the structural genes that encode proteins involved in a particular metabolic pathway are often found sequentially grouped on the chromosome along with the cis-acting elements that regulate the transcription of these genes. The transcription product is a single polycistronic messenger RNA ([mRNA] see p. 434). The genes are, thus, coordinately regulated (that is, turned on or off as a unit). This entire package is referred to as an operon.

B. Operators in bacterial operons

Bacterial operons contain an operator, a segment of DNA that regulates the activity of the structural genes of the operon by reversibly binding a protein known as the repressor. If the operator is not bound by the repressor, *RNA polymerase* (*RNA pol*) binds the promoter, passes over the operator, and reaches the protein-coding genes that it transcribes to mRNA. If the repressor is bound to the operator, the *polymerase* is blocked and does not produce mRNA. As long as the repressor is bound to the operator, no mRNA (and, therefore, no proteins) are made. However, when an inducer molecule is present, it binds to the repressor, causing the repressor to change shape so that it no longer binds the operator. When this happens, *RNA pol* can initiate transcription. One of the best-understood examples is the inducible lactose (lac) operon of E. coli that illustrates both positive and negative regulation (Fig. 33.4).

C. Lactose operon

The lac operon contains the genes that code for three proteins involved in the catabolism of the disaccharide lactose: the lacZ gene codes for *β-galactosidase*, which hydrolyzes lactose to galactose and glucose; the lacY gene codes for a *permease*, which facilitates the movement of lactose into the cell; and the lacA gene codes for *thiogalactoside transacetylase*, which acetylates lactose. [Note: The

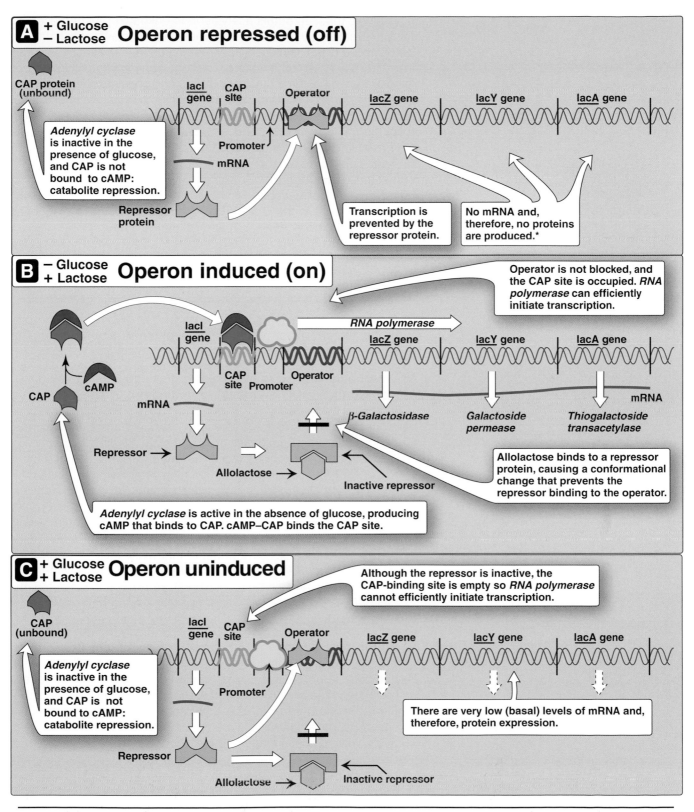

Figure 33.4

The lactose operon of <u>Escherichia coli</u> in the presence of A. only glucose, B. only lactose, and C. both sugars. *[Note: Even when the operon has been turned off, the repressor transiently dissociates from the operator at a slow rate, allowing a very low level of expression. The synthesis of a few molecules of *permease* (and *β-galactosidase*) allows the organism to respond rapidly should glucose become unavailable.] CAP = catabolite activator protein; cAMP = cyclic adenosine monophosphate; mRNA = messenger RNA.

physiologic function of this acetylation is unknown.] All of these proteins are maximally produced only when lactose is available to the cell and glucose is not. [Note: Bacteria use glucose, if available, as a fuel in preference to any other sugar.] The regulatory portion of the operon is upstream of the three structural genes and consists of the promoter region where *RNA pol* binds and two additional sites, the operator (O) and the catabolite activator protein (CAP) sites, where regulatory proteins bind. The lacZ, lacY, and lacA genes are maximally expressed only when the O site is empty and the CAP site is bound by a complex of cyclic adenosine monophosphate ([cAMP] see p. 94) and the CAP, sometimes called the cAMP regulatory protein (CRP). A regulatory gene, the lacI gene, codes for the repressor protein (a trans-acting factor) that binds to the O site with high affinity. [Note: The lacI gene has its own promoter and is not part of the lac operon.]

1. **When only glucose is available:** In this case, the lac operon is repressed (turned off). Repression is mediated by the repressor protein binding via a helix-turn-helix motif (Fig. 33.5) to the O site, which is downstream of the promoter (see Fig. 33.4A). Binding of the repressor interferes with the binding of *RNA pol* to the promoter, thereby inhibiting transcription of the structural genes. This is an example of negative regulation.

2. **When only lactose is available:** In this case, the lac operon is induced (maximally expressed, or turned on). A small amount of lactose is converted to an isomer, allolactose. This compound is an inducer that binds to the repressor protein, changing its conformation so that it can no longer bind to the O site. In the absence of glucose, *adenylyl cyclase* is active, and cAMP is made and binds to the CAP. The cAMP–CAP trans-acting complex binds to the CAP site, causing *RNA pol* to initiate transcription with high efficiency at the promoter site (see Fig. 33.4B). This is an example of positive regulation. The transcript is a single polycistronic mRNA molecule that contains three sets of start and stop codons. Translation of the mRNA produces the three proteins that allow lactose to be used for energy production by the cell. [Note: In contrast to the inducible lacZ, lacY, and lacA genes, whose expression is regulated, the lacI gene is constitutive. Its gene product, the repressor protein, is always made and is active unless the inducer is present.]

3. **When both glucose and lactose are available:** In this case, the lac operon is uninduced, and transcription is negligible, even if lactose is present at a high concentration. *Adenylyl cyclase* is inhibited in the presence of glucose (a process known as catabolite repression) so no cAMP–CAP complex forms, and the CAP site remains empty. Therefore, the *RNA pol* is unable to effectively initiate transcription, even though the repressor is not bound to the O site. Consequently, the three structural genes of the operon are expressed only at a very low (basal) level (see Fig. 33.4C). [Note: Induction causes a 50-fold enhancement over basal expression.]

D. **Tryptophan operon**

The tryptophan (trp) operon contains five structural genes that code for enzymes required for the synthesis of the amino acid tryptophan. As

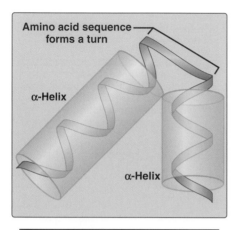

Figure 33.5
Helix-turn-helix motif of the lac repressor protein.

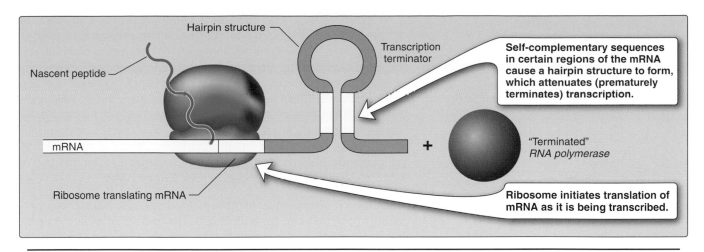

Figure 33.6
Attenuation of transcription of the trp operon when tryptophan is plentiful. mRNA = messenger RNA.

with the lac operon, the trp operon is subject to negative control. However, for the repressible trp operon, negative control includes Trp itself binding to a repressor protein and facilitating the binding of the repressor to the operator: Trp is a corepressor. Because repression by Trp is not always complete, the trp operon, unlike the lac operon, is also regulated by a process known as attenuation. With attenuation, transcription is initiated but is terminated well before completion (Fig. 33.6). If Trp is plentiful, transcription initiation that escaped repression by Trp is attenuated (stopped) by the formation of an attenuator, a hairpin (stem-loop) structure in the mRNA similar to that seen in rho-independent termination (see p. 437). [Note: Because transcription and translation are temporally linked in prokaryotes (see p. 454), attenuation also results in the formation of a truncated, nonfunctional peptide product that is rapidly degraded.] If Trp becomes scarce, the operon is expressed. The 5'-end of the mRNA contains two adjacent codons for Trp. The lack of Trp causes ribosomes to stall at these codons, covering regions of the mRNA required for formation of the attenuation hairpin. This prevents attenuation and allows transcription to continue.

> Transcriptional attenuation can occur in prokaryotes because translation of an mRNA begins before its synthesis is complete. This does not occur in eukaryotes because the presence of a membrane-bound nucleus spatially and temporally separates transcription and translation.

E. Coordination of transcription and translation

Although transcriptional regulation of mRNA production is primary in bacteria, regulation of ribosomal RNA (rRNA) and protein synthesis plays important roles in adaptation to environmental stress.

1. **Stringent response:** E. coli has seven operons that synthesize the rRNA needed for ribosome assembly, and each is regulated in response to changes in environmental conditions. Regulation in response to amino acid starvation is known as the stringent response. The binding of an uncharged transfer RNA (tRNA) to the A site of

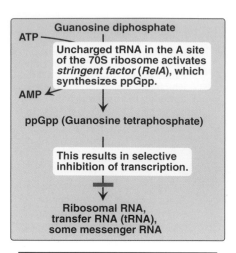

Figure 33.7
Regulation of transcription by the stringent response to amino acid starvation. S = Svedberg unit.

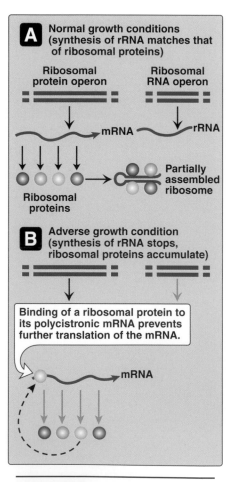

Figure 33.8
Regulation of translation by an excess of ribosomal proteins. mRNA = messenger RNA; rRNA = ribosomal RNA.

a ribosome (see p. 452) triggers a series of events that leads to the production of the alarmone guanosine tetraphosphate (ppGpp). The synthesis of this unusual derivative of guanosine diphosphate (GDP) is catalyzed by *stringent factor* (*RelA*), an enzyme physically associated with ribosomes. Elevated levels of ppGpp result in inhibition of rRNA synthesis (Fig. 33.7). [Note: In addition to rRNA synthesis, tRNA synthesis and some mRNA synthesis (for example, for ribosomal proteins) are also inhibited. However, synthesis of mRNA for enzymes required for amino acid biosynthesis is not inhibited. ppGpp binds *RNA pol* and alters promoter selection through use of different sigma factors for the *polymerase* (see p. 435).]

2. **Regulatory ribosomal proteins:** Operons for ribosomal proteins (r-proteins) can be inhibited by an excess of their own protein products. For each operon, one specific r-protein functions in the repression of translation of the polycistronic mRNA from that operon (Fig. 33.8). The r-protein does so by binding to the Shine-Dalgarno (SD) sequence located on the mRNA just upstream of the first initiating AUG codon (see p. 448) and acting as a physical impediment to the binding of the small ribosomal subunit to the SD sequence. Thus, one r-protein inhibits synthesis of all the r-proteins of the operon. This same r-protein also binds to rRNA and with a higher affinity than for mRNA. If the concentration of rRNA falls, the r-protein then is available to bind its own mRNA and inhibit its translation. This coordinated regulation keeps the synthesis of r-proteins in balance with the transcription of rRNA, so that each is present in appropriate amounts for the formation of ribosomes.

IV. REGULATION OF EUKARYOTIC GENE EXPRESSION

The higher degree of complexity of eukaryotic genomes, as well as the presence of a nuclear membrane, necessitates a wider range of regulatory processes. As with the prokaryotes, transcription is the primary site of regulation. Again, the theme of trans-acting factors binding to cis-acting elements is seen. Operons, however, are not found in eukaryotes, which must use alternate strategies to solve the problem of how to coordinately regulate all the genes required for a specific response. In eukaryotes, gene expression is also regulated at multiple levels other than transcription. For example, the major modes of posttranscriptional regulation at the mRNA level are alternative mRNA splicing and polyadenylation, control of mRNA stability, and control of translational efficiency. Additional regulation at the protein level occurs by mechanisms that modulate stability, processing, or targeting of the protein.

A. Coordinate regulation

The need to coordinately regulate a group of genes to cause a particular response is of key importance in organisms with more than one chromosome. An underlying theme occurs repeatedly: A trans-acting protein functions as a specific transcription factor (STF) that binds to a cis-acting regulatory consensus sequence (see p. 415) on each of the genes in the group even if they are on different chromosomes. [Note: The STF has a DNA-binding domain (DBD) and a transcription activation domain (TAD). The TAD recruits coactivators, such as *histone acetyltransferases* (see p. 438), and the general transcription factors (see p. 439) that, along with *RNA pol*, are required for formation of the transcription initiation complex at the promoter. Although the TAD recruits a variety of proteins, the specific effect of any one of them is dependent upon the protein composition of the complex. This is known as combinatorial control.] Examples of coordinate regulation in eukaryotes include the galactose circuit and the hormone response system.

1. **Galactose circuit:** This regulatory scheme allows for the use of galactose when glucose is not available. In yeast, a unicellular organism, the genes required to metabolize galactose are on different chromosomes. Coordinated expression is mediated by the protein Gal4 (Gal – galactose), a STF that binds to a short regulatory DNA sequence upstream of each of the genes. The sequence is called the upstream activating sequence Gal (UAS$_{Gal}$). Binding of Gal4 to UAS$_{Gal}$ through zinc fingers in its DBD occurs in both the absence and presence of galactose. When the sugar is absent, the regulatory protein Gal80 binds Gal4 at its TAD, thereby inhibiting gene transcription (Fig. 33.9A). When present, galactose activates the Gal3 protein. Gal3 binds Gal80, thereby allowing Gal4 to activate transcription (Fig. 33.9B). [Note: Glucose prevents the use of galactose by inhibiting expression of Gal4 protein.]

2. **Hormone response system:** Hormone response elements (HRE) are DNA sequences that bind trans-acting proteins and regulate

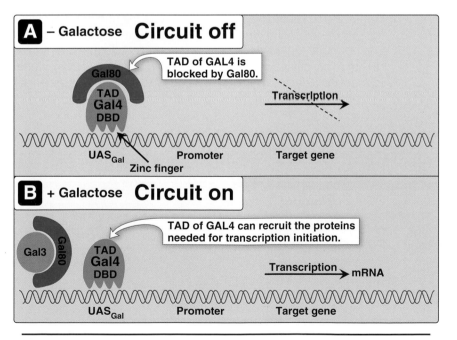

Figure 33.9
Regulation of galactose (gal) circuit in yeast in the A. absence and B. presence of galactose. [Note: Target genes, whether on the same or a different chromosome, each have an upstream activating sequence galactose (UAS$_{Gal}$).] TAD = transcription activation domain; DBD = DNA-binding domain; mRNA = messenger RNA.

gene expression in response to hormonal signals in multicellular organisms. Hormones bind to either intracellular (nuclear) receptors (for example, steroid hormones; see p. 240) or cell-surface receptors (for example, the peptide hormone glucagon; see p. 314).

a. **Intracellular receptors:** Members of the nuclear receptor superfamily, which includes the steroid hormone (glucocorticoids, mineralocorticoids, androgens, and estrogens), vitamin D, retinoic acid, and thyroid hormone receptors, function as STF. In addition to domains for DNA-binding and transcriptional activation, these receptors also contain a ligand-binding domain. For example, the steroid hormone cortisol (a glucocorticoid) binds intracellular receptors at the ligand-binding domain (Fig. 33.10). Binding causes a conformational change in the receptor that activates it. The receptor–hormone complex enters the nucleus, dimerizes, and binds via a zinc finger motif to DNA at a regulatory element, the glucocorticoid response element (GRE) that is an example of a HRE. Binding allows recruitment of coactivators to the TAD and results in expression of cortisol-responsive genes, each of which is under the control of its own GRE. Binding of the receptor–hormone complex to the GRE allows coordinate expression of a group of target genes, even though these genes are on different chromosomes. The GRE can be located upstream or downstream of the genes it regulates and at great distances from them. The GRE, then, can function as a true enhancer (see p. 440). [Note: If associated with repressors, hormone–receptor complexes inhibit transcription.]

b. **Cell-surface receptors:** These receptors include those for insulin, epinephrine, and glucagon. Glucagon, for example, is a peptide hormone that binds its G protein–coupled plasma membrane receptor on glucagon-responsive cells. This extracellular signal is then transduced to intracellular cAMP, a second messenger

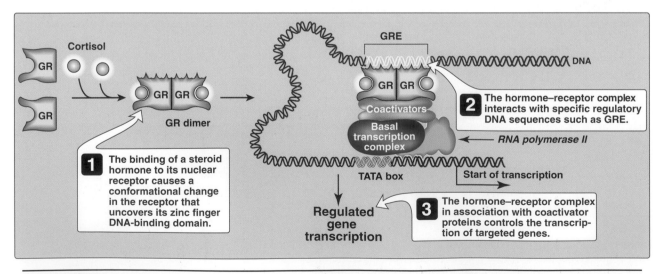

Figure 33.10
Transcriptional regulation by intracellular steroid hormone receptors. GRE = glucocorticoid response element; GR = glucocorticoid receptor.

(Fig. 33.11; also see Fig. 8.7 on p. 95), which can affect protein expression (and activity) through *protein kinase A*–mediated phosphorylation. In response to a rise in cAMP, a trans-acting factor (cAMP response element–binding [CREB] protein) is phosphorylated and activated. Active CREB protein binds via a leucine zipper motif to a cis-acting regulatory element, the cAMP response element (CRE), resulting in transcription of target genes with CRE in their promoters. [Note: The genes for *phosphoenolpyruvate carboxykinase* and *glucose 6-phosphatase*, key enzymes of gluconeogenesis (see p. 122), are examples of genes upregulated by the cAMP/CRE/CREB system.]

B. Messenger RNA processing and use

Eukaryotic mRNA undergoes several processing events before it is exported from the nucleus to the cytoplasm for use in protein synthesis. Capping at the 5′-end (see p. 441), polyadenylation at the 3′-end (see p. 442), and splicing (see p. 442) are essential for the production of a functional eukaryotic messenger from most pre-mRNA. Variations in splicing and polyadenylation can affect gene expression. In addition, messenger stability also affects gene expression.

1. **Alternative splicing:** Tissue-specific protein isoforms can be made from the same pre-mRNA through alternative splicing, which can involve exon skipping (loss), intron retention, and use of alternative splice-donor or -acceptor sites (Fig. 33.12). For example, the pre-mRNA for tropomyosin (TM) undergoes tissue-specific alternative splicing to yield a number of TM isoforms (see p. 443). [Note: Over 90% of all human genes undergo alternative splicing.]

2. **Alternative polyadenylation:** Some pre-mRNA transcripts have more than one site for cleavage and polyadenylation. Alternative polyadenylation (APA) generates mRNA with different 3′-ends, altering the untranslated region (UTR) or the coding (translated) sequence. [Note: APA is involved in the production of the membrane-bound and secreted forms of immunoglobulin M.]

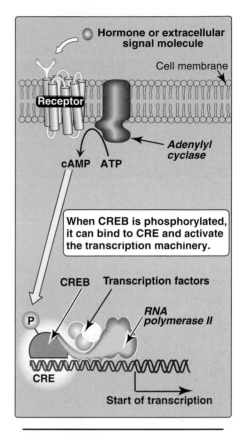

Figure 33.11
Transcriptional regulation by receptors located in the cell membrane. [Note: Cyclic adenosine monophosphate (cAMP) activates *protein kinase A* that phosphorylates cAMP response element–binding (CREB) protein.] CRE = cAMP response element.

> The use of alternative splicing and polyadenylation sites, as well as alternative transcription start sites explains, at least in part, how the ~20,000 to 25,000 genes in the human genome can give rise to well over 100,000 proteins.

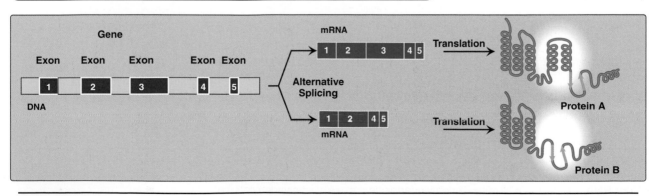

Figure 33.12
Tissue-specific alternative splicing produces different proteins, or isoforms, from a single gene. mRNA = messenger RNA.

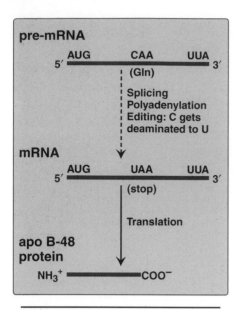

Figure 33.13
Editing of apolipoprotein (apo) B
pre-mRNA in the intestine and
generation of the apo B-48 protein
needed for chylomicron synthesis.
Gln = glutamine; mRNA = messenger
RNA; A = adenine; C = cytosine;
G = guanine; U = uracil.

3. **Messenger RNA editing:** Even after mRNA has been fully processed, it may undergo an additional posttranscriptional modification in which a base in the mRNA is altered. This is known as RNA
editing. An important example in humans occurs with the transcript
for apolipoprotein (apo) B, an essential component of chylomicrons (see p. 228) and very-low-density lipoproteins ([VLDL] see
p. 230). Apo B mRNA is made in the liver and the small intestine.
However, in the intestine only, the cytosine (C) base in the CAA
codon for glutamine is enzymatically deaminated to uracil (U),
changing the sense codon to the nonsense or stop codon UAA,
as shown in Figure 33.13. This results in a shorter protein (apo
B-48, representing 48% of the message) being made in the intestine (and incorporated into chylomicrons) than is made in the liver
(apo B-100, full-length, incorporated into VLDL).

4. **Messenger RNA stability:** How long an mRNA remains in the
cytosol before it is degraded influences how much protein product can be produced from it. Regulation of iron metabolism and
the gene-silencing process of RNA interference (RNAi) illustrate the importance of mRNA stability in the regulation of gene
expression.

a. **Iron metabolism:** Transferrin (Tf) is a plasma protein that
transports iron. Tf binds to cell-surface receptors (transferrin
receptors [TfR]) that get internalized and provide cells, such
as erythroblasts, with iron. The mRNA for the TfR has several cis-acting iron-responsive elements (IRE) in its 3'-UTR.
IRE have a short stem-loop structure that can be bound
by trans-acting iron regulatory proteins (IRP), as shown in
Figure 33.14. When the iron concentration in the cell is low,
the IRP bind to the 3'-IRE and stabilize the mRNA for TfR,
allowing TfR synthesis. When intracellular iron levels are high,

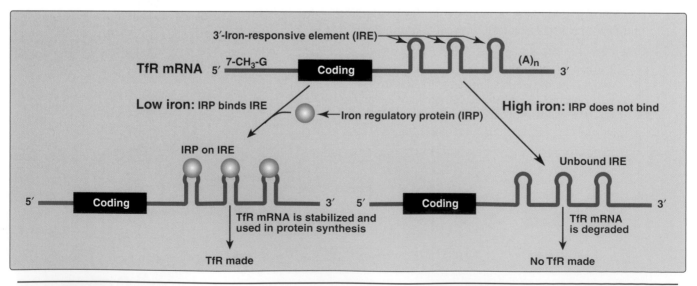

Figure 33.14
Regulation of transferrin receptor (TfR) synthesis. [Note: The IRE are located in the 3'-UTR (untranslated region) of TfR
messenger RNA (mRNA).] 7-CH₃-G = 7-methylguanosine cap; (A)ₙ = polyadenylate tail.

the IRP dissociate. The lack of IRP bound to the mRNA hastens its destruction, resulting in decreased TfR synthesis. [Note: The mRNA for ferritin, an intracellular protein of iron storage, has a single IRE in its 5′-UTR. When iron levels in the cell are low, IRP bind the 5′-IRE and prevent the use of the mRNA, and less ferritin is made. When iron accumulates in the cell, the IRP dissociate, allowing synthesis of ferritin molecules to store the excess iron. *Aminolevulinic acid synthase 2*, the regulated enzyme of heme synthesis (see p. 278) in erythroblasts, also contains a 5′-IRE.] (See Chapter 29 for a discussion of iron metabolism.)

b. RNA interference: RNAi is a mechanism of gene silencing through decreased expression of mRNA, either by repression of translation or by increased degradation. It plays a key role in such fundamental processes as cell proliferation, differentiation, and apoptosis. RNAi is mediated by short (~22 nucleotides), noncoding RNA called microRNA (miRNA). The miRNA arise from far longer, genomically encoded nuclear transcripts, primary miRNA (pri-miRNA), that are partially processed in the nucleus to pre-miRNA by an *endonuclease* (*Drosha*) then transported to the cytoplasm. There, an *endonuclease* (*Dicer*) completes the processing and generates short, double-stranded miRNA. A single strand (the guide or antisense strand) of the miRNA associates with a cytosolic protein complex known as the RNA-induced silencing complex (RISC). The guide strand hybridizes with a complementary sequence in the 3′-UTR of a full-length target mRNA, bringing RISC to the mRNA. This can result in repression of translation of the mRNA or its degradation by an *endonuclease* (*Argonaute/Ago/Slicer*) of the RISC. The extent of complementarity appears to be the determining factor (Fig. 33.15). RNAi can also be triggered by the introduction of exogenous double-stranded short interfering RNA (siRNA) into a cell, a process that has enormous therapeutic potential.

1) RNA interference–based therapeutics: The first clinical trial of RNAi-based therapy involved the neovascular form of age-related macular degeneration (AMD), which is triggered by overproduction of vascular endothelial growth factor (VEGF), leading to the sprouting of excess blood vessels behind the retina. The vessels leak, clouding and often entirely destroying vision (therefore, neovascular AMD is also referred to as wet AMD). An siRNA was designed to target the mRNA of VEGF and promote its degradation. Although considerable effort and resources have been expended to develop RNAi-based therapeutics, especially for the treatment of cancer, no products have gone from trials to the market. The research applications of RNAi, however, have grown rapidly.

5. Messenger RNA translation: Regulation of gene expression can also occur at the level of mRNA translation. One mechanism by which translation is regulated is through phosphorylation

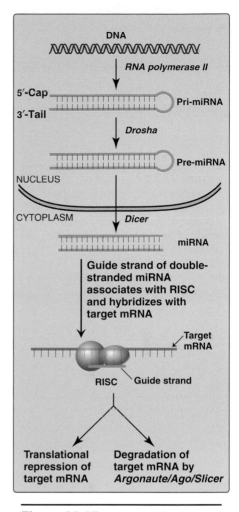

Figure 33.15
Biogenesis and actions of microRNA (miRNA). [Note: The extent of complementarity between the target messenger RNA (mRNA) and the miRNA determines the final outcome, with perfect complementarity resulting in mRNA degradation.] Pri = primary; RISC = RNA-induced silencing complex.

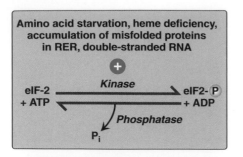

Figure 33.16
Regulation of translation initiation in eukaryotes by phosphorylation of eukaryotic translation initiation factor, eIF-2. RER = rough endoplasmic reticulum; ADP = adenosine diphosphate; P$_i$ = inorganic phosphate; ⓟ = phosphate.

of the eukaryotic translation initiation factor, eIF-2 (Fig. 33.16). Phosphorylation of eIF-2 inhibits its function and so inhibits translation at the initiation step (see p. 459). [Note: Phosphorylation of eIF-2 prevents its reactivation by inhibiting GDP-GTP exchange.] Phosphorylation is catalyzed by *kinases* that are activated in response to environmental conditions, such as amino acid starvation, heme deficiency in erythroblasts, the presence of double-stranded RNA (signaling viral infection), and the accumulation of misfolded proteins in the rough endoplasmic reticulum (see p. 460).

C. Regulation through variations in DNA

Gene expression in eukaryotes is also influenced by the accessibility of DNA to the transcriptional apparatus, the amount of DNA, and the arrangement of DNA. [Note: Localized transitions between the B and Z forms of DNA (see p. 414) can also affect gene expression.]

1. **Access to DNA:** In eukaryotes, DNA is found complexed with histone and nonhistone proteins to form chromatin (see p. 425). Transcriptionally active, decondensed chromatin (euchromatin) differs from the more condensed, inactive form (heterochromatin) in a number of ways. Active chromatin contains histone proteins that have been covalently modified at their amino terminal ends by reversible methylation, acetylation, or phosphorylation (see p. 438 for a discussion of histone acetylation/deacetylation by *histone acetyltransferase* and *histone deacetylase*). Such modifications decrease the positive charge of these basic proteins, thereby decreasing the strength of their association with negatively charged DNA. This relaxes the nucleosome (see p. 425), allowing transcription factors access to specific regions on the DNA. Nucleosomes can also be repositioned, an ATP-requiring process that is part of chromatin remodeling. Another difference between transcriptionally active and inactive chromatin is the extent of methylation of cytosine bases in CG-rich regions (CpG islands) in the promoter region of many genes. Methylation is by *methyltransferases* that use S-adenosylmethionine as the methyl donor (Fig. 33.17). Transcriptionally active genes are less methylated (hypomethylated) than their inactive counterparts, suggesting that DNA hypermethylation silences gene expression. Modification of histones and methylation of DNA are epigenetic in that they are heritable changes in DNA that alter gene expression without altering the base sequence.

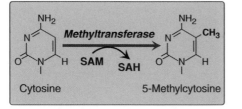

Figure 33.17
The methylation of cytosine in eukaryotic DNA. SAM = S-adenosylmethionine; SAH = S-adenosylhomocysteine.

2. **Amount of DNA:** A change up or down in the number of copies of a gene can affect the amount of gene product produced. An increase in copy number (gene amplification) has contributed to increased genomic complexity and is still a normal developmental process in certain nonmammalian species. In mammals, however, gene amplification is seen with some diseases and in response to particular chemotherapeutic drugs such as methotrexate, an inhibitor of the enzyme *dihydrofolate reductase* (*DHFR*), required for the synthesis of thymidine triphosphate (TTP) in the pyrimidine biosynthetic pathway (see p. 303). TTP is essential for DNA synthesis. Gene amplification results in an increase in the number of *DHFR* genes and resistance to the drug, allowing TTP to be made.

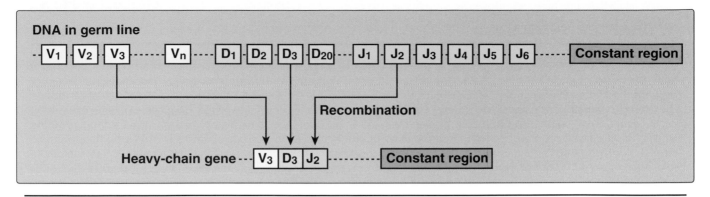

Figure 33.18
DNA rearrangements in the generation of immunoglobulins. V= variable; D = diversity; J = joining.

3. **Arrangement of DNA:** The process by which immunoglobulins (antibodies) are produced by B lymphocytes involves permanent rearrangements of the DNA in these cells. The immunoglobulins (for example, IgG) consist of two light and two heavy chains, with each chain containing regions of variable and constant amino acid sequence. The variable region is the result of somatic recombination of segments within both the light- and the heavy-chain genes. During B-lymphocyte development, single variable (V), diversity (D), and joining (J) gene segments are brought together through gene rearrangement to form a unique variable region (Fig. 33.18). This process allows the generation of 10^9–10^{11} different immunoglobulins from a single gene, providing the diversity needed for the recognition of an enormous number of antigens. [Note: Pathologic DNA rearrangement is seen with translocation, a process by which two different chromosomes exchange DNA segments.]

4. **Mobile DNA elements:** Transposons (Tn) are mobile segments of DNA that move in an essentially random manner from one site to another on the same or a different chromosome. Movement is mediated by *transposase*, an enzyme encoded by the Tn itself. Movement can be direct, in which *transposase* cuts out and then inserts the Tn at a new site, or replicative, in which the Tn is copied and the copy inserted elsewhere while the original remains in place. In eukaryotes, including humans, replicative transposition frequently involves an RNA intermediate made by a *reverse transcriptase* (see p. 424), in which case the Tn is called a retrotransposon. Transposition has contributed to structural variation in the genome but also has the potential to alter gene expression and even to cause disease. Tn comprise ~50% of the human genome, with retrotransposons accounting for 90% of Tn. Although the vast majority of these retrotransposons have lost the ability to move, some are still active. Their transposition is thought to be the basis for some rare cases of hemophilia A and Duchenne muscular dystrophy. [Note: The growing problem of antibiotic-resistant bacteria is a consequence, at least in part, of the exchange of plasmids among bacterial cells. If the plasmids contain Tn-carrying antibiotic resistance genes, the recipient bacteria gain resistance to one or more antimicrobial drugs.]

V. CHAPTER SUMMARY

Gene expression results in the production of a functional gene product (either RNA or protein) through the processes of transcription and translation (Fig. 33.19). **Genes** can be either **constitutive** (always expressed, housekeeping genes) or **regulated** (expressed only under certain conditions in all cells or in a subset of cells). The ability to appropriately **induce** (**positively regulate**) or **repress** (**negatively regulate**) genes is essential in all organisms. Regulation of gene expression occurs primarily at **transcription** in both prokaryotes and eukaryotes and is mediated through **trans-acting proteins** binding to **cis-acting regulatory DNA elements**. In **eukaryotes**, regulation also occurs through DNA **modifications** and through **posttranscriptional** and **posttranslational processing**. In **prokaryotes**, such as <u>Escherichia</u> <u>coli</u>, the coordinate regulation of genes whose protein products are required for a particular process is achieved through **operons** (groups of genes sequentially arranged on the chromosome along with the regulatory elements that determine their transcription). The **lac operon** contains the <u>Z</u>, <u>Y</u>, and <u>A</u> structural genes, the protein products of which are needed for the catabolism of lactose. It is subject to negative and positive regulation. When **glucose** is available, the operon is repressed by the binding of the **repressor protein** (the product of the <u>lacI</u> gene) to the **operator**, thus preventing transcription. When only **lactose** is present, the operon is induced by an isomer of lactose (**allolactose**) that binds the repressor protein, preventing it from binding to the operator. In addition, **cyclic adenosine monophosphate** (**cAMP**) binds the **catabolite activator protein** (**CAP**), and the complex binds the DNA at the **CAP site**. This increases **promoter** efficiency and results in the expression of the structural genes through the production of a **polycistronic messenger RNA** (**mRNA**). When both **glucose and lactose** are present, glucose prevents formation of cAMP, and transcription of these genes is negligible. The **trp operon** contains genes needed for the synthesis of tryptophan (Trp), and, like the lac operon, it is regulated by **negative control**. Unlike the lac operon, it is also regulated by **attenuation**, in which mRNA synthesis that escaped repression by Trp is terminated before completion. Transcription of **ribosomal RNA** and **transfer RNA** is selectively inhibited in prokaryotes by the **stringent response** to amino acid starvation. **Translation** is also a site of prokaryotic gene regulation: Excess ribosomal proteins bind the **Shine-Dalgarno sequence** on their own polycistronic mRNA, preventing ribosomes from binding. Gene regulation is more complex in **eukaryotes**. Operons are not present, but coordinate regulation of the transcription of genes located on different chromosomes can be achieved through the binding of trans-acting proteins to cis-acting elements as seen in the **galactose circuit** in unicellular yeast. In multicellular organisms, **hormones** can cause coordinated regulation, either through the binding of the **hormone receptor–hormone complex** to the DNA (as with steroid hormones) or through the binding of a protein that is activated in response to a **second messenger** (as with glucagon). In each case, binding to DNA is mediated through structural motifs such as the **zinc finger**. **Co-** and **posttranscriptional regulation** is also seen in eukaryotes and includes **alternative mRNA splicing** and **polyadenylation**, mRNA **editing**, and variations in mRNA **stability** as seen with **transferrin receptor** synthesis and with **RNA interference**. Regulation at the **translational level** can be caused by the **phosphorylation** and inhibition of **eukaryotic initiation factor-2**. Gene expression in eukaryotes is also influenced by **accessibility** of DNA to the transcriptional apparatus (as seen with **epigenetic** changes to histone proteins), the **amount** of DNA, and the **arrangement** of the DNA.

Study Questions

Choose the ONE best answer.

33.1 Which of the following mutations is most likely to result in reduced expression of the lac operon?

  A. cya⁻ (no adenylyl cyclase made)
  B. i⁻ (no repressor protein made)
  C. Oᶜ (operator cannot bind repressor protein)
  D. One resulting in impaired glucose uptake

Correct answer = A. In the absence of glucose, adenylyl cyclase makes cyclic adenosine monophosphate (cAMP), which forms a complex with the catabolite activator protein (CAP). The cAMP–CAP complex binds the CAP site on the DNA, causing RNA polymerase to bind more efficiently to the lac operon promoter, thereby increasing expression of the operon. With cya⁻ mutations, adenylyl cyclase is not made, and so the operon is unable to be maximally expressed even when glucose is absent and lactose is present. The absence of a repressor protein or decreased ability of the repressor to bind the operator results in constitutive (essentially constant) expression of the lac operon.

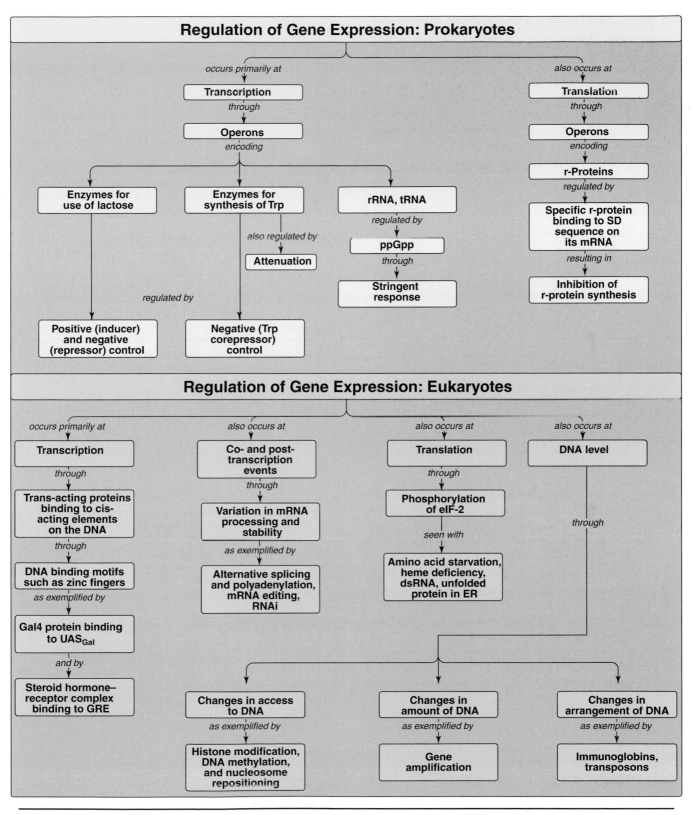

Figure 33.19

Summary of key concepts for the regulation of gene expression. Trp = tryptophan; rRNA, tRNA, mRNA = ribosomal, transfer, and messenger RNA, respectively; ppGpp; guanosine tetraphosphate; r-protein = ribosomal protein; SD = Shine-Dalgarno; Gal = galactose; UAS = upstream activating sequence; GRE = glucocorticoid response element; RNAi = RNA interference; eIF = eukaryotic initiation factor; ds = double stranded; ER = endoplasmic reticulum.

33.2 Which of the following is best described as cis-acting?

A. Cyclic adenosine monophosphate response element–binding protein

B. Operator

C. Repressor protein

D. Thyroid hormone nuclear receptor

Correct answer = B. The operator is part of the DNA itself, and so is cis-acting. The cyclic adenosine monophosphate response element–binding protein, repressor protein, and thyroid hormone nuclear receptor protein are molecules that diffuse (transit) to the DNA, bind, and affect the expression of that DNA and so are trans-acting.

33.3 Which of the following is the basis for the intestine-specific expression of apolipoprotein B-48?

A. DNA rearrangement and loss

B. DNA transposition

C. RNA alternative splicing

D. RNA editing

E. RNA interference

Correct answer = D. The production of apolipoprotein (apo) B-48 in the intestine and apo B-100 in liver is the result of RNA editing in the intestine, where a sense codon is changed to a nonsense codon by posttranscriptional deamination of cytosine to uracil. DNA rearrangement and transposition, as well as RNA interference and alternative splicing, do alter gene expression but are not the basis of apo B-48 tissue-specific production.

33.4 Which of the following is most likely to be true in hemochromatosis, a disease of iron accumulation?

A. The messenger RNA for the transferrin receptor is stabilized by the binding of iron regulatory proteins to its 3′-iron-responsive elements.

B. The messenger RNA for the transferrin receptor is not bound by iron regulatory proteins and is degraded.

C. The messenger RNA for ferritin is not bound by iron regulatory proteins at its 5′-iron-responsive element and is translated.

D. The messenger RNA for ferritin is bound by iron regulatory proteins and is not translated.

E. Both B and C are correct.

Correct answer = E. When iron levels in the body are high, as is seen with hemochromatosis, there is increased synthesis of the iron-storage molecule, ferritin, and decreased synthesis of the transferrin receptor (TfR) that mediates iron uptake by cells. These effects are the result of cis-acting iron-responsive elements not being bound by trans-acting iron regulatory proteins, resulting in degradation of the messenger RNA (mRNA) for TfR and increased translation of the mRNA for ferritin.

33.5 Patients with estrogen receptor–positive (hormone responsive) breast cancer may be treated with the drug tamoxifen, which binds the estrogen nuclear receptor without activating it. Which of the following is the most logical outcome of tamoxifen use?

A. Increased acetylation of estrogen-responsive genes

B. Increased growth of estrogen receptor–positive breast cancer cells

C. Increased production of cyclic adenosine monophosphate

D. Inhibition of the estrogen operon

E. Inhibition of transcription of estrogen-responsive genes

Correct answer = E. Tamoxifen competes with estrogen for binding to the estrogen nuclear receptor. Tamoxifen fails to activate the receptor, preventing its binding to DNA sequences that upregulate expression of estrogen-responsive genes. Tamoxifen, then, blocks the growth-promoting effects of these genes and results in growth inhibition of estrogen-dependent breast cancer cells. Acetylation increases transcription by relaxing the nucleosome. Cyclic adenosine monophosphate is a regulatory signal mediated by cell-surface rather than nuclear receptors. Mammalian cells do not have operons.

33.6 The ZYA region of the lac operon will be maximally expressed if:

A. cyclic adenosine monophosphate levels are low.

B. glucose and lactose are both available.

C. the attenuation stem-loop is able to form.

D. the CAP site is occupied.

Correct answer = D. It is only when glucose is gone, cyclic adenosine monophosphate (cAMP) levels are increased, the cAMP–catabolite activator protein (CAP) complex is bound to the CAP site, and lactose is available that the operon is maximally expressed (induced). If glucose is present, the operon is off as a result of catabolite repression. The lac operon is not regulated by attenuation, a mechanism for stopping transcription in some operons such as the trp operon.

33.7 X chromosome inactivation is a process by which one of two X chromosomes in mammalian females is condensed and inactivated to prevent overexpression of X-linked genes. What would most likely be true about the degree of DNA methylation and histone acetylation on the inactivated X chromosome?

Cytosines in CpG islands would be hypermethylated, and histone proteins would be deacetylated. Both conditions are associated with decreased gene expression, and both are important in maintaining X inactivation.

Biotechnology and Human Disease

34

I. OVERVIEW

In the past, efforts to understand genes and their expression have been confounded by the immense size and complexity of human deoxyribonucleic acid (DNA). The human genome contains ~3 billion (10^9) base pairs (bp) that encode 20,000–25,000 protein-coding genes located on 23 chromosomes in the haploid genome. It is now possible to determine the nucleotide sequence of long stretches of DNA, and the entire human genome has been sequenced. This effort (called the Human Genome Project and completed in 2003) was made possible by several tools that have already contributed to our understanding of many genetic diseases (Fig. 34.1). These include 1) the discovery of *restriction endonucleases* that permit the cleavage of huge DNA molecules into defined fragments, 2) the development of cloning techniques that provide a mechanism for amplification of specific nucleotide sequences, and 3) the ability to synthesize specific probes, which has allowed the identification and manipulation of nucleotide sequences of interest. These and other experimental approaches have permitted the identification of both normal and mutant nucleotide sequences in DNA. This knowledge has led to the development of methods for the diagnosis of genetic diseases and some successes in the treatment of patients by gene therapy. [Note: The genomes of several viruses, prokaryotes, and nonhuman eukaryotes have also been sequenced.]

II. RESTRICTION ENDONUCLEASES

One of the major obstacles to molecular analysis of genomic DNA is the immense size of the molecules involved. The discovery of a special group of bacterial enzymes, called *restriction endonucleases* (restriction enzymes), which cleave double-stranded DNA (dsDNA) into smaller, more manageable fragments, opened the way for DNA analysis. Because each enzyme cleaves dsDNA at a specific nucleotide sequence (restriction site), restriction enzymes are used experimentally to obtain precisely defined DNA segments called restriction fragments.

A. Specificity

Restriction endonucleases recognize short stretches of dsDNA (4–8 bp) that contain specific nucleotide sequences. These sequences, which differ for each restriction enzyme, are palindromes, that is, they

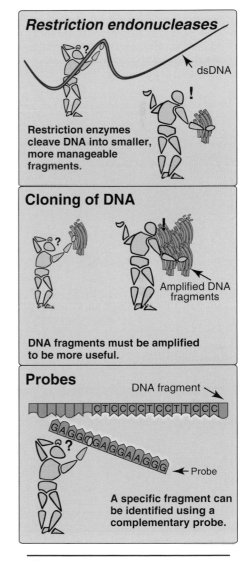

Figure 34.1
Three tools that facilitate analysis of human DNA. dsDNA = double-stranded DNA.

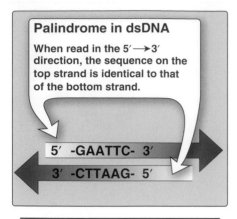

Palindrome in dsDNA

When read in the 5′→3′ direction, the sequence on the top strand is identical to that of the bottom strand.

5′ -GAATTC- 3′
3′ -CTTAAG- 5′

Figure 34.2
Recognition sequence of *restriction endonuclease Eco*RI shows twofold rotational symmetry. dsDNA = double-stranded DNA; A = adenine; C = cytosine; G = guanine; T = thymine.

exhibit twofold rotational symmetry (Fig. 34.2). This means that, within a short region of the dsDNA, the nucleotide sequence on the two strands is identical if each is read in the 5′→3′ direction. Therefore, if you turn the page upside down (that is, rotate it 180° around its axis of symmetry) the sequence remains the same.

> In bacteria, *restriction endonucleases* limit (restrict) the expression of nonbacterial (foreign) DNA through cleavage. Bacterial DNA is protected from cleavage by methylation of adenine at the restriction site.

B. Nomenclature

A restriction enzyme is named according to the organism from which it was isolated. The first letter of the name is from the genus of the bacterium. The next two letters are from the name of the species. An additional letter indicates the type or strain (as needed), and a number (Roman numeral) is appended to indicate the order in which the enzyme was discovered in that particular organism. For example, *Hae*III is the third *restriction endonuclease* isolated from the bacterium <u>Hae</u>mophilus <u>ae</u>gyptius.

C. Sticky and blunt ends

Restriction enzymes cleave dsDNA so as to produce a 3′-hydroxyl group on one end and a 5′-phosphate group on the other. Some *restriction endonucleases*, such as *Taq*I, form staggered cuts that produce sticky or cohesive ends (that is, the resulting DNA fragments have single-stranded regions that are complementary to each other), as shown in Figure 34.3. Other *restriction endonucleases*, such as *Hae*III, produce fragments that have blunt ends that are entirely double stranded and, therefore, do not form hydrogen bonds with each other. Using the enzyme *DNA ligase* (see p. 418), sticky ends of a DNA fragment of interest can be covalently joined with other DNA fragments that have sticky ends produced by cleavage with the same *restriction endonuclease* (Fig. 34.4). [Note: A *ligase* encoded by bacteriophage T4 can covalently join blunt-ended fragments.]

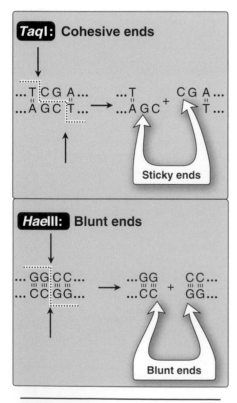

*Taq*I: **Cohesive ends**

...T CG A...
...A GC T... → ...T   CG A...
                ...A GC +   T...

Sticky ends

*Hae*III: **Blunt ends**

... GG CC...
... CC GG... → ...GG   CC...
               ...CC + GG...

Blunt ends

Figure 34.3
Specificity of *Taq*I and *Hae*III *restriction endonucleases*. A = adenine; C = cytosine; G = guanine; T = thymine.

D. Restriction sites

A DNA sequence that is recognized and cut by a restriction enzyme is called a restriction site. *Restriction endonucleases* cleave dsDNA into fragments of different sizes depending upon the size of the sequence recognized. For example, an enzyme that recognizes a specific 4-bp sequence produces many cuts in the DNA molecule, one every 4^4 bp. In contrast, an enzyme requiring a unique sequence of 6 bp produces fewer cuts (one every 4^6 bp) and, therefore, longer pieces. Hundreds of these enzymes, each having different cleavage specificities (varying in both nucleotide sequences and length of recognition sites), are commercially available.

III. DNA CLONING

Introduction of a foreign DNA molecule into a replicating cell permits the cloning or, amplification (that is, the production of many identical copies) of that DNA. [Note: Human DNA for cloning can be obtained from blood, saliva, and solid tissue.] In some cases, a single DNA fragment can be isolated and purified prior to cloning. More commonly, to clone a nucleotide sequence of interest, the total cellular DNA is first cleaved with a specific restriction enzyme, creating hundreds of thousands of fragments. Each of the resulting DNA fragments is joined to a DNA vector molecule (referred to as a cloning vector) to form a hybrid, or recombinant, DNA molecule. Each recombinant molecule carries its inserted DNA fragment into a single host cell (for example, a bacterium), where it is replicated. [Note: The process of introducing foreign DNA into a cell is called transformation for bacteria and yeast and transfection for higher eukaryotes.] As the host cell multiplies, it forms a clone in which every bacterium contains copies of the same inserted DNA fragment, hence the name "cloning." The cloned DNA can be released from its vector by cleavage (using the appropriate *restriction endonuclease*) and isolated. By this mechanism, many identical copies of the DNA of interest can be produced. [Note: An alternative to amplification by biologic cloning, the polymerase chain reaction (PCR), is described on p. 495.]

A. Vectors

A vector is a molecule of DNA to which the fragment of DNA to be cloned is joined. Essential properties of a vector include the 1) capacity for autonomous replication within a host cell, 2) presence of at least one specific nucleotide sequence recognized by a *restriction endonuclease*, and 3) presence of at least one gene (such as an antibiotic resistance gene) that confers the ability to select for the vector. Commonly used vectors include plasmids and viruses.

1. **Prokaryotic plasmids:** Prokaryotic organisms typically contain single, large, circular chromosomes. In addition, most species of bacteria also normally contain small, circular, extrachromosomal DNA molecules called plasmids (Fig. 34.5). Plasmid DNA undergoes replication that may or may not be synchronized to chromosomal division. Plasmids may carry genes that convey antibiotic resistance to the host bacterium and may facilitate the transfer of genetic information from one bacterium to another. They can be readily isolated from bacterial cells, their circular DNA cleaved at specific sites by *restriction endonucleases*, and up to 15 kb (kilobases) of foreign DNA (cut with the same restriction enzyme) inserted. The recombinant plasmid vector can be introduced into a bacterium, producing large numbers of copies of the plasmid. The bacteria are grown in the presence of antibiotics, thus selecting for cells containing the hybrid plasmids, which provide antibiotic resistance (Fig. 34.6). Artificial plasmids are routinely constructed. An example is the classic pBR322 (see Fig. 34.5), which contains an origin of replication, two antibiotic resistance genes, and >40 unique restriction sites. Use of plasmids is limited by the size of the DNA that can be inserted.

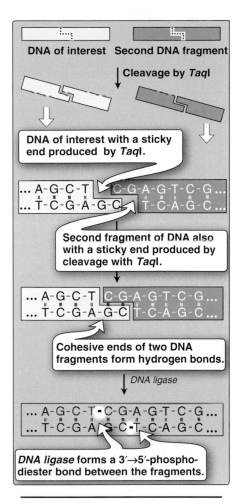

Figure 34.4
Formation of recombinant DNA from restriction fragments with sticky ends. A = adenine; C = cytosine; G = guanine; T = thymine.

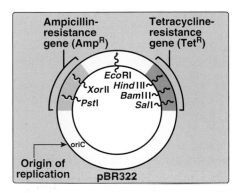

Figure 34.5
A partial map of pBR322 indicating the positions of its antibiotic resistance genes and 6 of the >40 unique sites recognized by specific *restriction endonucleases*. p = plasmid.

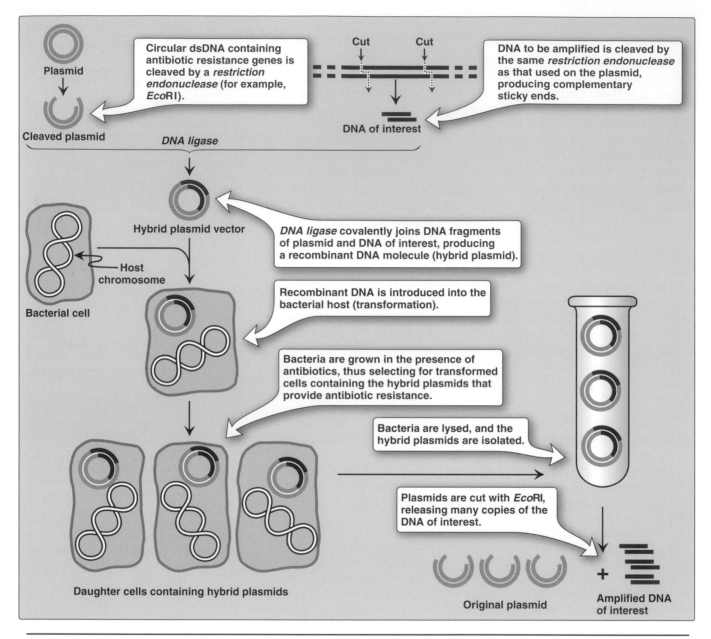

Figure 34.6

Summary of biologic gene cloning. [Note: Transformation is inefficient in that only a small percentage of the cells will contain the recombinant plasmid.] dsDNA = double-stranded DNA.

2. **Other vectors:** The development of improved vectors that can more efficiently accommodate larger DNA segments, or express the passenger genes in different cell types, has aided molecular genetics research and therapeutics. In addition to the prokaryotic plasmids described above, naturally occurring viruses that infect bacteria (bacteriophage λ, for example) or mammalian cells (retroviruses, for example), as well as artificial constructs such as cosmids and bacterial or yeast artificial chromosomes (BAC or YAC, respectively), are currently used as cloning vectors. [Note: BAC and YAC can accept DNA inserts of 100–300 kb and 250–1,000 kb, respectively.]

B. DNA libraries

A DNA library is a collection of cloned restriction fragments of the DNA of an organism. Two kinds of libraries are commonly used: genomic libraries and complementary DNA (cDNA) libraries. Genomic libraries ideally contain a copy of every DNA nucleotide sequence in the genome. In contrast, cDNA libraries contain those DNA sequences that only appear as processed messenger RNA (mRNA) molecules, and these differ according to cell type and environmental conditions. [Note: cDNA lacks introns and the control regions of the genes, whereas these are present in genomic DNA.]

1. **Genomic DNA libraries:** A genomic library is created by digestion of the total DNA of an organism with a *restriction endonuclease* and subsequent ligation to an appropriate vector. The recombinant DNA molecules replicate within host bacteria. Thus, the amplified DNA fragments collectively represent the entire genome of the organism and are called a genomic library. Regardless of the restriction enzyme used, the chances are good that the gene of interest contains more than one restriction site recognized by that enzyme. If this is the case, and if the digestion is allowed to go to completion, the gene of interest is fragmented (that is, it is not contained in any one clone in the library). To avoid this usually undesirable result, a partial digestion is performed in which either the amount or the time of action of the enzyme is limited. This results in cleavage occurring at only a fraction of the restriction sites on any one DNA molecule, thus producing fragments of ~20 kb. Enzymes that cut very frequently (that is, those that recognize 4-bp sequences) are generally used for this purpose so that the result is an almost random collection of fragments. This insures a high degree of probability that the gene of interest is contained, intact, in some fragment.

2. **Complementary DNA libraries:** If a protein-coding gene of interest is expressed at a high level in a particular tissue, the mRNA transcribed from that gene is likely also present at high concentrations in the cells of that tissue. For example, reticulocyte mRNA is composed largely of molecules that code for the α-globin and β-globin chains of hemoglobin A (HbA). This mRNA can be used as a template to make a cDNA molecule using the enzyme *reverse transcriptase* (Fig. 34.7). Therefore, the resulting cDNA is a double-stranded copy of mRNA. [Note: The template mRNA is isolated from transfer RNA and ribosomal RNA by the presence of its poly-A tail.] cDNA can be amplified by biologic cloning or by PCR. It can be used as a probe to locate the gene that encodes the original mRNA (or fragments of the gene) in mixtures containing many unrelated DNA fragments. If the mRNA used as a template is a mixture of many different size species, the resulting cDNA is heterogeneous. These mixtures can be cloned to form a cDNA library. Because cDNA has no introns, it can be cloned into an expression vector for the synthesis of eukaryotic proteins by bacteria (Fig. 34.8). These special plasmids contain a bacterial promoter for transcription of the cDNA and a Shine-Dalgarno (SD) sequence (see p. 454) that allows the bacterial ribosome to initiate translation of the resulting mRNA molecule. The cDNA is inserted

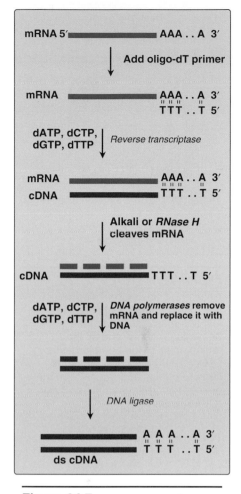

Figure 34.7
Synthesis of complementary DNA (cDNA) from messenger RNA (mRNA) using *reverse transcriptase*. Ligation of double-stranded (ds) DNA sequences containing a restriction site to each end allows biologic cloning of cDNA. [Note: DNA is resistant to alkaline hydrolysis.] dATP, dCTP, dGTP, dTTP = deoxyadenosine, deoxycytidine, deoxyguanosine, and deoxythymidine triphosphates.

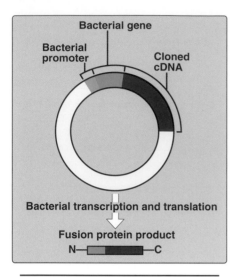

Figure 34.8
An expression vector. The product is a fusion protein that contains just some amino acids of the bacterial protein ■ and all the amino acids of the complementary DNA (cDNA)-encoded protein ■. [Note: Proteins are written from the amino (N)-terminus to the carboxy (C)-terminus.]

downstream of the promoter and within a gene for a protein that is expressed in the bacterium (for example, lacZ; see p. 466), such that the mRNA produced contains an SD sequence, a few codons for the bacterial protein, and all the codons for the eukaryotic protein. This allows for more efficient expression and results in the production of a fusion protein. [Note: Therapeutic human insulin is made in bacteria through this technology. However, the extensive co- and posttranslational modifications required for most other human proteins (for example, blood clotting factors) necessitates the use of eukaryotic, even mammalian, hosts.]

C. Sequencing cloned DNA fragments

The base sequence of DNA fragments that have been cloned can be determined. The original procedure for this purpose was the Sanger dideoxy chain termination method illustrated in Figure 34.9. In this method, the single-stranded DNA (ssDNA) to be sequenced is used as the template for DNA synthesis by *DNA polymerase* (*DNA pol*). A radiolabeled primer complementary to the 3′-end of the target DNA is added, along with the four deoxyribonucleoside triphosphates (dNTP). The sample is divided into four reaction tubes, and a small amount of one of the four dideoxyribonucleoside triphosphates (ddNTP) is added to each tube. Because it contains no 3′-hydroxyl group, incorporation of a ddNMP terminates elongation at that point. The products of this reaction, then, consist of a mixture of DNA strands of different lengths, each terminating at a specific base. Separation of the various DNA products by size in an electric field using polyacrylamide gel electrophoresis, followed by autoradiography, yields a pattern of bands from which the DNA base sequence can be read. [Note: The shorter the fragment, the farther it travels on the gel, with the shortest fragment representing that which was made first (that is, the 5′-end).] In place of a labeled primer, a mixture of the four ddNTP linked to different fluorescent dyes and in a single reaction tube is now commonly used. The mixture is separated by capillary electrophoresis, the fluorescent labels are detected, and a color readout of the sequence is generated (Fig. 34.10). [Note: The Human Genome Project used variations of this technique to sequence the human genome.] Advances in sequencing technology, so-called next generation, or high-throughput sequencing, now allow the rapid sequencing of an entire genome with increased fidelity and decreased cost through the simultaneous (parallel) sequencing of many DNA pieces. [Note: Sequencing of the exome, that portion of the genome that encodes proteins, is now possible.]

IV. PROBES

Cleavage of large DNA molecules by restriction enzymes produces an enormous array of fragments. How can the DNA sequence of interest be picked out of such a mixture? The answer lies in the use of a probe, a short piece of ssDNA or RNA, labeled with a radioisotope, such as ^{32}P, or with a nonradioactive molecule, such as biotin or a fluorescent dye. The sequence of a probe is complementary to a sequence in the DNA of interest, called the target DNA. Probes are used to identify which band on a gel or which clone in a library contains the target DNA, a process called screening.

A. Hybridization to DNA

The utility of probes hinges on the process of hybridization (or annealing) in which a probe containing a complementary sequence binds a single-stranded sequence of a target DNA. ssDNA, produced by alkaline denaturation of dsDNA, is first bound to a solid support, such as a nitrocellulose membrane. The immobilized DNA strands are prevented from self-annealing but are available for hybridization to the exogenous, radiolabeled, single-stranded probe. The extent of hybridization is measured by the retention of radioactivity on the membrane. Excess probe molecules that do not hybridize are removed by washing the membrane.

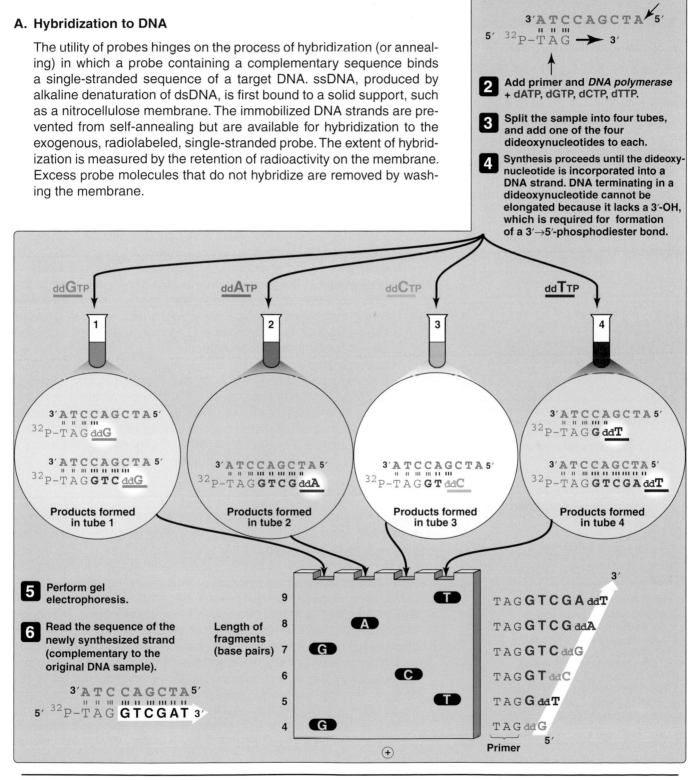

1 Single-stranded DNA of unknown sequence is used as a template.

2 Add primer and *DNA polymerase* + dATP, dGTP, dCTP, dTTP.

3 Split the sample into four tubes, and add one of the four dideoxynucleotides to each.

4 Synthesis proceeds until the dideoxynucleotide is incorporated into a DNA strand. DNA terminating in a dideoxynucleotide cannot be elongated because it lacks a 3′-OH, which is required for formation of a 3′→5′-phosphodiester bond.

5 Perform gel electrophoresis.

6 Read the sequence of the newly synthesized strand (complementary to the original DNA sample).

Figure 34.9

DNA sequencing by the Sanger dideoxy method. [Note: The original method utilized a radiolabeled primer. Fluorescent dye-labeled dideoxyribonucleoside triphosphates are now commonly used.] A = adenine; C = cytosine; G = guanine; T = thymine; d = deoxy; dd = dideoxy.

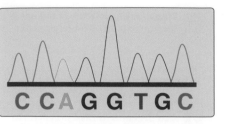

Figure 34.10
Color readout of a DNA sequence.

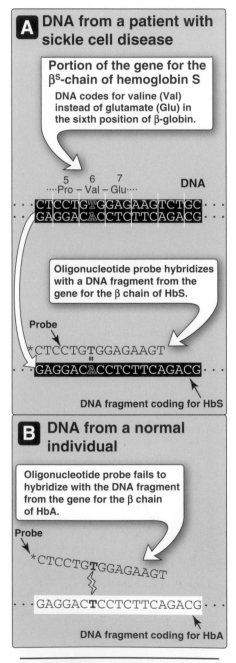

Figure 34.11
Allele-specific oligonucleotide probe detects hemoglobin (Hb) S allele. [Note: The * indicates ^{32}P radiolabel.]

B. Synthetic oligonucleotide probes

If the sequence of all or part of the target DNA is known, short, single-stranded oligonucleotide probes can be synthesized that are complementary to a small region of the gene of interest. If the sequence of the gene is unknown, the amino acid sequence of the protein, the final gene product, may be used to construct a nucleic acid probe using the genetic code as a guide. Because of the degeneracy of the genetic code (see p. 449), it is necessary to synthesize several oligonucleotides. [Note: Oligonucleotides can be used to detect single-base changes in the sequence to which they are complementary. In contrast, cDNA probes contain many thousands of bases, and their binding to a target DNA with a single-base change is unaffected.]

1. **Detecting the β^S-globin mutation:** A synthetic allele-specific oligonucleotide (ASO) probe can be used to detect the presence of the sickle cell mutation in the β-globin gene (Fig. 34.11). DNA, isolated from white blood cells (WBC) and amplified, is denatured and applied to a membrane. A radiolabeled oligonucleotide probe, complementary to the point mutation (GAG → GTG, glutamate → valine) at codon 6 in patients with the β^S gene, is applied to the membrane. DNA isolated from a heterozygous individual (sickle cell trait) or a homozygous patient (sickle cell anemia) contains a sequence that is complementary to the probe and a double-stranded hybrid form can be detected. In contrast, DNA obtained from normal individuals is not complementary at this position and, therefore, does not form a hybrid (see Fig. 34.11). Use of a pair of such ASO probes (one specific for the normal allele and one specific for the mutant allele) allows all three possible genotypes (homozygous normal, heterozygous, and homozygous mutant) to be distinguished (Fig. 34.12). [Note: ASO probes are useful only if the mutation and its location are known.]

C. Biotinylated probes

Because the disposal of radioactive waste is becoming increasingly expensive, nonradiolabeled probes have been developed. One of the most successful is based on the vitamin biotin (see p. 385), which can be chemically linked to the nucleotides used to synthesize the probe. Biotin was chosen because it binds very tenaciously to avidin, a readily available protein contained in chicken egg whites. Avidin can be attached to a fluorescent dye detectable optically with great sensitivity. Thus, a DNA fragment (displayed, for example, by gel electrophoresis) that hybridizes with the biotinylated probe can be made visible by immersing the gel in a solution of dye-coupled avidin. After washing away the excess avidin, the DNA fragment that binds the probe is fluorescent. [Note: Labeled probes can allow detection and localization of DNA or RNA sequences in cell or tissue preparations, a process called in situ hybridization (ISH). If the probe is fluorescent (F), the technique is called FISH.]

D. Antibodies

If no amino acid sequence information is available to guide the synthesis of a probe for direct detection of the DNA of interest, a gene can be identified indirectly by cloning cDNA in an expression vector that allows the cloned cDNA to be transcribed and translated. A labeled antibody is used to identify which bacterial colony produces the protein and, therefore, contains the cDNA of interest.

V. SOUTHERN BLOTTING

Southern blotting is a technique that combines the use of restriction enzymes, electrophoresis, and DNA probes to generate, separate, and detect pieces of DNA.

A. Procedure

This method, named after its inventor, Edward Southern, involves the following steps (Fig. 34.13). First, DNA is extracted from cells, for example, a patient's WBC. Second, the DNA is cleaved into many fragments using a restriction enzyme. Third, the resulting fragments (all of which are negatively charged) are separated on the basis of size by electrophoresis. [Note: Because the large fragments move more slowly than the smaller ones, the lengths of the fragments, usually expressed as the number of base pairs, can be calculated from comparison of the position of the band relative to standard fragments of known size.] The DNA fragments in the gel are denatured and transferred (blotted) to a nitrocellulose membrane for analysis. If the original DNA represents the individual's entire genome, the enzymic digest contains $\geq 10^6$ fragments. The gene of interest is on only one (or a few if the gene itself was fragmented) of these pieces of DNA. If all the DNA fragments were visualized by a nonspecific technique, they would appear as an unresolved blur of overlapping bands. To avoid this, the last step in Southern blotting uses a probe to identify the DNA fragments of interest. The patterns observed on Southern blot analysis depend both on the specific *restriction endonuclease* and on the probe used to visualize the restriction fragments. [Note: Variants of the Southern blot have been facetiously named northern if RNA is being studied (see p. 499) and western if protein is being studied (see p. 500), neither of which relates to anyone's name or to points of the compass.]

B. Mutation detection

Southern blotting can detect DNA mutations such as large insertions or deletions, trinucleotide repeat expansions, and rearrangements of nucleotides. It can also detect point mutations (replacement of one nucleotide by another; see p. 449) that cause the loss or gain of restriction sites. Such mutations cause the pattern of bands to differ from those seen with a normal gene. Longer fragments are generated if a restriction site is lost. For example, in Figure 34.13, person 2 lacks a restriction site present in person 1. Alternatively, the point mutation may create a new cleavage site with the production of shorter fragments. [Note: Most sequence differences at restriction sites are harmless variations in the DNA.]

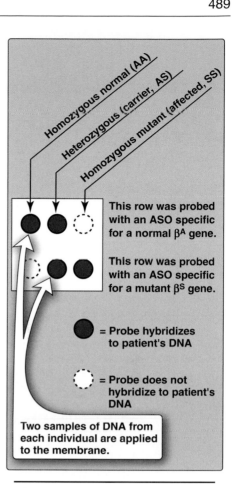

This row was probed with an ASO specific for a normal β^A gene.

This row was probed with an ASO specific for a mutant β^S gene.

● = Probe hybridizes to patient's DNA

◌ = Probe does not hybridize to patient's DNA

Two samples of DNA from each individual are applied to the membrane.

Figure 34.12
Allele-specific oligonucleotide (ASO) probes used to detect the sickle cell mutation and differentiate between sickle cell trait and disease.

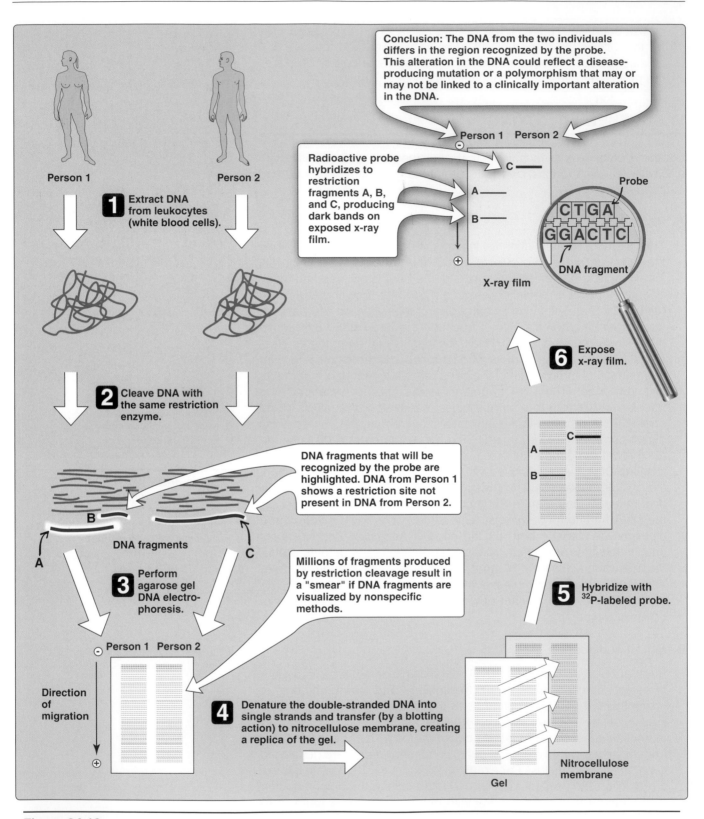

Figure 34.13
Southern blotting procedure. [Note: Nonradiolabeled probes are now commonly used.]

VI. RESTRICTION FRAGMENT LENGTH POLYMORPHISM

It has been estimated that the genomes of any two unrelated people are 99.5% identical. With 6 billion bp in the diploid human genome, that represents variation in ~30 million bp. These genome variations are the result of mutations that lead to polymorphisms. A polymorphism is a change in genotype that can result in no change in phenotype or a change in phenotype that is harmless, causes increased susceptibility to a disease, or, rarely, causes the disease. It is traditionally defined as a sequence variation at a given locus (allele) in >1% of a population. Polymorphisms primarily occur in the 98% of the genome that does not encode proteins (that is, in introns and intergenic regions). A restriction fragment length polymorphism (RFLP) is a genetic variant that can be observed by cleaving the DNA into fragments (restriction fragments) with a *restriction endonuclease*. The length of the restriction fragments is altered if the variant alters the DNA so as to create or abolish a restriction site. RFLP can be used to detect human genetic variations, for example, in prospective parents or in fetal tissue.

A. DNA variations resulting in RFLP

Two types of DNA variations commonly result in RFLP: single-base changes in the DNA sequence and tandem repeats of DNA sequences.

1. **Single-base changes:** About 90% of human genome variation comes in the form of single nucleotide polymorphisms (SNPs, pronounced "snips"), that is, variations that involve just one base (Fig. 34.14). The substitution of one nucleotide at a restriction site can render the site unrecognizable by a particular *restriction endonuclease*. A new restriction site can also be created by the same mechanism. In either case, cleavage with an *endonuclease* results in fragments of lengths that differ from the normal and can be detected by DNA hybridization (see Fig. 34.13). The altered restriction site can be either at the site of a disease-causing mutation (rare) or at a site some distance from the mutation. [Note: The HapMap, developed by The International Haplotype Map Project, is a catalog of common SNP in the human genome. The data are being used in genome-wide association studies (GWAS) to identify those alleles that affect health and disease.]

2. **Tandem repeats:** Polymorphisms in chromosomal DNA can also arise from the presence of a variable number of tandem repeats (VNTR), as shown in Figure 34.15. These are short sequences of DNA at scattered locations in the genome, repeated in tandem (one after another). The number of these repeat units varies from person to person but is unique for any given individual and, therefore, serves as a molecular "fingerprint." Cleavage by restriction enzymes yields fragments that vary in length depending on how many repeated segments are contained in the fragment (see Fig. 34.15). Many different VNTR loci have been identified and are extremely useful for DNA fingerprint analysis, such as in forensic and paternity cases. It is important to emphasize that

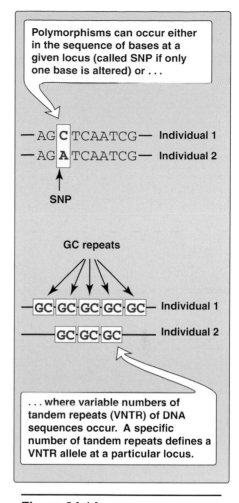

Figure 34.14
Common forms of genetic polymorphism. SNP = single nucleotide polymorphism; A = adenine; C = cytosine; G = guanine; T = thymine.

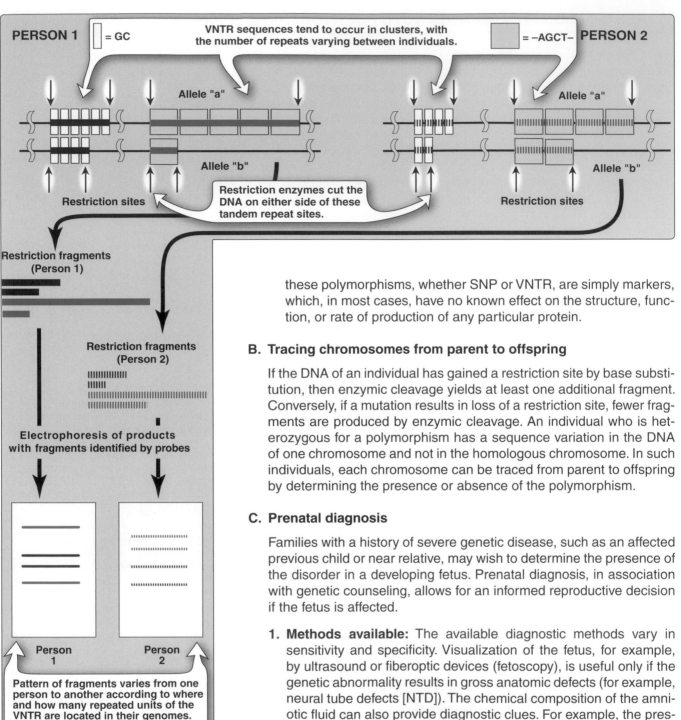

Figure 34.15
Restriction fragment length polymorphism of variable number tandem repeats (VNTR). For each person, a pair of homologous chromosomes is shown.

these polymorphisms, whether SNP or VNTR, are simply markers, which, in most cases, have no known effect on the structure, function, or rate of production of any particular protein.

B. Tracing chromosomes from parent to offspring

If the DNA of an individual has gained a restriction site by base substitution, then enzymic cleavage yields at least one additional fragment. Conversely, if a mutation results in loss of a restriction site, fewer fragments are produced by enzymic cleavage. An individual who is heterozygous for a polymorphism has a sequence variation in the DNA of one chromosome and not in the homologous chromosome. In such individuals, each chromosome can be traced from parent to offspring by determining the presence or absence of the polymorphism.

C. Prenatal diagnosis

Families with a history of severe genetic disease, such as an affected previous child or near relative, may wish to determine the presence of the disorder in a developing fetus. Prenatal diagnosis, in association with genetic counseling, allows for an informed reproductive decision if the fetus is affected.

1. **Methods available:** The available diagnostic methods vary in sensitivity and specificity. Visualization of the fetus, for example, by ultrasound or fiberoptic devices (fetoscopy), is useful only if the genetic abnormality results in gross anatomic defects (for example, neural tube defects [NTD]). The chemical composition of the amniotic fluid can also provide diagnostic clues. For example, the presence of high levels of α-fetoprotein is associated with NTD. Fetal cells obtained from amniotic fluid or from biopsy of the chorionic villi can be used for karyotyping, which assesses the morphology of metaphase chromosomes. Staining and cell sorting techniques permit the rapid identification of trisomies and translocations that produce an extra chromosome or chromosomes of abnormal lengths. However, molecular analysis of fetal DNA provides the most detailed genetic picture.

2. **DNA sources:** DNA may be obtained from blood cells, amniotic fluid, or chorionic villi (Fig. 34.16). For amniotic fluid, it was formerly necessary to grow cells in culture for 2–3 weeks in order to have sufficient DNA for analysis. The ability to amplify DNA by PCR has dramatically shortened the time needed for a DNA analysis.

3. **Direct diagnosis of sickle cell anemia using RFLP:** The genetic disorders of Hb are the most common genetic diseases in humans. In the case of sickle cell anemia (Fig. 34.17), the point mutation that gives rise to the disease (see p. 35) is actually one and the same mutation that gives rise to the polymorphism. However, direct detection by RFLP of diseases that result from point mutations is limited to only a few genetic diseases.

   a. **Early diagnostic efforts:** In the past, prenatal diagnosis of sickle cell anemia involved the determination of the amount and kinds of Hb synthesized in the nucleated red cells obtained from fetal blood. However, the invasive procedures to obtain fetal blood have a high mortality rate (~5%), and analysis cannot be carried out until late in the second trimester of pregnancy when HbA (and its HbS variant) begins to be produced.

   b. **RFLP analysis:** In sickle cell anemia, the sequence alteration caused by the point mutation abolishes the recognition site of the *restriction endonuclease Mst*II: CCTNAGG (where N is any nucleotide; see Fig. 34.17). Thus, the A-to-T mutation in codon 6 of the β^S-globin gene eliminates a cleavage site for the enzyme. Normal DNA digested with *Mst*II yields a 1.15-kb fragment, whereas a 1.35-kb fragment is generated from the β^S gene as a result of the loss of one *Mst*II cleavage site. Diagnostic techniques that allow analysis of fetal DNA from amniotic cells or chorionic villus sampling rather than fetal blood have proved valuable because they provide safe, early detection of sickle cell anemia as well as other genetic diseases. [Note: Genetic disorders caused by insertions or deletions between two restriction sites, rather than by the creation or loss of cleavage sites, will also display RFLP.]

4. **Indirect diagnosis of phenylketonuria using RFLP:** The gene for *phenylalanine hydroxylase (PAH)*, the enzyme deficient in phenylketonuria ([PKU] see p. 270), is located on chromosome 12. It spans ~90 kb of genomic DNA and contains 13 exons separated by introns (Fig. 34.18; see p. 442 for a description of exons and introns). Mutations in the *PAH* gene usually do not directly affect any *restriction endonuclease* recognition site. To establish a diagnostic protocol for PKU, DNA from family members of the affected individual must be analyzed. The goal is to identify genetic markers (RFLP) that are tightly linked to the disease trait. Once these markers are identified, RFLP analysis can be used to carry out prenatal diagnosis.

   a. **Mutant gene identification:** Determining the presence of the mutant gene by identifying the polymorphism marker can be done if two conditions are satisfied. First, if the polymorphism is closely linked to a disease-producing mutation, the defective

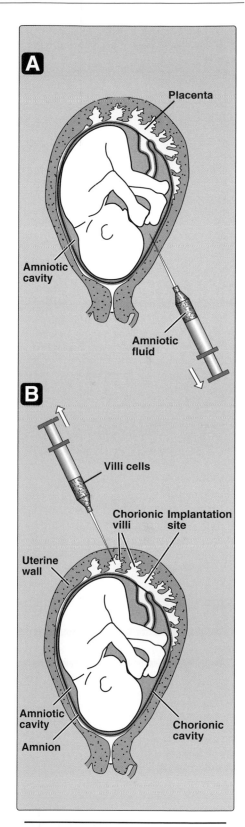

Figure 34.16
Sampling of fetal cells. A. Amniotic fluid. B. Chorionic villus.

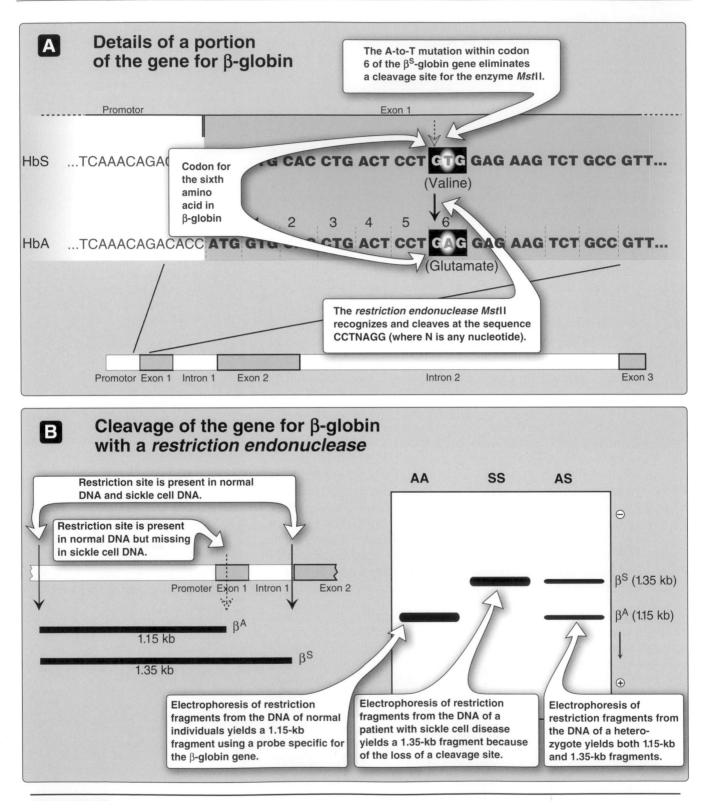

Figure 34.17
Detection of β^S-globin mutation. kb = kilobase (1 kb = 1,000 base pairs in double-stranded DNA); Hb = hemoglobin.

gene can be traced by detection of the RFLP. For example, if DNA from a family carrying a disease-causing gene is examined by restriction enzyme cleavage and Southern blotting, it is sometimes possible to find an RFLP that is consistently associated with that gene (that is, they show close linkage and are coinherited). It is then possible to trace the inheritance of the gene within a family without knowledge of the nature of the genetic defect or its precise location in the genome. [Note: The polymorphism may be known from the study of other families with the disorder or may be discovered to be unique in the family under investigation.] Second, for autosomal-recessive disorders, such as PKU, the presence of an affected individual in the family would aid in the diagnosis. This individual would have the mutation present on both chromosomes, allowing identification of the RFLP associated with the genetic disorder.

b. **RFLP analysis:** The presence of abnormal genes for *PAH* can be shown using DNA polymorphisms as markers to distinguish between normal and mutant genes. For example, Figure 34.19 shows a typical pattern obtained when DNA from members of an affected family is cleaved with an appropriate restriction enzyme and subjected to electrophoresis. The vertical arrows represent the cleavage sites for the restriction enzyme used. The presence of a polymorphic site creates fragment "b" in the autoradiogram (after hybridization with a labeled *PAH*-cDNA probe), whereas the absence of this site yields only fragment "a." Note that subject II-2 demonstrates that the polymorphism, as shown by the presence of fragment "b," is associated with the mutant gene. Therefore, in this particular family, the appearance of fragment "b" corresponds to the presence of a polymorphic site that marks the abnormal gene for *PAH*. The absence of fragment "b" corresponds to having only the normal gene. In Figure 34.19, examination of fetal DNA shows that the fetus inherited two abnormal genes from the parents and, therefore, has PKU.

c. **Value of DNA testing:** DNA-based testing is useful not only in determining if an unborn fetus is affected by PKU but also in detecting unaffected carriers of the mutated gene to aid in family planning. [Note: PKU is treatable by dietary restriction of phenylalanine. Early diagnosis and treatment are essential in preventing severe neurologic damage in affected individuals.]

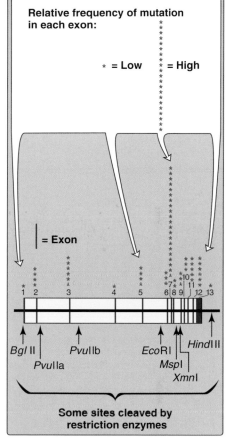

Figure 34.18
The gene for *phenylalanine hydroxylase* showing 13 exons, restriction sites, and some of the >500 mutations causing phenylketonuria.

VII. POLYMERASE CHAIN REACTION

PCR is an in vitro method for amplifying a selected DNA sequence that does not rely on the biologic (in vivo) cloning method described on p. 483. PCR permits the synthesis of millions of copies of a specific nucleotide sequence in a few hours. It can amplify the sequence, even when the targeted sequence makes up less than one part in a million of the total initial sample. The method can be used to amplify DNA sequences from any source, including viral, bacterial, plant, or animal. The steps in PCR are summarized in Figures 34.20 and 34.21.

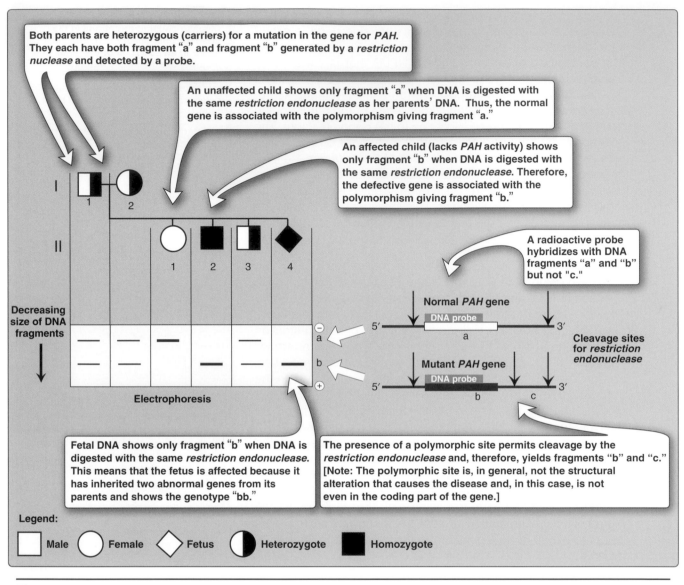

Figure 34.19
Analysis of restriction fragment length polymorphism in a family with a child affected by phenylketonuria (PKU), an autosomal-recessive disease. The molecular defect in the gene for *phenylalanine hydroxylase* (*PAH*) in the family is not known. The family wanted to know if the current pregnancy would be affected by PKU.

A. Procedure

PCR uses *DNA pol* to repetitively amplify targeted portions of genomic or cDNA. Each cycle of amplification doubles the amount of DNA in the sample, leading to an exponential increase (2^n, where n = cycle number) in DNA with repeated cycles of amplification. The amplified DNA products can then be separated by gel electrophoresis, detected by Southern blotting and hybridization, and sequenced.

1. **Constructing primer:** It is not necessary to know the nucleotide sequence of the target DNA in the PCR method. However, it is necessary to know the nucleotide sequence of short segments on each side of the target DNA. These stretches, called flanking sequences, bracket the DNA sequence of interest. The nucleotide

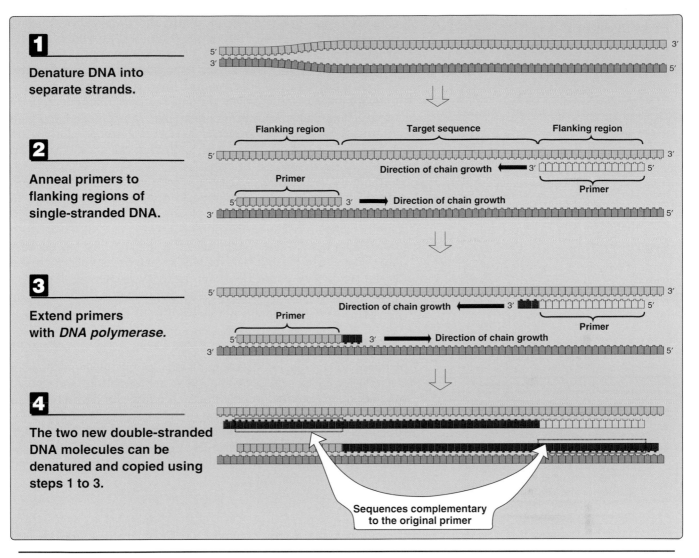

Figure 34.20
Steps (denature, anneal, extend) in one cycle of the polymerase chain reaction.

sequences of the flanking regions are used to construct two, single-stranded oligonucleotides, usually 20–35 nucleotides long, which are complementary to the respective flanking sequences. The 3′-hydroxyl end of each oligonucleotide points toward the target sequence (see Fig. 34.20). These synthetic oligonucleotides function as primers in PCR.

2. **Denaturing DNA:** The target DNA to be amplified is heated to ~95°C to separate the dsDNA into single strands.

3. **Annealing primers:** The separated strands are cooled to ~50°C and the two primers (one for each strand) anneal to a complementary sequence on the ssDNA.

4. **Extending primers:** *DNA pol* and dNTP (in excess) are added to the mixture (~72°C) to initiate the synthesis of two new strands complementary to the original DNA strands. *DNA pol* adds nucleotides to the 3′-hydroxyl end of the primer, and strand growth

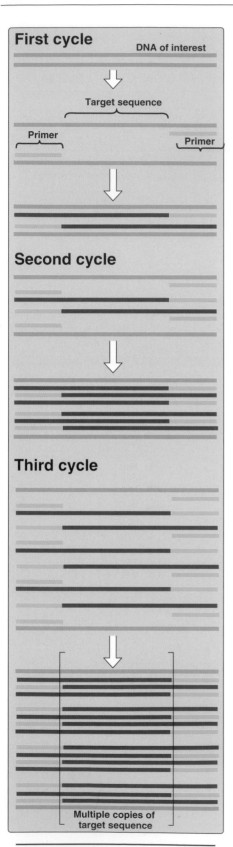

Figure 34.21
Multiple cycles of the polymerase chain reaction.

extends in the $5' \rightarrow 3'$ direction across the target DNA, making complementary copies of the target. [Note: PCR products can be several thousand base pairs long.] At the completion of one cycle of replication, the reaction mixture is heated again to separate the strands (of which there are now four). Each strand binds a complementary primer, and the step of primer extension is repeated. By using a heat-stable *DNA pol* (for example, *Taq* from the bacterium Thermus aquaticus that normally lives at high temperatures), the *polymerase* is not denatured and, therefore, does not have to be added at each successive cycle. However, *Taq* lacks proofreading activity. Typically, 20–30 cycles are run during this process, amplifying the DNA by a million-fold (2^{20}) to a billion-fold (2^{30}). [Note: Each extension product includes a sequence at its $5'$-end that is complementary to the primer (see Fig. 34.20). Thus, each newly synthesized strand can act as a template for the successive cycles (see Fig. 34.21). This leads to an exponential increase in the amount of target DNA with each cycle, hence, the name "polymerase chain reaction."] Probes can be made during PCR by adding labeled nucleotides to the last few cycles.

B. Advantages

The major advantages of PCR over biologic cloning as a mechanism for amplifying a specific DNA sequence are sensitivity and speed. DNA sequences present in only trace amounts can be amplified to become the predominant sequence. PCR is so sensitive that DNA sequences present in an individual cell can be amplified and studied. Isolating and amplifying a specific DNA sequence by PCR is faster and less technically difficult than traditional cloning methods using recombinant DNA techniques.

C. Applications

PCR has become a very common tool in research, forensics, and clinical diagnostics.

1. **Comparison of a normal gene to its mutant form:** PCR allows the synthesis of mutant DNA in sufficient quantities for a sequencing protocol without laborious biologic cloning of the DNA.

2. **Forensic analysis of DNA samples:** DNA fingerprinting by means of PCR has revolutionized the analysis of evidence from crime scenes. DNA isolated from a single human hair, a tiny spot of blood, or a sample of semen is sufficient to determine whether the sample comes from a specific individual. The DNA markers analyzed for such fingerprinting are most commonly a type of polymorphism known as short tandem repeats. These are very similar to the VNTR described previously (see p. 491) but are smaller in size. [Note: Paternity testing uses the same techniques.]

3. **Detection of low-abundance nucleic acid sequences:** Viruses that have a long latency period, such as human immunodeficiency virus (HIV), are difficult to detect at the early stage of infection using conventional methods. PCR offers a rapid and sensitive method for detecting viral DNA sequences even when only a small proportion of cells harbors the virus. [Note: Quantitative PCR (qPCR), also

known as real-time PCR, allows quantification of the amount (copy number) of the target nucleic acid after each cycle of amplification (that is, in real time) rather than at the end and is useful in determining viral load (the amount of virus).]

4. **Prenatal diagnosis and carrier detection of cystic fibrosis:** Cystic fibrosis is an autosomal-recessive genetic disease resulting from mutations in the gene for the cystic fibrosis transmembrane conductance regulator (CFTR) protein. The most common mutation is a three-base deletion that results in the loss of a phenylalanine residue from the CFTR protein (see p. 450). Because the mutant allele is three bases shorter than the normal allele, it is possible to distinguish them from each other by the size of the PCR products obtained by amplifying that portion of the DNA. Figure 34.22 illustrates how the results of such a PCR test can distinguish between homozygous normal, heterozygous (carriers), and homozygous mutant (affected) individuals.

|| The simultaneous amplification of multiple regions of a target DNA using multiple primer pairs is known as multiplex PCR. It allows detection of the loss of ≥1 exons in a gene with many exons such as the gene for CFTR, which has 27 exons.

VIII. GENE EXPRESSION ANALYSIS

The tools of biotechnology not only allow the study of gene structure, but also provide ways of analyzing the mRNA and protein products of gene expression.

A. Determining messenger RNA levels

mRNA levels are usually determined by the hybridization of labeled probes to either mRNA itself or to cDNA produced from mRNA. [Note: Amplification by PCR of cDNA made from mRNA by retroviral *reverse transcriptase* (*RT*) is referred to as RT-PCR.]

1. **Northern blots:** Northern blots are similar to Southern blots (see Fig. 34.13), except that the sample contains a mixture of mRNA molecules that are separated by electrophoresis, then transferred to a membrane and hybridized with a radiolabeled probe. The bands obtained by autoradiography give a measure of the amount and size of the mRNA molecules in the sample.

2. **Microarrays:** DNA microarrays contain thousands of immobilized ssDNA sequences organized in an area no larger than a microscope slide. These microarrays are used to analyze a sample for the presence of gene variations or mutations (genotyping) or to determine the patterns of mRNA production (gene expression analysis), analyzing thousands of genes at the same time. For genotyping analysis, the sample is from genomic DNA. For

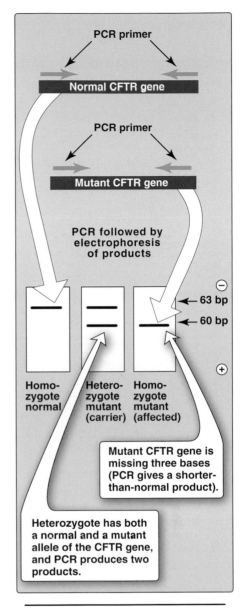

Figure 34.22
Genetic testing for cystic fibrosis (CF) using the polymerase chain reaction (PCR). [Note: CF is also diagnosed using allele-specific oligonucleotide analysis (see p. 488).] CFTR = cystic fibrosis transmembrane conductance regulator; bp = base pairs.

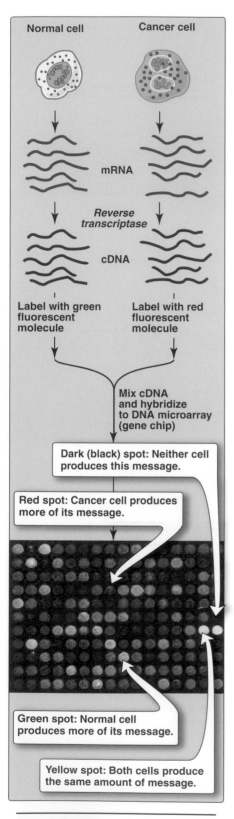

Figure 34.23

Microarray analysis of gene expression using DNA (gene) chips. [Note: Protein chips are also used.] mRNA = messenger RNA; cDNA = complementary DNA.

expression analysis, the population of mRNA molecules from a particular cell type is converted to cDNA and labeled with a fluorescent tag (Fig. 34.23). This mixture is then exposed to a gene (or, DNA) chip, which is a glass slide or membrane containing thousands of tiny spots of DNA, each corresponding to a different gene. The amount of fluorescence bound to each spot is a measure of the amount of that particular mRNA in the sample. DNA microarrays are used to determine the differing patterns of gene expression in two different types of cell (for example, normal and cancer cells; see Fig. 34.23). They can also be used to subclassify cancers, such as breast cancer, to optimize treatment. [Note: Microarrays involving proteins and the antibodies or other proteins that recognize them are being used to identify biomarkers to aid in the diagnosis, prognosis, and treatment of disease based on a patient's protein expression profile. Protein (and DNA) microarrays are important tools in the development of personalized (precision) medicine in which the treatment and/or prevention strategies consider the genetic, environmental, and lifestyle variations among individuals.]

B. Protein analysis

The kinds and amounts of proteins in cells do not always directly correspond to the amounts of mRNA present. Some mRNA are translated more efficiently than others, and some proteins undergo posttranslational modification. When analyzing the abundance and interactions of a large number of proteins, automated methods involving a variety of techniques, such as mass spectrometry and two-dimensional electrophoresis, are used. When investigating one, or a limited number of proteins, labeled antibodies (Ab) are used to detect and quantify specific proteins and to determine posttranslational modifications.

1. **Enzyme-linked immunosorbent assays:** These assays (known as ELISA) are performed in the wells of a microtiter dish. The antigen (protein) is bound to the plastic of the dish. The probe used consists of an Ab specific for the protein (such as troponin, see p. 66) to be measured. The Ab is covalently bound to an enzyme, which will produce a colored product when exposed to its substrate. The amount of color produced is proportional to the amount of Ab present and, indirectly, to the amount of protein in a test sample.

2. **Western blots:** Western blots (also called immunoblots) are similar to Southern blots, except that it is protein molecules in the sample that are separated by electrophoresis and blotted (transferred) to a membrane. The probe is a labeled Ab, which produces a band at the location of its antigen.

3. **Detecting exposure to human immunodeficiency virus:** ELISA and western blots are commonly used to detect exposure to HIV by measuring the amount of anti-HIV Ab present in a patient's blood sample. ELISA are used as the primary screening tool because they are very sensitive. Because these assays sometimes give false positives, however, western blots, which are more specific,

are often used as a confirmatory test (Fig. 34.24). [Note: ELISA and western blots can only detect HIV exposure after anti-HIV Ab appear in the bloodstream. PCR-based testing for HIV is more useful in the first few months after exposure.]

C. Proteomics

The study of the proteome, or all the proteins expressed by a genome, including their relative abundance, distribution, posttranslational modifications, functions, and interactions with other macromolecules, is known as proteomics. The 20,000–25,000 protein-coding genes of the human genome translate into well over 100,000 proteins when posttranscriptional and posttranslational modifications are considered. Although a genome remains essentially unchanged, the amounts and types of proteins in any particular cell change dramatically as genes are turned on and off. [Note: Proteomics (and genomics) required the parallel development of bioinformatics, the computer-based organization, storage, and analysis of biologic data.] Figure 34.25 compares some of the analytic techniques discussed in this chapter.

IX. GENE THERAPY

The goal of gene therapy is to treat disease through delivery of the normal, cloned DNA for a gene into the somatic cells of a patient who has a defect in that gene as a result of a disease-causing mutation. Because somatic gene therapy changes only the targeted somatic cells, the change is not passed on to the next generation. [Note: In germline gene therapy, the germ cells are modified, and so the change is passed on. A long-standing moratorium on germline gene therapy is in effect worldwide.] There are two types of gene transfer: 1) ex vivo, in which cells from the patient are removed, transduced, and returned, and 2) in vivo, in which the cells are directly transduced. Both types require use of a viral vector to deliver the DNA. Challenges of gene therapy include development of vectors, achievement of long-lived expression, and prevention of side effects such as an immune response. The first successful gene therapy involved two patients with severe combined immunodeficiency disease (SCID) caused by mutations to the gene for *adenosine deaminase* (*ADA*, see p. 301). It utilized mature T lymphocytes transduced ex vivo with a retroviral vector (Fig. 34.26). [Note: Human *ADA* cDNA is now used.] Since 1990, only a small number of patients (with a variety of disorders, such as hemophilia, cancers, and certain types of blindness) have been treated with gene therapy, with varying degrees of success.

Gene editing, as opposed to gene addition, allows a mutated gene to be repaired. Combinations of DNA-binding molecules (proteins or RNA) and *endonucleases* are used to identify and cleave the mutated sequence. Cleavage activates homologous recombination repair of dsDNA breaks (see p. 429) that integrates DNA containing the correct sequence into the gene. [Note: An *endonuclease* guided to a specific DNA sequence by a custom-designed RNA has been used in gene editing in human cell lines. The technique is based on (and named for) the prokaryotic CRISPR-*Cas9* (clustered regularly interspaced short palindromic repeats [CRISPR]-associated protein) system that identifies and cleaves foreign DNA in bacterial cells. CRISPR is currently used in the laboratory but not in the clinic.]

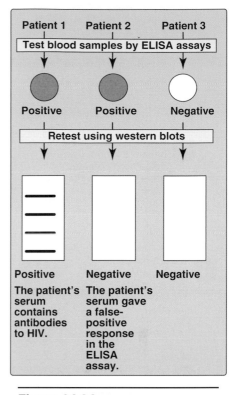

Figure 34.24
Testing for human immunodeficiency virus (HIV) exposure by enzyme-linked immunosorbent assays (ELISA) and western blots.

TECHNIQUE	SAMPLE ANALYZED
Southern blot	DNA
Northern blot	RNA
Western blot	Protein
ASO	DNA
Microarray	cDNA or genomic DNA
	Protein
ELISA	Protein

Figure 34.25
Techniques used to analyze DNA, RNA, and proteins. [Note: The three blotting techniques involve the use of a gel.] ASO = allele-specific oligonucleotides. ELISA = enzyme-linked immunosorbent assay; cDNA = complementary DNA.

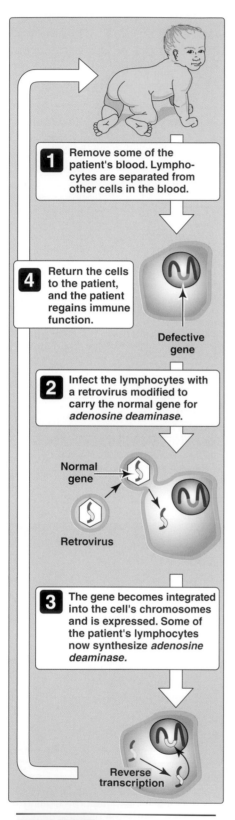

1 Remove some of the patient's blood. Lymphocytes are separated from other cells in the blood.

4 Return the cells to the patient, and the patient regains immune function.

Defective gene

2 Infect the lymphocytes with a retrovirus modified to carry the normal gene for *adenosine deaminase*.

Normal gene

Retrovirus

3 The gene becomes integrated into the cell's chromosomes and is expressed. Some of the patient's lymphocytes now synthesize *adenosine deaminase*.

Reverse transcription

Figure 34.26

Gene therapy for severe combined immunodeficiency disease caused by *adenosine deaminase* deficiency. [Note: Bone marrow stem cells and a modified retroviral vector are now used.]

X. TRANSGENIC ANIMALS

Transgenic animals can be produced by injecting a cloned foreign gene (a transgene) into a fertilized egg. If the gene randomly and stably integrates into a chromosome, it will be present in the germline of the resulting animal and can be passed from generation to generation. A giant mouse called "Supermouse" was produced in this way by injecting the gene for rat growth hormone into a fertilized mouse egg. [Note: Transgenic animals have been designed that produce therapeutic human proteins in their milk, a process called "pharming." Antithrombin, an anticlotting protein (see online Chapter 35), was produced by transgenic goats and approved for clinical use in 2009.] If the functional transgene undergoes targeted (not random) insertion, a knockin (KI) mouse that expresses the gene is created. Targeted insertion of a nonfunctional version of the transgene creates a knockout (KO) mouse that does not express the gene. Such genetically engineered animals can serve as models for the study of a corresponding human disease.

XI. CHAPTER SUMMARY

Restriction endonucleases are bacterial enzymes that cleave double-stranded DNA (dsDNA) into smaller fragments. Each enzyme cleaves at a specific 4–8 base-pair sequence (a restriction site), producing DNA segments called **restriction fragments**. The sequences that are recognized are **palindromic**. Restriction enzymes form either **staggered cuts (sticky ends)** or **blunt-end cuts** on the DNA. Bacterial ***DNA ligases*** can join two DNA fragments from different sources if they have been cut by the same *restriction endonuclease*. This hybrid combination of two fragments is called a **recombinant DNA molecule**. Introduction of a foreign DNA molecule into a replicating cell permits the **amplification** (production of many copies) of the DNA, a process called **cloning**. A **vector** is a molecule of DNA to which the fragment of DNA to be cloned is joined. Vectors must be capable of **autonomous replication** within the host cell, must contain at least one specific nucleotide sequence recognized by a *restriction endonuclease*, and must carry at least one gene that confers the ability to select for the vector such as an **antibiotic resistance gene**. Prokaryotic organisms normally contain small, circular, extrachromosomal DNA molecules called **plasmids** that can serve as vectors. They can be readily isolated from the bacterium (or artificially constructed), joined with the DNA of interest, and reintroduced into the bacterium, which will replicate, thus making multiple copies of the **hybrid** plasmid. A **DNA library** is a collection of cloned restriction fragments of the DNA of an organism. A **genomic library** is a collection of fragments of dsDNA obtained by digestion of the total DNA of the organism with a *restriction endonuclease* and subsequent ligation to an appropriate vector. It ideally contains a copy of every DNA nucleotide sequence in the genome. In contrast, **complementary DNA (cDNA) libraries** contain only those DNA sequences that are complementary to **processed messenger RNA (mRNA)** molecules present in a cell and differ according to cell type and environmental conditions. Because cDNA has no introns, it can be cloned into an **expression vector** for the synthesis of human proteins by bacteria or eukaryotes. Cloned, then purified, fragments of DNA can be sequenced, for example, using the **Sanger dideoxy chain termination method**. A **probe** is a small piece of RNA or single-stranded DNA (usually labeled with a radioisotope, such as ^{32}P, or another identifiable compound, such as biotin or a fluorescent dye) that has a nucleotide sequence complementary to the DNA molecule of interest (target DNA). Probes can be used to identify which clone of a library or which band on a gel contains the target DNA. **Southern blotting** is a technique that can be used to detect specific sequences present in DNA. The DNA is cleaved using a *restriction endonuclease*, after which the pieces are separated by **gel electrophoresis** and are denatured and transferred (blotted) to a **nitrocellulose membrane** for analysis. The fragment of interest is detected using a probe. The human genome contains many thousands of **polymorphisms** (DNA sequence variations at a given locus). Polymorphisms can arise from single-base changes and from tandem repeats. A polymorphism can serve as a genetic marker that can be followed through families. A **restriction fragment length polymorphism** (**RFLP**) is a genetic variant that can be observed by cleaving the DNA into restriction fragments using a restriction enzyme. A base substitution in one or more nucleotides at a restriction site can render the site unrecognizable by a particular *restriction endonuclease*. A new restriction site also can be created by the same mechanism. In either case, cleavage with the *endonuclease* results in fragments of lengths differing from the normal that can be detected by **hybridization** with a probe. **RFLP analysis** can be used to diagnose genetic diseases early in the gestation of a fetus. The **polymerase chain reaction** (**PCR**), another method for **amplifying** a selected DNA sequence, does not rely on the biologic cloning method. PCR permits the synthesis of millions of copies of a specific nucleotide sequence in a few hours. It can amplify the sequence, even when the targeted sequence makes up less than one part in a million of the total initial sample. The method can be used to amplify DNA sequences from any source. Applications of the PCR technique include 1) efficient comparison of a normal gene with a mutant form of the gene, 2) forensic analysis of DNA samples, 3) detection of low-abundance nucleic acid sequences, and 4) prenatal diagnosis and carrier detection (for example, of cystic fibrosis). The products of gene expression (mRNA and proteins) can be measured by techniques such as **northern blots**, which are like Southern blots except that the sample contains a mixture of **mRNA** molecules that are separated by electrophoresis, then hybridized to a radiolabeled probe; **microarrays** are used to determine the differing patterns of gene expression in two different types of cells (for example, normal and cancer cells); **enzyme-linked immunosorbent assays** (**ELISA**); and **western blots** (**immunoblots**) are used to detect specific proteins. **Proteomics** is the study of all the proteins expressed by a genome. The goal of **gene therapy** is the insertion of a normal cloned gene to replace a defective gene in a **somatic cell**, whereas the goal of **gene editing** is the repair of a mutated gene. Insertion of a foreign gene (transgene) into the germline of an animal creates a **transgenic animal** that can produce therapeutic proteins or serve as gene **knockin** or **knockout** models for human diseases.

Study Questions

Choose the ONE best answer.

34.1 HindIII is a restriction endonuclease. Which of the following is most likely to be the recognition sequence for this enzyme?

    A. AAGAAG
    B. AAGAGA
    C. AAGCTT
    D. AAGGAA
    E. AAGTTC

Correct answer = C. The vast majority of restriction endonucleases recognize palindromes in double-stranded DNA, and AAGCTT is the only palindrome among the choices. Because the sequence of only one DNA strand is given, the base sequence of the complementary strand must be determined. To be a palindrome, both strands must have the same sequence when read in the $5'\rightarrow3'$ direction. Thus, the complement of 5'-AAGCTT-3' is also 5'-AAGCTT-3'.

34.2 An Ashkenazi Jewish couple has their 6-month-old son evaluated for listlessness, poor head control, and a fixed gaze. Tay-Sachs disease, an autosomal-recessive disease of lipid degradation, is diagnosed. The couple also has a daughter. The family's pedigree is shown to the right, along with Southern blots of a restriction fragment length polymorphism very closely linked to the gene for hexosaminidase A, which is defective in Tay-Sachs disease. Which of the statements below is most accurate with respect to the daughter?

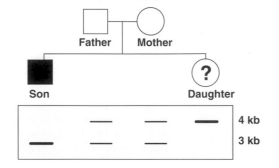

A. She has a 25% chance of having Tay-Sachs disease.
B. She has a 50% chance of having Tay-Sachs disease.
C. She has Tay-Sachs disease.
D. She is a carrier for Tay-Sachs disease.
E. She is homozygous normal.

Correct answer = E. Because they have an affected son, both the biological father and mother must be carriers for this disease. The affected son must have inherited a mutant allele from each parent. Because he shows only the 3-kilobase (kb) band on the Southern blot, the mutant allele for this disease must be linked to the 3-kb band. The normal allele must be linked to the 4-kb band, and because the daughter inherited only the 4-kb band, she must be homozygous normal for the hexosaminidase A gene.

34.3 A physician would like to determine the global patterns of gene expression in two different types of tumor cells in order to develop the most appropriate form of chemotherapy for each patient. Which of the following techniques would be most appropriate for this purpose?

A. Enzyme-linked immunosorbent assay
B. Microarray
C. Northern blot
D. Southern blot
E. Western blot

Correct answer = B. Microarray analysis allows the determination of messenger RNA (mRNA) production (gene expression) from thousands of genes at once. A northern blot only measures mRNA production from one gene at a time. Western blots and enzyme-linked immunosorbent assay measure protein production (also gene expression) but only from one gene at a time. Southern blots are used to analyze DNA, not the products of DNA expression.

34.4 A 2-week-old infant is diagnosed with a urea cycle defect. Enzymic analysis showed no activity for ornithine transcarbamoylase (OTC), an enzyme of the cycle. Molecular analysis revealed that the messenger RNA (mRNA) product of the gene for OTC was identical to that of a control. Which of the techniques listed below was most likely used to analyze mRNA?

A. Dideoxy chain termination
B. Northern blot
C. Polymerase chain reaction
D. Southern blot
E. Western blot

Correct answer = B. Northern blot allows analysis of the messenger RNA present (expressed) in a particular cell or tissue. Southern blot is used for DNA analysis, whereas western blot is used for protein analysis. Dideoxy chain termination is used to sequence DNA. Polymerase chain reaction is used to generate multiple, identical copies of a DNA sequence in vitro.

34.5 For the patient above, which phase of the central dogma was most likely affected?

Correct answer = Translation. The gene is present and is able to be expressed as evidenced by normal production of messenger RNA. The lack of enzymic activity means that some aspect of protein synthesis is affected.

APPENDIX
Clinical Cases

I. INTEGRATIVE CASES

Metabolic pathways, initially presented in isolation, are, in fact, linked to form an interconnected network. The following four integrative case studies illustrate how a perturbation in one process can result in perturbations in other processes of the network.

CASE 1: CHEST PAIN

Patient Presentation: BJ, a 35-year-old man with severe substernal chest pain of ~2 hours' duration, is brought by ambulance to his local hospital at 5 AM. The pain is accompanied by dyspnea (shortness of breath), diaphoresis (sweating), and nausea.

Focused History: BJ reports episodes of exertional chest pain in the last few months, but they were less severe and of short duration. He smokes (2–3 packs per day), drinks alcohol only rarely, eats a "typical" diet, and walks with his wife most weekends. His blood pressure has been normal. Family history reveals that his father and paternal aunt died of heart disease at age 45 and 39 years, respectively. His mother and younger (age 31 years) brother are said to be in good health.

Physical Examination (Pertinent Findings): BJ is pale and clammy and is in distress due to chest pain. Blood pressure and respiratory rate are elevated. Lipid deposits are noted on the periphery of his corneas (corneal arcus; see left image) and under the skin on and around his eyelids (xanthelasmas; see right image). No deposits on his tendons (xanthomas) are detected.

Corneal arcus   **Xanthelasmas**

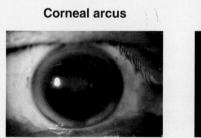
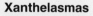
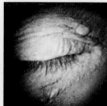

Pertinent Test Results: BJ's electrocardiogram is consistent with a myocardial infarction (MI). Angiography reveals areas of severe stenosis (narrowing) of several coronary arteries. Initial results from the clinical laboratory include the following:

	Patient	Reference Range
Troponin	+	0
Total cholesterol	365 mg/dl (**H**)	<200
Low-density lipoprotein (LDL)-cholesterol	304 mg/dl (**H**)	<130
High-density lipoprotein (HDL)-cholesterol	38 mg/dl (**L**)	>45
Triglycerides (triacylglycerols)	115 mg/dl	<150

H = High; **L** = Low. [Note: BJ had not eaten for ~8 hours prior to the blood draw.]

Diagnosis: MI, the irreversible necrosis (death) of heart muscle secondary to ischemia (decreased blood supply), is caused by the occlusion (blockage) of a blood vessel most commonly by a blood clot (thrombus). BJ subsequently is determined to have heterozygous familial hypercholesterolemia (FH), also known as type IIa hyperlipidemia.

Immediate Treatment: BJ is given O_2, a vasodilator, pain medication, and drugs to dissolve blood clots (thrombolytics) and reduce clotting (antithrombotics).

Long-Term Treatment: Lipid-lowering drugs (for example, high-potency statins, bile acid [BA] sequestrants, and niacin); daily aspirin; β-blockers; and counseling on nutrition, exercise, and smoking cessation would be part of the long-term treatment plan.

Prognosis: Patients with heterozygous FH have ~50% of the normal number of functional LDL receptors and a hypercholesterolemia (two to three times normal) that puts them at high risk (>50% risk) for premature coronary heart disease (CHD). However, <5% of patients with hypercholesterolemia have FH.

Nutrition Nugget: Dietary recommendations for individuals with heterozygous FH include limiting saturated fats to <7% of total calories and cholesterol to <200 mg/day, substituting unsaturated fats for saturated fats, and adding soluble fiber (10–20 g/day) and plant sterols (2 g/day) for their hypocholesterolemic effects. Fiber increases BA excretion. This results in increased hepatic uptake of cholesterol-rich LDL to supply the substrate for BA synthesis. Plant sterols decrease cholesterol absorption in the intestine.	**Genetics Gem:** FH is caused by hundreds of different mutations in the gene for the LDL receptor (on chromosome 19) that affect receptor amount and/or function. FH is an autosomal-dominant disease in which homozygotes are more seriously affected than heterozygotes. Heterozygous FH has an incidence of ~1:500 in the general population. It is associated with increased risk of cardiovascular disease. Genetic screening of the first-degree relatives of BJ would identify affected individuals for treatment.

REVIEW QUESTIONS: Choose the ONE best answer.

RQ1. Triacylglycerols are glycerol-based lipids. Which of the following is also a glycerol-based lipid?

    A. Ganglioside GM_2

    B. Phosphatidylcholine

    C. Prostaglandin PGI_2

    D. Sphingomyelin

    E. Vitamin D

RQ2. Statins are of benefit to patients with hypercholesterolemia because they:

    A. decrease a rate-limiting and regulated step of de novo cholesterol biosynthesis by inhibiting hydroxymethylglutaryl coenzyme A (HMG CoA) reductase.

    B. decrease expression of the gene for the LDL receptor by preventing the movement of the sterol regulatory element–binding protein-2 (SREBP-2) in complex with SREBP cleavage–activating protein (SCAP) from the membrane of the endoplasmic reticulum to the membrane of the Golgi.

    C. increase the oxidation of cholesterol to $CO_2 + H_2O$.

    D. interfere with the absorption of bile salts in the enterohepatic circulation, thereby causing the liver to take up cholesterol from the blood for use in BA synthesis.

    E. reduce cholesterol by increasing steroid hormone and vitamin D synthesis.

RQ3. Statins are competitive inhibitors of HMG CoA reductase. Which of the following statements about competitive inhibitors is correct?

    A. Competitive inhibitors are examples of irreversible inhibitors.

    B. Competitive inhibitors increase both the apparent Michaelis constant (K_m) and the apparent maximal velocity (V_{max}).

    C. Competitive inhibitors increase the apparent K_m and have no effect on the V_{max}.

    D. Competitive inhibitors decrease both the apparent K_m and the apparent V_{max}.

    E. Competitive inhibitors have no effect on the K_m and decrease the apparent V_{max}.

RQ4. In an MI, a blood clot forms as a result of injury to a blood vessel that leads to production of a platelet plug and a fibrin meshwork. The clot occludes the blood vessel, preventing blood flow and, therefore, delivery of O_2. Destruction of the clot (thrombolysis) restores blood flow. Which one of the following is an example of a thrombolytic agent?

    A. Activated protein C complex

    B. Antithrombin III

    C. Aspirin

    D. Factor XIII

    E. Heparin

    F. Tissue plasminogen activator

    G. Vitamin K

    H. Warfarin

RQ5. Decreased tissue perfusion results in hypoxia (decreased O_2 availability). Relative to normoxia, in hypoxia the:

    A. electron transport chain will be upregulated to provide protons for ATP synthesis.

    B. ratio of the oxidized form of nicotinamide adenine dinucleotide (NAD^+) to the reduced form (NADH) will increase.

    C. pyruvate dehydrogenase complex will be active.

    D. process of substrate-level phosphorylation will be increased in the cytosol.

    E. tricarboxylic acid cycle will be upregulated to provide the reducing equivalents needed for oxidative phosphorylation to occur.

RQ6. Genetic screening of BJ's first-degree relatives would be accomplished by mutation analysis via polymerase chain reaction–based amplification followed by automated sequencing of the promoter region and the 18 exons of the LDL receptor gene. This process would involve the:

    A. generation and use of complementary DNA (cDNA).

    B. initiation of DNA synthesis with dideoxynucleotides.

    C. isolation of genomic DNA from germ cells.

    D. use of fluorescently labeled nucleotides.

THOUGHT QUESTIONS

TQ1. Relative to an individual with familial defective LDL receptors, what would be the expected phenotype in an individual with familial defective apolipoprotein B-100? With apolipoprotein E-2, the isoform that only poorly binds its receptor?

TQ2. Why was aspirin prescribed? **Hint:** What pathway of lipid metabolism is affected by aspirin?

TQ3. Heart muscle normally uses aerobic metabolism to meet its energy needs. However, in hypoxia, anaerobic glycolysis is increased. What allosteric activator of glycolysis is responsible for this effect? With hypoxia, what will be the end product of glycolysis?

TQ4. One of the reasons for encouraging smoking cessation and exercise for BJ is that these changes raise the level of HDL, and elevated HDL reduces the risk for CHD. How does a rise in HDL reduce the risk for CHD?

CASE 2: SEVERE FASTING HYPOGLYCEMIA

Patient Presentation: JS is a 4-month-old boy whose mother is concerned about the "twitching" movements he makes just before feedings. She tells the pediatrician that the movements started ~1 week ago, are most apparent in the morning, and disappear shortly after eating.

Focused History: JS is the product of a normal pregnancy and delivery. He appeared normal at birth. On his growth charts, he has been at the 30th percentile for both weight and length since birth. His immunizations are up to date. JS last ate a few hours ago.

Physical Examination (Pertinent Findings): JS appears sleepy and feels clammy to the touch. His respiratory rate is elevated. His temperature is normal. JS has a protuberant, firm abdomen that appears to be nontender. His liver is palpable 4 cm below the right costal margin and is smooth. His kidneys are enlarged and symmetrical.

Pertinent Test Results:

	Patient	Pediatric Reference Range
Glucose	50 mg/dl (**L**)	60–105
Lactate	3.4 mmol/l (**H**)	0.6–3.2
Urate	5.6 mg/dl (**H**)	2.4–5.4
Total cholesterol	220 mg/dl (**H**)	<170
Triglycerides (triacylglycerols)	280 mg/dl (**H**)	<90
pH	7.30 (**L**)	7.35–7.45
HCO_3^-	12 mEq/l (**L**)	19–25

H = High; **L** = Low.

JS is sent to the regional children's hospital for further evaluation. Ultrasound studies confirm hepatomegaly and renomegaly and show no evidence of tumors. A liver biopsy is performed. The hepatocytes are distended. Staining reveals large amounts of lipid (primarily triacylglycerol) and carbohydrate. Liver glycogen is elevated in amount and normal in structure. Enzyme assay using liver homogenate treated with detergent reveals <10% of the normal activity of *glucose 6-phosphatase*, an enzyme of the endoplasmic reticular (ER) membrane in the liver and the kidneys.

Diagnosis: JS has *glucose 6-phosphatase* deficiency (glycogen storage disease [GSD] type Ia, von Gierke disease).

Treatment (Immediate): JS was given glucose intravenously, and his blood glucose level rose into the normal range. However, as the day progressed, it fell to well below normal. Administration of glucagon had no effect on blood glucose levels but increased blood lactate. JS's blood glucose levels were able to be maintained by constant infusion of glucose.

Prognosis: Individuals with *glucose 6-phosphatase* deficiency develop hepatic adenomas starting in the second decade of life and are at increased risk for hepatic carcinoma. Kidney glomerular function is impaired and can result in kidney failure. Patients are at increased risk for developing gout, but this rarely occurs before puberty.

Nutrition Nugget Long-term medical nutrition therapy for JS is designed to maintain his blood glucose levels in the normal range. Frequent (every 2–3 hours) daytime feedings rich in carbohydrate (provided by uncooked cornstarch that is slowly hydrolyzed) and nighttime nasogastric infusion (pump assisted) of glucose are advised. Avoidance of fructose and galactose is recommended because they are metabolized to glycolytic intermediates and lactate, which can exacerbate the metabolic problems. Calcium and vitamin D supplements are prescribed.

Genetics Gem GSD Ia is an autosomal-recessive disorder caused by >100 known mutations to the gene for *glucose 6-phosphatase* located on chromosome 17. It has an incidence of 1:100,000 and accounts for ~25% of all cases of GSD in the United States. It is one of the few genetic causes of hypoglycemia in newborns. GSD Ia is not routinely screened for in newborns. [Note: Deficiency of the translocase that moves glucose 6-phosphate into the ER is the cause of GSD Ib. Hypoglycemia and neutropenia are seen.]

REVIEW QUESTIONS: Choose the ONE best answer.

RQ1. JS is hypoglycemic because:

A. free (nonphosphorylated) glucose cannot be produced from either glycogenolysis or gluconeogenesis as a result of the deficiency in glucose 6-phosphatase.

B. glycogen phosphorylase is dephosphorylated and inactive, and glycogen cannot be degraded.

C. hormone-sensitive lipase is dephosphorylated and inactive, and fatty acid substrates for gluconeogenesis cannot be generated.

D. the decrease in the insulin/glucagon ratio upregulates glucose transporters in the liver and kidneys, resulting in increased uptake of blood glucose.

RQ2. JS was prescribed calcium supplements because chronic acidosis can cause bone demineralization, resulting in osteopenia. Vitamin D (1,25-diOH-D₃) was also prescribed because vitamin D:

A. binds G_q protein–coupled membrane receptors and causes a rise in inositol trisphosphate with release of calcium from intracellular stores.

B. cannot be synthesized by humans and, therefore, must be supplied in the diet.

C. is a fat-soluble vitamin that increases intestinal absorption of calcium.

D. is the coenzyme-prosthetic group for calbindin, a calcium transporter in the intestine.

RQ3. The hepatomegaly and renomegaly seen in JS are primarily the result of an increase in the amount of glycogen stored in these organs. What is the basis for glycogen accumulation in these organs?

    A. Glycolysis is downregulated, which pushes glucose to glycogenesis.

    B. Increased oxidation of fatty acids spares glucose for glycogenesis.

    C. Glucose 6-phosphate is an allosteric activator of glycogen synthase b.

    D. The rise in the insulin/glucagon ratio favors glycogenesis.

RQ4. Glucose 6-phosphatase is an integral protein of the ER membrane. Which of the following statements about such proteins is correct?

    A. If glycosylated, the carbohydrate is on the portion of the protein that extends into the cytosol.

    B. They are synthesized on ribosomes that are free in the cytosol.

    C. The membrane-spanning domain consists of hydrophilic amino acids.

    D. The initial targeting signal is an amino terminal hydrophobic signal sequence.

THOUGHT QUESTIONS

TQ1. What is the likely reason for JS's twitching movements?

TQ2. Why was the liver homogenate treated with detergent? **Hint:** Think about where the enzyme is located.

TQ3. Why is JS's blood glucose level unaffected by glucagon? **Hint:** What is the role of glucagon in normal individuals who experience a drop in blood glucose?

TQ4. Why are urate and lactate elevated in a disorder of glycogen metabolism? **Hint:** It is the result of a decrease in inorganic phosphate (P_i), but why is P_i decreased?

TQ5. A. Why are triacylglycerols and cholesterol elevated? **Hint:** Glucose is the primary carbon source for their synthesis.

    B. Why are ketone bodies not elevated?

CASE 3: HYPERGLYCEMIA AND HYPERKETONEMIA

Patient Presentation: MW, a 40-year-old woman, was brought to the hospital in a disoriented, confused state by her husband.

Focused History: As noted on her medical alert bracelet, MW has had type 1 diabetes (T1D) for the last 24 years. Her husband reports that this is her first medical emergency in 2 years.

Physical Examination (Pertinent Findings): MW displayed signs of dehydration (such as dry mucous membranes and skin, poor skin turgor, and low blood pressure) and acidosis (such as deep, rapid breathing [Kussmaul respiration]). Her breath had a faintly fruity odor. Her temperature was normal.

Pertinent Test Results: Rapid, bedside tests were strongly positive for glucose and acetoacetate and negative for protein. Results on blood tests performed by the clinical laboratory are shown below:

	Patient	Reference Range
Glucose	414 mg/dl (23 mmol/l) (**H**)	70–99 (3.9–5.5)
Blood urea nitrogen	8 mmol/l (**H**)	2.5–6.4
3-Hydroxybutyrate	350 mg/dl (**H**)	0–3
HCO_3^-	12 mmol/l (**L**)	22–28
Na^+	136 mmol/l	138–150
K^+	5.3 mmol/l	3.5–5.0
Cl^-	102 mmol/l	95–105
pH	7.1 (**L**)	7.35–7.45

H = High; **L** = Low.

Microscopic examination of her urine revealed a urinary tract infection (UTI).

Diagnosis: MW is in diabetic ketoacidosis (DKA) that was precipitated by a UTI. [Note: Diabetes increases the risk for infections such as UTI.]

Immediate Treatment: MW was rehydrated with normal saline given intravenously (IV). She also was given insulin IV. Blood glucose, ketone bodies, and electrolytes were measured periodically. Antibiotic treatment of her UTI was started.

Long-Term Treatment: Diabetes increases the risk for macrovascular complications (such as coronary artery disease and stroke) and microvascular complications (such as retinopathy, nephropathy, and neuropathy). Ongoing monitoring for these complications will be continued.

Prognosis: Diabetes is the seventh leading cause of death by disease in the United States. Individuals with diabetes have a reduced life expectancy relative to those without diabetes.

Nutrition Nugget Monitoring total intake of carbohydrates is primary in blood glucose control. Carbohydrates should come from whole grains, vegetables, legumes, and fruits. Low-fat dairy products and nuts and fish rich in ω-3 fatty acids are encouraged. Intake of saturated and trans fats should be minimized.	**Genetics Gem** Autoimmune destruction of pancreatic β cells is characteristic of T1D. Of the genetic loci that confer risk for T1D, the human-leukocyte antigen (HLA) region on chromosome 6 has the strongest association. The majority of genes in the HLA region are involved in the immune response.

REVIEW QUESTIONS: Choose the ONE best answer.

RQ1. Which of the following statements concerning T1D is correct?

    A. Diagnosis can be made by measuring the level of glucose or glycated hemoglobin (HbA_{1c}) in the blood.

    B. During periods of physiologic stress, the urine of an individual with T1D would likely test negative for reducing sugars.

    C. T1D is associated with obesity and a sedentary lifestyle.

    D. The characteristic metabolic abnormalities seen in T1D result from insensitivity to both insulin and glucagon.

    E. Treatment with exogenous insulin allows normalization of blood glucose (euglycemia).

RQ2. DKA occurs when the rate of ketone body production is greater than the rate of utilization. Which of the following statements concerning ketone body metabolism is correct? Ketone bodies:

    A. are made in mitochondria from acetyl coenzyme A (CoA) primarily produced by the oxidation of glucose.

    B. are utilized by many tissues, particularly the liver, after conversion to acetyl CoA.

    C. include acetoacetate, which can impart a fruity odor to the breath.

    D. require albumin for transport through the blood.

    E. utilized in energy metabolism are organic acids that can add to the proton load of the body.

RQ3. Adipose lipolysis followed by β-oxidation of the fatty acid (FA) products is required for the generation of ketone bodies. Which of the following statements concerning the generation and use of FA is correct?

    A. Mitochondrial β-oxidation of FA is inhibited by malonyl CoA.

    B. Production of FA from adipose lipolysis is upregulated by insulin.

    C. The acetyl CoA product of FA β-oxidation favors the use of pyruvate for gluconeogenesis by activating the pyruvate dehydrogenase complex.

    D. The β-oxidation of FA utilizes reducing equivalents generated by gluconeogenesis.

    E. The FA produced by lipolysis are taken up by the brain and oxidized for energy.

THOUGHT QUESTIONS

TQ1. At admission, MW was hypoinsulinemic, and she was given insulin. Why did MW's hypoinsulinemia result in hyperglycemia? **Hint:** What is the role of insulin in glucose metabolism?

TQ2. Why is there glucose in MW's urine (glucosuria)? How is the glucosuria related to her dehydrated state?

TQ3. Why is the majority of the acetyl CoA from FA β-oxidation being used for ketogenesis rather than being oxidized in the tricarboxylic acid cycle?

TQ4. Was MW in positive or negative nitrogen balance when she was brought to the hospital?

TQ5. What response to the DKA is apparent in MW? What response is likely occurring in the kidney? **Hint:** In addition to conversion to urea, how is toxic ammonia removed from the body?

TQ6. What would be true about the levels of ketone bodies and glucose during periods of physiologic stress in individuals with impaired FA oxidation?

CASE 4: HYPOGLYCEMIA, HYPERKETONEMIA, AND LIVER DYSFUNCTION

Patient Presentation: AK, a 59-year-old male with slurred speech, ataxia (loss of skeletal muscle coordination), and abdominal pain, was dropped off at the Emergency Department (ED).

Focused History: AK is known to the ED staff from previous visits. He has a 6-year history of chronic, excessive alcohol consumption. He is not known to take illicit drugs. At this ED visit, AK reports that he has been drinking heavily in the past day or so. He cannot recall having eaten anything in that time. There is evidence of recent vomiting, but no blood is apparent.

Physical Examination (Pertinent Findings): The physical examination was remarkable for AK's emaciated appearance. (His body mass index was later determined to be 17.5, which put him in the underweight category.) His facial cheeks were erythematous (red in color) due to dilated blood vessels in the skin (telangiectasia). Eye movement was normal. Neither icterus (jaundice) nor edema (swelling due to fluid retention) was seen. The liver was slightly enlarged. Bedside tests revealed hypoglycemia and hyperketonemia (as acetoacetate). Blood was drawn and sent to the clinical laboratory.

Pertinent Test Results:

	Patient	Reference Range
Ethanol	180 mg/dl (**H**)	(>80 considered positive for DUI)
Glucose	58 mg/dl (**L**)	70–99
Lactate	23 mg/dl (**H**)	5–15
Uric acid	7.0 mg/dl	2.5–8.0
3-Hydroxybutyrate	50 mg/dl (**H**)	0–3.0
Total bilirubin	1.5 mg/dl (**H**)	0.3–1.0
Direct (conjugated) bilirubin	0.5 mg/dl (**H**)	0.1–0.3
Albumin	3.0 g/dl (**L**)	3.5–5.8
Aspartate transaminase (AST)	130 U/l (**H**)	0–35
Alanine transaminase (ALT)	75 U/l (**H**)	0–35
Prothrombin time	15.5 s (**H**)	11.0–13.2

DUI = driving under the influence; **H** = High; **L** = Low.

Additional Tests: Complete blood count (CBC) and blood smear revealed a macrocytic anemia (see right image). Folate and B_{12} levels were ordered.

Diagnosis: AK is diagnosed with alcoholism.

Treatment (Immediate): Thiamine and glucose were given intravenously.

Prognosis: Alcoholism (alcohol dependence) is the third most common cause of preventable death in the United States. People with alcoholism are at increased risk for liver cirrhosis, pancreatitis, gastrointestinal bleeding, and some cancers.

Normocytic red blood cells   Macrocytic red blood cells

Nutrition Nugget Those with alcoholism are at risk for vitamin deficiencies as a result of decreased intake and absorption. Thiamine (vitamin B₁) deficiency is common and can have serious consequences such as Wernicke-Korsakoff syndrome with its neurologic effects. Thiamine pyrophosphate (TPP), the coenzyme form, is required for the *dehydrogenase*-mediated oxidation of α-keto acids (such as pyruvate) as well as the transfer of two-carbon ketol groups by *transketolase* in the reversible sugar interconversions in the pentose phosphate pathway.

Genetics Gem Acetaldehyde, the product of ethanol oxidation by the hepatic, cytosolic, nicotinamide adenine dinucleotide (NAD^+)-requiring enzyme *alcohol dehydrogenase* (*ADH*), is oxidized to acetate by the mitochondrial, NAD^+-requiring *aldehyde dehydrogenase* (*ALDH2*). The majority of individuals of East Asian (but not European or African) heritage have a single nucleotide polymorphism (SNP) that renders *ALDH2* essentially inactive. This results in aldehyde-induced facial flushing and mild to moderate intoxication after consumption of small amounts of ethanol.

REVIEW QUESTIONS: Choose the ONE best answer.

RQ1. Many of the metabolic consequences of chronic excessive alcohol consumption seen in AK are the result of an increase in the ratio of reduced nicotinamide adenine dinucleotide (NADH) to its oxidized form (NAD$^+$) in both the cytoplasm and mitochondria. Which of the following statements concerning the effects of the rise in mitochondrial NADH is correct?

A. Fatty acid oxidation is increased.

B. Gluconeogenesis is increased.

C. Lipolysis is inhibited.

D. The tricarboxylic acid cycle is inhibited.

E. The reduction of malate to oxaloacetate in the malate–aspartate shuttle is increased.

RQ2. Ethanol can also be oxidized by cytochrome P450 (CYP) enzymes, and CYP2E1 is an important example. CYP2E1, which is ethanol inducible, generates reactive oxygen species (ROS) in its metabolism of ethanol. Which of the following statements concerning the CYP proteins is correct?

A. CYP proteins are heme-containing dioxygenases.

B. CYP proteins of the inner mitochondrial membrane are involved in detoxification reactions.

C. CYP proteins of the smooth endoplasmic reticular membrane are involved in the synthesis of steroid hormones, bile acids, and calcitriol.

D. ROS such as hydrogen peroxide generated by CYP2E1 can be oxidized by glutathione peroxidase.

E. The pentose phosphate pathway is an important source of the nicotinamide adenine dinucleotide phosphate (NADPH) that provides the reducing equivalents needed for activity of CYP proteins and the regeneration of functional glutathione.

RQ3. Alcohol is known to modulate the levels of serotonin in the central nervous system, where the monoamine functions as a neurotransmitter. Which of the following statements about serotonin is correct? Serotonin is:

A. associated with anxiety and depression.

B. degraded via methylation by monoamine oxidase, which also degrades the catecholamines.

C. released by activated platelets.

D. synthesized from tyrosine in a two-step process that utilizes a tetrahydrobiopterin-requiring hydroxylase and a pyridoxal phosphate–requiring carboxylase.

RQ4. Chronic, excessive consumption of alcohol is a leading cause of acute pancreatitis, a painful inflammatory condition that results from autodigestion of the gland by premature activation of pancreatic enzymes. Which of the following statements concerning the pancreas is correct?

A. Autodigestion of the pancreas would be expected to result in a decrease in pancreatic proteins in the blood.

B. In individuals who progress from acute to chronic pancreatitis, with the characteristic structural changes that result in decreased pancreatic function, diabetes and steatorrhea are expected findings.

C. In response to secretin, the exocrine pancreas secretes protons to lower the pH in the intestinal lumen.

D. Pancreatitis may also be seen in individuals with hypercholesterolemia.

THOUGHT QUESTIONS

TQ1. A. What effect does the rise in cytosolic NADH seen with ethanol metabolism have on glycolysis? **Hint:** What coenzyme is required in glycolysis?

B. How does this relate to the fatty liver (hepatic steatosis) commonly seen in alcohol-dependent individuals?

TQ2. Why might individuals with a history of gouty attacks be advised to reduce their consumption of ethanol?

TQ3. Why might prothrombin time be affected in alcohol-dependent individuals?

TQ4. Folate and vitamin B$_{12}$ deficiencies cause a macrocytic anemia that may be seen in those with alcoholism. Why is it advisable to measure vitamin B$_{12}$ levels before supplementing with folate in an individual with macrocytic anemia?

II. INTEGRATIVE CASE ANSWERS

CASE 1: Answers to Review Questions

RQ1. Answer = B. Phosphatidylcholine is a glycerol-based phospholipid derived from diacylglycerol phosphate (phosphatidic acid) and cytidine diphosphate-choline. Gangliosides are derived from ceramides, lipids with a sphingosine backbone. Prostaglandins of the 2 series (such as PGI$_2$) are derived from the 20-carbon polyunsaturated fatty acid arachidonic acid. Sphingomyelin is a sphingophospholipid derived from ceramide. Vitamin D is derived from an intermediate in the biosynthetic pathway for the sterol cholesterol.

RQ2. Answer = A. Statins inhibit hydroxymethylglutaryl coenzyme A (HMG CoA) reductase, thereby preventing the nicotinamide adenine dinucleotide phosphate (NADPH)-dependent reduction of HMG CoA to mevalonate and decreasing cholesterol biosynthesis (see figure below). The decrease in cholesterol content caused by statins results in movement of the sterol regulatory element–binding protein-2 (SREBP-2) in complex with SREBP cleavage–activating protein (SCAP) from the endoplasmic reticular membrane to the Golgi membrane. SREBP-2 is cleaved, generating a transcription factor that moves to the nucleus and binds to the sterol regulatory element upstream of the genes for HMG CoA reductase and the low-density lipoprotein (LDL) receptor, increasing their expression. Humans are unable to degrade the steroid nucleus to CO_2 + H_2O. Bile acid (BA) sequestrants, such as cholestyramine, prevent the absorption of bile salts by the liver, thereby increasing their excretion. The liver then takes up cholesterol via the LDL receptor and uses it to make BA, thereby reducing blood cholesterol levels. Steroid hormones are synthesized from cholesterol, and vitamin D is synthesized in skin from an intermediate (7-dehydrocholesterol) in the cholesterol biosynthetic pathway. Therefore, inhibition of cholesterol synthesis would be expected to decrease their production as well.

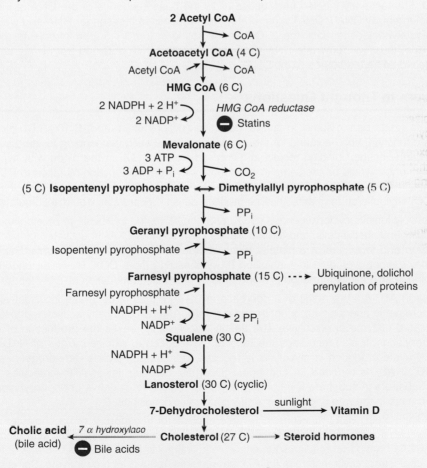

RQ3. Answer = C. Competitive inhibitors bind to the same site as the substrate (S) and prevent the S from binding. This results in an increase in the apparent K_m (Michaelis constant, or that S concentration that gives one half of the maximal velocity [V_{max}]). However, because the inhibition can be reversed by adding additional substrate, the V_{max} is unchanged (see figure at right). It is noncompetitive inhibitors that decrease the apparent V_{max} and have no effect on K_m.

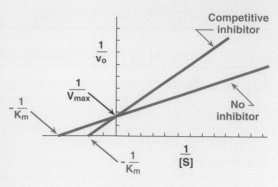

RQ4. Answer = F. Tissue plasminogen activator (TPA) converts plasminogen to plasmin that degrades fibrin (fibrinolysis), thereby degrading the clot (thrombolysis). Aspirin, an inhibitor of cyclooxygenase, is an antiplatelet drug. Antithrombin III (ATIII) removes thrombin from the blood, and its action is potentiated by heparin. Activated protein C (APC) complex cleaves the accessory proteins factor (F)Va and FVIIIa. ATIII and APC are involved in anticoagulation. FXIII is a transglutaminase that crosslinks the fibrin meshwork. Vitamin K is a fat-soluble vitamin required for the γ-carboxylation of FII, FVII, FIX, and FX. Warfarin prevents regeneration of the functional, reduced form of vitamin K.

RQ5. Answer = D. In hypoxia, substrate-level phosphorylation in glycolysis provides ATP. Oxidative phosphorylation is inhibited by the lack of O_2. Because the rate of ATP synthesis by oxidative phosphorylation controls the rate of cellular respiration, electron transport is inhibited. The resulting rise in the ratio of the reduced form of nicotinamide adenine dinucleotide (NADH) to the oxidized form (NAD^+) inhibits the tricarboxylic acid cycle and the pyruvate dehydrogenase complex.

RQ6. Answer = D. Fluorescently labeled nucleotides allow the base sequence of the DNA of interest to be determined. Complementary DNA (cDNA) is generated from processed messenger RNA and would not contain the promoter. Dideoxynucleotides lack the 3′-OH needed to form the 3′→5′-phosphodiester bond that joins the nucleotides and, thus, will terminate DNA synthesis. Genomic DNA obtained from white cells isolated from a blood sample would be the source of the DNA.

CASE 1: Answers to Thought Questions

TQ1. The phenotype would be the same. In familial defective apolipoprotein (apo) B-100, LDL receptors are normal in number and function, but the ligand for the receptor is altered such that binding to the receptor is decreased. Decreased ligand–receptor binding results in increased levels of LDL in the blood with hypercholesterolemia. [Note: The phenotype would be the same in individuals with a gain-of-function mutation to PCSK9, the protease that decreases recycling of the LDL receptor, thereby increasing its degradation.] With the apo E-2 isoform, cholesterol-rich chylomicron remnants and intermediate-density lipoproteins would accumulate in blood.

TQ2. Aspirin irreversibly inhibits cyclooxygenase (COX) and, therefore, the synthesis of prostaglandins (PG), such as PGI_2 in vascular endothelial cells, and thromboxanes (TX), such as TXA_2 in activated platelets. TXA_2 promotes vasoconstriction and formation of a platelet plug, whereas PGI_2 inhibits these events. Because platelets are anucleate, they cannot overcome this inhibition by synthesizing more COX. However, endothelial cells have a nucleus. Aspirin, then, inhibits formation of blood clots by preventing production of TXA_2 for the life of the platelet.

TQ3. The decrease in ATP (as the result of a decrease in O_2 and, thus, a decrease in oxidative phosphorylation) causes an increase in adenosine monophosphate (AMP). AMP allosterically activates phosphofructokinase-1, the key regulated enzyme of glycolysis. The rise in glycolysis increases the production of ATP by substrate-level phosphorylation. It also increases the ratio of the reduced to oxidized forms of NAD. Under anaerobic conditions, pyruvate produced in glycolysis is reduced to lactate by lactate dehydrogenase as NADH is oxidized to NAD^+. NAD^+ is required for continued glycolysis. Because fewer ATP molecules are produced per molecule of substrate in substrate-level phosphorylation relative to oxidative phosphorylation, there is a compensatory increase in the rate of glycolysis under anaerobic conditions.

TQ4. High-density lipoprotein (HDL) functions in reverse cholesterol transport. It takes cholesterol from nonhepatic (peripheral) tissues (for example, the endothelial layer of arteries) and brings it to the liver (see figure on the next page). The ABCA1 transporter mediates the efflux of cholesterol to HDL. The cholesterol is esterified by extracellular lecithin–cholesterol acyltransferase (LCAT) that requires apo A-1 as a coenzyme. Some cholesteryl ester is transferred to very-low-density lipoproteins (VLDL) by cholesteryl ester transfer protein (CETP) in exchange for triacylglycerol. The remainder is taken up by a scavenger receptor (SR-B1) on the surface of hepatocytes. The liver can use the cholesterol from HDL in the synthesis of bile acids. Removal of cholesterol from endothelial cells prevents its accumulation (as cholesterol or cholesteryl ester), decreasing the risk of heart disease. [Note: In contrast, LDL carries cholesterol from the liver to peripheral tissues or back to the liver.]

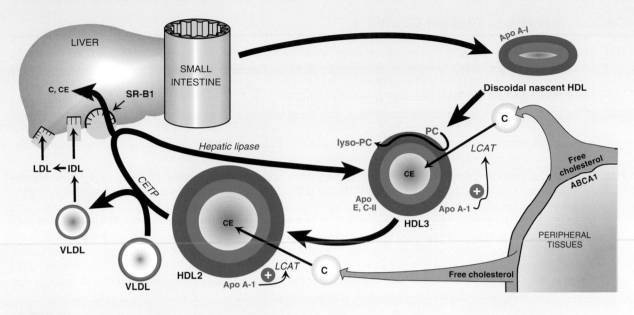

CASE 2: Answers to Review Questions

RQ1. Answer = A. Deficiency of glucose 6-phosphatase prevents the glucose 6-phosphate generated by glycogenolysis and gluconeogenesis from being dephosphorylated and released into the blood (see figure below). Blood glucose levels fall, and a severe, fasting hypoglycemia results. [Note: JS's symptoms appeared only recently because, at age 4 months, his feedings are less frequent.] Hypoglycemia stimulates release of glucagon, which leads to phosphorylation and activation of glycogen phosphorylase kinase that phosphorylates and activates glycogen phosphorylase. Epinephrine is also released and leads to phosphorylation and activation of hormone-sensitive lipase. However, typical fatty acids (FA) cannot serve as substrates for gluconeogenesis. The glucose transporters in the liver and kidneys are insulin insensitive.

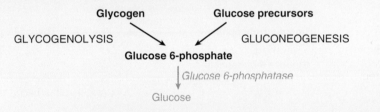

RQ2. Answer = C. Vitamin D is a fat-soluble vitamin that functions as a steroid hormone. In complex with its intracellular nuclear receptor, it increases transcription of the gene for calbindin, a calcium (Ca^{2+}) transporter protein in the intestine (see figure at right). Vitamin D does not bind to a membrane receptor and does not produce second messengers. It can be synthesized in the skin by the action of ultraviolet light on an intermediate of cholesterol synthesis, 7-dehydrocholesterol. Of the fat-soluble vitamins (A, D, E, and K), only K functions as a coenzyme.

RQ3. Answer = C. Glucose 6-phosphate is a positive allosteric effector of the covalently inhibited (phosphorylated) glycogen synthase b. With the rise in glucose 6-phosphate, glycogen synthesis is activated, and glycogen stores are increased in both the liver and the kidneys. The increased availability of glucose 6-phosphate also drives glycolysis. The increase in glycolysis provides substrates for lipogenesis, thereby increasing synthesis of FA and triacylglycerols (TAG). In hypoglycemia, the insulin/glucagon ratio is low, not high.

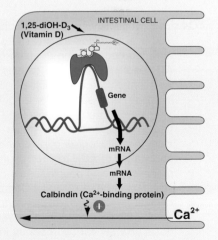

RQ4. Answer = D. Membrane proteins are initially targeted to the endoplasmic reticulum (ER) by an amino terminal hydrophobic signal sequence. Glycosylation is the most common posttranslational modification found in proteins. The glycosylated portion of membrane proteins is found on the extracellular face of the membrane. The membrane-spanning domain consists of ~22 hydrophobic amino acids. Proteins destined for secretion or for membranes, the ER lumen, Golgi, or lysosomes are synthesized on ribosomes associated with the ER.

CASE 2: Answers to Thought Questions

TQ1. The twitching is the result of the adrenergic response to hypoglycemia and is mediated by the rise in epinephrine. The adrenergic response includes tremor and sweating. Neuroglycopenia (impaired delivery of glucose to the brain) results in impairment of brain function that can lead to seizures, coma, and death. Neuroglycopenic symptoms develop if the hyperglycemia persists.

TQ2. Detergents are amphipathic molecules (that is, they have both hydrophilic [polar] and hydrophobic [nonpolar] regions). Detergents solubilize membranes, thereby disrupting membrane structure. If the problem were the translocase needed to move the glucose 6-phosphate substrate into the ER, rather than the phosphatase, disruption of the ER membrane would allow the substrate access to the phosphatase.

TQ3. Glucagon, a peptide hormone released from pancreatic α cells in hypoglycemia, binds its plasma membrane G protein–coupled receptor on hepatocytes. The α_s subunit of the associated trimeric G protein is activated (guanosine diphosphate is replaced by guanosine triphosphate), separates from the β and γ subunits, and activates adenylyl cyclase that generates cyclic adenosine monophosphate (cAMP) from ATP. cAMP activates protein kinase A (PKA) that phosphorylates and activates glycogen phosphorylase kinase, which phosphorylates and activates glycogen phosphorylase. The phosphorylase degrades glycogen, generating glucose 1-phosphate that is converted to glucose 6-phosphate. With glucose 6-phosphatase deficiency, the degradative process stops here (see figure below). Consequently, administration of glucagon is unable to cause a rise in blood glucose. [Note: Epinephrine would be similarly ineffective.]

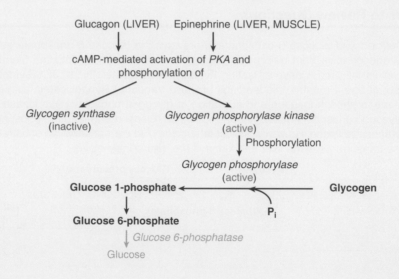

TQ4. The availability of inorganic phosphate (P_i) is decreased because it is trapped as phosphorylated glycolytic intermediates as a result of the upregulation of glycolysis by the rise in glucose 6-phosphate. Urate is elevated because the trapping of P_i decreases the ability to phosphorylate adenosine diphosphate (ADP) to ATP, and the fall in ATP causes a rise in adenosine monophosphate (AMP). The AMP is degraded to urate. Additionally, the availability of glucose 6-phosphate drives the pentose phosphate pathway, resulting in a rise in ribose 5-phosphate (from ribulose 5-phosphate) and, consequently, a rise in purine synthesis. Nicotinamide adenine dinucleotide phosphate (NADPH) also rises. Purines made beyond need are degraded to urate (see figure on the next page). [Note: The decrease in P_i reduces the activity of glycogen phosphorylase, resulting in increased storage of glycogen with a normal structure.] Lactate is elevated because the decrease in phosphorylation of ADP to ATP results in a decrease in cellular respiration (respiratory control) as a result of these processes being coupled. As a consequence, reduced nicotinamide adenine dinucleotide (NADH) from glycolysis cannot be oxidized by Complex I of the electron transport chain. Instead, it is oxidized by cytosolic lactate dehydrogenase with its coenzyme NADH as pyruvate is reduced to lactate. [Note: Pyruvate is increased as a result of the increase in glycolysis.] The lactate ionizes, releasing protons (H^+) and leading to a metabolic acidosis (low pH caused here by increased production of acid). Respiratory compensation causes an increased respiratory rate.

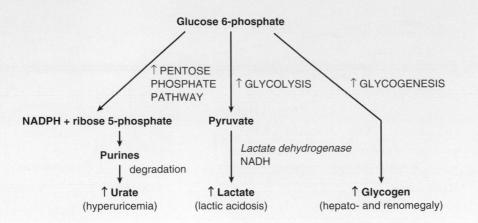

TQ5. Increased glycolysis results in increased availability of glycerol 3-phosphate for hepatic TAG synthesis. Additionally, some of the pyruvate generated in glycolysis will be oxidatively decarboxylated to acetyl coenzyme A (CoA). However, the tricarboxylic acid cycle is inhibited by the rise in NADH, and the acetyl CoA is transported to the cytosol as citrate. The rise of acetyl CoA in the cytosol results in increased fatty acid (FA) synthesis. Recall that citrate is an allosteric activator of acetyl CoA carboxylase (ACC). The malonyl product of ACC inhibits FA oxidation at the carnitine palmitoyltransferase I step. Because mitochondrial FA oxidation generates the acetyl CoA substrate for hepatic ketogenesis, ketone body levels do not rise. The FA gets esterified to the glycerol backbone, resulting in an increase in TAG that gets sent out of the liver as components of very-low-density lipoproteins (VLDL). [Note: The hypoglycemia results in release of epinephrine and the activation of TAG lipolysis with release of free FA into the blood. The FA are oxidized, with the excess used in hepatic TAG synthesis.] The acetyl CoA is also a substrate for cholesterol synthesis. Thus, the increase in glycolysis results in the hyperlipidemia seen in JS (see figure below).

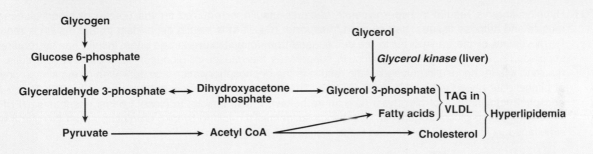

CASE 3: Answers to Review Questions

RQ1. Correct answer = A. Diabetes is characterized by hyperglycemia. Chronic hyperglycemia can result in the nonenzymatic glycosylation (glycation) of hemoglobin (Hb), producing HbA_{1c}. Therefore, measurement of glucose or HbA_{1c} in the blood is used to diagnose diabetes. In response to physiologic stress (for example, a urinary tract infection), secretion of counterregulatory hormones (such as the catecholamines) results in a rise in blood glucose. Glucose is a reducing sugar. It is type 2 diabetes (T2D) that is associated with obesity and a sedentary lifestyle and is caused by insensitivity to insulin (insulin resistance). T1D is caused by lack of insulin as a result of the autoimmune destruction of pancreatic β cells. Even individuals on a program of tight glycemic control do not achieve euglycemia.

RQ2. Correct answer = E. The ketone bodies 3-hydroxybutyrate and acetoacetate are organic acids, and their ionization contributes to the proton load of the body. Ketone bodies are made in the mitochondria of liver cells using acetyl coenzyme A (CoA) generated primarily from the β-oxidation of fatty acids ([FA]; see figure on the next page). Because they are water soluble, they do not require a transporter. The liver cannot use them because it lacks the enzyme thiophorase, which moves CoA from succinyl CoA to acetoacetate for conversion to two molecules of acetyl CoA. It is the acetone released in the breath that can impart a fruity odor.

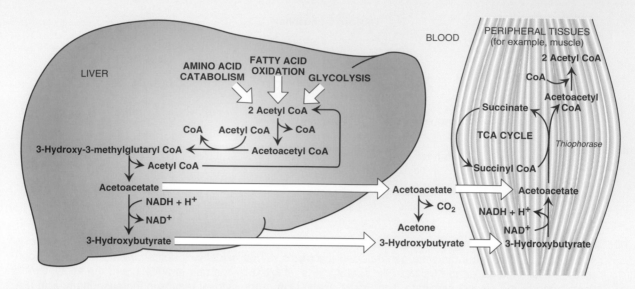

RQ3. Correct answer = A. Malonyl CoA, an intermediate of FA synthesis, inhibits FA β-oxidation through inhibition of carnitine palmitoyltransferase I. Lipolysis occurs when the insulin/counterregulatory hormone ratio decreases. Acetyl CoA, the product of FA β-oxidation, inhibits the pyruvate dehydrogenase (PDH) complex through activation of PDH kinase and activates pyruvate carboxylase. Acetyl CoA, then, pushes pyruvate to gluconeogenesis. β-Oxidation generates reduced nicotinamide adenine dinucleotide (NADH), the reducing equivalent required for gluconeogenesis. FA are not readily catabolized for energy by the brain.

CASE 3: Answers to Thought Questions

TQ1. Hypoinsulinemia results in hyperglycemia because insulin is required for the uptake of blood glucose by muscle and adipose tissue. Their glucose transporter (GLUT-4) is insulin dependent in that insulin is required for movement of the transporter to the cell surface from intracellular storage sites. Insulin is also required to suppress hepatic gluconeogenesis. Insulin suppresses the release of glucagon from pancreatic α cells. The resulting rise in the insulin/glucagon ratio results in the dephosphorylation and activation of the kinase domain of bifunctional phosphofructokinase-2 (PFK-2). The fructose 2,6-bisphosphate produced by PFK-2 activates phosphofructokinase-1 of glycolysis (see figure below). It also inhibits fructose 1,6-bisphosphatase (FBP-2), thereby inhibiting gluconeogenesis. With hypoinsulinemia, the failure to take up glucose from the blood while simultaneously sending it out into the blood results in hyperglycemia.

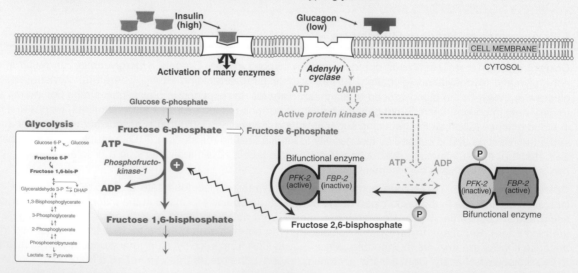

TQ2. The blood glucose level has exceeded the capacity of the kidney to reabsorb glucose (via a sodium-dependent glucose transporter [SGLT]). The high concentration of glucose in the urine osmotically draws water from the body. This causes increased urination (polyuria) with loss of water that results in dehydration.

TQ3. The NADH generated in FA β-oxidation inhibits the tricarboxylic acid (TCA) cycle at the three NADH-producing dehydrogenase steps. This shifts acetyl CoA away from oxidation in the TCA cycle and toward use as a substrate in hepatic ketogenesis.

TQ4. MW was in negative nitrogen balance: More nitrogen was going out than coming in. This is reflected in the elevated blood urea nitrogen (BUN) level seen in the patient (see figure at top right). [Note: The BUN value also reflects dehydration.] Muscle proteolysis and amino acid catabolism are occurring as a result of the fall in insulin. (Recall that skeletal muscle does not express the glucagon receptor.) Amino acid catabolism produces ammonia (NH_3), which is converted to urea by the hepatic urea cycle and sent into the blood. [Note: Urea in the urine is reported as urinary urea nitrogen.]

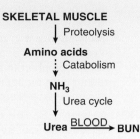

SKELETAL MUSCLE
↓ Proteolysis
Amino acids
⋮ Catabolism
NH_3
↓ Urea cycle
Urea $\xrightarrow{\text{BLOOD}}$ **BUN**

TQ5. The Kussmaul respiration seen in MW is a respiratory response to the metabolic acidosis. Hyperventilation blows off CO_2 and water, reducing the concentration of protons (H^+) and bicarbonate (HCO_3^-) as reflected in the following equation:

$$H^+ + HCO_3^- \leftrightarrow H_2CO_3 \text{ (carbonic acid)} \leftrightarrow CO_2 + H_2O.$$

The renal response includes, in part, the excretion of H^+ as ammonium (NH_4^+). Degradation of branched-chain amino acids in skeletal muscle results in the release of large amounts of glutamine (Gln) into the blood. The kidneys take up and catabolize the Gln, generating NH_3 in the process. The NH_3 is converted to NH_4^+ by secreted H^+ and is excreted (see figure at middle right). [Note: When ketone bodies are plentiful, enterocytes shift to using them as a fuel instead of Gln. This increases the amount of Gln going to the kidney.]

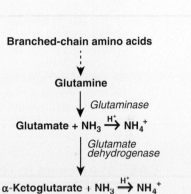

Branched-chain amino acids
⋮
↓
Glutamine
↓ *Glutaminase*
Glutamate + NH_3 $\xrightarrow{H^+}$ NH_4^+
↓ *Glutamate dehydrogenase*
α-Ketoglutarate + NH_3 $\xrightarrow{H^+}$ NH_4^+

TQ6. Because FA β-oxidation supplies the acetyl CoA substrate for ketogenesis, impaired β-oxidation decreases the ability to make ketone bodies. Ketone bodies are an alternate to the use of glucose, and, thus, dependence on glucose increases. Because FA β-oxidation supplies the NADH and the nucleoside triphosphates needed for gluconeogenesis, glucose production decreases. The result is a hypoketotic hypoglycemia. Recall that this was seen with medium-chain acyl CoA dehydrogenase (MCAD) deficiency.

CASE 4: Answers to Review Questions

RQ1. Answer = D. The rise in reduced nicotinamide adenine dinucleotide (NADH) in the mitochondria decreases the tricarboxylic acid (TCA) cycle, fatty acid (FA) oxidation, and gluconeogenesis. NADH inhibits the isocitrate dehydrogenase reaction, the key regulated step of the TCA cycle, and the α-ketoglutarate dehydrogenase reaction (see figure at bottom right). It also favors the reduction of oxaloacetate (OAA) to malate (not malate to OAA), decreasing the availability of OAA for condensation with acetyl coenzyme A (CoA) in the TCA cycle and for gluconeogenesis. FA oxidation requires the oxidized form of nicotinamide adenine dinucleotide (NAD^+) for the 3-hydroxyacyl CoA dehydrogenase step and, thus, is inhibited by the rise in NADH. The decrease in FA oxidation decreases the production of ATP and acetyl CoA (the allosteric activator of pyruvate carboxylase) needed for gluconeogenesis. Lipolysis is activated in fasting as a consequence of the fall in insulin and the rise in catecholamines that result in activation of hormone-sensitive lipase.

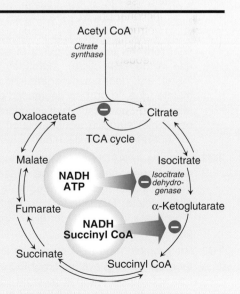

Acetyl CoA
Citrate synthase
Oxaloacetate ⊖ Citrate
TCA cycle
Malate   Isocitrate
NADH ATP   *Isocitrate dehydrogenase* ⊖
Fumarate   α-Ketoglutarate
NADH Succinyl CoA ⊖
Succinate   Succinyl CoA

RQ2. Answer = E. The irreversible, oxidative portion of the pentose phosphate pathway provides the nicotinamide adenine dinucleotide phosphate (NADPH) that supplies the reducing equivalents needed for activity of cytochrome P450 (CYP) proteins and for the regeneration of functional (reduced) glutathione. It is also an important source of NADPH for reductive biosynthetic processes in the cytosol, such as FA and cholesterol synthesis. [Note: Malic enzyme is another source.] CYP proteins are monooxygenases (mixed-function oxidases). They incorporate one O atom from O_2 into the substrate as the other is reduced to water. It is the CYP proteins of the smooth endoplasmic reticular membrane that are involved in detoxification reactions. Those of the inner mitochondrial membrane are involved in the synthesis of steroid hormones, bile acids, and vitamin D. Reactive oxygen species are reduced by glutathione peroxidase as glutathione is oxidized.

RQ3. Answer = C. Serotonin is released by activated platelets and causes vaso-constriction and platelet aggregation. [Note: Platelets do not synthesize sero-tonin, but they take up that which was made in the intestine and secreted into the blood.] Serotonin is associated with a feeling of well-being. It is degraded to 5-hydroxyindoleacetic acid by monoamine oxidase that catalyzes oxidative deamination. It is catechol-O-methyltransferase that catalyzes the methyla-tion step in the degradation of the catecholamines. Serotonin is synthesized from tryptophan in a two-step process that utilizes tetrahydrobiopterin (BH$_4$)-requiring tryptophan hydroxylase and a pyridoxal phosphate (PLP)-requiring decarboxylase (see figure at right).

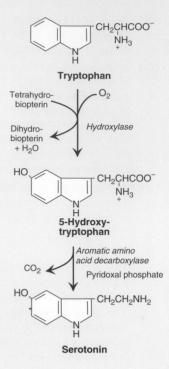

RQ4. Answer = B. The exocrine pancreas secretes enzymes required for the digestion of dietary carbohydrate, protein, and fat. The endocrine pancreas secretes the peptide hormones insulin and glucagon. Damage that affects the functions of the pancreas would lead to diabetes (decreased insulin) and steatorrhea (fatty stool), with the latter the consequence of maldigestion of dietary fat. As was seen with the rise of troponins in a myocardial infarction and transaminases in liver damage, loss of cellular integrity (as would be seen in autodigestion of the pancreas) results in proteins that normally are intracel-lular being found in higher-than-normal concentrations in the blood. Secretin causes the pancreas to release bicarbonate to raise the pH of the chyme com-ing to the intestine from the stomach. Pancreatic enzymes work best at neutral or slightly alkaline pH. Pancreatitis is seen in individuals with hypertriglyceri-demia as a result of a deficiency in lipoprotein lipase or its coenzyme, apolipo-protein C-II.

CASE 4: Answers to Thought Questions

TQ1. A. The rise in cytosolic NADH seen with ethanol metabolism inhibits gly-colysis. The glyceraldehyde 3-phosphate dehydrogenase step requires NAD$^+$, which gets reduced as glyceraldehyde 3-phosphate gets oxidized. With the rise in NADH, glyceraldehyde 3-phosphate accumulates.

B. Glyceraldehyde 3-phosphate from glycolysis is converted to glycerol 3-phosphate, the initial acceptor of FA in triacylglycerol (TAG) synthesis (see figure at right). FA are available because of increased synthesis (from acetyl CoA, which is increased as a result of both increased produc-tion from the acetate product of acetaldehyde oxidation and decreased use in the TCA cycle), increased availability from lipolysis in adipose tissue, and decreased degradation. The TAG produced in the liver accu-mulate (due, in part, to decreased production of very-low-density lipopro-teins) and cause fatty liver (steatosis). Hepatic steatosis is an early (and reversible) stage in alcohol-related liver disease. Subsequent stages are alcohol-related hepatitis (sometimes reversible) and cirrhosis (irreversible).

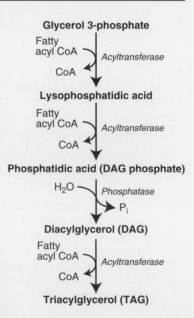

TQ2. The rise in NADH favors the reduction of pyruvate to lactate by lactate dehydrogenase. Lactate decreases the renal excretion of uric acid, thereby causing hyperuricemia, a necessary step in an acute gouty attack. [Note: The shift from pyruvate to lactate decreases the availability of pyruvate, a substrate for gluconeogenesis. This contributes to the hypo-glycemia seen in AK.]

TQ3. Prothrombin time (PT) measures the time it takes for plasma to clot after the addition of tissue factor (FIII), thereby allowing evaluation of the extrinsic (and common) pathways of coagulation. In the extrinsic pathway, FIII activates FVII in a calcium (Ca^{2+})- and phospholipid (PL)-dependent process (see figure at bottom right). FVII, like most of the proteins of clotting, is made by the liver. Alcohol-induced liver damage can decrease its synthesis. Additionally, FVII has a short half-life, and, as a γ-carboxyglutamate (Gla)-containing pro-tein, its synthesis requires vitamin K. Poor nutrition can result in decreased availability of vitamin K and, therefore, decreased abil-ity to clot. [Note: Severe liver disease results in prolonged PT and activated partial thromboplastin time, or aPPt.]

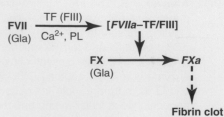

TQ4. Administration of folate can mask a deficiency in vitamin B_{12} by reversing the hematologic manifestation (macrocytic anemia) of the deficiency. However, folate has no effect on the neurologic damage caused by B_{12} deficiency. Over time, then, the neurologic effects can become severe and irreversible. Thus, folate can mask a deficiency of B_{12} and prevent treatment until the neuropathy is apparent.

III. FOCUSED CASES

CASE 1: MICROCYTIC ANEMIA

Patient Presentation: ME is a 24-year-old man who is being evaluated as a follow-up to a preplacement medical evaluation he had prior to starting his new job.

Focused History: ME has no significant medical issues. His family history is unremarkable, but he knows little of the health status of those family members who remain in Greece.

Pertinent Findings: The physical examination was normal. Routine analysis of his blood included the following results:

	Patient	Reference Range
Red blood cells	$4.8 \times 10^{6}/mm^{3}$	4.3–5.9
Hemoglobin	9.6 g/dl **(L)**	13.5–7.5 (men)
Mean corpuscular volume	70 μm^{3} **(L)**	80–100
Serum iron	150 μg/dl	50–170

Based on the data, hemoglobin (Hb) electrophoresis was performed. The results are as follows:

	Patient	Reference Range
HbA	90% **(L)**	96–98
HbA$_2$	6% **(H)**	<3
HbF	4% **(H)**	<2

H = High; **L** = Low. [Note: HbA includes HbA$_{1c}$.]

Diagnosis: ME has β-thalassemia trait (β-thalassemia minor) that is causing a microcytic anemia (see image at right). Ethnicity (such as being of Mediterranean origin) influences the risk for thalassemia.

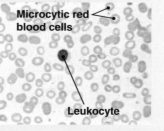

Microcytic red blood cells

Leukocyte

Treatment: None is required at this time. Patients are advised that iron supplements will not prevent their anemia.

Prognosis: β-Thalassemia trait does not cause mortality or significant morbidity. Patients should be informed of the genetic nature of their autosomal-recessive condition for family planning considerations because homozygous β-thalassemia (Cooley anemia) is a serious disorder.

CASE-RELATED QUESTIONS: Choose the ONE best answer.

Q1. Mutations to the gene for β globin that result in decreased production of the protein are the cause of β-thalassemia. The mutations primarily affect gene transcription or posttranscriptional processing of the messenger RNA (mRNA) product. Which of the following statements concerning mRNA is correct?

A. Eukaryotic mRNA is polycistronic.

B. mRNA synthesis involves trans-acting factors binding to cis-acting elements.

C. mRNA synthesis is terminated at the DNA base sequence thymine adenine guanine (TAG).

D. Polyadenylation of the 5′-end of eukaryotic mRNA requires a methyl donor.

E. Splicing of eukaryotic mRNA involves removal of exons and joining of introns by the proteasome.

Q2. HbA, a tetramer of 2 α and 2 β globin chains, delivers O_2 from the lungs to the tissues and protons and CO_2 from the tissues to the lungs. Increased concentration of which of the following will result in decreased O_2 delivery by HbA?

A. 2,3-Bisphosphoglycerate

B. Carbon dioxide

C. Carbon monoxide

D. Protons

Q3. What is the basis for the increase in HbA$_2$ and HbF (fetal Hb) in the β-thalassemias?

Q4. Why is the allele-specific oligonucleotide (ASO) hybridization technique useful in the diagnosis of all cases of sickle cell anemia but not all cases of β-thalassemia?

CASE 2: SKIN RASH

Patient Presentation: KL is a 34-year-old woman who presents with a red, nonitchy rash on her left thigh and flu-like symptoms.

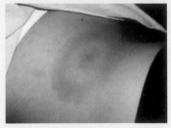

Focused History: KL reports that the rash first appeared a little over 2 weeks ago. It started out small but has gotten larger. She also thinks she is getting the flu because her muscles and joints ache (myalgia and arthralgia, respectively), and she has had a headache for the last few days. Upon questioning, KL reports that she and her husband took a camping trip through New England last month.

Pertinent Findings: The physical examination is remarkable for the presence of a red, circular, flat lesion ~11 cm in size that resembles a bullseye (erythema migrans) (see image at right). KL also has a low-grade fever.

Diagnosis: KL has Lyme disease caused by the bacterium Borrelia burgdorferi, which is transmitted by the bite of a tick in the genus Ixodes. Infected ticks are endemic in the Northeast region of the United States.

Treatment: KL is prescribed doxycycline, an antibiotic in the tetracycline family. Monitoring of KL will continue until all symptoms have completely resolved. Blood is drawn for clinical laboratory tests.

Prognosis: Patients treated with the appropriate antibiotic in the early stages of Lyme disease typically recover quickly and completely.

CASE-RELATED QUESTIONS: Choose the ONE best answer.

Q1. Antibiotics in the tetracycline class inhibit protein synthesis (translation) at the initiation step. Which of the following statements about translation is correct?

    A. In eukaryotic translation, the initiating amino acid is formylated methionine.

    B. Only the charged initiating transfer RNA goes directly to the ribosomal A site.

    C. Peptidyltransferase is a ribozyme that forms the peptide bond between two amino acids.

    D. Prokaryotic translation can be inhibited by the phosphorylation of initiation factor 2.

    E. Termination of translation is independent of guanosine triphosphate hydrolysis.

    F. The Shine-Dalgarno sequence facilitates the binding of the large ribosomal subunit to eukaryotic messenger RNA (mRNA).

Q2. The Centers for Disease Control and Prevention recommends a two-tier testing procedure for Lyme disease that involves a screening enzyme-linked immunosorbent assay (ELISA) followed by a confirmatory western blot analysis on any sample with a positive or equivocal ELISA result. Which of the following statements about these testing procedures is correct?

    A. Both techniques are used to detect specific mRNA.

    B. Both techniques involve the use of antibodies.

    C. ELISA requires the use of electrophoresis.

    D. Western blots require use of the polymerase chain reaction.

Q3. Why are eukaryotic cells unaffected by antibiotics in the tetracycline class?

CASE 3: BLOOD ON THE TOOTHBRUSH

Patient Presentation: LT is an 84-year-old man whose gums have been bleeding for several months.

Focused History: LT is a widower and lives alone in a suburban community on the East Coast. He no longer drives. His two children live on the West Coast and come east infrequently. Since the death of his wife 11 months ago, he has been isolated and finds it hard to get out of the house. His appetite has changed, and he is content with cereal, coffee, and packaged snacks. Chewing is difficult.

Pertinent Findings: The physical examination was remarkable for the presence of swollen dark-colored gums (see image at right). Several of LT's teeth were loose, including one that anchors his dental bridge. Several black and blue marks (ecchymoses) were noted on the legs, and an unhealed sore was present on the right wrist. Inspection of his scalp revealed tiny red spots (petechiae) around some of the hair follicles. Blood was drawn for testing.

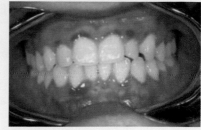

Results of tests on LT's blood:

	Patient	Reference Range
Red blood cells	$4.0 \times 10^6/mm^3$ (**L**)	4.3–5.9
Hemoglobin	10 g/dl (**L**)	13.5–17.5 (men)
Mean corpuscular volume	78 μm^3 (**L**)	80–100
Serum iron	40 $\mu g/dl$ (**L**)	50–170
Serum ferritin	23 $\mu g/l$ (**L**)	40–160 $\mu g/l$
Total iron-binding capacity	375 $\mu g/dl$ (**H**)	300–360 $\mu g/dl$
Platelets	$250 \times 10^9/l$	150–350×10^9

The test for blood in his stool (occult blood test) was negative.

Results of follow-up tests (obtained several days after the appointment) included the following:

	Patient	Reference Range
Vitamin C (plasma)	0.16 mg/dl (**L**)	0.2–2

H = High; **L** = Low.

Diagnosis: LT has vitamin C deficiency with a microcytic, hypochromic anemia secondary to the deficiency.

Treatment: LT was prescribed vitamin C (as oral ascorbic acid) and iron (as oral ferrous sulfate) supplements. He will also be referred to social services.

Prognosis: The prognosis for recovery is excellent.

CASE-RELATED QUESTIONS: Choose the ONE best answer.

Q1. Which of the following statements about vitamin C is correct? Vitamin C is:

A. a competitor of iron absorption in the intestine.

B. a fat-soluble vitamin with a 3-month supply typically stored in adipose tissue.

C. a coenzyme in several enzymic reactions such as the hydroxylation of proline.

D. required for the cross-linking of collagen.

Q2. In contrast to the microcytic anemia characteristic of iron deficiency (common in older adults), a macrocytic anemia is seen with deficiencies of vitamin B_{12} and/or folic acid. These vitamin deficiencies are also common in older adults. Which of the following statements concerning these vitamins is correct?

A. An inability to absorb B_{12} results in pernicious anemia.

B. Both vitamins cause changes in gene expression.

C. Folic acid plays a key role in energy metabolism in most cells.

D. Treatment with methotrexate can result in toxic levels of the coenzyme form of folic acid.

E. Vitamin B_{12} is the coenzyme for enzymes catalyzing amino acid deaminations, decarboxylations, and transaminations.

Q3. How do hemolytic anemias differ from nutritional anemias?

CASE 4: RAPID HEART RATE, HEADACHE, AND SWEATING

Patient Presentation: BE is a 45-year-old woman who presents with concerns about sudden (paroxysmal), intense, brief episodes of headache, sweating (diaphoresis), and a racing heart (palpitations).

Focused History: BE reports that the attacks started ~3 weeks ago. They last from 2 to 10 minutes, during which time she feels quite anxious. During the attacks, it feels as though her heart is skipping beats (arrhythmia). At first, she thought the attacks were related to recent stress at work and maybe even menopause. The last time it happened, she was in a pharmacy and had her blood pressure taken. She was told it was 165/110 mm Hg. BE notes that she has lost weight (~8 lbs) in this period even though her appetite has been good.

Pertinent Findings: The physical examination was remarkable for BE's thin, pale appearance. Blood pressure was elevated (150/100 mm Hg), as was the heart rate (110–120 beats/minute). Based on BE's history, blood levels of normetanephrine and metanephrine were ordered. They were found to be elevated.

Diagnosis: BE has a pheochromocytoma, a rare catecholamine-secreting tumor of the adrenal medulla.

Treatment: Imaging studies of the abdomen were done to locate the tumor. Surgical resection of the tumor was performed. The tumor was found to be nonmalignant. Follow-up measurement of plasma metanephrines was performed 2 weeks later and was in the normal range.

Prognosis: The 5-year survival rate for nonmalignant pheochromocytomas is >95%.

CASE-RELATED QUESTIONS: Choose the ONE best answer.

Q1. Pheochromocytomas secrete norepinephrine (NE) and epinephrine. Which of the following statements concerning the synthesis and degradation of these two biogenic amines is correct?

    A. The substrate for their synthesis is tryptophan, which is hydroxylated to 3,4-dihydroxyphenylalanine (DOPA) by tetrahydrobiopterin-requiring tryptophan hydroxylase.

    B. The conversion of DOPA to dopamine utilizes a pyridoxal phosphate–requiring carboxylase.

    C. The conversion of NE to epinephrine requires vitamin C.

    D. Degradation involves methylation by catechol-O-methyltransferase and produces normetanephrine from NE and metanephrine from epinephrine.

    E. Normetanephrine and metanephrine are oxidatively deaminated to homovanillic acid by monoamine oxidase.

Q2. Which of the following statements concerning the actions of epinephrine and/or NE are correct?

    A. NE functions as a neurotransmitter and a hormone.

    B. They are initiated by autophosphorylation of select tyrosine residues in their receptors.

    C. They are mediated by binding to adrenergic receptors, which are a class of nuclear receptors.

    D. They result in the activation of glycogen and triacylglycerol synthesis.

Q3. NE bound to certain receptors causes vasoconstriction and an increase in blood pressure. Why might NE be used clinically in the treatment of septic shock?

CASE 5: SUN SENSITIVITY

Patient Presentation: AZ is a 6-year-old boy who is being evaluated for freckle-like areas of hyperpigmentation on his face, neck, forearms, and lower legs.

Focused History: AZ's father reports that the boy has always been quite sensitive to the sun. His skin turns red (erythema) and his eyes hurt (photophobia) if he is exposed to the sun for any period of time.

Pertinent Findings: The physical examination was remarkable for the presence of thickened, scaly areas (actinic keratosis) and hyperpigmented areas on skin exposed to ultraviolet (UV) radiation from the sun. Small dilated blood vessels (telangiectasia) were also seen. Tissue from several sites on his face was biopsied, and two were later determined to be squamous cell carcinomas.

Diagnosis: AZ has xeroderma pigmentosum, a rare defect in nucleotide excision repair of DNA.

Treatment: Protection from sunlight through use of sunscreens such as protective clothing that reflect UV radiation and chemicals that absorb it is essential. Frequent skin and eye examinations are recommended.

Prognosis: Most patients with xeroderma pigmentosum die at an early age from skin cancers. However, survival beyond middle age is possible.

CASE-RELATED QUESTIONS: Choose the ONE best answer.

Q1. Which of the following statements about DNA repair mechanisms is correct? DNA repair:

    A. is performed only by eukaryotes.

    B. of double-strand breaks is error free.

    C. of mismatched bases involves repair of the parental strand.

    D. of UV radiation–induced pyrimidine dimers involves removal of a short oligonucleotide containing the dimer.

    E. of uracil produced by the deamination of cytosine requires the actions of endo- and exonucleases to remove the uracil base.

Q2. Which one of the following statements about DNA synthesis (replication) is correct? Replication:

    A. in both eukaryotes and prokaryotes requires an RNA primer.

    B. in eukaryotes requires condensation of chromatin.

    C. in prokaryotes is accomplished by a single DNA polymerase.

    D. is initiated at random sites in the genome.

    E. produces a polymer of deoxyribonucleoside monophosphates linked by $5' \rightarrow 3'$-phosphodiester bonds.

Q3. What is the difference between DNA proofreading and repair?

CASE 6: DARK URINE AND YELLOW SCLERAE

Patient Presentation: JF is a 13-year-old boy who presents with fatigue and yellow sclerae.

Focused History: JF began treatment ~4 days ago with a sulfonamide antibiotic and a urinary analgesic for a urinary tract infection. He had been told that his urine would change color (become reddish) with the analgesic, but he reports that it has gotten darker (more brownish) over the last 2 days. Last night, his mother noticed that his eyes had a yellow tint. JF says he feels as though he has no energy.

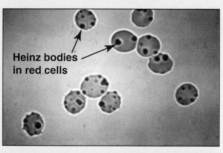

Heinz bodies in red cells

Pertinent Findings: The physical examination was remarkable for JF's pale appearance, mild scleral icterus (jaundice), mild splenomegaly, and increased heart rate (tachycardia). JF's urine tested positive for hemoglobin (hemoglobinuria). A peripheral blood smear reveals a lower-than-normal number of red blood cells (RBC), with some containing precipitated hemoglobin (Heinz bodies; see image at right), and a higher-than-normal number of reticulocytes (immature RBC). Results of the complete blood count (CBC) and blood chemistry tests are pending.

Diagnosis: JF has *glucose 6-phosphate dehydrogenase* (*G6PD*) deficiency, an X-linked disorder that causes hemolysis (RBC lysis).

Treatment: *G6PD* deficiency can result in a hemolytic anemia in affected individuals exposed to oxidative agents. JF will be switched to a different antibiotic. He will be advised that he is susceptible to certain drugs (for example, sulfa drugs), foods (fava or broad beans), and certain chemicals (for example, naphthalene), and must avoid exposure to them.

Prognosis: In the absence of exposure to oxidative agents, *G6PD* deficiency does not cause mortality or significant morbidity.

CASE-RELATED QUESTIONS: Choose the ONE best answer.

Q1. G6PD catalyzes the regulated step in the pentose phosphate pathway. Which of the following statements concerning G6PD and the pentose phosphate pathway is correct?

    A. Deficiency of G6PD occurs only in RBC.

    B. Deficiency of G6PD results in an inability to keep glutathione in its functional, reduced form.

    C. The pentose phosphate pathway includes one reversible reductive reaction followed by a series of phosphorylated sugar interconversions.

    D. The reduced nicotinamide adenine dinucleotide phosphate (NADPH) product of the pentose phosphate pathway is utilized in processes such as fatty acid oxidation.

Q2. The results of JF's CBC were consistent with a hemolytic anemia. Blood chemistry tests revealed an elevation in the bilirubin level. Which of the following statements concerning bilirubin is correct?

A. Hyperbilirubinemia can cause deposition of bilirubin in the skin and sclerae resulting in jaundice.

B. The solubility of bilirubin is increased by conjugating it with two molecules of ascorbic acid in the liver.

C. The conjugated form of bilirubin increases in the blood with a hemolytic anemia.

D. Phototherapy can increase the solubility of the excess bilirubin generated in the porphyrias.

Q3. Why is urinary urobilinogen increased relative to normal in hemolytic jaundice and absent in obstructive jaundice?

CASE 7: JOINT PAIN

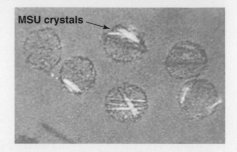

MSU crystals

Patient Presentation: IR is a 22-year-old male who presents for follow-up 10 days after having been treated in the Emergency Department (ED) for severe inflammation at the base of his thumb.

Focused History: This was IR's first occurrence of severe joint pain. In the ED, he was given an anti-inflammatory medication. Fluid aspirated from the carpometacarpal joint of the thumb was negative for organisms but positive for needle-shaped monosodium urate (MSU) crystals (see image at right). The inflammatory symptoms have since resolved. IR reports he is in good health otherwise, with no significant past medical history. His body mass index (BMI) is 31. No tophi (deposits of MSU crystals under the skin) were detected in the physical examination.

Pertinent Findings: Results on a 24-hour urine specimen and blood tests requested in advance of this visit reveal that IR is not an undersecretor of uric acid. His blood urate was 8.5 mg/dl (reference = 2.5–8.0). The unusually young age of presentation is suggestive of an enzymopathy of purine metabolism, and additional blood tests are ordered.

Diagnosis: IR has gout (MSU crystal deposition disease), a type of inflammatory arthritis.

Treatment: IR was given prescriptions for allopurinol and colchicine. The treatment goals are to reduce his blood urate levels to <6.0 mg/dl and prevent additional attacks. He was advised to lose weight because being overweight or obese is a risk factor for gout. His BMI of 31 puts him in the obese category. He was also given written information on the association between diet and gout.

Prognosis: Gout increases the risk of developing renal stones. It is also associated with hypertension, diabetes, and heart disease.

CASE-RELATED QUESTIONS: Choose the ONE best answer.

Q1. Allopurinol is converted in the body to oxypurinol, which functions as a noncompetitive inhibitor of an enzyme in purine metabolism. Which of the following statements concerning purine metabolism and its regulation is correct?

A. As a noncompetitive inhibitor, oxypurinol increases the apparent Michaelis constant (K_m) of the target enzyme.

B. Colchicine inhibits xanthine oxidase, an enzyme of purine degradation.

C. Glutamate provides two of the nitrogen atoms of the purine ring.

D. In purine nucleotide synthesis, the ring system is first constructed and then attached to ribose 5-phosphate.

E. Oxypurinol inhibits the amidotransferase that initiates degradation of the purine ring system.

F. Partial or complete enzymic deficiencies in the salvage of purine bases are characterized by hyperuricemia.

Q2. Purines are one type of nitrogenous base found in nucleotides. Pyrimidines are the other. Which of the following statements is true of the pyrimidines?

A. Carbamoyl phosphate synthetase I is the regulated enzymic activity in pyrimidine ring synthesis.

B. Methotrexate decreases synthesis of the pyrimidine nucleotide thymidine monophosphate.

C. Orotic aciduria is a pathology of pyrimidine degradation.

D. Pyrimidine nucleotide synthesis is independent of 5-phosphoribosyl-1-pyrophosphate (PRPP).

Q3. IR is subsequently shown to have a form of PRPP synthetase that shows increased enzymic activity. Why does this result in hyperuricemia?

CASE 8: NO BOWEL MOVEMENT

Patient Presentation: DW is a 48-hour-old female who has not yet had a bowel movement.

Focused History: DW is the full-term product of a normal pregnancy and delivery. She appeared normal at birth. DW is the first child of parents of Northern European ethnicity. The parents are both in good health, and their family histories are unremarkable.

Pertinent Findings: DW has a distended abdomen. She recently vomited small amounts of bilious (green-colored) material.

Diagnosis: Meconium ileus (obstruction of the ileum by meconium, the first stool produced by newborns) was confirmed by abdominal x-rays. About 98% of full-term newborns with meconium ileus have cystic fibrosis (CF). Diagnosis of CF was subsequently confirmed with a chloride sweat test.

Treatment: The ileus was successfully treated nonsurgically. For management of the CF, the family was referred to the CF center at the regional children's hospital.

Prognosis: CF is the most common life-limiting autosomal-recessive disease in Caucasians.

CASE-RELATED QUESTIONS: Choose the ONE best answer.

Q1. CF is the result of mutations to the gene that encodes the CF transmembrane conductance regulator (CFTR) protein that functions as a chloride channel in the apical membrane of epithelial cells on a mucosal surface. Which of the following statements concerning CF is correct?

  A. Clinical manifestations of CF are the consequence of chloride retention with increased water reabsorption that causes mucus on the epithelial surface to be excessively thick and sticky.

  B. Excessive pancreatic secretion of insulin in CF commonly results in hypoglycemia.

  C. Genetic testing for CF may involve the use of a set of probes for the most common mutations, a technique known as restriction fragment length polymorphism analysis.

  D. Some mutations result in premature degradation of the CFTR protein through tagging with ubiquinone followed by proteasome-mediated proteolysis.

  E. The most common mutation, ΔF508, results in the loss of a codon for phenylalanine (F) and is classified as a frameshift mutation.

Q2. The CFTR protein is an intrinsic plasma membrane glycoprotein. Targeting of proteins destined to function as components of membranes:

  A. includes transport to and through the Golgi.

  B. involves an amino-terminal signal sequence that is retained in the functional protein.

  C. occurs after the protein has been completely synthesized (that is, posttranslationally).

  D. requires the presence of mannose 6-phosphate residues on the protein.

Q3. Why might steatorrhea be seen with CF?

CASE 9: ELEVATED AMMONIA

Patient Presentation: RL is a 40-hour-old male with signs of cerebral edema.

Focused History: RL is the full-term product of a normal pregnancy and delivery. He appeared normal at birth. At age 36 hours, he became irritable, lethargic, and hypothermic. He fed only poorly and vomited. He also displayed tachypneic (rapid) breathing and neurologic posturing. At age 38 hours, he had a seizure.

Pertinent Findings: Respiratory alkalosis (increased pH, decreased CO_2 [hypocapnia]), increased ammonia, and decreased blood urea nitrogen were found. An amino acid screen revealed that argininosuccinate was increased >60-fold over baseline, and citrulline was increased 4-fold. Glutamine was elevated, and arginine (Arg) was decreased relative to normal.

Diagnosis: RL has a urea cycle enzyme defect with neonatal onset.

Treatment: Hemodialysis was performed to remove ammonia. Sodium phenylacetate and sodium benzoate were administered to aid in excretion of waste nitrogen, as was Arg. Long-term treatment will include lifelong limitation of dietary protein; supplementation with essential amino acids; and administration of Arg, sodium phenylacetate, and sodium phenylbutyrate.

Prognosis: Survival into adulthood is possible. The degree of neurologic impairment is related to the degree and extent of the hyperammonemia.

CASE-RELATED QUESTIONS: Choose the ONE best answer.

Q1. Based on the findings, which enzyme of the urea cycle is most likely to be deficient in this patient?

A. Arginase

B. Argininosuccinate lyase

C. Argininosuccinate synthetase

D. Carbamoyl phosphate synthetase I

E. Ornithine transcarbamoylase

Q2. Why is Arg supplementation helpful in this case?

Q3. In individuals with partial (milder) deficiency of urea cycle enzymes, the level of which one of the following would be expected to be decreased during periods of physiologic stress?

A. Alanine

B. Ammonia

C. Glutamine

D. Insulin

E. pH

CASE 10: CALF PAIN

Patient Presentation: CR is a 19-year-old female who is being evaluated for pain and swelling in her right calf.

Focused History: Ten days ago, CR had her spleen removed following a bicycle accident in which she fractured her tibial eminence, necessitating immobilization of the right knee. She has had a good recovery from the surgery. CR is no longer taking pain medication but has continued her oral contraceptives (OCP).

Pertinent Findings: CR's right calf is reddish in color (erythematous) and warm to the touch. It is visibly swollen. The left calf is normal in appearance and is without pain. An ultrasound is ordered.

Diagnosis: CR has a deep venous thrombosis (DVT). OCP are a risk factor for DVT, as are surgery and immobilization.

Treatment (Immediate): Heparin and warfarin are administered.

Prognosis: In the 10 years following a DVT, about one third of individuals have a recurrence.

CASE-RELATED QUESTIONS: Choose the ONE best answer.

Q1. A DVT is a blood clot that occludes the lumen of a deep vein, most commonly in the leg. Which of the following statements about the clotting cascade is correct?

A. A deficiency in factor (F)IX of the intrinsic pathway results in hemophilia A.

B. FIII of the extrinsic pathway is a serine protease.

C. Formation of the fibrin meshwork is referred to as primary hemostasis.

D. Thrombin proteolytically activates components of the extrinsic, intrinsic, and common pathways.

E. Vitamin K is required for the activation of fibrinogen.

Q2. Which one of the following would increase the risk of thrombosis?

A. Excess production of antithrombin

B. Excess production of protein S

C. Expression of FV Leiden

D. Hypoprothrombinemia

E. von Willebrand disease

Q3. Compare and contrast the actions of heparin and warfarin.

IV. FOCUSED CASES: ANSWERS TO CASE-BASED QUESTIONS

CASE 1: Anemia with β-Thalassemia Minor

Q1. **Answer = B.** Transcription (synthesis of single-stranded RNA from the template strand of double-stranded DNA) requires the binding of proteins (trans-acting factors) to sequences on the DNA (cis-acting elements). Eukaryotic messenger RNA (mRNA) is monocistronic because it contains information from just one gene (cistron). The base sequence TAG (thymine adenine guanine) in the coding strand of DNA is U(uracil)AG in the mRNA. UAG is a signal that terminates translation (protein synthesis), not transcription. It is formation of the 5′-cap of eukaryotic mRNA that requires methylation (using S-adenosylmethionine), not 3′-end polyadenylation. Splicing is the spliceosome-mediated process by which introns are removed from eukaryotic mRNA and exons joined.

Q2. **Answer = C.** Carbon monoxide (CO) increases the affinity of hemoglobin (Hb)A for O_2, thereby decreasing the ability of HbA to offload O_2 in the tissues. CO stabilizes the R (relaxed) or oxygenated form and shifts the O_2 dissociation curve to the left, decreasing O_2 delivery (see figure at top right). The other choices decrease the affinity for O_2, stabilize the T (tense) or deoxygenated form, and cause a right shift in the curve.

Q3. HbA_2 and fetal Hb (HbF) do not contain β globin. As β globin production decreases, synthesis of HbA_2 ($\alpha_2\delta_2$) and HbF ($\alpha_2\gamma_2$) increases.

Q4. Sickle cell anemia is caused by a single point mutation (A→T) in the gene for β globin that results in the replacement of glutamate by valine at the sixth amino acid position in the protein. Mutational analysis using allele-specific oligonucleotide (ASO) probes for that mutation (β^S) and for the normal sequence (β^A) is used in diagnosis (see figure at lower right). β-Thalassemia, in contrast, is caused by hundreds of different mutations. Mutational analysis using ASO probes can assess common mutations, including point mutations, in at-risk populations (for example, those of Greek ancestry). However, less common mutations are often not included in the panel and can be detected only by DNA sequencing.

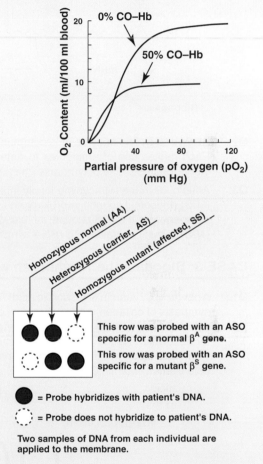

CASE 2: Skin Rash with Lyme Disease

Q1. **Answer = C.** Peptide-bond formation between the amino acid in the A site of the ribosome and the amino acid last added to the growing peptide in the P site is catalyzed by an RNA of the large ribosomal subunit. Any RNA with catalytic activity is referred to as a ribozyme (see figure on the next page). Formylated methionine is used to initiate prokaryotic translation. The charged initiating transfer RNA (tRNAi) is the only tRNA that goes directly to the P site, leaving the A site available for the tRNA carrying the next amino acid of the protein being made. Eukaryotic translation is inhibited by the phosphorylation of initiation factor 2 (eIF-2). The Shine-Dalgarno sequence is found in prokaryotic messenger RNA (mRNA) and facilitates the interaction of the mRNA with the small ribosomal subunit. In eukaryotes, the cap-binding proteins perform that task.

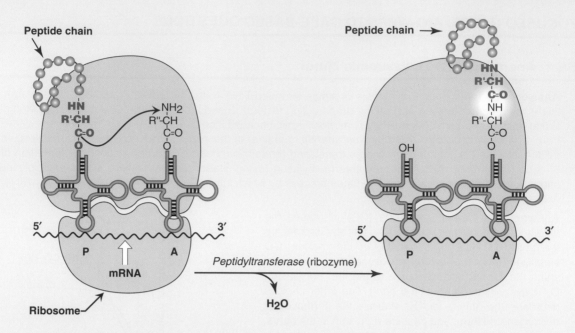

Q2. **Answer = B.** The enzyme-linked immunosorbent assay (ELISA) and western blot are used to analyze proteins. Each makes use of antibodies to detect and quantify the protein of interest. It is western blots that utilize electrophoresis. The polymerase chain reaction (PCR) is used to amplify DNA.

Q3. Antibiotics in the tetracycline family inhibit protein synthesis by binding to and blocking the A site of the small (30S) ribosomal subunit in prokaryotes. Tetracycline specifically interacts with the 16S ribosomal RNA (rRNA) component of the 30S subunit, inhibiting translation initiation. Eukaryotes do not contain 16S rRNA. Their small (40S) subunit contains 18S rRNA, which does not bind tetracycline.

CASE 3: Blood on the Toothbrush with Vitamin C Deficiency

Q1. **Answer = C.** Vitamin C (ascorbic acid) functions as a coenzyme in the hydroxylation of proline and lysine in the synthesis of collagen, a fibrous protein of the extracellular matrix. Vitamin C is also the coenzyme for duodenal cytochrome b (Dcytb) that reduces dietary iron from the ferric (Fe^{3+}) to the ferrous (Fe^{2+}) form that is required for absorption via the divalent metal transporter (DMT) of enterocytes (see figure below). With a deficiency of vitamin C, uptake of dietary iron is impaired and results in a microcytic, hypochromic anemia. As a water-soluble vitamin, vitamin C is not stored. Cross-linking of collagen by lysyl oxidase requires copper, not vitamin C.

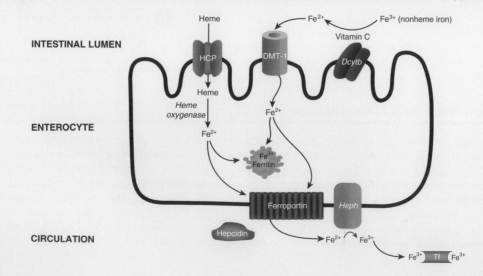

Q2. **Answer = A.** An inability to absorb vitamin B_{12} leads to pernicious anemia and is most commonly caused by decreased production of intrinsic factor (IF) by the parietal cells of the stomach (see figure at right). Vitamins D and A, in complex with their receptors, bind to DNA and alter gene expression. Thiamine (vitamin B_1) is a coenzyme in the oxidative decarboxylation of pyruvate and α-ketoglutarate and, therefore, is important in energy metabolism in most cells. Methotrexate inhibits dihydrofolate reductase, the enzyme that reduces dihydrofolate to tetrahydrofolate (THF), the functional coenzyme form of folate. This results in decreased availability of THF. It is pyridoxine (vitamin B_6) as pyridoxal phosphate that is the coenzyme for most reactions involving amino acids. [Note: Tetrahydrobiopterin is required by aromatic amino acid hydroxylases and nitric oxide synthases.]

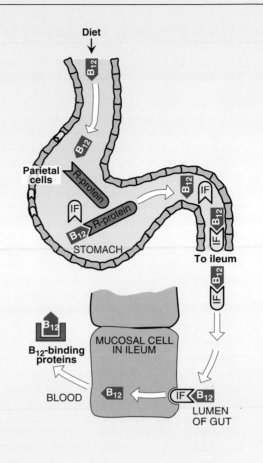

Q3. Nutritional anemias are characterized by either increased red blood cell (RBC) size (folate and B_{12} deficiencies) or decreased RBC size (iron and vitamin C deficiencies). In hemolytic anemias, such as is seen in glucose 6-phosphate dehydrogenase and pyruvate kinase deficiencies and in sickle cell anemia, RBC size typically is normal, and RBC number is decreased.

CASE 4: Rapid Heart Rate, Headache, and Sweating with a Pheochromocytoma

Q1. **Answer = D.** Degradation of both epinephrine and norepinephrine (NE) involves methylation by catechol-O-methyltransferase (COMT) that produces normetanephrine from NE and metanephrine from epinephrine (see figure at right). Both of these products are deaminated to vanillylmandelic acid by monoamine oxidase (MAO). The substrate for the synthesis of the catecholamines is tyrosine, which gets hydroxylated to 3,4-dihydroxyphenylalanine (DOPA) by tetrahydrobiopterin-requiring tyrosine hydroxylase. DOPA is converted to dopamine by a pyridoxal phosphate–requiring decarboxylase. [Note: Most carboxylases require biotin.] NE is converted to epinephrine by methylation, and S-adenosylmethionine provides the methyl group.

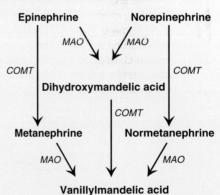

Q2. **Answer = A.** NE released from the sympathetic nervous system functions as a neurotransmitter that acts on postsynaptic neurons and causes, for example, increased heart rate. It is also released from the adrenal medulla and, along with epinephrine, functions as a counterregulatory hormone that results in mobilization of stored fuels (for example, glucose and triacylglycerols). These actions are mediated by the binding of NE to adrenergic receptors, which are G protein–coupled receptors of the plasma membrane, and not to nuclear receptors like those of steroid hormones or membrane tyrosine kinase receptors like that of insulin.

Q3. Septic shock is vasodilatory hypotension (low blood pressure caused by blood vessel dilation) resulting from the production of large amounts of nitric oxide by inducible nitric oxide synthase in response to infection. NE bound to receptors on smooth muscle cells causes vasoconstriction and, thus, raises blood pressure.

CASE 5: Sun Sensitivity with Xeroderma Pigmentosum

Q1. **Answer = D.** Pyrimidine dimers are the characteristic DNA lesions caused by ultraviolet (UV) radiation. Their repair involves the excision of an oligonucleotide containing the dimer and replacement of that oligonucleotide, a process known as nucleotide excision repair (NER). (See figure at right for a representation of the process in prokaryotes.) DNA repair systems are found in prokaryotes and eukaryotes. Nothing is error free, but the homologous recombination (HR) method of double-strand break repair is much less prone to error than is the nonhomologous end joining (NHEJ) method because any DNA that was lost is replaced. Mismatched-base repair (MMR) involves identification and repair of the newly synthesized (daughter) strand. In prokaryotes, the extent of strand methylation is used to discriminate between the strands. Base excision repair (BER), the mechanism by which uracil is removed from DNA, utilizes a glycosylase to remove the base, creating an apyrimidinic or apurinic (AP) site. The sugar-phosphate is then removed by the actions of an endo- and exonuclease.

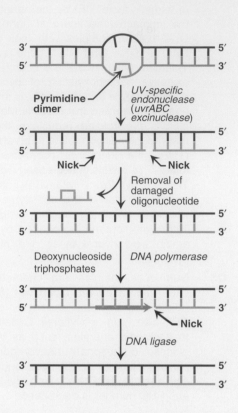

Q2. **Answer = A.** All replication requires an RNA primer because DNA polymerases (pol) cannot initiate DNA synthesis. The chromatin of eukaryotes gets decondensed (relaxed) for replication. Relaxation can be accomplished, for example, by acetylation via histone acetyltransferases. Prokaryotes have more than one DNA pol. For example, pol III extends the RNA primer with DNA, and pol I removes the primer and replaces it with DNA. Replication is initiated at specific locations (one in prokaryotes, many in eukaryotes) that are recognized by proteins (for example, DnaA in prokaryotes). Deoxynucleoside monophosphates (dNMP) are joined by a phosphodiester bond that links the 3′-hydroxyl group of the last dNMP added with the 5′-phosphate group of the incoming nucleotide, thereby forming a 3′→5′-phosphodiester bond as pyrophosphate is released.

Q3. Proofreading occurs during replication in the S (synthesis of DNA) phase of the cell cycle and involves the 3′→5′ exonuclease activity possessed by some DNA pol (see figure below). Because repair can occur independently of replication, it can be performed outside of the S phase.

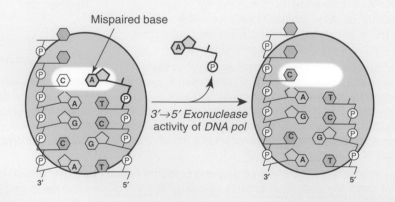

Mispaired base

3′→5′ Exonuclease activity of DNA pol

CASE 6: Dark Urine and Yellow Sclerae with Glucose 6-Phosphate Dehydrogenase Deficiency

Q1. **Answer = B.** Glutathione in its reduced form (G-SH) is an important antioxidant. The selenium-containing enzyme glutathione peroxidase reduces hydrogen peroxide (H_2O_2, a reactive oxygen species) to water as glutathionine is oxidized (G-S-S-G). Reduced nicotinamide adenine dinucleotide phosphate (NADPH)-requiring glutathionine reductase regenerates G-SH from G-S-S-G (see Figure A). The NADPH is supplied by the oxidative reactions of the pentose phosphate pathway (see Figure B), which is regulated by the availability of NADPH at the glucose 6-phosphate dehydrogenase (G6PD)-catalyzed step (the first step). Deficiency of G6PD occurs in all cells, but the effects are seen in red blood cells where the pentose phosphate pathway is the only source of NADPH. The pathway involves two irreversible oxidative reactions, each of which generates NADPH. The NADPH is used in reductive processes such as fatty acid synthesis (not oxidation) as well as steroid hormone and cholesterol synthesis.

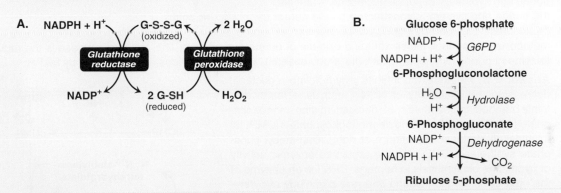

Q2. **Answer = A.** Jaundice (icterus) refers to the yellow color of the skin, nail beds, and sclerae that results from bilirubin deposition when the bilirubin level in the blood is elevated (hyperbilirubinemia; see Image C). Bilirubin has low solubility in aqueous solutions, and its solubility is increased by conjugation with uridine diphosphate–glucuronic acid in the liver, forming bilirubin diglucuronide or conjugated bilirubin (CB). In hemolytic conditions, such as G6PD deficiency, both CB and unconjugated bilirubin (UCB) are increased, but it is UCB that is found in the blood. CB is sent into the intestine. Phototherapy is used to treat unconjugated hyperbilirubinemia because it converts bilirubin to isomeric forms that are more water soluble. Bilirubin is the product of heme degradation in cells of the mononuclear phagocyte system, particularly in the liver and the spleen. The porphyrias are pathologies of heme synthesis and, therefore, are not characterized by hyperbilirubinemia.

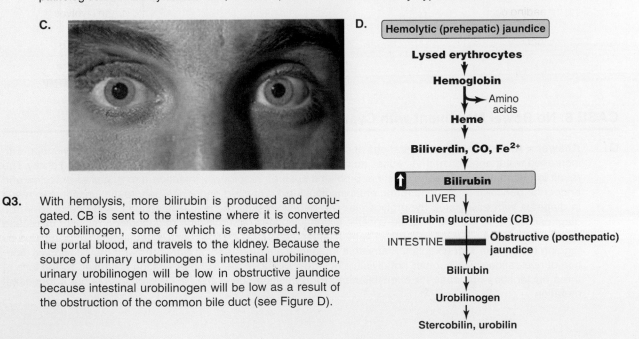

Q3. With hemolysis, more bilirubin is produced and conjugated. CB is sent to the intestine where it is converted to urobilinogen, some of which is reabsorbed, enters the portal blood, and travels to the kidney. Because the source of urinary urobilinogen is intestinal urobilinogen, urinary urobilinogen will be low in obstructive jaundice because intestinal urobilinogen will be low as a result of the obstruction of the common bile duct (see Figure D).

CASE 7: Joint Pain with Gout

Q1.   Answer = F. Salvage of the purine bases hypoxanthine and guanine to the purine nucleotides inosine monophosphate (IMP) and guanosine monophosphate (GMP) by hypoxanthine-guanine phosphoribosyltransferase (HGPRT) requires 5-phosphoribosyl-1-pyrophosphate (PRPP) as the source of the ribose 1-phosphate. Salvage decreases the amount of substrate available for degradation to uric acid. Therefore, a deficiency in salvage results in hyperuricemia (see figure at right).

Noncompetitive inhibitors such as oxypurinol have no effect on the Michaelis constant (K_m) but decrease the apparent maximal velocity (V_{max}). Colchicine is an anti-inflammatory drug. It has no effect on the enzymes of purine synthesis or degradation. Glutamine (not glutamate) is a nitrogen source for purine ring synthesis. In purine nucleotide synthesis, the purine ring system is constructed on the ribose 5-phosphate provided by PRPP. Allopurinol and its

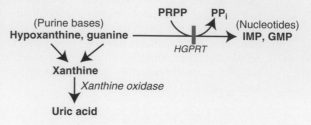

metabolite, oxypurinol, inhibit xanthine oxidase of purine degradation. The amidotransferase is the regulated enzyme of purine synthesis. Its activity is decreased by purine nucleotides and increased by PRPP.

Q2.   Answer = B. Methotrexate inhibits dihydrofolate reductase, decreasing the availability of N^5,N^{10}-methylene tetrahydrofolate needed for synthesis of deoxythymidine monophosphate (dTMP) from deoxyuridine monophosphate (dUMP) by thymidylate synthase (see figure at right). Carbamoyl phosphate synthetase (CPS) II is the regulated enzymic activity of pyrimidine biosynthesis in humans. CPS I is an enzyme of the urea cycle. Orotic aciduria is a rare pathology of pyrimidine synthesis caused by a deficiency in one or both enzymic activities of bifunctional uridine monophosphate synthase. Pyrimidine nucleotide synthesis, like purine synthesis and salvage, requires PRPP.

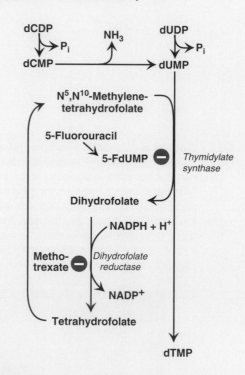

Q3. Increased activity of PRPP synthetase results in increased synthesis of PRPP. This results in an increase in purine nucleotide synthesis beyond need. The excess purine nucleotides get degraded to uric acid, thereby causing hyperuricemia.

CASE 8: No Bowel Movement with Cystic Fibrosis

Q1.   Answer = A. The clinical manifestations of cystic fibrosis (CF) are the consequence of chloride retention with increased water absorption that causes mucus on an epithelial surface to be excessively thick and sticky. The result is pulmonary and gastrointestinal problems such as respiratory infection and impaired exocrine and endocrine pancreatic functions (pancreatic insufficiency). Impaired endocrine pancreatic function can result in diabetes with associated hyperglycemia. The genetic testing technique described, and one used in the diagnosis of CF, is the use of allele-specific oligonucleotides (ASO). Some mutations do result in increased degradation of the CF transmembrane conductance regulator (CFTR) protein, but degradation is initiated by tagging the protein with ubiquitin. Frameshift mutations alter the reading frame through the addition or deletion of nucleotides by a number not divisible by three. Because the ΔF509 mutation is caused by the loss of three nucleotides that code for phenylalanine (F) at position 509 in the CFTR protein, it is not a frameshift mutation.

Q2. Answer = A. Targeting of proteins destined to function as components of the plasma membrane is an example of cotranslational targeting. It involves the initiation of translation on cytosolic ribosomes; recognition of the amino (N)-terminal signal sequence in the protein by the signal recognition particle; movement of the protein-synthesizing complex to the outer face of the membrane of the endoplasmic reticulum (ER); and continuation of protein synthesis, such that the protein is threaded into the lumen of the ER and packaged into vesicles that travel to and through the Golgi and eventually fuse with the plasma membrane. The N-terminal signal sequence is removed by a peptidase in the lumen of the ER. Mannose 6-phosphate is the signal that cotranslationally targets proteins to the matrix of the lysosome where they function as acid hydrolases.

Q3. The pancreatic insufficiency seen in some patients with CF results in a decreased ability to digest food, and digestion is required for absorption. Dietary fats move through the intestine and are excreted in the stool (see figure at right), which is foul-smelling and bulky and may float. Patients are at risk for malnutrition and deficiencies in fat-soluble vitamins. Oral supplementation of pancreatic enzymes is the treatment.

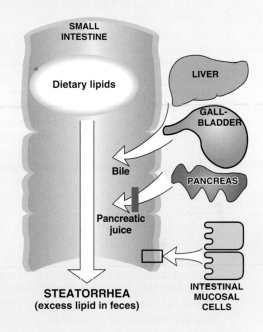

CASE 9: Hyperammonemia with a Urea Cycle Defect

Q1. **Answer = B.** Argininosuccinate lyase (ASL) cleaves argininosuccinate to arginine (Arg) and fumarate. The increase in argininosuccinate and citrulline and the decrease in Arg seen in RL indicate a deficiency in ASL (see figure below). With arginase deficiency, Arg would be increased, not decreased. Additionally, with arginase deficiency, the hyper-ammonemia would be less severe because two nitrogens are excreted. Deficiency of argininosuccinate synthetase (ASS) would also cause an increase in citrulline, but argininosuc-cinate would be low to absent. Deficiency of carbamoyl phos-phate synthetase (CPS) I is characterized by low levels of Arg and citrulline. Deficiency of ornithine transcarbamoylase (OTC), the only X-linked enzyme of the urea cycle, would result in low levels of Arg and citrulline and elevated levels of urinary orotic acid. [Note: The orotic acid is elevated because the carbamoyl phosphate (CP) substrate of OTC is being used in the cytosol as a substrate for pyrimidine synthesis.]

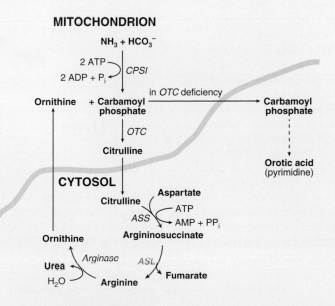

Q2. Arg supplementation is helpful because the Arg will be hydrolyzed to urea + ornithine by arginase. The ornithine will be combined with CP to form citrulline (see figure above). With ASL (and ASS) deficiency, citrulline accumulates and is excreted, thereby carrying waste nitrogen out of the body.

Q3.   Answer = D. In individuals with milder (partial) deficiencies in the enzymes of the urea cycle, hyperammonemia may be triggered by physiologic stress (for example, an illness or prolonged fasting) that decreases the insulin/counterregulatory hormone ratio. [Note: The degree of the hyperammonemia is usually less severe than that seen in the neonatal onset forms.] The shift in the ratio results, in part, in skeletal muscle proteolysis, and the amino acids that are released get degraded. Degradation involves transamination by pyridoxal phosphate–requiring aminotransferases that generate the α-keto acid derivative of the amino acid + glutamate. The glutamate undergoes oxidative deamination to α-ketoglutarate and ammonia (NH_3) by glutamate dehydrogenase (GDH; see figure at right). [Note: GDH is unusual in that it uses both nicotinamide adenine dinucleotide (NAD) and nicotinamide adenine dinucleotide phosphate (NADP) as coenzymes.]

The NH_3, which is toxic, can be transported to the liver as glutamine (Gln) and alanine (Ala). The Gln is generated by the amination of glutamate by ATP-requiring glutamine synthetase. In the liver, the enzyme glutaminase removes the NH_3, which can be converted to urea by the urea cycle or excreted as ammonium (NH_4^+) (see figure at right). Gln, then, is a nontoxic vehicle of NH_3 transport in the blood. Ala is generated in skeletal muscle from the catabolism of the branched-chain amino acids (BCAA). In the liver, Ala is transaminated by alanine transaminase (ALT) to pyruvate (used in gluconeogenesis) and glutamate. Thus, Ala carries nitrogen to the liver for conversion to urea (see figure below). Therefore, defects in the urea cycle would result in an elevation in NH_3, Gln, and Ala. The

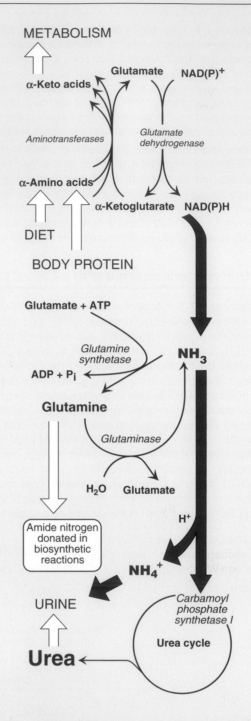

elevated NH_3 drives respiration, and the hyperventilation causes a rise in pH (respiratory alkalosis). [Note: Hyperammonemia is toxic to the nervous system. Although the exact mechanisms are not completely understood, it is known that the metabolism of large amounts of NH_3 to Gln (in the astrocytes of the brain) results in osmotic effects that cause the brain to swell. Additionally, the rise in Gln decreases the availability of glutamate, an excitatory neurotransmitter.]

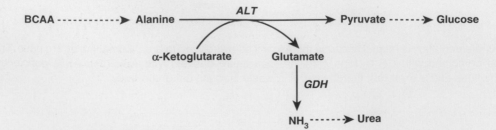

CASE 10: Swollen, Painful Calf with Deep Venous Thrombosis

Q1. **Answer = D.** Thrombin, a serine protease, is activated by the prothrombinase complex of factor (F)Xa + FVa. Once formed, activated thrombin (FIIa) proteolytically activates components of the extrinsic (FVII) and intrinsic (FXI, FVIII) pathways, generating FXa. Thrombin can also activate FV, FI, and FXIII of the common pathway (see figure below). Hemophilia A is caused by a deficiency in FVIII. FIX deficiency results in hemophilia B. FIII, also known as tissue factor (TF), is a transmembrane glycoprotein of the vascular endothelium. It functions as an accessory protein and not a protease. Formation of the platelet plug is primary hemostasis, and formation of the fibrin meshwork is secondary hemostasis. Vitamin K is required for the activation (γ-carboxylation) of FII, FVII, FIX, and FX (proteases that require calcium [Ca^{2+}] and phospholipids [PL]) but not for FI (fibrinogen).

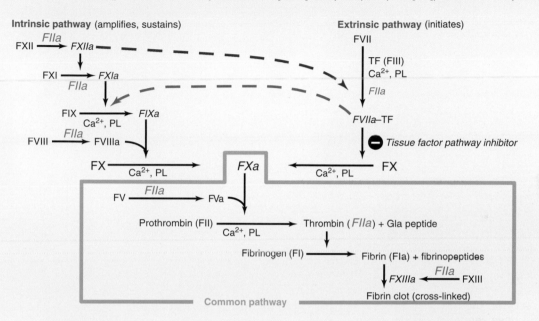

Q2. **Answer = C.** FV Leiden is a mutant form of FV that is resistant to proteolysis by the activated protein C complex. Decreased ability to degrade FV allows continued production of activated thrombin and leads to an increased risk of clot formation or thrombophilia. Antithrombin III (ATIII) and protein S are proteins of anticoagulation. Increased, not decreased, production of prothrombin would result in thrombophilia. Deficiency of von Willebrand factor causes a coagulopathy or a deficiency in clotting through effects on FVIII and platelets.

Q3. Heparin and warfarin are anticoagulants. Heparin, a glycosaminoglycan, increases the affinity of ATIII for thrombin. Binding of ATIII removes thrombin from the blood and prevents it from converting fibrinogen to fibrin. Warfarin, a synthetic analog of vitamin K, inhibits vitamin K epoxide reductase and prevents the regeneration of the functional hydroquinone form of the vitamin that is required for the γ-carboxylation of glutamate residues to γ-carboxyglutamate (Gla) residues in FII, FVII, FIX, and FX (see figures below).

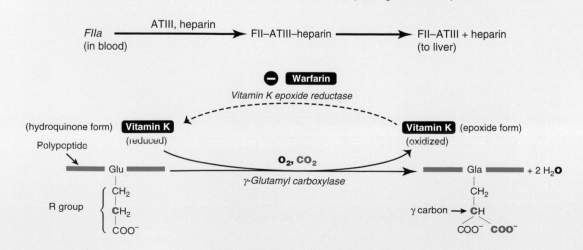

Index

Figure Sources

Figure 2.12: Modified from Garrett RH, Grisham CM. *Biochemistry*. Philadelphia, PA: Saunders College Publishing, 1995. Figure 6.36, p. 193.

Figure 2.13 (panel C, top): Horizon Symposium on Protein Folding and Disease, Italy. Stuttgart, Germany: Nature Publishing Group, Macmillan Publishers, 2002.

Figure 3.1A: Illustration: Irving Geis. Rights owned by Howard Hughes Medical Institute. Not to be used without permission.

Figure 3.21: Photo courtesy of Photodyne Incorporated, Hartland, WI.

Figure 4.3: Electron micrograph of collagen: Natural Toxin Research Center. Texas A&M University Kingsville. Collagen molecule modified from Mathews CK, van Holde KE, Ahern KG. *Biochemistry*, 3rd ed. Boston, MA: Addison Wesley Longman, Inc., 2000:175. Figure 6.13.

Figure 4.4: Modified from Yurchenco PD, Birk DE, Mecham RP, eds. *Extracellular Matrix Assembly and Structure*. San Diego, CA: Academic Press, 1994.

Figure 4.8: From Buhler K. Images in clinical medicine. *N Engl J Med*. 1995;332(24):1611.

Figure 4.10: Photo from Web site Derma.de.

Figure 4.11: From Jorde LB, Carey JC, Bamshad MJ, et al. *Medical Genetics*, 2nd ed. Mosby, St. Louis, MO, 1999. http://medgen.genetics.utah.edu/Index.htm

Chapter 4, Question 4.3: From Berge LN, Marton V, Tranebjaerg L, et al. Prenatal diagnosis of osteogenesis imperfecta. *Acta Obstet Gynecol Scand*. 1995;74(4):321–323.

Figure 13.11: The Crookston Collection, University of Toronto.

Figure 17.13: *Urbana Atlas of Pathology*, University of Illinois College of Medicine at Urbana-Champaign. Image number 26.

Figure 17.19: Interactive Case Study Companion to Robbins Pathologic Basis of Disease.

Figure 18.12: Custom Medical Stock Photo.

Figure 20.21: Success in MRCO path: http://www.mrcophth.com/iriscases/albinism.html.

Figure 20.23A: Rubin E, Farber JL. *Pathology*, 2nd ed. Philadelphia, PA: J. B. Lippincott, 1994:244. Figure 6-30.

Figure 20.23B: Gilbert-Barness E, Barness L. *Metabolic Disease*. Natick, MA: Eaton Publishing, 2000:42. Figure 15.

Figure 21.6: Rich MW. Porphyria cutanea tarda. *Postgrad Med*. 1999;105:208–214.

Figure 21.7: Department of Dermatology, University of Pittsburgh. http://www.upmc.edu/dermatology/MedStudentInfo/introLecture/enlarged/vespct.htm.

Figure 21.11: Custom Medical Stock Photo, Inc.

Figure 21.14: Phototake.

Figure 22.16: Wuthrich DA, Lebowitz AL. Tophaceous gout. Images in clinical medicine. *N Engl J Med*. 1995;332:646.

Figure 22.18: WebMD Inc. http://www.samed.com/sam/forms/index.htm.

Figure 23.2: Childs G. http://www.cytochemistry.net/.

Figure 23.13: Modified from Cryer PE, Fisher JN, Shamoon H. Hypoglycemia . *Diabetes Care*. 1994;17:734–753.

Figure 24.5: Phototake.

Figure 26.5: Corbis.

Figure 26.6: Gibson W, et al. Hypoglycemia. *J Clin Endocrinol Metab*. 2004;89(10):4821.

Figure 27.22 A, B: Centers for Disease Control and Prevention Public Health Image Library, Atlanta, GA.

Figure 28.4: Matthews JH. Queen's University Department of Medicine, Division of Hematology/Oncology, Kingston, Canada.

Figure 30.7: Nolan J. Department of Biochemistry, Tulane University, New Orleans, LA.

Figure 35.10: Foerster J, Lee G, Lukens J, et al. *Wintrobe's Clinical Hematology*, 10th ed. Philadelphia, PA: Lippincott Williams & Wilkins, 1998.

Figure 35.20: Cohen BJ, Taylor JJ. *Memmler's the Human Body in Health and Disease*, 10th ed. Baltimore, MD: Lippincott Williams & Wilkins, 2005.

Appendix, p. 505: Gold DH, Weingeist TA. *Color Atlas of the Eye in Systemic Disease*. Baltimore, MD: Lippincott Williams & Wilkins, 2001.

Appendix, p. 522: Goodheart HP. *Goodheart's Photographs of Common Skin Disorders*, 2nd ed. Philadelphia, PA: Lippincott Williams & Wilkins, 2003.

Appendix, p. 526: McConnell TH. *The Nature of Disease Pathology for the Health Professions*. Philadelphia, PA: Lippincott Williams & Wilkins, 2007.